Practical Neonatal Echocardiography

Edited by

Bijan Siassi, MD, FACC
Associate Professor of Pediatrics and Radiology
Keck School of Medicine
University of Southern California
Los Angeles, California

Shahab Noori, MD, MS CBTI, RDCS
Associate Professor of Pediatrics
Keck School of Medicine
University of Southern California
Fetal and Neonatal Institute
Division of Neonatology
Children's Hospital Los Angeles
Los Angeles, California

Ruben J. Acherman, MD
Professor of Pediatric Cardiology
University of Nevada, Las Vegas Director, Fetal Cardiology
Children's Heart Center Nevada
Las Vegas, Nevada

Pierre C. Wong, MD
Associate Professor of Pediatrics
Keck School of Medicine
University of Southern California
Director, Echocardiography Lab and Cardiac Pathology Registry
Children's Hospital Los Angeles
Los Angeles, California

Mc Graw Hill Education

New York Chicago San Francisco Lisbon London Madrid Mexico City
Milan New Delhi San Juan Seoul Singapore Sydney Toronto

Practical Neonatal Echocardiography

2 3 4 5 6 7 8 9 DSS 23

ISBN 978-1-260-12313-5
MHID 1-260-12313-8

Notice

Medicine is an ever-changing science. As new research and clinical experience broaden our knowledge, changes in treatment and drug therapy are required. The editors and the publisher of this work have checked with sources believed to be reliable in their efforts to provide information that is complete and generally in accord with the standards accepted at the time of publication. However, in view of the possibility of human error or changes in medical sciences, neither the editors nor the publisher nor any other party who has been involved in the preparation or publication of this work warrants that the information contained herein is in every respect accurate or complete, and they disclaim all responsibility for any errors or omissions or for the results obtained from use of the information contained in this work. Readers are encouraged to confirm the information contained herein with other sources. For example and in particular, readers are advised to check the product information sheet included in the package of each drug they plan to administer to be certain that the information contained in this work is accurate and that changes have not been made in the recommended dose or in the contraindications for administration. This recommendation is of particular importance in connection with new or infrequently used drugs.

This book was set in Minion Pro by MPS Limited.
The editors were Andrew Moyer and Christie Naglieri.
The production supervisor was Richard Ruzycka.
Project management was provided by Poonam Bisht, MPS Limited.
The cover designer was W2 Design.

This book is printed on acid-free paper.

Library of Congress Cataloging-in-Publication Data

Names: Siassi, Bijan, editor. | Noori, Shahab, editor. | Wong, Pierre C., editor. | Acherman, Ruben, editor.
Title: Practical neonatal echocardiography / editors, Bijan Siassi, Shahab Noori, Pierre C. Wong, Ruben Acherman.
Description: New York : McGraw-Hill, [2018] | Includes bibliographical references and index.
Identifiers: LCCN 2018015020| ISBN 9781260123135 (hardcover sewn : alk. paper) | ISBN 1260123138 (hardcover sewn : alk. paper) | ISBN 9781260123142 (e-ISBN)
Subjects: | MESH: Echocardiography—methods | Infant, Newborn | Heart Defects, Congenital—diagnostic imaging | Fetal Heart—diagnostic imaging
Classification: LCC RJ423.5.U46 | NLM WG 141.5.E2 | DDC 618.92/1207543—dc23 LC record available at https://na01.safelinks.protection.outlook.com/?url=https%3A%2F%2Flccn.loc.gov%2F2018015020&data=01%7C01%7Cleah.carton%40mheducation.com%7C6ca77527b4254cc5260b08d5964c7da4%7Cf919b1efc0c347358fca0928ec39d8d5%7C0&sdata=6Oq2Qy9A9EhiQsNzhULZmZQ2vBTIjgrCuZ6%2B4XJaMpU%3D&reserved=0

The editors would like to dedicate this book to the many trainees and attendees of our *Functional Echocardiography* for *Neonatologists* course that we have had the honor and privilege of teaching over the past 15 years. Your interest and enthusiasm provided us with the strong motivation we need to write this book, and they continue to fuel our passion for teaching.

Contents

Contributors .... *vii*
Preface .... *ix*

Chapter 1
Basic Principles of Echocardiography 1
Apichai Khongphatthanayothin

Chapter 2
Echocardiographic Scanners and Transducers 19
Mahmood Ebrahimi

Chapter 3
Cross-Sectional Neonatal Cardiac Anatomy as Depicted by Standard Two-Dimensional Echocardiography 33
Bijan Siassi, Mahmood Ebrahimi, Shilpa Patil, and Ruben J. Acherman

Chapter 4
Application of Echocardiographic Simulators in Training for Neonatal Echocardiography 61
Bijan Siassi, Mahmood Ebrahimi, and Shahab Noori

Chapter 5
M-Mode Echocardiography and 2D Cardiac Measurements.. 71
Merujan Uzunyan and Lindsey Miller

Chapter 6
Pulsed Wave, Continuous-Wave, and Color Flow Doppler in Assessment of Regurgitant Flow and Measurement of Pressure Gradients 85
Merujan Uzunyan and Lindsey Miller

Chapter 7
Application of Pulsed Wave and Continuous-Wave Doppler in the Assessment and Measurement of Cardiac and Systemic Blood Flow 101
Shahab Noori

Chapter 8
Assessment of Systolic, Diastolic, and Global Cardiac Function 121
Shahab Noori

Chapter 9
Shunts Through a Patent Foramen Ovale 139
Bijan Siassi

Chapter 10
Shock, Myocardial Dysfunction, and Heart Failure 151
Shahab Noori and Tai Wei Wu

Chapter 11
Patent Ductus Arteriosus 161
Shahab Noori

Chapter 12
Persistent Pulmonary Hypertension in Newborn Infants: Assessment of Pulmonary Artery Pressure... 177
Tina A. Leone

Chapter 13
Desaturation and Cyanosis in the Newborn Infant without Congenital Heart Disease.................. 191
Tina A. Leone

Chapter 14
Aneurysm of Ductus Arteriosus, Cardiomyopathies, and Aortopulmonary Collaterals..................... 217
Ruben J. Acherman and William N. Evans

Chapter 15
Suspecting Congenital Heart Disease........... 235
Bijan Siassi, Mahmood Ebrahimi, and Ruben J. Acherman

Chapter 16
Overview of Fetal Echocardiography 259
Ruben J. Acherman and William N. Evans

Index *279*

Contributors

Apichai Khongphatthanayothin, MD
Pediatric Cardiologist, LAC-USC Medical Center
Professor of Clinical Pediatrics
Keck School of Medicine, University of Southern California
Los Angeles, California
Chief of Paediatric Cardiology
Bangkok General Hospital
Professor of Pediatrics
Chulalongkorn University
Bangkok, Thailand

Bijan Siassi, MD
Associate Professor of Pediatrics and Radiology
Keck School of Medicine, University of Southern California
Los Angeles, California

Lindsey Miller, MD
Clinical Assistant Professor of Pediatrics
Keck School of Medicine, University of Southern California
Los Angeles, California

Mahmood Ebrahimi, MD, RDCS
Instructor of Clinical Pediatrics
Keck School of Medicine, University of Southern California
Los Angeles, California

Merujan Uzunyan, MD
Assistant Professor of Clinical Pediatrics
Keck School of Medicine, University of Southern California
Director, Pediatric Cardiology
LAC+USC Medical Center
Los Angeles, California

Pierre C. Wong, MD
Associate Professor of Pediatrics
Keck School of Medicine, University of Southern California
Director, Echocardiography Lab and Cardiac Pathology Registry
Children, Echocardiography Lab
Los Angeles, California

Ruben J. Acherman, MD
Professor of Clinical Pediatrics
University of Nevada, Las Vegas School of Medicine
Director of Fetal Cardiology
Childrens Heart Center Nevada
Las Vegas, Nevada

Shahab Noori, MD, MS CBTI, RDCS
Associate Professor of Pediatrics
Keck School of Medicine
University of Southern California
Fetal and Neonatal Institute
Division of Neonatology
Children's Hospital Los Angeles
Los Angeles, California

Shilpa Patil, MD
Attending Neonatologist
East Bay Newborn Specialists
UCSF Benioff Children's Hospital Oakland
Oakland, California

Tai Wei Wu, MD
Assistant Professor of Pediatrics
Keck School of Medicine, University of Southern California
Fetal and Neonatal Institute
Division of Neonatology
Children's Hospital Los Angeles
Los Angeles, California

Tina A. Leone, MD
Associate Professor of Pediatrics
Columbia University, College of Physicians and Surgeons
New York-Presbyterian, Morgan Stanley Children's Hospital
New York, New York

William N. Evans, MD
Professor of Clinical Pediatrics
University of Nevada, Las Vegas School of Medicine
Co-Director
Childrens Heart Center Nevada
Las Vegas, Nevada

Preface

Echocardiography is the predominant bedside, noninvasive method of assessing cardiac structure and function. Although originally developed as a diagnostic tool for cardiologists, recently it has been increasingly used across different specialties for acute patient care. The utility of point-of-care echocardiography has been demonstrated by neonatologists in neonatal intensive care units. Training in echocardiography is a complex process that, in addition to thorough theoretical knowledge, requires extensive hands-on training to acquire the all-important technical skills.

Over the past 18 years, our group has been involved in presenting an annual course on functional echocardiography for neonatologists. The lectures and presentations in these courses provide the basis of this work. The book is extensively illustrated, and relevant video clips of echocardiograms are included: (available at http://PracticalNeonatalEcho.com). In this book, we present the core knowledge relevant to training physicians in point-of-care echocardiography for neonates. Although the book is primarily intended for neonatologists, it can serve as a resource for other professionals interested in neonatal echocardiography.

We dedicate this work to the neonatologists who in spite of many obstacles have the passion to pursue the learning of this technique.

Bijan Siassi
Shahab Noori
Ruben J. Acherman
Pierre C. Wong

CHAPTER 1

Basic Principles of Echocardiography

Apichai Khongphatthanayothin

- INTRODUCTION
- WHAT IS ULTRASOUND?
- HOW IS AN ECHOCARDIOGRAPHIC IMAGE (M-MODE, 2D, AND 3D) CREATED?
- M-MODE ECHOCARDIOGRAPHY
- TWO-DIMENSIONAL (2D) ECHOCARDIOGRAPHY
- THREE-DIMENSIONAL (3D) ECHOCARDIOGRAPHY
- HOW TO OPTIMIZE THE QUALITY OF 2D ECHOCARDIOGRAPHIC IMAGES
  - Image Resolution
  - Artifacts
- DOPPLER ECHOCARDIOGRAPHY
  - Pulsed Wave (PW) Doppler
  - Continuous-Wave (CW) Doppler
  - Color Flow Imaging (Color Doppler)
- PITFALLS WHEN USING DOPPLER ECHOCARDIOGRAPHY
  - Angle Correction
  - Gain Settings for Doppler Measurement
  - Adjusting Nyquist Limit, Transducer Frequency, and Depth Setting
  - How to Measure a Velocity That Is Higher Than the Nyquist Limit
- REFERENCES

INTRODUCTION

Echocardiography utilizes ultrasound to produce images of the heart and vascular structures (using M-mode, two-dimensional [2D], and and three-dimensionall [3D] echocardiography) and to provide information about the direction and velocity of blood flow within these structures (using spectral Doppler and color flow Doppler mapping). This chapter presents a basic review of the physics of ultrasound and the principles of cardiovascular ultrasonic imaging for all clinicians and medical personnel who perform echocardiography.

WHAT IS ULTRASOUND?

Ultrasound refers to sound waves with a frequency well beyond the range of human hearing (the normal human range is 20-20,000 Hz). Because the ability of ultrasound waves to penetrate human tissue carries an inverse relationship to the frequency of the transmitted ultrasound (as shown in Table 1-1), the range of frequencies that are suitable for transthoracic echocardiography generally falls between 2 to 10 MHz,[1] which corresponds to an image depth of 6 cm in premature neonates (using a 10-MHz probe) down to 30 cm in adults (using a 2-MHz transducer). High

TABLE 1-1. Penetration (imaging Depth) and Axial Resolution (using Two-Cycle Pulse) of Transducer Used in Echocardiography

Subject	Frequency (MHz)	Imaging Depth (cm)	Axial Resolution (mm)
Adult	2	30	0.77
Child	5	12	0.31
Infant	7.5	8	0.21
Newborn	10	6	0.15

Modified with permission from Kremkau FW. *Diagnostic Ultrasound: Principles and Instruments, 5th ed.* Philadelphia: W.B. Saunders Company; 1998.

ultrasonic frequencies are required to produce the necessary resolution for diagnostic imaging of small cardiovascular structures in newborns (Table 1-1). Because image resolution is directly related to the ultrasound frequency, the highest frequency that can penetrate to the structure of interest is generally preferred for M-mode, 2D, and 3D echocardiography. The opposite is true for Doppler and color flow mapping, in which lower ultrasonic frequencies generally provide better information.

HOW IS AN ECHOCARDIOGRAPHIC IMAGE (M-MODE, 2D, AND 3D) CREATED?

Echocardiography utilizes properties of sound wave interaction with human tissue called **reflection** and **scattering** (Figure 1-1). The human body consists of various tissues, each with a different composition and density, that result in a sound-related property called **acoustic impedance** that is specific to the tissue. When sound propagates through a smooth and long interface between homogeneous tissues with two different acoustic impedances (such as between blood and endocardium), both transmission and reflection of the sound wave occur; the degree of transmission versus reflection depends upon the degree of matching between the two acoustic impedances (the greater the degree of mismatch, the greater the amount of reflection). Reflection of sounds waves is similar to reflection of light upon a mirror or a flat and smooth surface. Most human tissues, however, are either irregular or inhomogeneous. Reflection of sound in these irregular surfaces occurs in all directions, called "scattering," similar to the reflection of light upon a ground glass or a wall with an irregular surface. Depending on the intensity of sound waves that reflects. or scatters, back to the transducer (we will call this "echo signals"), numerical values can be calculated and displayed as shades of gray on the display monitor. To obtain an echocardiographic image, ultrasound is created by a **transducer**, a device containing a material possessing **piezoelectric properties** (such as quartz or titanate ceramics) that enables the conversion from electrical to mechanical energy (and vice versa).[2,3] When stimulated by electric current, these materials vibrate and produce an ultrasonic wave of predictable frequency. Therefore, through the use of brief electrical stimulation followed by immediate dampening of the transducer, a short pulse of ultrasonic energy can be emitted (each pulse is composed of several wavelengths of sound). Ultrasound pulses from the transducer travel through the tissue, and

$$D = \frac{C \times T}{2}$$

when different tissue interfaces are encountered, various sound signals reflect or scatter (echo) back to the transducer. Because the speed that sound travels in human tissues is relatively constant (approximately 1,540 m/s),[1] the distance to each tissue interface can then be calculated according to the time that the pulse of ultrasound travels to and from each tissue interface, using the formula where

D = distance to tissue interface (such as between endocardium and the blood in the heart chamber, between subcutaneous tissue and pericardium, etc.)

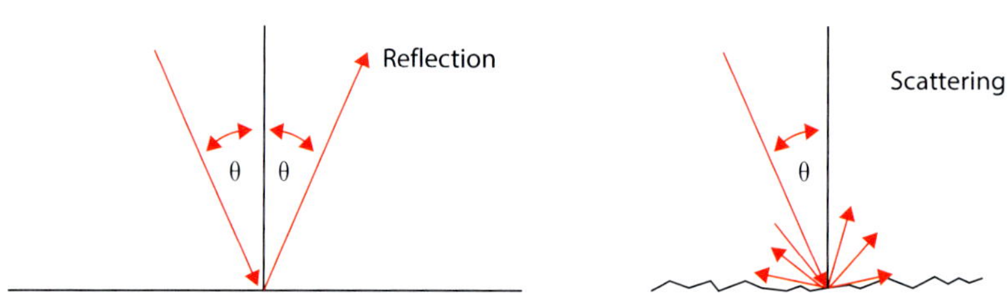

FIGURE 1-1. Reflection and scattering of a sound wave.

T = time from the beginning of ultrasound pulse initiation to the return of the echo signal

C = speed of sound in human tissue (1,540 m/s)

Returning echo signals from the various tissue interfaces produces vibration of the piezoelectric material in the transducer, which in turn creates electric currents. The computer plots these currents as shades of gray to represent the intensity of the echo signals on the vertical axis according to the calculated distance between the transducer and each tissue interface.

M-MODE ECHOCARDIOGRAPHY

M-mode, short for motion mode, is one of the oldest ultrasound techniques. It allows for assessment of motion of various structures of the heart along a single line. In a structurally normal heart, because the anatomy of the heart is known, each echo signal (gray dot) produced by the M-mode can be read as representing a certain interface between various structures (Figure 1-2). Because the heart is a moving organ, it is of interest to see the relative movement of these parts with time. For example, the relative movement of intraventricular septum to left ventricular (LV) posterior wall in systole compared to diastole provides information on LV systolic function (see Chapter 5). The M-mode images are created by repetitively sending and receiving ultrasound signals through the same path. To do so, the transducer will have to send an ultrasound signal, wait to listen for echo signals for a finite time, and then send another signal and listen once more. Because the speed of sound in the human tissue is relatively constant, there would be a specific amount of time, depending upon the depth of tissue, that an echo signal can be sent and received by the transducer before it can emit the next ultrasound pulse. The relationship between time (T) and depth (D) can be calculated using the formula given in the previous section, $D=\frac{C \times T}{2}$.

In reality, when an M-mode echocardiogram is performed, one does not choose the time between each pulse (T), or how often to send the ultrasound pulse in 1 second, also known as **pulse repetition frequency** (**PRF**). Instead, the machine has a user-defined depth adjustment that it uses to calculate the PRF. The image of M-mode echocardiography is made by putting the new "column" of gray dots to the right of the previous one (Figure 1-2). As such, the x-axis on an M-mode image represents time and the y-axis represents distance from the transducer, with the nearest distance on the top and the farthest distance on the bottom. It can also be seen that, for M-mode as well as other forms of echocardiographic imaging, the time that the machine sends and receives an ultrasound pulse has an inverse relationship to the depth of imaging: the deeper the depth, the longer it will take to obtain each line, and the lower the maximum PRF (**Maximum PRF = 1/T**). This has the potential to lower time (temporal) resolution. However, because the speed of sound is very fast relative

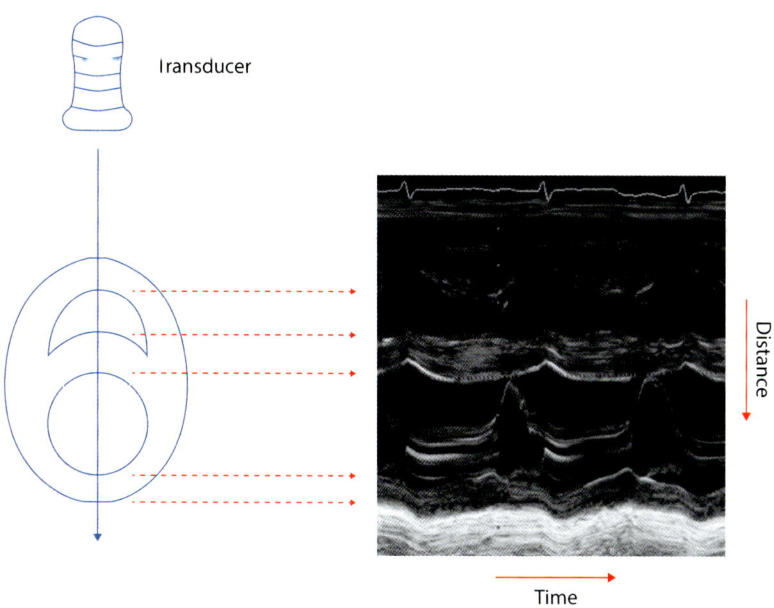

FIGURE 1-2. Location of the cursor on a 2D echocardiogram to generate an M-mode image.

to the depth of the human body, temporal resolution is excellent for M-mode echocardiography.[1,3] This might not be the case in 2D or 3D echocardiography, especially when color flow mapping is also used, as will be discussed later in this chapter.

TWO-DIMENSIONAL (2D) ECHOCARDIOGRAPHY

For M-mode echocardiography, a single unit of piezoelectric material is used to send and receive ultrasound to create an image which is essentially a one-dimensional plot of cardiac or vascular structures against time (Figure 1-2). It can give a good amount of information on the length of cardiac structures (such as wall thickness and chamber size) and how each structure moves in relation to other structures (such as the shortening fraction and ejection fraction). However, M-mode does not give any information on what each structure looks like unless one has a great imaginary capability (and most people do not).

With the advances in the computing technology, two-dimensional (2D) echocardiography (previously known as B-mode echocardiography) has now become the standard for cardiac imaging. For this form of echocardiography, images are created by sending and receiving multiple lines of ultrasound beams arranged in a fan-shape orientation, wide enough to visualize the area of interest. In the past, this was produced by automatically rotating the transducer back and forth (**mechanical transducer**), but currently it is performed by having an array of separate piezoelectric elements sending and receiving ultrasound signals at the same time or using a tiny fraction of time difference in the stimulation of the individual elements.[2] In the transducer, piezoelectric materials are placed in a linear array such that successive ultrasound beams are directed with a very small change in angle (**phased-array transducer**). Each column of returning signals is then assembled with the previous column to create a "sector" scan (a collection of scan lines) that looks like a piece of pie (Figure 1-3). This image represents a 2D image of the heart along the scan plane at a particular point in time. When the transducer completes its round of sending and receiving echo signals throughout the sector, it begins the next cycle and the new image is created when the previous image disappears, in the same fashion as in a movie. Similar to a movie, when the images are created at a high enough frequency (frame rate), the motion appears continuous.

THREE-DIMENSIONAL (3D) ECHOCARDIOGRAPHY

In 2D echocardiography, an operator can gain more complete information of the three-dimensional (3D) nature of a cardiac structure by moving (sweeping) the transducer and creating a mental picture of the 3D cardiac structure. Using this method, with adequate training, the diagnosis and understanding of 3D cardiac structure and function can be achieved with a high degree of accuracy. However, in certain circumstances, a true 3D rendering of a cardiac structure is desirable, such as when presenting the heart valve pathology to a cardiovascular surgeon in preparation for cardiac surgery. Similar to how a 2D image is obtained by putting together multiple lines of echo signals from a small linear array, a 3D echocardiogram is obtained by sending and receiving multiple scan lines from a 2D array containing a large number of elements arranged a tiny

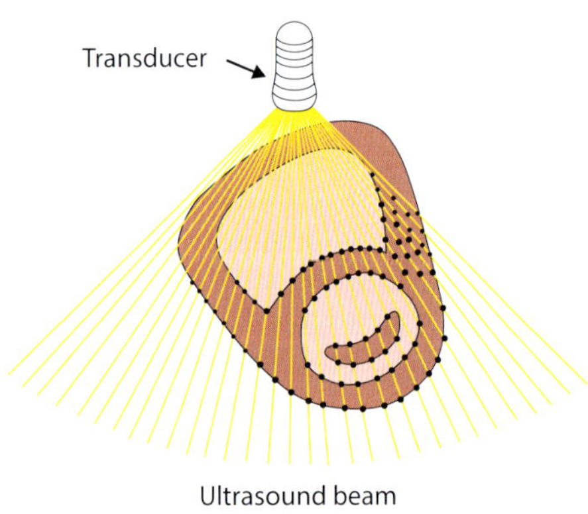

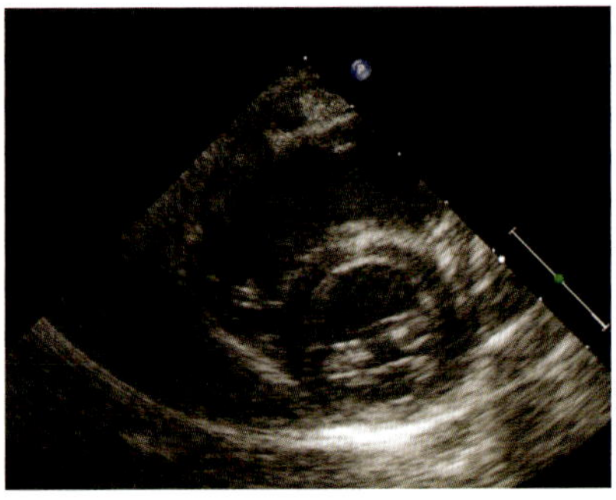

FIGURE 1-3. Sector scan in the generation of 2D echocardiographic image.

distance apart on a square or rectangular matrix. A pyramidal volume of gray-scale dots is then created for each time frame, resulting in a 3D rendered image. As with 2D imaging, the process is repeated continuously and rapidly to give the appearance of real-time motion (also known as four-dimensional, or 4D echocardiography). Because one cannot fully appreciate complex spatial relationships on a rendered 3D image displayed on a 2D computer monitor, it is often necessary to post-process the 3D dataset (using such maneuvers as image cropping and rotation) in order to develop a more complete 3D understanding of the structure of interest (such as a heart valve or a septal defect). Imaging with 3D echocardiography is beyond the scope of this book and will be omitted for simplicity.

HOW TO OPTIMIZE THE QUALITY OF 2D ECHOCARDIOGRAPHIC IMAGES

Image Resolution

Resolution of a 2D image is further divided into (1) **detail resolution**, which is the ability of the echocardiography to differentiate two adjacent points (or structures) as separate; (2) **contrast resolution**, which is the ability of the machine to differentiate between two tissue densities; and (3) **temporal (time) resolution**, or the ability to display a moving cardiac structure with a smooth transition between frames.

Detail Resolution

Detail resolution is further divided into resolution along the ultrasound beam, or **axial resolution,** and resolution between ultrasound beams, or **lateral resolution** (Figure 1-4). For most ultrasound images including echocardiography, axial resolution is better than lateral resolution.

Axial resolution of echocardiography is largely dependent on the frequency of the ultrasound used to obtain the image (Table 1-1). The higher the frequency, the shorter the wavelength of the sound wave, resulting in better axial resolution. This is because when the transducer sends out an ultrasound beam, it does so by creating a short train of sound waves (2-5 wavelengths) and then waits to listen for the echo signals. Hence, the shortest distance between two points that can reflect the sound back and be resolved by the transducer as different points is equal to the length of the ultrasound pulse divided by 2.[2] If the pulse consists of two wavelengths, the resolution will be equal to the wavelength of ultrasound wave (Table 1-1). As a result, the shorter the wavelength (the higher the frequency), the shorter the pulse duration can be made, and the better the resolution. However, since the higher-frequency sound penetrates tissue less than lower-frequency sound, there is a trade-off between the ability to obtain better resolution 2D images and the decreased penetration from the higher frequency. Consequently, one should use the highest frequency that will penetrate to the structure of interest. In general, a transducer with sound frequencies of 2 to 4 MHz is used in adults, 4 to 6 MHz in children, and 6 to 12 MHz in neonates. The more premature the newborn, the higher the frequency of a transducer that can be used because of smaller chest size (and resultant smaller depth of penetration).

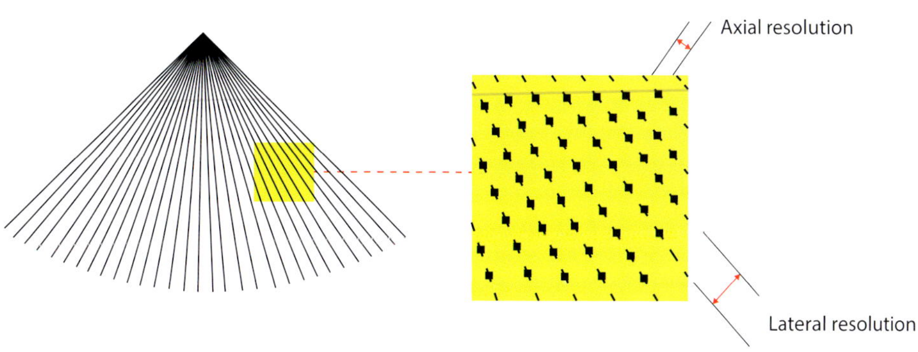

FIGURE 1-4. Axial resolution and lateral resolution. Axial resolution is the ability to distinguish between two structures in axial dimension and therefore measured parallel to the ultrasound beam. Lateral resolution is the ability to distinguish between two structures in lateral dimension and therefore measured perpendicular to the path of ultrasound beam.

Lateral resolution of 2D echocardiography is largely dependent on the width of the ultrasound beam. When the beam of the ultrasound is wide, two different points separated by a small distance can reflect the same beam of sound wave, thus the reflected wave is received by the transducer and interpreted as a single point. Therefore, the narrower the ultrasound beam, the more likely that two closely spaced points can be discerned separately, resulting in greater lateral resolution. Because ultrasound beams diverge at longer distances, lateral resolution of a 2D echocardiography image tend to degrade at farther distances from the transducer (far field) compared to the shorter distance (near field). To improve resolution, the operator can focus the ultrasound beam (to narrow the width) by using a concaved piezoelectric element or by using an acoustic lens (in the same way that an optical lens focuses a light beam). This will result in a better lateral resolution at the region of interest (Figure 1-5).[1,3] Higher-frequency sound can also be more tightly focused than lower-frequency sound,[1] thus giving better lateral resolution, again at the expense of lesser penetration and lesser depth of tissue that can be imaged. Usually, beam width is predefined in each echocardiography machine and is not adjustable. However, with modern phased array transducers, an operator can electronically adjust the focus of the ultrasound beam to the area of interest, in order to obtain a better lateral resolution (Figure 1-6).

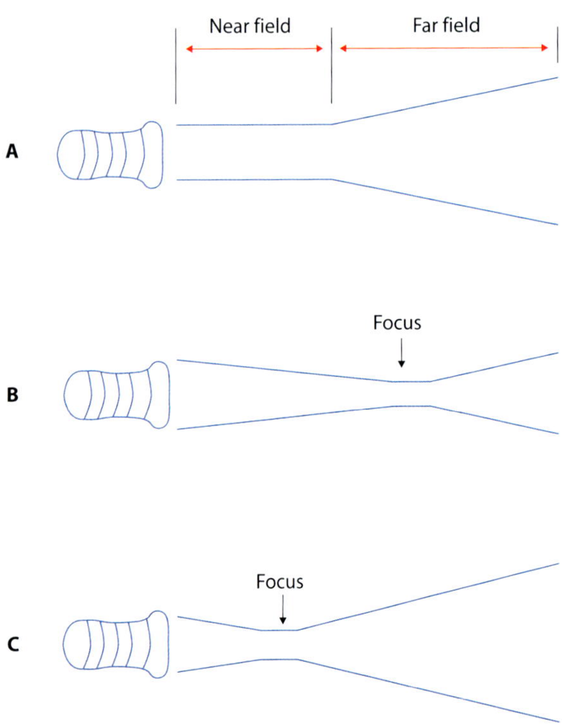

FIGURE 1-5. Near and far field zones in an unfocused (5A) and focused (5B and 5C) transducer. With modern phased array transducers, focusing of the ultrasound beam can be adjusted by the operator to enhance lateral resolution.

Contrast Resolution

Contrast resolution refers to the ability to differentiate between interfaces of tissues with various densities. A pure black-and-white echo image is said to have worse contrast resolution than a grayscale image. Good contrast resolution has clinical relevance, since one would like to differentiate tissues with different densities as being pericardium, myocardium, endocardium, moving blood, blood clot, tumor or scar, and so on.

Contrast between tissues with different densities is commonly displayed on an echo monitor as gray scale. The scale is dependent on the amplitude of echo signals that scatter or reflect back from each tissue interface and can be adjusted by the **gain** control, **log compression or dynamic range** control, and **depth gain compensation (DGC)** control on the echocardiography machine.

The basic technical details of how contrast resolution can be improved with machine design are complex and the echocardiographic operator does not usually have control over it. Detail contrast resolution, however, can be improved by adjusting the gain control and/or grayscale control (log compression or dynamic range) such that the weakest echo signals have gray scale that is just a little brighter than the area that should have no echo signal (totally dark, such as normal blood flow inside the cardiac cavity) and the brightest cardiac echo (such as the pericardium) is just below the maximum (totally bright white). Adjusting the gain too low makes most structures look dark, with some thin structures (such as atrial septum or membranous part of the interventricular septum) artifactually disappearing. Adjusting the gain too high creates "noise" or artifacts in the area that should have no echo signal and may saturate the image such that the distinction between less bright and brighter tissues (such as normal myocardium and blood clot) is difficult. In some instances, however, deviation from this practice can give better clinical information. For example, when trying to visualize coronary arteries, the operator must use his or her own judgment and experience to determine how best to image the structure of interest.

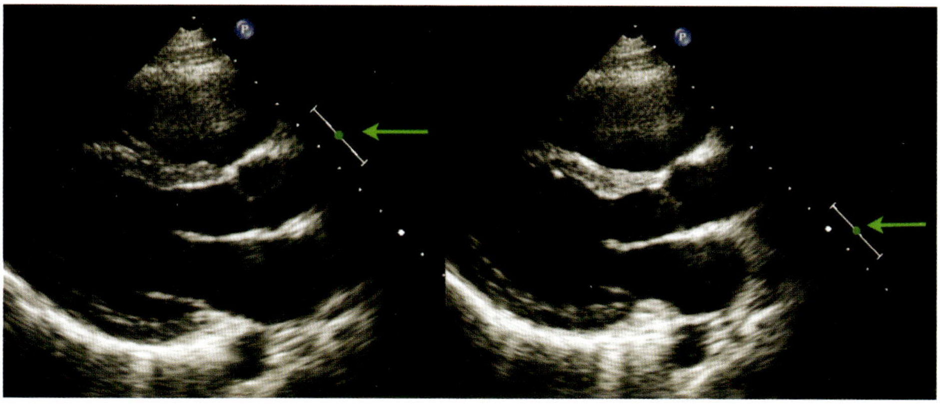

FIGURE 1-6. Image focus on 2D echocardiography. The arrows demonstrate that the focus can be varied for different regions of interest.

Depth gain compensation (DGC) or **time gain compensation** (TGC) refer to multiple gain controls that can be separately adjusted for different depths. This is useful because as sound travels deeper into the tissue, it loses power (amplitude) due to **scattering** and **attenuation** (absorption) of its energy. Hence, the echo signals are normally weaker from the tissue interfaces that are farther away from the transducer. In order to compensate for this energy loss, higher gain is generally required for echo signals from deeper structures. By adjusting DGC, the user is able to compensate for this loss and make the overall image more homogeneous.

Temporal Resolution

Temporal resolution refers to how smooth the movement of the 2D image appears, and it is dependent on the frame rate. The factors that affect frame rate include (1) the depth of the 2D scan, (2) the density of echo lines used to produce the 2D image, and (3) the number of focal zones.[2]

As discussed earlier, in order to complete each scan line, the ultrasound pulse has to travel to the maximal depth of interest and then back to the transducer. The deeper the depth, the longer the wait time before sending the next ultrasound pulse such that it takes more time to complete the multiple lines that compose the sector of a 2D image. The density of scan lines also affects the frame rate, as a greater number of scan lines per sector requires time to complete one sector image. Multiple focal zones also decrease frame rate. Similar to a movie, which is a series of pictures moving at high speed, movement of cardiac structures will appear smoother with a higher frame rate. In general, a frame rate of 30 frames/second or greater is desirable for echocardiography.[3]

Artifacts

Dropout Artifacts

Dropout artifacts usually occur when a thin, smooth structure is imaged at the angle that is parallel to the axis of ultrasound beam. One notable example is the dropout of a part of interatrial septum when the transducer is placed at cardiac apex (ie, in an apical four-chamber view, Figure 1-7, left). This is explained by the fact that the atrial septum is a long, thin, smooth structure; thus most of the ultrasound beam will be transmitted and little information from the septum will be reflected back to the transducer when imaged from the apex. Conversely, when the image is obtained from the subcostal views (Figure 1-7, right) where the ultrasound beam is perpendicular to the atrial septum, much more information is reflected back to the transducer, and it is apparent that the atrial septum is actually intact.

Shadowing from Echo-dense Structures

When an ultrasound beam is directed to a structure that largely reflects the sound back (such as air, prosthetic valve, or bone), that structure will appear very bright and no detail of the distal structure can be imaged because no sound can penetrate further. For example, a heart may not be seen when an echocardiogram is obtained from precordial regions in a newborn with pneumopericardium, because air in the pericardial sac reflects all the sound back to the transducer (due to significant acoustic impedance

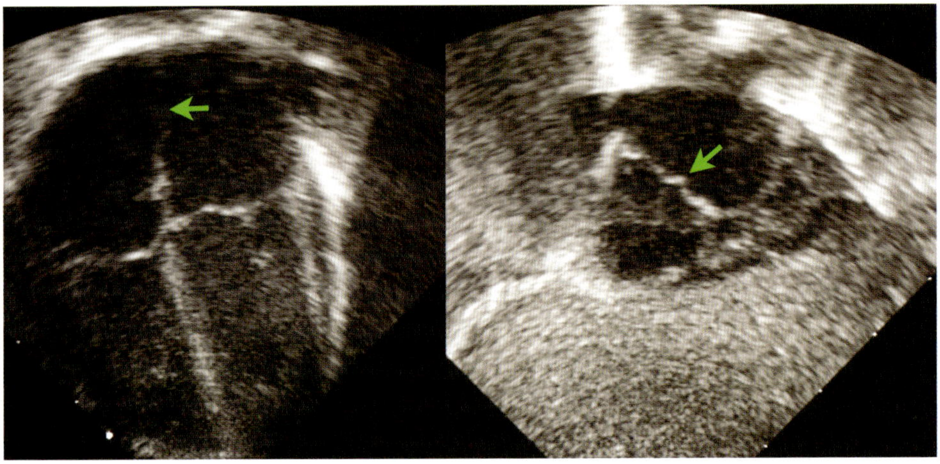

FIGURE 1-7. Dropout artifact of an atrial septum. Left: Atrial septum (arrow) is imaged from the cardiac apex (apical four-chamber view) with dropout artifact. The path of ultrasound beam is parallel to the atrial septum. The artifact produces the appearance of an atrial septal defect. Right: Atrial septum (arrow) from the same patient as viewed from subcostal region. The path of ultrasound beam is perpendicular to the plane of atrial septum, and from this perspective, the atrial septum appears intact.

mismatch between air and soft tissue) and does not permit transmission of the ultrasound, thereby precluding visualization of the underlying heart. In such cases, echocardiography from the subcostal region might be the only way to visualize the heart because air generally rises to the top in a patient lying supine on a bed. Another example of shadowing is from a prosthetic mechanical valve, in which the metal/carbon components of the valve reflect all incident ultrasound, thereby prohibiting visualization of the structures behind it.

DOPPLER ECHOCARDIOGRAPHY

Doppler echocardiography is the ultrasonic modality used to measure **direction** and **velocity** of blood flow. In addition to 2D imaging, it can give a great deal of information on a patient's hemodynamic status. **Color flow imaging** uses multiple points of Doppler data to produce a color-mapped image of mean Doppler velocities superimposed upon the concurrent 2D echo image, suitable for an overall assessment of the direction and velocity of blood flow inside vascular structures.

Originating from the work of Christian Doppler, an Austrian physicist, Doppler echocardiography is based upon the **Doppler principle**, which holds that the observed frequency of a wave depends not just on the actual frequency of the wave originating from the source, but also on the relative speed between the source and observer of that wave. When an observer is static (not moving), a sound wave received by him or her will have the same frequency as what was emitted by the source. However, when the source of the echo signal moves relative to the transducer (such as echo signals that scatter back from moving red blood cells inside a blood vessel), a frequency shift of the echo signals occurs. Because frequency changes of the echo signals are dependent upon the relative speed (and direction) of the red blood cells compared to the transducer, the difference in frequencies between incident and returning sound waves can be measured and compared, and with the use of the **Doppler equation**, the speed of red blood cells (or speed of blood flow) inside the area of interest can be calculated. The **Doppler equation** is given as follows.[1]

$$V = \frac{C \times fd}{2 \times f0 \times \cos\theta}$$

where

v = Velocity of blood flow

f0 = Transmitted frequency

fd = Frequency difference or observed Doppler frequency

C = Velocity of sound in human tissue at 37 C

θ = Intercept angle between the ultrasound beam and the blood flow directions

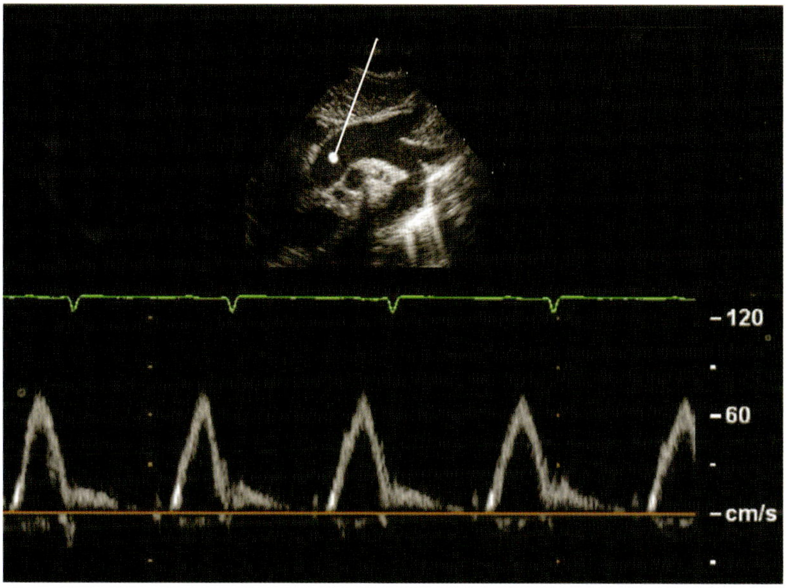

FIGURE 1-8. Pulsed wave (PW) Doppler spectral display from ascending aorta obtained with a transducer in the suprasternal notch position (normal laminar flow).

For echocardiography, two different modes of Doppler are commonly used to calculate velocity and direction: (1) pulsed wave Doppler (PW) and (2) continuous-wave Doppler (CW). These are described below.

Pulsed Wave (PW) Doppler

Pulsed wave (PW) Doppler uses a single piezoelectric crystal to send and receive echo signals one cycle at a time. The machine measures the frequency shift of the sound waves that return (echo) from a particular moving structure in the heart or blood vessel to calculate the velocity and create a display of velocity over time. If one wanted to measure the velocity of blood flow at a point in ascending aorta from a transducer placed at suprasternal notch (Figure 1-8), a pulse of ultrasound wave is sent in that direction (usually guided by 2D imaging) to the area of interest, known as a **sample volume**. The location (depth) of the sample volume is determined from the calculated time that it takes for the ultrasound pulse to travel to and echo back from that depth (using 1540 m/s as the speed of sound in soft tissue). At the end of this time period, the frequency of the returning echo signals is measured and, based upon the frequency shift of the echo signals, the velocity of the moving structure (eg, red blood cells) is calculated and plotted (versus time) on the screen. Because blood flow in the ascending aorta is directed toward the transducer, the frequency of the returning echoes will produce a shift toward a higher frequency, which by convention is plotted on the positive side (above) the zero velocity line (Figure 1-8). The same procedure is then repeated, and a new velocity is plotted next to the previous one, and so forth.

The graph of velocity versus time is called a **Doppler spectral display** and is shown in Figure 1-8 with the y-axis as the velocity and the x-axis as the time. In the case of the descending aorta, the Doppler spectral tracing is negative because blood flow in this area is directed away from the transducer (Figure 1-9). The highest frequency shift (and thus the highest velocity in each direction) that can be measured by PW Doppler is dependent upon how frequently the ultrasound pulse is sent (**pulse repetitive frequency**, or **PRF**). The highest frequency shift that can be measured with each PRF is equal to PRF/2, and the highest velocity obtainable from the maximum measurable frequency shift is known as the **Nyquist limit**. At deeper locations, more time is required to complete the journey to and from the sample volume location, thus the maximum obtainable PRF is lower, resulting in a lower maximal velocity that can be measured. The other factor that influences the Nyquist limit is the frequency

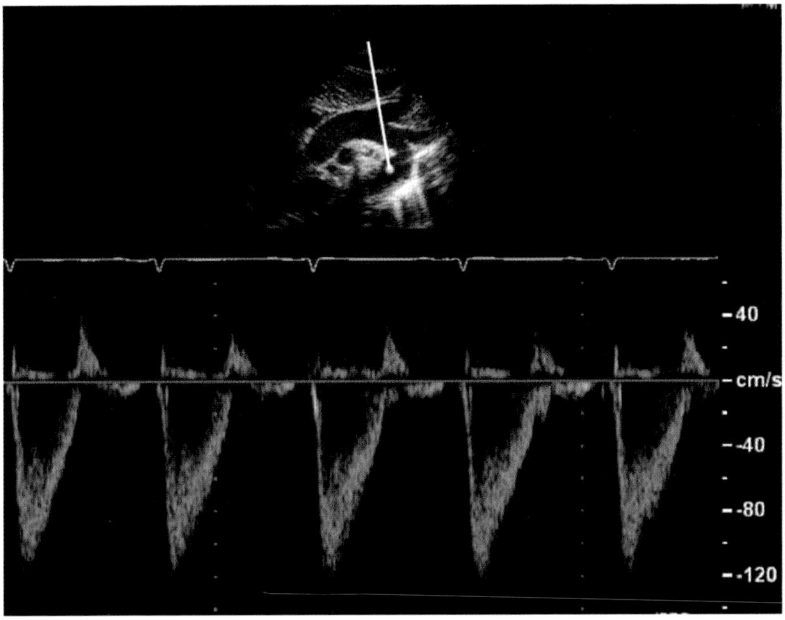

FIGURE 1-9. Pulsed wave (PW) Doppler spectral display from descending aorta obtained with a transducer in the suprasternal notch position (normal laminar flow).

of ultrasound, which holds the same inverse relationship as for 2D imaging—the higher the ultrasound frequency used for Doppler, the lower the Nyquist limit. When the velocity of blood flow exceeds the Nyquist limit, the machine interprets it as having the opposite direction, and the Doppler spectral tracing "wraps around" to the opposite side. This process is known as **velocity aliasing** (Figure 1-10).

When using PW Doppler to measure frequency shift and blood flow velocity, the user moves the sample volume to the area of interest. The sample volume has a finite length called a **receiving gate** which defines the area that Doppler measurements will be made. The receiving gate usually has a length of around 3 mm but can be decreased to get a better resolution or increased to get a better Doppler signal intensity.[3] Because there are many blood cells flowing through this region of interest with different velocities, the spectral Doppler tracing is not usually displayed as a straight thin line, but instead as a bright white line with some thickness (a band) on a black background. The brightness of an echo spectral display of a particular velocity is dependent upon the number of red blood cells with that velocity, and the thickness of the spectral display band is dependent upon the variation of red blood cell velocities that are being sampled. If blood flow is laminar (which characterizes most normal blood flow in the human body), the difference of velocity and direction of red blood cells will be small (small variance), and a relatively thin band of spectral Doppler velocities is seen (Figures 1-8 and 1-9). The range of difference in velocities is called **variance** and is shown as the thickness of this Doppler spectral band. Variance can give information on whether blood flow is laminar or turbulent.

In addition to the spectral Doppler display, most echocardiographic machines also can emit an audible sound, delivered at the same frequency as the frequency shift, that is produced by the sampled moving reflectors. Laminar flow results in a tonal or music-like sound, as opposed to turbulent flow, which produces a harsh sound from the audio output.

In certain pathologic conditions, such as a patient with a stenotic valve, blood flow accelerates at the stenotic point and causes turbulence distal to the area of stenosis. Blood flow in this area will have many directions and velocities and is called **disturbed** or **turbulent flow** (as opposed to **laminar flow**). When a Doppler signal is obtained from this area, different velocity vectors in the direction of the transducer will be recorded (increased variance) and thus

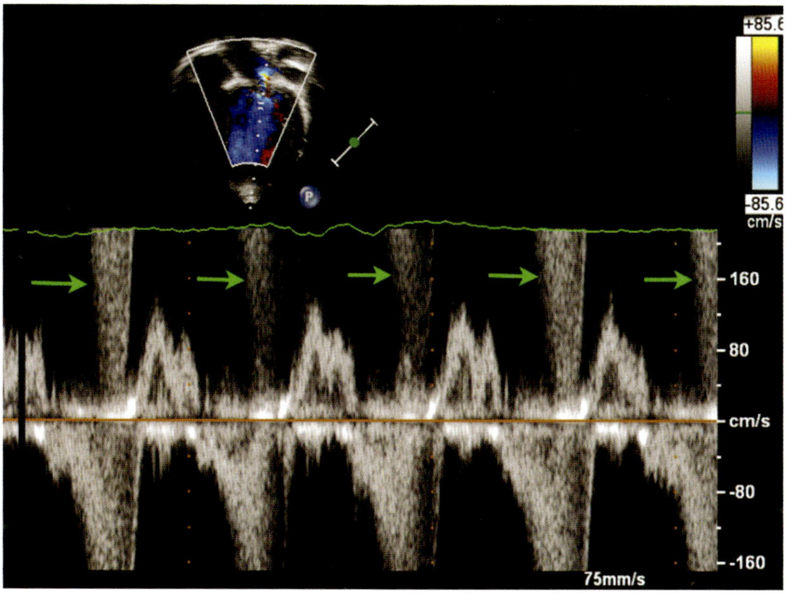

FIGURE 1-10. Doppler spectral display when the velocity is higher than the Nyquist limit in a patient with mitral regurgitation. Note the "wraparound" signifying aliasing of the Doppler spectral display because the velocity was higher than the Nyquist limit (arrows). Also, compare PW Doppler spectral display of a turbulence flow in this patient to a laminar flow in Figures 1-8 and 1-9.

the thickness of Doppler spectral band will be increased, with a harsh quality of the audio output.

PW Doppler can give information on the direction and velocity of blood flow at the region of interest, but it is limited by a maximum frequency shift and velocity that can be measured. This is usually not a problem in normal circulation with blood flow velocities < 1.5 m/s but can present a problem when the velocity of blood flow is higher, such as when measuring the degree of pulmonary hypertension or valve stenosis.

Continuous-wave (CW) Doppler

In general, continuous-wave (CW) Doppler is used when the Nyquist limit has been reached on PW Doppler and an accurate measurement of peak blood flow velocity (and thus the peak pressure gradient) is needed. It can also be helpful if one wants to record blood flow from more than one region at the same time, such as to record the timing of inflow and outflow of left ventricle to calculate isovolumic relaxation time (see Chapter 8).

To obtain CW Doppler, two separate piezoelectric crystals in the transducer continuously send and receive ultrasound signals along the path of interest. Doppler shifts from any point along the echo beam are recorded and displayed; there is no limitation to the highest velocity that can be measured. However, there is no discrete sample volume and therefore no information on the origin/location of the highest frequency shift (highest flow velocity) is available. Therefore, CW Doppler is said to have **range ambiguity**. Because the frequency shift of the echo signals occurs from blood flow at any depth along the line of ultrasound path, the CW spectral Doppler display is generally a solid white column consisting of both low- and high-velocity signals (Figure 1-11). In case of a stenotic valve, a low-velocity blood flow proximal to stenosis can also be seen as a shadow inside the high-velocity signals. The maximal velocity proximal (V1) and distal to the stenosis (V2) can then be used to calculate the pressure gradient (see arrows in Figure 1-11). The method of calculating pressure gradients from Doppler velocities will be discussed in Chapter 6.

Color Flow Imaging (Color Doppler)

Color flow Doppler imaging uses Doppler information from many small adjacent regions of interest to demonstrate the direction and velocity of blood flow within that

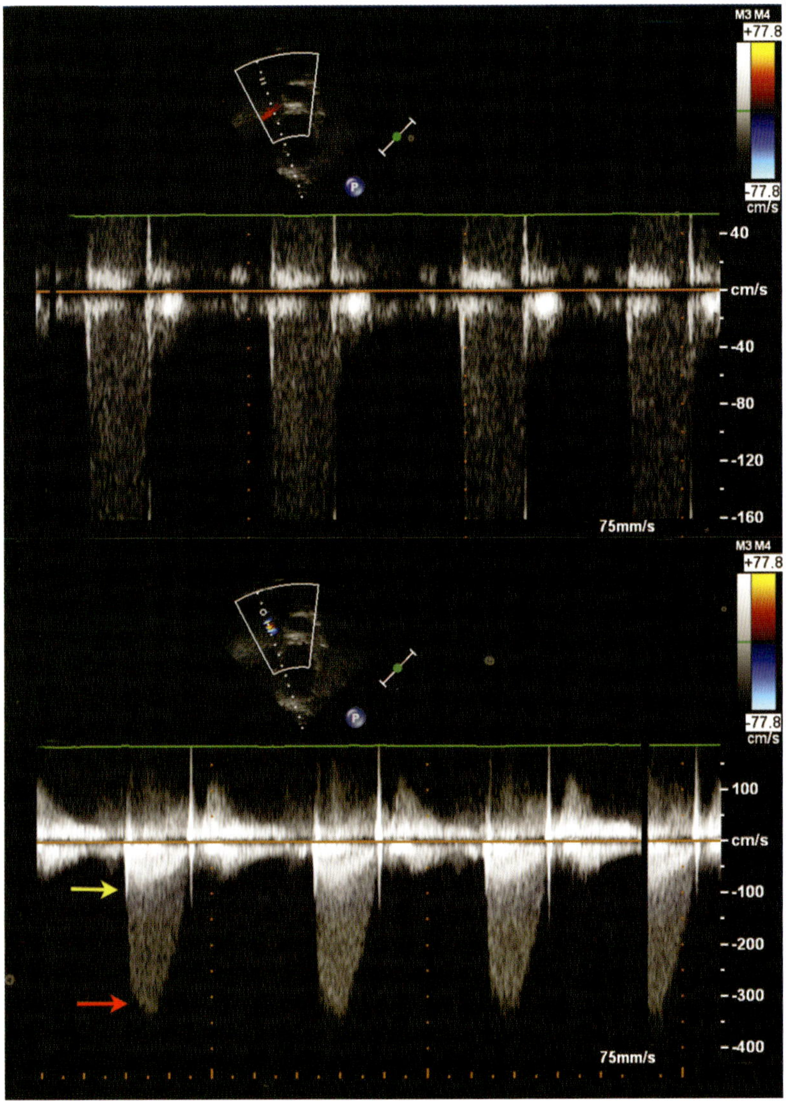

FIGURE 1-11. Top: Pulsed wave (PW) Doppler in a patient with aortic valve stenosis demonstrates higher maximal flow velocity than the Nyquist limit. Bottom: Continuous-wave (CW) Doppler in the same patient demonstrates its ability to measure high flow velocity. Note the peak blood flow velocity proximal to the stenosis (V1, yellow arrow) and distal to the stenosis (V2, red arrow).

region. The information is color-coded and superimposed on a 2D image to give the operator an easy and quick way to visualize the cardiac structure and blood flow at the same time (Figure 1-12, top). For more detailed information of the direction and velocity of blood flow, the operator can then use the color flow map to choose a specific area to interrogate with PW Doppler (by placing a sample volume, Figure 1-12, bottom) or a general direction to interrogate flow velocities using CW Doppler (by placing a line over the blood flow of interest).

To obtain color Doppler flow imaging, the computer divides user-defined areas of interest into several pixels, obtaining PW-derived mean velocity (± variance) in those areas and plotting them with color codes. By convention, velocity in the positive direction (toward the transducer) is generally plotted in red and in the negative direction (away

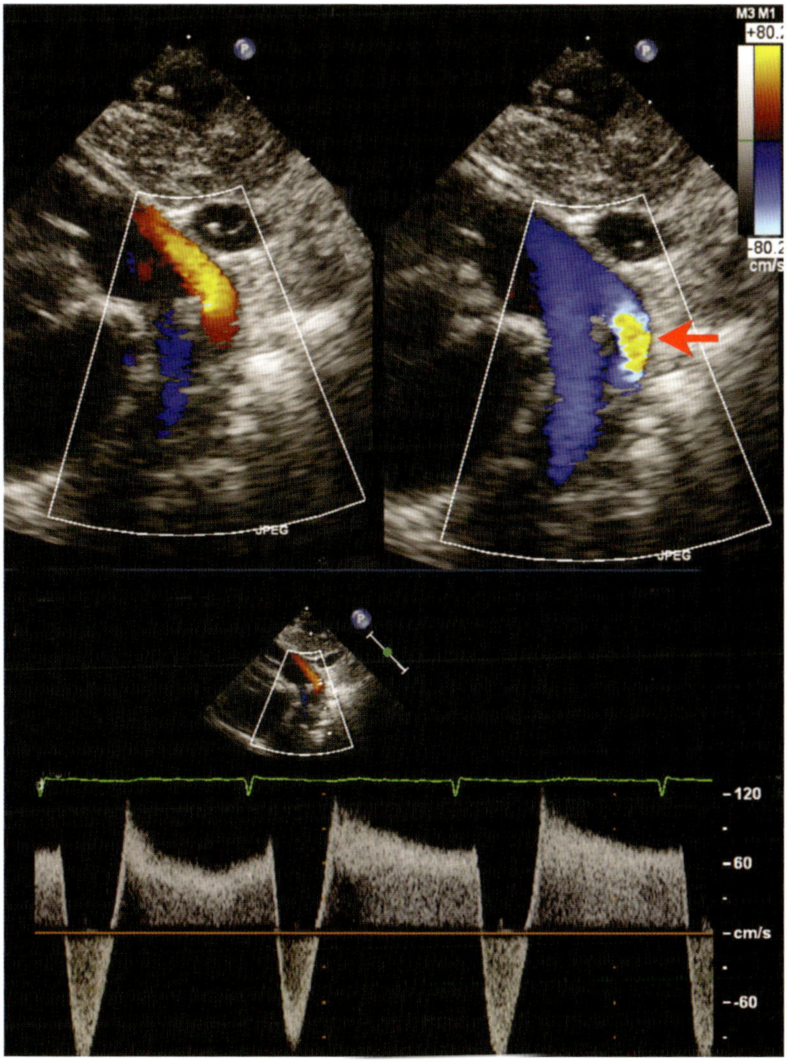

FIGURE 1-12. Color flow mapping and spectral Doppler of a patent ductus arteriosus (PDA) in a patient with pulmonary hypertension showing bidirectional flow. Top, left: Left-to-right shunt in late systole and throughout diastole (descending aorta to pulmonary artery). Top, right: Right-to-left shunt (pulmonary artery to descending aorta) in early systole. Note the aliasing of R to L shunt flow during systole resulting in color changing from blue to yellow (arrow). Bottom: Pulsed wave Doppler with sample volume at PDA showing spectral Doppler tracing of the bidirectional shunt.

from the transducer) in blue. A brighter color (red or blue) would signify a higher velocity such that fast-moving blood flow will appear brighter than slowly moving blood flow. The color flow map can also be adjusted to include the variance—which conveys information on how turbulent the flow is—usually as a green hue on the red/blue color map.

Because color flow mapping utilizes PW Doppler principles to obtain multiple velocities from a specific, defined region of interest, it is subject to the same limitations as PW Doppler. This includes the limit of the highest positive and negative velocities obtainable with each ultrasound frequency at certain depths (Nyquist limit). As discussed earlier, **aliasing** occurs when the velocity of flow exceeds the Nyquist limit, and this is represented by the color converting from red to blue or blue to red, and/or a mosaic pattern including other colors such as green and yellow

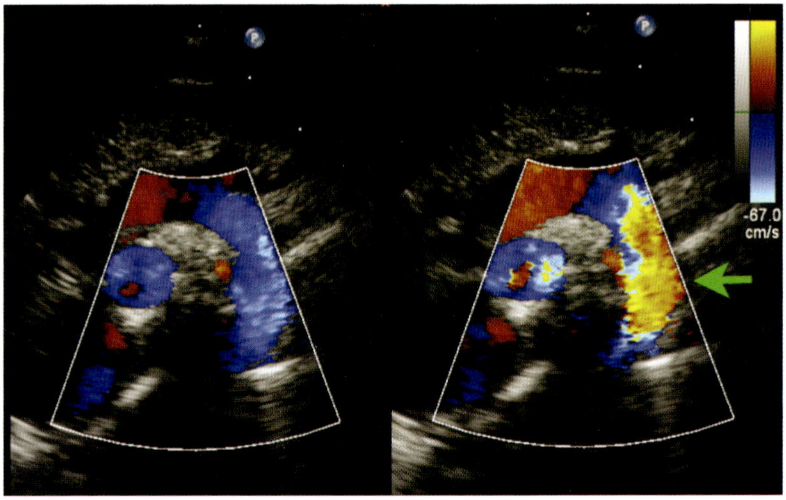

FIGURE 1-13. Color flow aliasing in descending aorta in a patient with a normal heart. Left: The color of flow mapping in the descending aorta is blue in late systole, and no aliasing is seen. Right: During early systole, the flow has higher velocity and exceeds the Nyquist limit (67 cm/s in this picture), which results in aliasing, displayed as a bright red color mixed with the blue and yellow (arrow).

(Figures 1-12 and 1-13). To reduce or sometimes eliminate the aliasing, users can shift the zero line to increase the Nyquist limit. However, doing so would potentially cause the color flow image to lose directional information for blood flow.

Color flow imaging demands a great deal from echocardiography computational resources. Not only does the machine have to produce the 2D image, it also has to send and receive multiple PW Doppler pulses to obtain all the velocity information that makes up the superimposed color flow image. If the region of interest for the color flow image is too large, or must be expanded, a reduction in frame rates will occur. Therefore, the user should always adjust the color flow data area of interest to the smallest acceptable size and least amount of depth necessary to yield the desired information. Using this approach, color flow velocity information of a particular structure can be obtained without compromising the frame rate (ie, temporal resolution is optimized). Once enough information has been obtained, the color window can be moved to other areas of interest.

PITFALLS WHEN USING DOPPLER ECHOCARDIOGRAPHY

Angle Correction

Because velocity is a vector value with directional information as well as amplitude, Doppler measurement of any blood flow velocity will result in frequency shift only for the velocity vector along the line of measurement. If there is any angle difference between the direction of ultrasound pulse and the direction of blood flow, the measured velocity will be different (lower) than the actual flow velocity. For any given angle between the ultrasound path and the direction of blood flow θ, the velocity of blood flow can be calculated using the Doppler equation discussed above:

$$V = \frac{C \times fd}{2 \times f0 \times \cos\theta}$$

As a consequence, the echo operator should attempt to obtain Doppler data from the angle that is most parallel to the direction of blood flow, which sometimes necessitates multiple transducer movements or obtaining the Doppler data from multiple views. For example, obtaining a pressure gradient in a patient with aortic valve stenosis can be performed from an apical 5-chamber view as well as from the suprasternal notch. Similarly, a right ventricular pressure can be obtained by measuring the velocity of tricuspid valve regurgitation from either an apical four-chamber view or a parasternal long-axis view with the transducer tilted toward the tricuspid valve (Figure 1-14). Chapter 6 discusses the noninvasive assessment of hemodynamic information utilizing Doppler echocardiography.

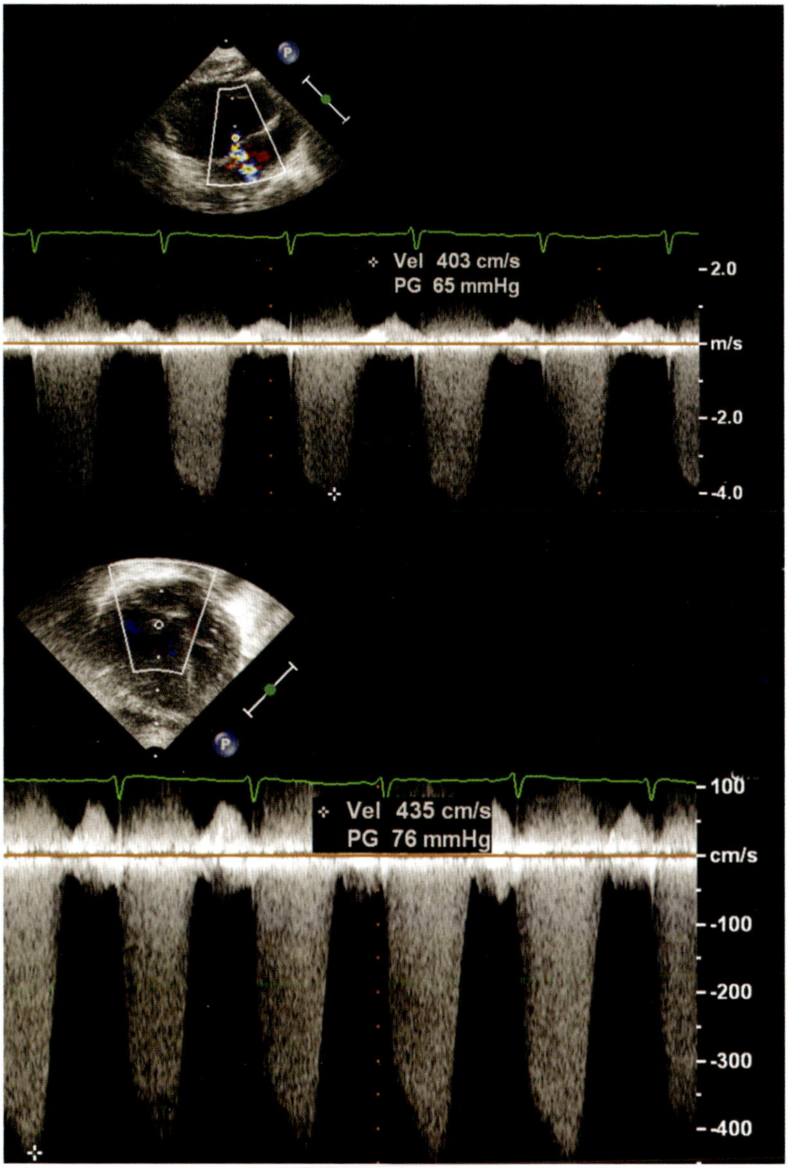

FIGURE 1-14. Continuous-wave (CW) Doppler measurement of the peak velocity of tricuspid valve regurgitation for evaluation of a newborn with pulmonary hypertension. Top: Measurement from long-axis parasternal view with transducer tilted towards the tricuspid valve. Bottom: Measurement from apical four-chamber view. Note the difference between the two measurements. In this case, the measurement from the parasternal long-axis view slightly underestimates the velocity from the other window. Both tracings have a good Doppler spectral envelope and absence of significant noise.

Gain Settings for Doppler Measurement

One of the common pitfalls when using Doppler to measure blood flow velocity is the improper adjustment of gain for the Doppler spectral image. Too high or too low gain can cause the measured pressure gradient to be higher or lower than the actual value, and at higher velocities the differences will be more pronounced because the measure velocity must be squared to obtain the pressure gradient (see Chapter 5). In general, adjustment of gain should be made such that the background remains black on the monitor, with no "noise," and there should be a complete and smooth "envelope" of the Doppler spectral image (Figure 1-14).

Adjusting Nyquist Limit, Transducer Frequency, and Depth Setting

The Nyquist limit can be adjusted for PW Doppler or color flow image to best visualize the blood flow of interest. For example, when blood flow ejected into the aorta or into the arterial system is evaluated, there are usually higher velocities (0.7–1.3 m/s) that will require higher Nyquist limit setting to avoid aliasing (wraparound) of the Doppler signals. On the other hand, lower Nyquist limits might be more appropriate in the use of PW Doppler or color flow image in areas with low velocity blood flow, such as in the pulmonary or systemic veins (Figure 1-15). It is also important to remember that Nyquist limit depends upon the frequency of the sound wave used (higher velocity limit for lower frequency) and the distance of measurement (higher velocity limit for lower depth). To obtain the highest Nyquist limit, one should then use the lowest frequency Doppler and limit the area of interest to the lowest depth possible to image the structure. With multifrequency transducers, the machine generally uses the lowest frequency for that particular transducer to make a Doppler assessment (such as using 5 MHz Doppler for 5 to 8 MHz transducer).

How to Measure a Velocity That Is Higher Than the Nyquist Limit

Increase the Nyquist Limit to the Maximum

This is usually done by increasing the scale control on the machine to the maximum possible value for PW Doppler at that depth/sound frequency.

Use a Lower Ultrasound Frequency

This is usually performed by changing to a lower frequency transducer, as the lowest frequency for a particular multifrequency probe is generally already selected for Doppler evaluation. This contrasts with 2D imaging, in which the user can change the frequency of the multifrequency probe higher or lower for better image resolution or penetration, respectively.

Use CW Doppler

The important advantage of CW Doppler is that there is no limit to the highest velocity that can be measured. However, as discussed earlier, this measurement will have complete range ambiguity. Therefore, it is often helpful to combine color flow Doppler and PW Doppler with CW Doppler in order to determine the likely area of aliasing and high velocity.

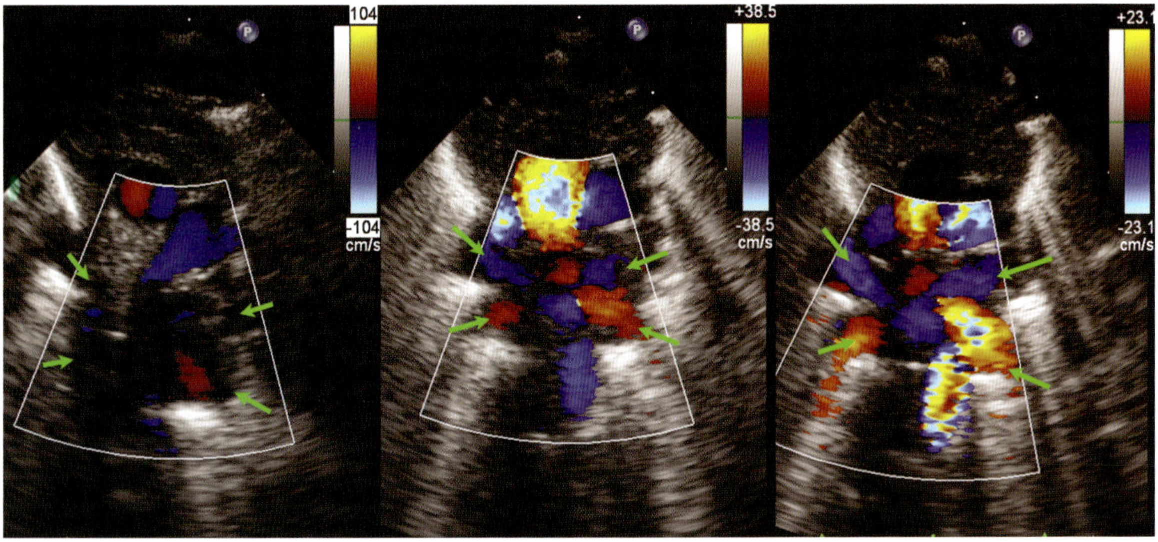

FIGURE 1-15. Color flow Doppler of pulmonary veins in a normal newborn. From left to right, the Nyquist limit is set at ± 104, 38.5, and 23.1 cm/s. Note that the pulmonary venous flows (arrows) are not well-visualized until the Nyquist limit is lowered to ± 38.5 cm/s.

Zero Line Shift

Zero line shift is achieved by shifting the zero line (baseline) up or down to get a higher limit of velocity for the direction of interest. The zero line can be shifted all the way down for a positive velocity and all the way up for a negative velocity (Figure 1-16). The location where the Doppler signal is obtained can still be precisely determined, but there is a limit to the highest velocity that can be measured, which is equal to twice the velocity limit without the zero shift.

High PRF PW Doppler

High PRF PW Doppler is performed by sending one (or more) pulse of ultrasound before waiting for the first pulse to return to the transducer, for example, at twice the PRF. In this example, the Nyquist limit is then doubled

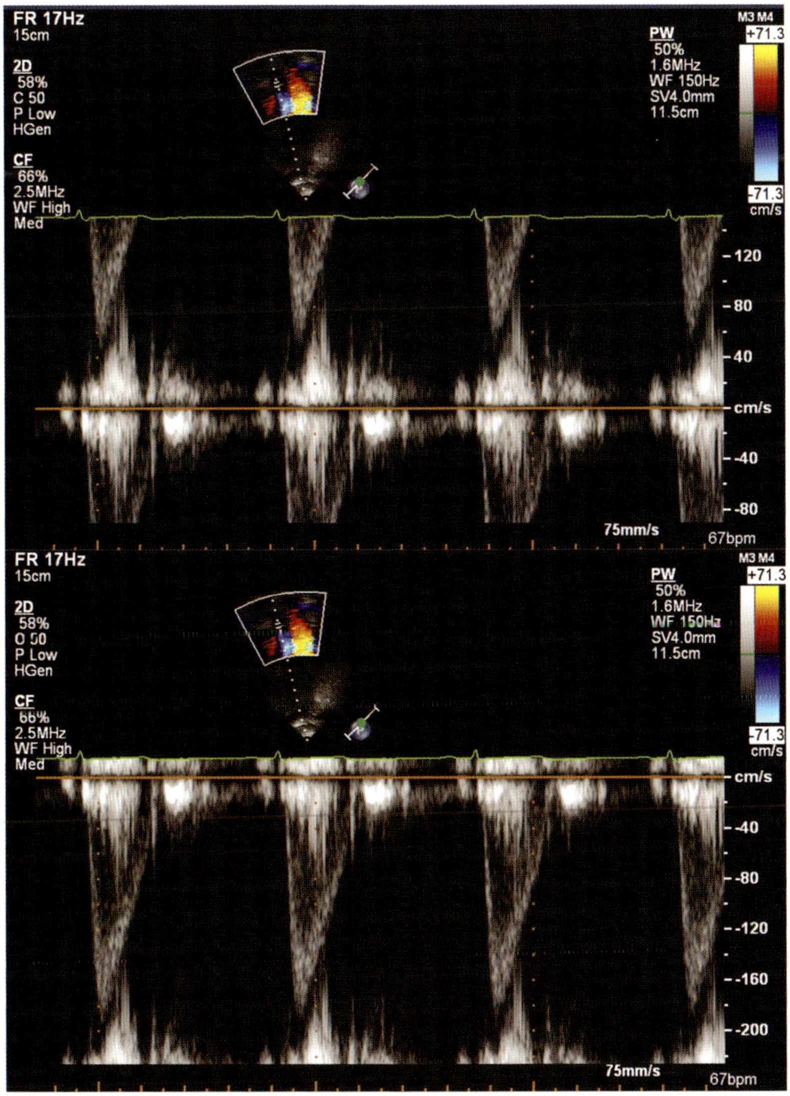

FIGURE 1-16. Top: Pulsed wave Doppler measurement of ascending aortic flow velocity showing aliasing (wraparound) of the Doppler spectral display because the peak flow velocity is higher than Nyquist limit. Bottom: "Zero shift" method is used to avoid aliasing of the Doppler spectral display.

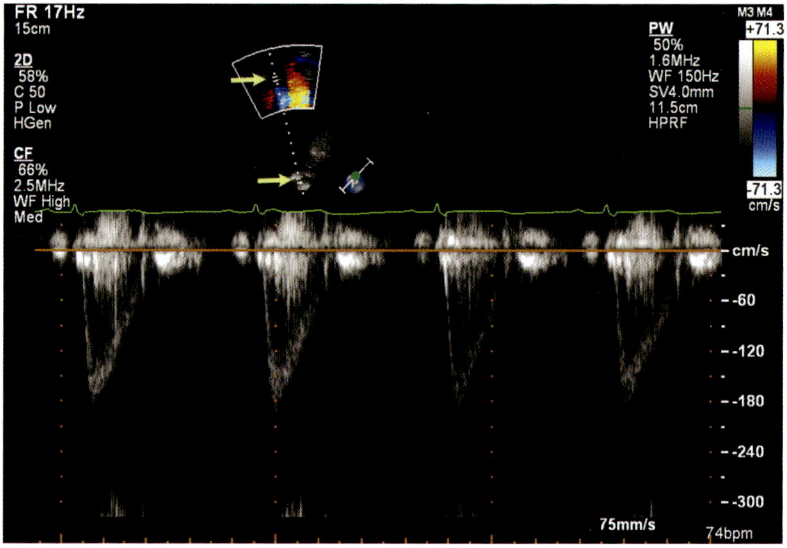

FIGURE 1-17. High pulse repetition frequency (PRF) pulsed wave Doppler is used to measure ascending aortic flow velocity in the same patient as shown in Figure 1-16. Note that the absolute highest velocity that can be measured increases from −200 cm/s to −300 cm/s using multiple sample volumes (arrows). However, there is range ambiguity, in that the recorded velocity can come from either sample gate.

(because the PRF is doubled). The disadvantage of this method is that the return of ultrasound from the second pulse returning from at lower depth (in this example, at the depth of 50% of the intended region of interest) can also be detected by the transducer and range ambiguity occurs from these two points. On the display, this is often shown as two (or more) sample volumes (Figure 1-17). This method can be thought of as an intermediate one between PW Doppler (one pulse at a time, one region of interest) and CW Doppler (continuous pulse, indefinite region of interest along the ultrasound beam).

REFERENCES

1. Armstrong WF, Ryan T. Chapter 2, Physics and instrumentation. In: *Feigenbaum's Echocardiography*. Philadelphia, PA: Lippincott, Williams, and Wilkins; 2010.
2. Kremkau FW. *Sonography Principles and Instruments*. 8th ed. Philadelphia, PA: Elsevier/Saunders; 2011.
3. Otto CM. *Textbook of Clinical Echocardiography*. Philadelphia, PA: Elsevier Saunders; 2009.

CHAPTER 2

Echocardiographic Scanners and Transducers

Mahmood Ebrahimi

- **TRANSDUCER**
- **MAIN UNIT**
  - Control Panel
  - Pulse Generator
  - Receiver
  - Amplification
  - Compensation
  - Compression
  - Demodulation
  - Reject
  - Memory and Storing Images
  - Display
- **THE INTEGRATED SYSTEM**
- **CONTROLS OF ECHOCARDIOGRAPHIC MODALITIES**
  - Two-Dimensional Controls
  - M-mode Controls
  - Doppler Controls
- **REFERENCES**

Ultrasound machines have greatly evolved during the last few decades. Bulky machines with limited capability have been transformed to much smaller units with enhanced capability of performing all modalities of echocardiography that we take for granted at present (Figure 2-1). Portable and even handheld devices have capabilities unimaginable 20 to 30 years ago. These units are technologically advanced, enabling performance of high-quality, complete studies. Regardless of their sizes, all have basically the same components and operate in the same manner.[1,2]

Ultrasound machines have two major components: the **transducer** (or **probe**) and the **main unit.**

TRANSDUCER

The transducer is the part of the system that generates and sends out ultrasound pulses, and then receives echoes coming back from the target (Figure 2-2). These sound waves are shaped via the transducer as beams that are focused and electronically scanned through tissues. This process is done by converting electrical energy into ultrasonic (mechanical) energy, and vice versa. The element that facilitates this conversion of energy is **PZT**, a ceramic plate made of lead, zirconium, and titanium. PZT has piezoelectric properties, which means that applied voltage deforms the material, causing it to vibrate and generate ultrasonic waves, and reflected ultrasound received by the PZT element(s) produces voltage changes that are processed and converted to echocardiographic images (Figure 2-2). Since transducer elements are solid and have high acoustic impedance, if no compensation is made for a much lower impedance of skin and tissues, most ultrasound energy will be reflected and little will be transmitted to the target organs, resulting in virtually no usable information (see Chapter 1). To prevent this, and to facilitate ultrasound transmission, the face of the transducer

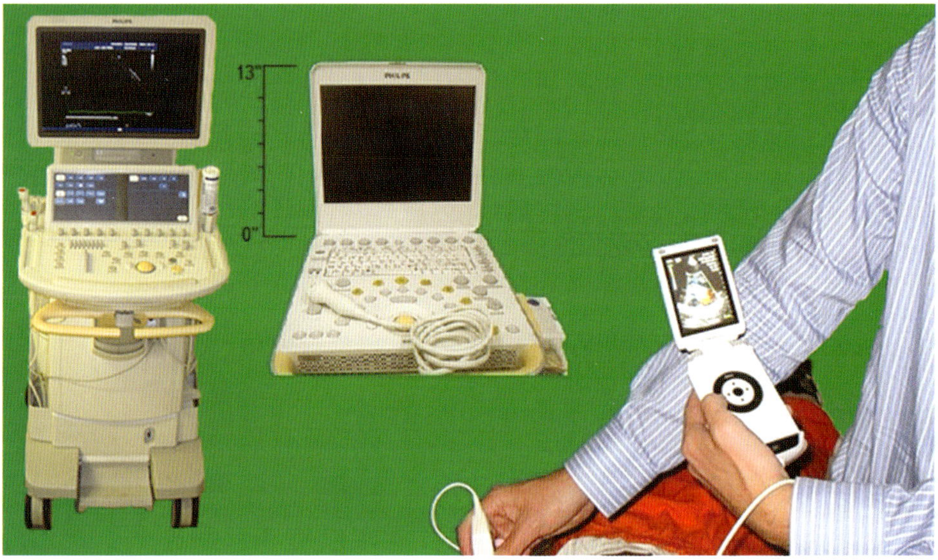

FIGURE 2-1. Three sizes of ultrasound systems, from a full-size system on the left to a handheld on the right and a portable system in the middle.

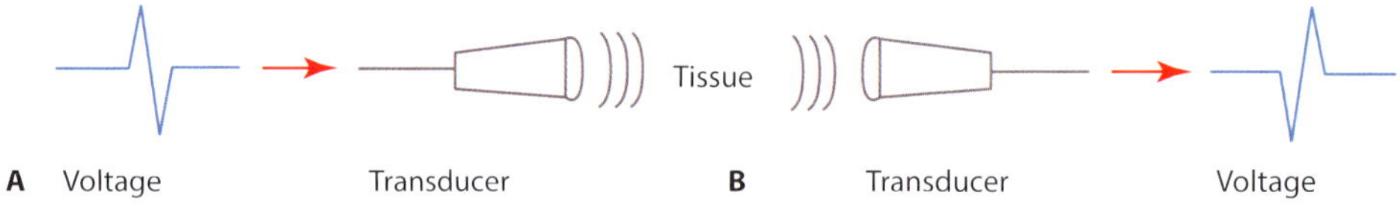

FIGURE 2-2. This figure demonstrates how a transducer works both as a transmitter and receiver at the same time. **A**. Electricity applied to the transducer produces ultrasound pulses. **B**. Echoes received by the transducer produces voltages that can be processed further.

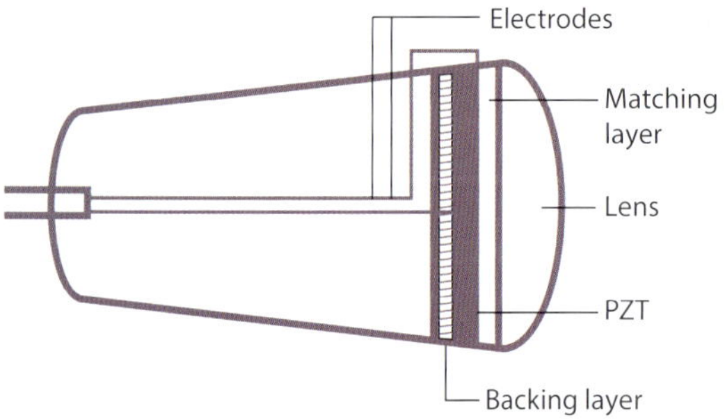

FIGURE 2-3. Basic structure of a single element transducer.

is covered by a matching layer with an impedance value intermediate to the transducer and tissue. A backing layer is also applied to absorb the extra sounds, thus keeping the pulses short. This will ease the transfer of pulses between the transducer and the patient, and vice versa. The transducer element is then placed in a casing and covered by a lens to enable more effective transmission and reception from a particular region. Figure 2-3 demonstrates the basic structure of a single-element transducer.

In older transducers, beam forming and scanning were done by rotating or swinging the transducer element inside the probe (mechanical transducers). For the new generation of transducers, multiple elements (arranged in an array) are used in each probe and the ultrasonic beam is formed electronically by delaying the signals to and from each element. These phased array scanners contain a large number of elements (up to 128) and come in a variety of shapes and sizes, depending upon the usage. For cardiac use, the elements are placed very close to each other and provide a sector scanning format, which yields a pie-shaped sector.

The operating frequency of the transducer is determined by the propagation speed and the thickness of

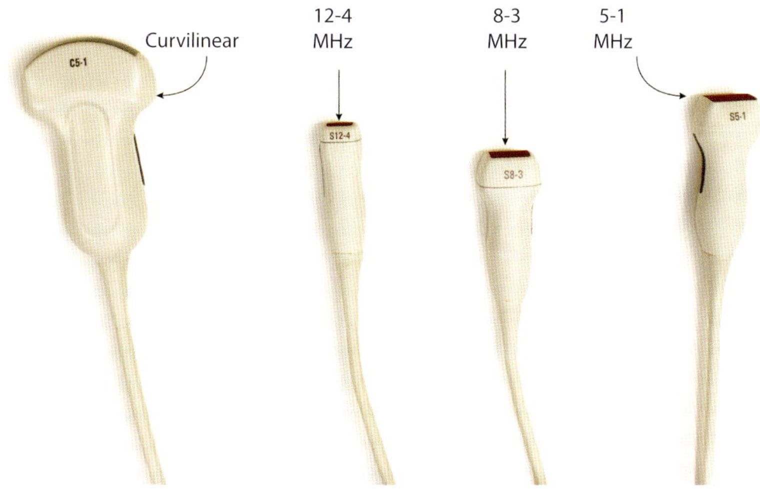

FIGURE 2-4. Different transducers mainly used in fetal, neonatal, and pediatric echocardiography. Curvilinear is used for fetal echocardiography, and sector transducers (S5 through S 12 and 3D) is used for neonatal and pediatric evaluation.

its element. For diagnostic ultrasound, the thickness is between 0.22 to 1.0 mm, with thinner elements yielding higher frequencies. Although a transducer should produce a frequency equal to its native operating frequency, in practice the ultrasound pulses produced can be composed of different frequencies. This range of frequencies is called **bandwidth**. Wide-bandwidth transducers give the operator the option of using the same transducer for different applications by selecting one of a range of available frequencies. If a higher frequency is chosen, better resolution can be achieved. However, if the penetration is insufficient, a lower frequency can be selected to obtain the desired penetration, although this will result in lower resolution (see Chapter 1). Each manufacturer provides a variety of transducers to be used for its ultrasound system for different applications (Figure 2-4). For pediatric and neonatal imaging, transducers with frequencies between 5 to 12 MHz are generally used, providing high-resolution imaging for neonates even less than 500g.

MAIN UNIT

As mentioned earlier, the ultrasound unit ranges from a handheld device to a full-sized machine. In this section, we will describe the components that are most commonly shared by all these machines. Some of these components (Figure 2-5) are integrated into the machine without any access by the operator, while others are controlled by different knobs, buttons, or touch screens. The core components of the main unit are as follows:

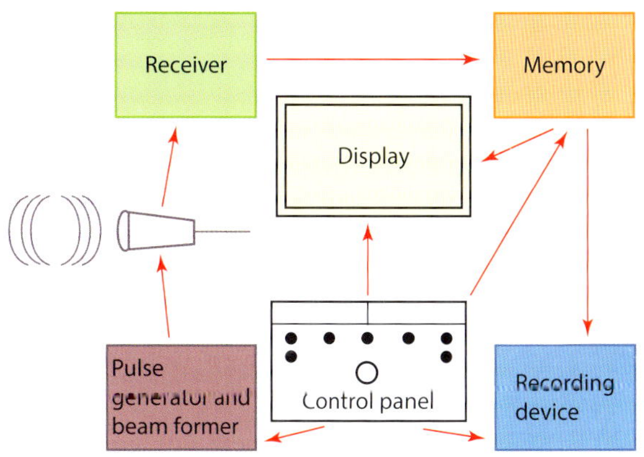

FIGURE 2-5. Near and far field zones in an unfocused (5a) and focused (5b and 5c) transducer. With modern phased array transducers, focusing of the ultrasound beam can be adjusted by the operator to enhance lateral resolution.

- Control panel
- Pulse generator and beam former
- Receiver
- Memory
- Recording device
- Display

Control Panel

The control panel is the part of the system that coordinates the action and interaction among other components; it is

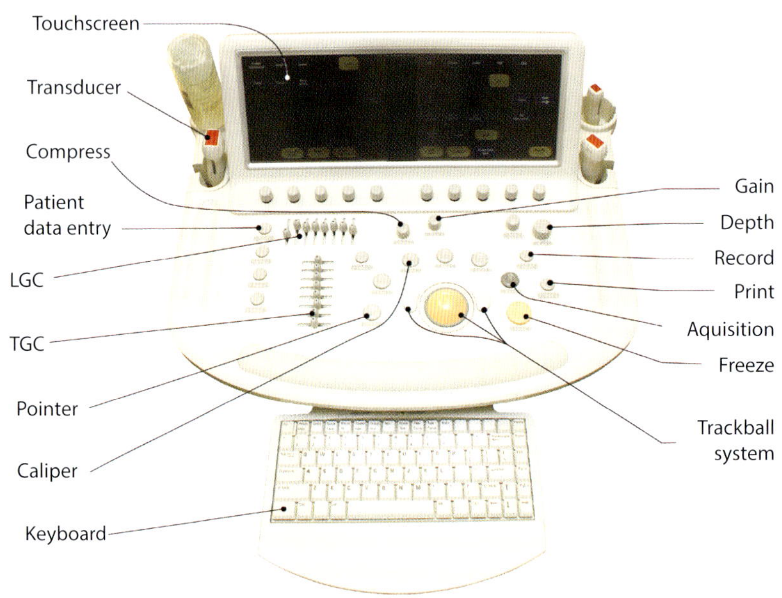

FIGURE 2-6. Control panel of a full-size ultrasound system. Buttons and knobs shown here are those of commonly shared in most of the systems. Abbreviations: LGC, lateral gain compensation; TGC, time gain compensation.

unique to each machine. It includes a keyboard for entering information and a trackball to control cursors. Knobs and touch-screen icons (Figure 2-6) are used to access various modalities used in the ultrasound machines.

Pulse Generator

The pulse generator (pulser) produces electrical pulses which in turn are changed to ultrasound pulses by the transducer. The pulser's job for a single-element transducer appears to be straightforward, but for phased array transducers, where sequencing and phasing are involved, it becomes much more complicated. In array transducers, switching, delays, and variation in pulse amplitudes (for multiple elements) are necessary for the electronic control of scanning, steering, transmission, and focusing of the beam of ultrasound pulses. These tasks are performed by the beam former.

The amplitude and intensity of the ultrasound pulse that is produced by the transducer is determined by the voltage amplitude produced by the pulser. The transducer output can be adjusted from the control panel by the sonographer, with the goal of achieving adequate ultrasound penetration while limiting the amount of ultrasonic energy that is directed at the patient. Transducer output is also called output gain, acoustic power, pulser power, energy output, and transmitter output. Output levels are often shown on the display in terms of percentage or decibel relative to maximum output. To the degree that output setting is increased, the amplitude of returning ultrasound pulses is enhanced. One should, however, be careful while using high power output, since the biological effects of ultrasound, such as peak negative acoustic pressure and intensity, could increase the likelihood of cavitation and tissue heating.

Receiver

Echoes returning from the tissue are received by the transducer and produce electric voltages in the transducer that are sent through the beam former to the receiver for further processing. The functions of the receiver include (1) amplification, (2) compensation, (3) compression, (4) demodulation, and (5) reject.

Amplification

Not all returning signals from the patient are suitable for further processing. Only frequencies around 100 kilohertz

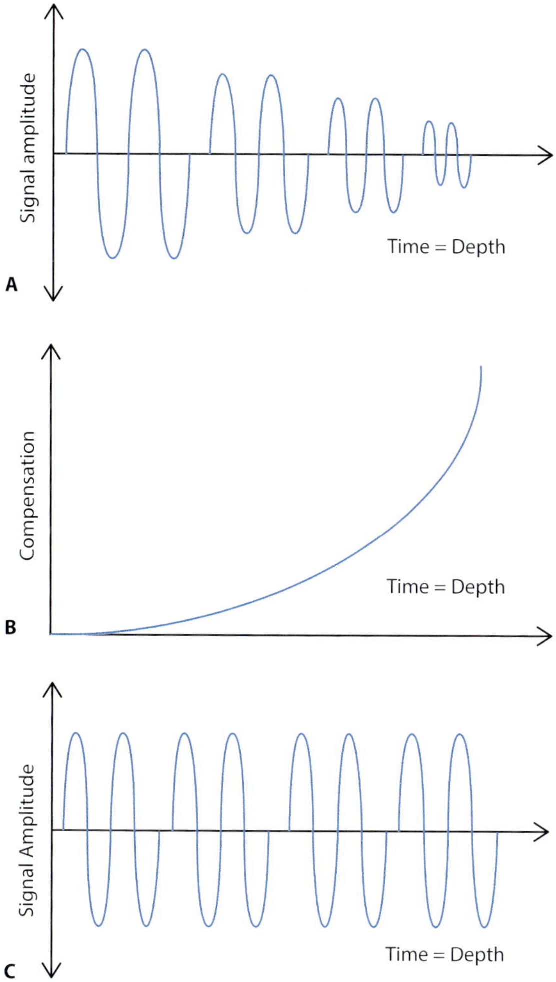

FIGURE 2-7. Compensation for attenuation. **A**. Echoes arriving from far field traveling for longer time are attenuated more and are weaker. **B**. To compensate, these weaker signals are amplified. **C**. All the amplitudes are equalized after compensation.

can be processed further, and these signals are often not strong enough. Therefore, a radiofrequency amplifier is used. Amplification is controlled by the operator and is also called **receiver gain**, or **overall gain**.

Compensation

The echoes received from greater depth are more attenuated than those from shallower depth. However, they have lower amplitudes and do not appear as bright. The receiver will make special compensations to make all echoes arising from similar tissue appear with the same brightness. This process is also called:

- Time gain compensation (TGC)
- Depth gain compensation (DGC)
- Swept gain compensation

TGC increases amplification of returning signals from increasing depths (Figure 2-7), in order to compensate for the progressive attenuation of the deeper echoes. The higher-frequency transducers usually need more compensation since they experience greater attenuation.

Some newer systems have lateral gain compensation (LGC, Figure 2-6). LGC amplifies the signals similar to TGC, but does so in the lateral aspect of the sector; hence, they become stronger and brighter. TGC and LGC are adjusted by the operator to optimize image quality. If compensation is properly used, all images of similar reflectors located at different depths will appear identical. Incorrect TGC settings affect only a portion of the image at a certain depth.

Compression

Ultrasound systems process a large range of the signals, with echo voltage amplitudes from smaller than 0.01 mV to greater than 1000 mV. Compression reduces the difference between the smallest and largest signals. This process is performed by special amplifiers called logarithmic amplifiers that do not alter the relationship between the signals. This means that weak inputs will be amplified more than strong ones, so that after compression (Figure 2-8) the largest signal is still the largest and the smallest signal is still the smallest. Dynamic range is the ratio of the largest to smallest amplitude that can be processed by an ultrasound system and is expressed in decibels. The dynamic range of an amplifier that is capable of processing between 0.01 mV to 1000 mV is 100 db. Although these amplifiers have a range of up to 160 dB, other electronic parts of the system might not have such a range. Typical displays have only about 20 dB of dynamic range, which means that the most powerful signal can only be 100 times larger than the smallest signal for display. Therefore, the compressor is generally used to change 50 dB, with an intensity ratio of 100,000, down to 20 db. This corresponds to an intensity ratio of 100, which is acceptable for the display.

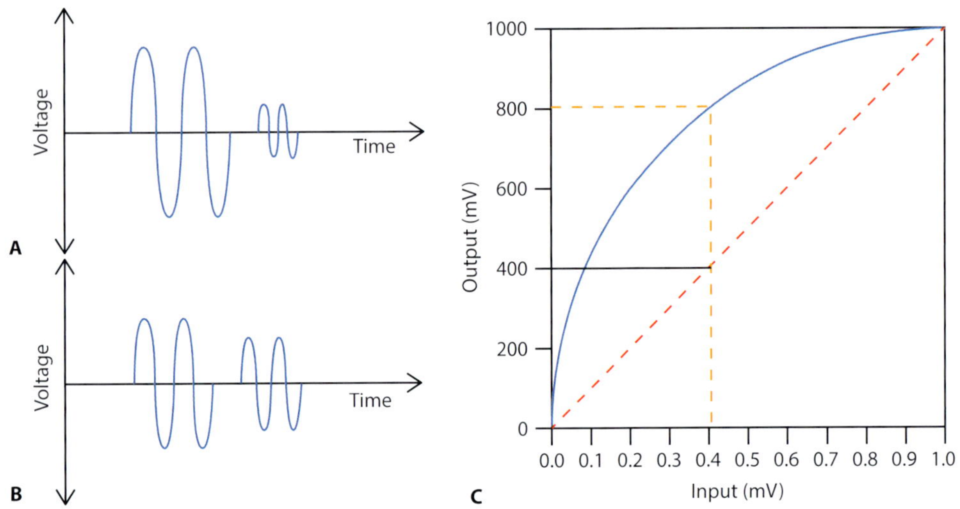

FIGURE 2-8. A logarithmic amplifier compresses the signals to decrease the difference between the largest and smallest voltage amplitude. **A**. Voltage amplitude before being compressed. **B**. Compressed voltages are shown; although they are smaller than before, the largest voltages are still the largest and the smallest voltages are still the smallest. **C**. This curve demonstrates how a logarithmic amplifier amplifies smaller voltages more than larger ones. A 0.4-mV input is amplified to 400 mV by a linear amplifier; however, the same input through a logarithmic amplifier results in signal amplification to 800 mV.

Demodulation

The ultrasound signals (voltages representing echoes) entering the receiver are in the form of radiofrequency (RF) and cannot be displayed on the screen. They must be converted to a video format (Figure 2-9). The conversion process used is called demodulation and consists of two steps:

1. Rectification
2. Smoothing

Rectification flips the negative half of the RF signal to a positive deflection. Smoothing evens out rough edges by putting an envelope around them, making square shapes of video format. Smoothing is also called filtering. Demodulation is done automatically within the system and is not operator-dependent.

Reject

The reject process is also called threshold suppression. Not all reflected echoes are suitable for processing. Some of the very low-level voltage pulses are weak echoes produced from scattering within the tissue ("acoustic noise"), and some from the electronic components within the system ("electronic noise"). These noises do not contribute to the quality of the image, and often interfere with display of useful information; therefore, they should be rejected from further processing (Figure 2-10). The reject control is activated and manipulated by the operator and eliminates all low-level signals from the entire field of view. However, improper use of this control could reject some low-level yet useful echo signals.

Memory and Storing Images

Up to this point, all the echo signals (voltage amplitudes) are in analog form. For electronic amplification, analog form is desired, but further processing and storing images is accomplished better in a digital format. The conversion of analog form to digital format is done by passing the signal through an analog-to-digital converter (ADC). Digital signals are then stored in computer memory. Digital signal processing can be performed prior to storage, called preprocessing, and after storage in the memory, called post-processing). How the computer digital memory works is beyond the scope of this discussion, but to put it simply, each echo amplitude leaving the ADC is assigned a discrete number based upon

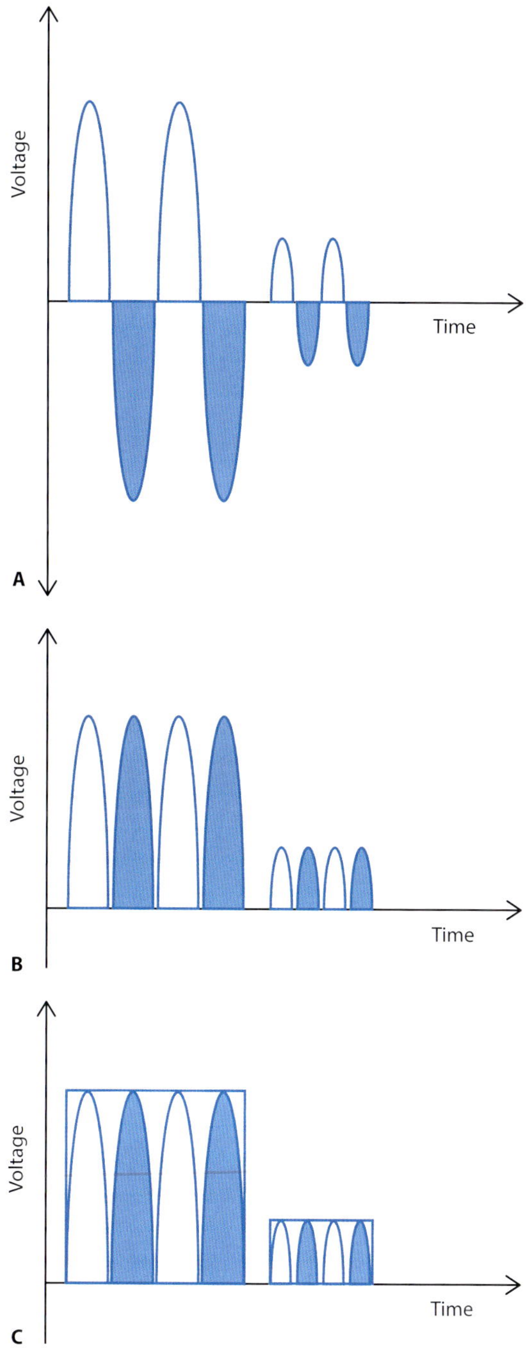

FIGURE 2-9. Demodulation process. **A**. Radiofrequency signal has positive and negative deflections. **B**. Rectification flips the negative half cycle to positive. **C**. Final stage of demodulation is smoothing or filtering by putting an envelope around the rectified signal.

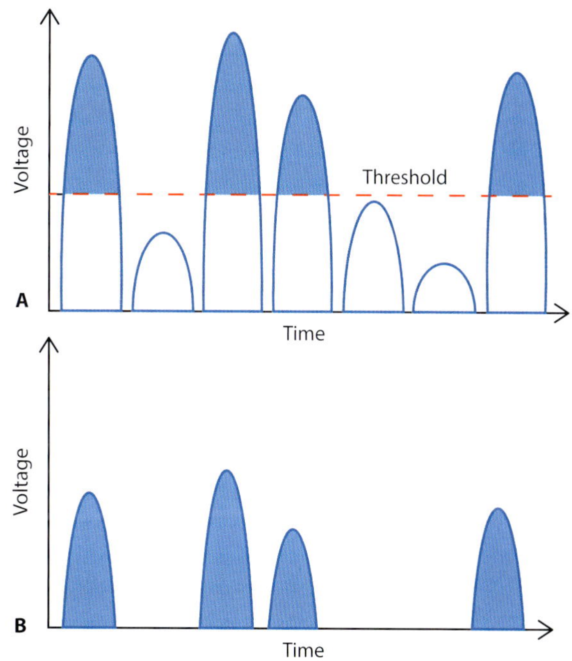

FIGURE 2-10. Rejection eliminates electronic noise and low-level signals. **A**. Setting a threshold or rejection level. **B**. Remaining signals after rejection.

a binary code (composed of 0s or 1s) that is stored in memory. In the memory, the information is written into the image plane or **matrix**, which is rectangular and divided into tiny squares (typically 512 x 512) called picture elements, or pixels, which make up the smallest elements of a digital picture. Each pixel has a horizontal (x) and a vertical (y) "address" that corresponds to the same address on the memory. Since echo data stored in the memory are in binary numbers (**b**inary dig**it** = **bit**), an image represented by a single bit would only produce a black-and-white picture (value of 0 vs. 1). Therefore, to depict digitally an image in grayscale, multiple layers must be used (Figure 2-11) to assign a group of bits to each pixel, thus creating different shades of gray. Higher numbers of bits provide better resolution and greater detail in the image; 8 bits per pixel allow for 2^8 or 256 shades of gray, which is the minimum number of bits utilized by most modern-day echocardiographic systems. A perfect example for preprocessing and post-processing is **write** and **read** magnification. **Write magnification**, also called write zoom, is a process that is performed prior

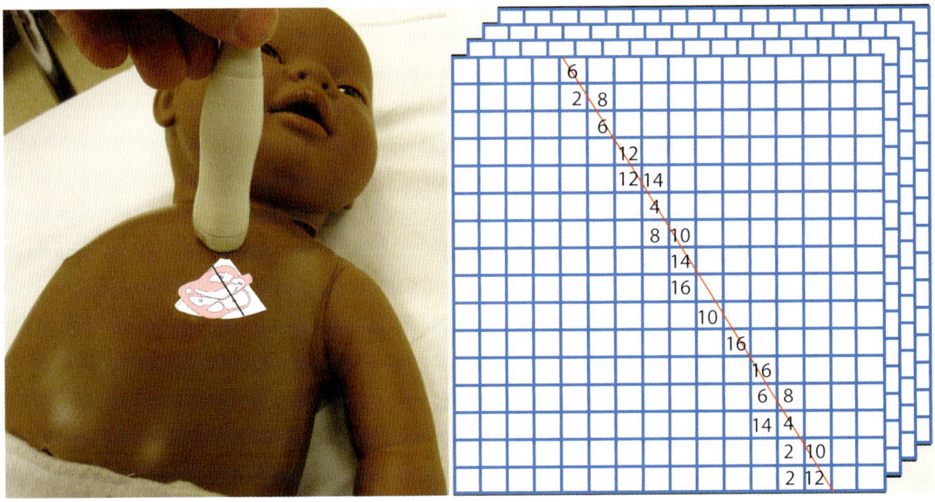

FIGURE 2-11. On the left, the cross section of the tissue to be scanned and imaged. On the right, a simplified four bits (four layer) per pixel digital memory capable of producing 16 shades of gray. Modern machines are 16 bits and produce 256 shades of gray.

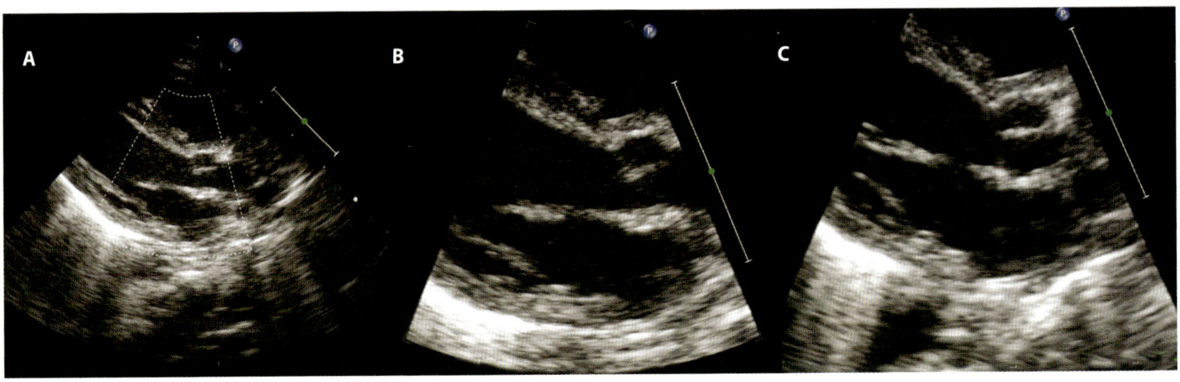

FIGURE 2-12. Write and Read zoom. **A**. Two-dimensional image with a zoom box set on the area of interest. **B**. Write zoom showing a larger picture with a high concentration of pixels, therefore resulting in a high resolution. **C**. Read zoom shows the magnified image with expanded pixels, thus yielding a lower resolution.

to storing the data and therefore is part of preprocessing. The operator will choose a region of interest from the image that needs to be magnified, and the system will scan only this area (Figure 2-12). Therefore, all the scan lines are concentrated in that region; hence, the line density is increased and the resolution is improved. The next step will store the information from this small area to the memory and from there will be displayed as a magnified image with good resolution. Write zoom allows information from a small anatomic field of view to be written into the entire memory, thus enlarging the image without enlarging the pixel size. **Read magnification**, or read zoom, is performed after the information is written to the memory (post-processing) and the image has already been created. Magnification merely enlarges the pixels, and the region of interest fills the entire screen. However, there is no improvement in image resolution. This is analogous to using a magnifying glass on a newspaper picture, in which the image is enlarged and might be seen more clearly, but image resolution remains unchanged.

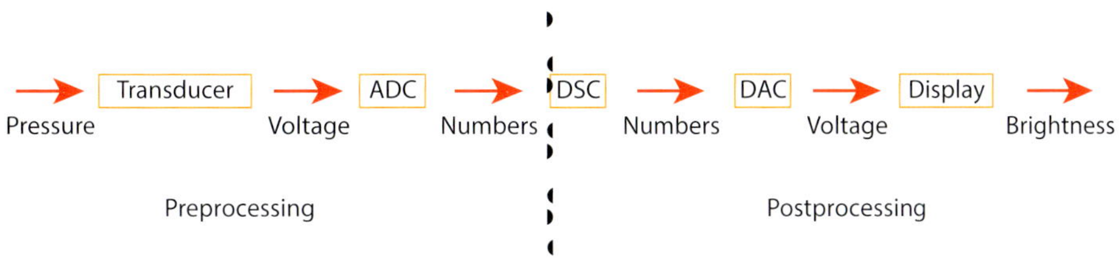

FIGURE 2-13. The process of displaying a 2D image on the screen. Pressure waves (echoes) entering the transducer produces a voltage which enters an analog-to-digital converter (A DC) resulting in binary numbers. Numbers are entered into a digital scan converter (DSC) of the computer memory. From here numbers are converted back to a voltage by passing through a digital to analog converter (DAC). In the next step voltages are applied to a display (TV screen) which produces brightness resulting in an image in the front of the screen.

Display

In order to display echo signals written to the computer memory as an image on the screen, the following steps must be performed:

1. The ultrasound beam needs to be scanned through the patient to produce cross-sectional "cuts" of the tissue.
2. Echoes received from all points are assigned binary numbers (analog to digital conversion) and stored to corresponding pixel locations in the memory (as described above).
3. This information can now be displayed on the monitor screen such as (cathode ray tube or CRT). The numbers are now displayed on the face of the screen as a bright spot corresponding to the pixel brightness. The brightness of the CRT, which is controlled by the voltages applied, is in analog form. Therefore, again, digital signals need to be converted to analog format for the image to be displayed on screen.

Figure 2-13 shows the summary of the actions that take place from the transducer to the displayed image. The new generation of ultrasound scanners use LCD screens which interface with the computer digitally. These displays can provide higher contrast and color definition by using large number of pixels. Therefore, digital to analog conversions are not needed. A rapid sequence of images (frames) is stored in the memory for producing a real-time two-dimensional video display from the cross section of the tissue (multiple frames per second). The ability to display each frame individually is called freeze-frame. Modern echocardiography systems have enough memory to store a few seconds of images and display them as a video loop. These loops can be displayed at a real-time rate, at a slower rate, or one frame at a time. This process is called image review, cine review, or more commonly cine-loop.

THE INTEGRATED SYSTEM

Echocardiography machines are available in different sizes and configurations (Figure 2-1). The full-sized machines have the advantage of being able to apply various ultrasound modalities—all with high quality—for different applications. These machines are powerful and versatile, and enable the use of a variety of different transducers and recording devices. Their disadvantages include large size, and the increased time required for these systems (essentially computers) to boot up and shut down between patients when the user is performing portable studies. In contrast, the smaller, more portable machines have some limitations, although the newer ones can perform most of the functions of the larger machines.[3,4] The advantages of these smaller machines include the following:

- They are lightweight and can be easily carried from patient to patient.
- They are battery operated so there is no need to shut down the machine completely between patients.

Following are the disadvantages:

- They might not have the wide selection of transducers available to a full-sized machine.
- Available transducers might have limitations such as penetration, color flow, and Doppler limitations.
- Battery life is limited (although this will likely this may be improved in the future).

The limitations in functionality of the smaller machines increase as the size of the equipment decreases. For example, handheld machines might have only one available transducer, and the available ultrasonic modalities might be limited to 2D echocardiography and color flow Doppler.

While all the above systems are different, they share many common operational features. Some of these might be named differently, depending upon the manufacturer, but they will still perform the same function. In this section, we will explain the basics as to which knob or button will operate a function of the system (also known as "knobology"). The control panel (Figure 2-6) is used by the operator to manipulate the knobs/buttons that perform different functions. However, some systems have touch screens that serve as part of their control panel. Some touch screens have different menus (Figure 2-14) that will change depending upon the ultrasonic modality being used (two-dimensional imaging, color flow Doppler, etc.). These are sometimes called "context-sensitive" menus, and generally they include buttons that can lead to other pages that provide additional functions. Some parts of the different touch-screen menus can also be operated by specific physical buttons and knobs on the control panel and their functions can be changed with their integrated menu. Thus, these buttons/knobs are termed *multifunction*.

After the machine is turned on, the system goes through a self-test and evaluation, initializing the software and loading the programs like any computer. This might take seconds to minutes, depending upon how powerful, advanced, and sophisticated the machine is. Upon finishing this process, the system is ready and the operator will start to work as follows:

1. Patient data and information related to the examination are entered, by using the keyboard on the control panel. If there is a worklist connected to a digital Picture Archive and Communications System (PACS), the patient's name can be selected from the worklist and patient information automatically populates the data fields.
2. The appropriate transducer for the patient is selected. Modern echocardiography machines can support multiple transducers (except for handheld machines, as noted above), but only one can be active at a time. Therefore, the appropriate transducer for the task at hand must be selected.
3. After selecting the desired probe, the user must select the appropriate echocardiographic application—for example, pediatric, adult, vascular, or fetal. These standard applications, usually preset by the manufacturer for tissue-specific imaging, can also be customized by manipulating and optimizing the image to the desired settings, and then saving it for future use as an individual preset.

From this point on, the user begins the examination, using several different modalities of ultrasound to perform a complete echocardiographic exam. It is customary to begin with 2D echocardiography, and to proceed to

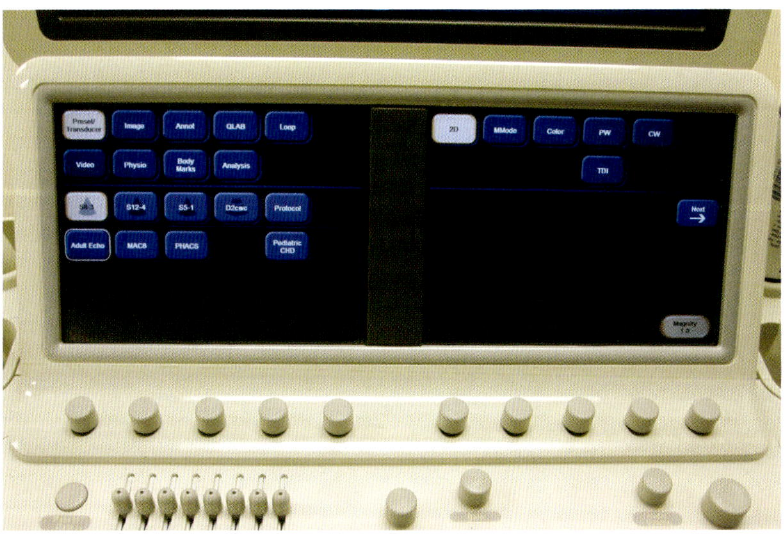

FIGURE 2-14. A touch-screen panel and multifunction knobs that enable the use of different menus ("context-sensitive menus") on the same screen.

other modalities such as M-mode, color flow Doppler, and spectral Doppler studies as needed. The actual performance of the echocardiogram is discussed at length throughout the remainder of this book, but in the following section we will discuss how to operate the echocardiography machine using the different modalities, and how to optimize the results.

CONTROLS OF ECHOCARDIOGRAPHIC MODALITIES

Two-dimensional Controls

The following controls are used to modify the field of view:

Depth

Decreases or increases the image depth to achieve the desired depth setting. The range of this control is determined by the transducer type and its frequency.

Sector width

Used to decrease the 2D sector width. The frame rate will increase when a narrower sector width is selected (because of the reduced number of scan lines required to produce the sector), which will lead to better temporal resolution.

Zoom

Concentrates all the imaging power into a user-defined area of interest, resulting in high resolution of a zoomed image (write zoom, see above). The operator will adjust the size and location of the region of interest, and the zoom function takes the image information from this area and rewrites the data to the new size of the zoom box. Since the image information within the zoom box is the only information being processed, this function provides zoomed images with a high spatial and temporal resolution. This function is only available in real time.

Magnification

This control is a read zoom (see above) and is used to magnify the existing 2D image in the entire sector. This function will work in a real-time or frozen image. Since this is a read zoom function, the frame rate will not change, but the resolution may appear decreased since the pixels are being spread across a larger region.

The quality of the received signals is optimized by the following controls:

Overall Gain

This control amplifies all frequencies received by the transducer from all depths, and to the same degree. Therefore, changing the overall gain affects the entire field of view.

Compress This control is used to adjust the range of gray shades (dynamic range) of the system. A broad/wide dynamic range displays more shades of gray, producing a smoother image; a small/narrow range displays fewer shades of gray, producing higher contrast. Once dynamic range is adjusted for a specific tissue, there is little or no further adjustment necessary.

Time gain compensation (TGC). The TGC slider (Figure 2-15A) applies gain selectively to compensate for the attenuation of the echoes returning from deeper areas in the tissue. Keeping the slider in the center can be used as an initial setting, but based upon image quality,

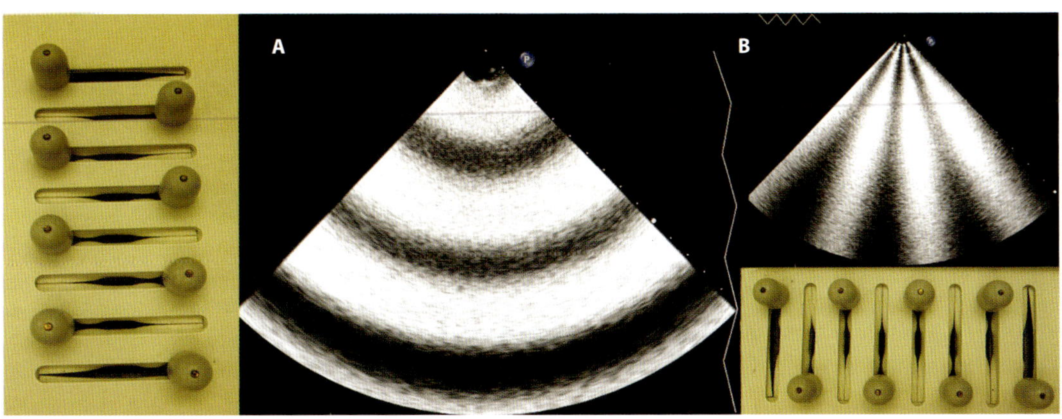

FIGURE 2-15. Compensation controls set in minimum and maximum positions to demonstrate their effect on the image. **A**. Time gain compensation (TGC) sliders. **B**. Lateral gain compensation (LGC) sliders.

the individual TGC sliders might have to be adjusted for specific tissue depths and acoustic windows.

Lateral gain compensation (LGC). These sliders operate like TGC but compensate for the attenuation of the echoes that occur across the image sector (Figure 2-15B). Returning echoes are usually weaker at the edges of the sector, and this is where LGC can be very useful.

Gray map settings. This function assigns different levels of gray shades to enhance the returning echo intensities. These maps are different in each system, and they can be changed in real time or on a frozen image.

Persistence. Also called frame averaging or smoking, this control is used to reduce the amount of speckle noise seen in 2D imaging. The process averages consecutive frames, causing the displayed image to appear smoother and less noisy. In cardiac imaging, higher settings of persistence produce very smooth images that appear to be moving at a slower rate.

Focus settings. This function has two controls. The first control positions the focal zone depth, and the second control changes the size or length of the focal area.

Speed. This control adjusts the sweep speed of EKG, M-mode, and Doppler tracings. The speed can be adjusted from a minimum of 25 mm/second to a maximum of 150 mm/second, depending upon the system.

Transmit or output power. This control determines the amount of acoustic power transmitted by the transducer. The safe limits of maximum acoustic power level for human use is set by Food and Drug Administration (FDA), and it is important for the operator to stay within these limits. Modern machines are designed in a way that if proper transducer and tissue specific image settings are used, one cannot exceed these limits. To utilize output power safely, always follow these important steps:

- Select the correct transducer and setting
- Set the output power to the lowest level possible to achieve adequate imaging.
- Optimize the 2D image by adjusting the gain, TGC and LGC, focal zone, and gray maps.
- Use output power only as the last control to be adjusted for improving the image.

There are other buttons and knobs on the control panel that are used for different modalities. They perform different functions and can vary significantly depending on the manufacturer and the capability of the system. The following are some of the more common ones:

The trackball system operates analogously to a computer mouse, with functions that will differ depending upon the modality being used. Some examples of these functions include moving/sizing the zoom box in 2D mode, moving/sizing the color box in color flow Doppler mode, steering the cursor in M-mode and spectral Doppler, and using calipers for measurement.

Record control is used to activate the recording device.

Digital acquisition is used to acquire images and video loops to store in the memory of the hard drive.

Freeze is used to activate cine-loop freeze-frame.

Calipers are used in different modalities (2D/M-mode/spectral Doppler) for measurements.

Print is used to print the images on a strip chart recorder in the older systems.

M-mode Controls

M-mode should be performed after completing the adjustments for 2D echocardiography, since image optimization for both modalities utilizes many of the same principal controls. After optimization, only a few more controls require manipulation. Specific controls used for M-mode are as follows:

Depth control to make sure all the structures are in the field of view for M-mode.

Trackball to bring the M-mode line to the desired area.

Compress to adjust dynamic range, to obtain a cleaner tracing.

Gain control to increase or decrease the intensities for all areas.

TGC to compensate for different depths.

Sweep speed should be adjusted according to the heart rate. For a normal heart rate, medium speed is suitable. However, for a faster heart rate, M-mode deflections will appear very close to each other, and therefore sweep speeds might need to be increased for easier measurement/calculations.

Doppler Controls

As previously noted, good 2D imaging should be obtained prior to Doppler evaluation. A correct acoustic window and view are the keys to optimizing the Doppler signals.

The controls for performing Doppler evaluation are as follows:

Color flow is the first option to be turned on. Newer machines have the option of simultaneous color flow and 2D side by side, also known as color compare. This option shows the color flow Doppler on one half of the display and the 2D image on the other half.

Trackball adjusts the size of the color box and moves it to the desired location. It also moves the Doppler cursor to the area of interest.

PW (pulsed wave Doppler) is the next function to be activated. The gate or sample volume can be adjusted at this time to the optimal size. By activating PW, a **spectral Doppler** tracing will appear on the screen.

Scale is used to adjust the velocities, therefore preventing aliasing. In color flow Doppler, this controller adjusts the Nyquist limit.

Baseline control moves the zero line on the spectral Doppler toward more positive or negative values, which also helps to prevent aliasing.

CW (continuous wave Doppler) is the next control to be used when the velocities are very high and PW adjustments cannot prevent aliasing. Most controls used in the pulsed wave Doppler have the same functions as in CW Doppler, except for sample volume, since CW is not range-specific.

Doppler gain is used to adjust the overall gain.

Speed control is used to adjust the sweep speed of the image. A faster speed is needed with higher heart rates to show the shape of some flow information, thereby making Doppler measurements easier.

Angle correction is used to better align the Doppler cursor and the flow for an improved Doppler signal. However, corrections greater than 15 inches will cause underestimation of the Doppler value.

Wall filter, compress, and reject controls are used to reduce extra noise (see above). **TDI** (tissue Doppler imaging) is used as needed when available.

REFERENCES

1. Kremkau FW. *Sonography Principles and Instruments*. 8th ed. Philadelphia, PA: Elsevier/Saunders; 2011.
2. Armstrong WF, Ryan T. Chapter 2, Physics and instrumentation. In: *Feigenbaum's Echocardiography*. Philadelphia, PA: Lippincott, Williams, and Wilkins; 2010.
3. Prinz C, Dohrmann J, van Buren F, et al. Diagnostic performance of handheld echocardiography for assessment of basic cardiac morphology and function: A validation study in routine cardiac patients. *Echocardiography*. 2012;29:887–894.
4. Spencer KT, Anderson AS, Bhargava A, et al. Physician performed point-of-care echocardiography using a laptop platform compared with physical examination in the cardiovascular patient. *J Am Coll Cardiol*. 2001;37:2013–2018.

CHAPTER 3

Cross-Sectional Neonatal Cardiac Anatomy as Depicted by Standard Two-Dimensional Echocardiography*

Bijan Siassi, Mahmood Ebrahimi, Shilpa Patil, and Ruben J. Acherman

- **CROSS-SECTIONAL NEONATAL ANATOMY**
  - Cardiac Orientation in the Fetus
  - Changes in Cardiac Orientation During Gestation
  - Differences Between Neonatal and Adult Heart
- **CARDIAC CHAMBERS, HEART VALVES AND GREAT VESSELS**
  - Location of the Heart Valves and Great Vessels
  - Imagining Planes of the Heart
- **OBTAINING NEONATAL ECHOCARDIOGRAM**
  - Preparing the Infant for Echocardiography
  - Selection and Manipulation of an Appropriate Probe
  - Display of 2D Images
- **HOW TO OBTAIN SPECIFIC SECTOR SCANS**
  - Parasternal Long Axis (Figure 3-15)
  - Parasternal Short Axis (Figure 3-16)
  - Apical Window (Figure 3-17)
  - Subcostal Coronal Views (Figure 3-18)
  - Subcostal Sagittal Views (Figure 3-19)
  - Infra-diaphragmatic Subcostal Views (Figure 3-20)
  - Suprasternal Window: Superior Vena Cava, Aortic Arch, Ductal Cut (Figure 3-21)
  - Suprasternal Window: Left Atrium and Pulmonary Veins (Figure 3-22)
  - Suprasternal Window: Innominate, Right Subclavian and Right Carotid Arteries (Figure 3-23)
- **REFERENCES**

CROSS-SECTIONAL NEONATAL CARDIAC ANATOMY

Cardiac anatomy is often taught on a heart excised from a cadaver, or on heart models that do not reflect the true spatial orientation of the heart as it lies in the chest cavity. However, with the advent of newer cardiac imaging techniques, diagnostic studies, and procedures on the heart, it is now essential that the structures of the heart be displayed and visualized as they lie in situ, and as they relate to the other contents of the thoracic cavity. In this chapter, we provide a comprehensive description of cardiac anatomy, particularly as depicted by echocardiography. Through the detailed use of drawings and representative

*Videos can be accessed at http://PracticalNeonatalEcho.com.

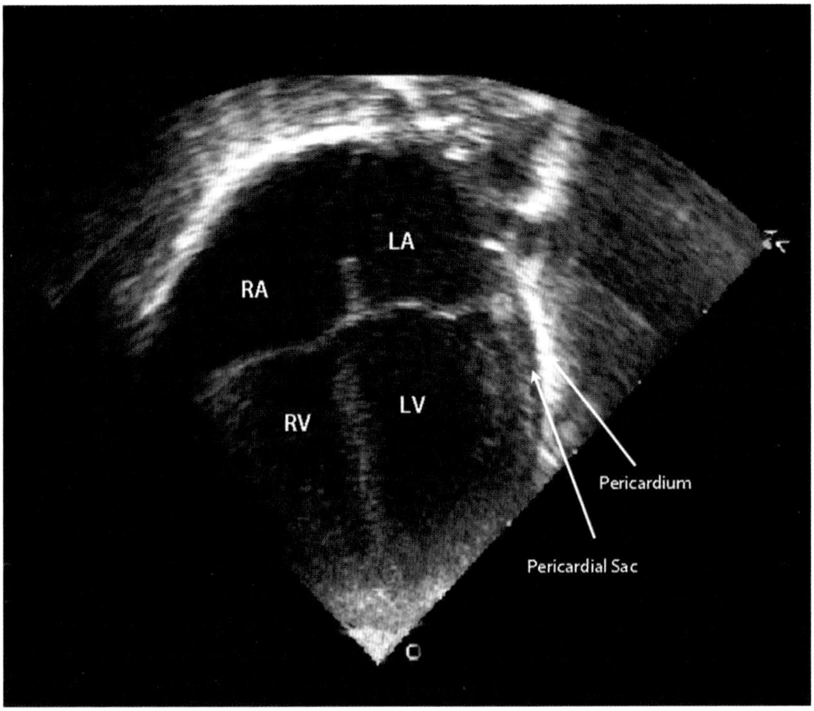

FIGURE 3-1. Apical four-chamber echocardiogram obtained from a 1-day-old neonate. Abbreviations: RA, right atrium; RV, right ventricle, LA, left atrium; LV, left ventricle.

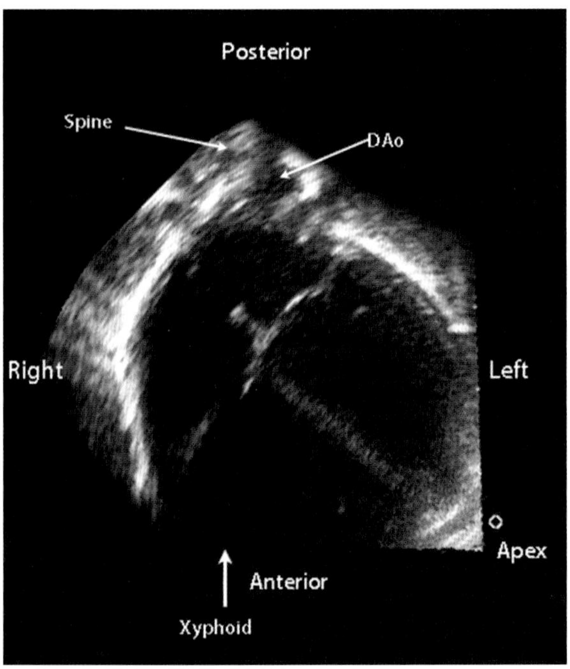

FIGURE 3-2. Apical four-chamber 2D transverse sector scan depicting accurate position of the heart in the thorax.

echocardiographic scans, we will focus on describing all cardiac structures, specifically as they are situated in the thoracic cavity.

Cardiac Orientation in the Fetus

Up to the fourth week of gestation, the heart is completely symmetrical, with the right atrium and ventricle located to the right and the left atrium and ventricle to the left of mid chest, as shown in Figure 3-1.[1] However, this echocardiographic image is obtained from the apex of the heart of a newborn and partially satisfies our preconception of how an ideal heart should appear, although this is not a realistic expectation. In this case, the transducer is placed at the apex of the heart and the cut is made mainly transversely, indicating the relationship of anterior and posterior structure of the heart (Figure 3-2). The rearrangement of cardiac position in the thoracic cavity occurs after fifth weeks of gestation and involves displacement and counterclockwise rotation (as viewed anteriorly) of the apex to the left and counterclockwise and displacement of posterior attachment of the atrial septum to the right. In this way, the posterior attachment of the atrial septum is located to the right of the spine, whereas the apex of the

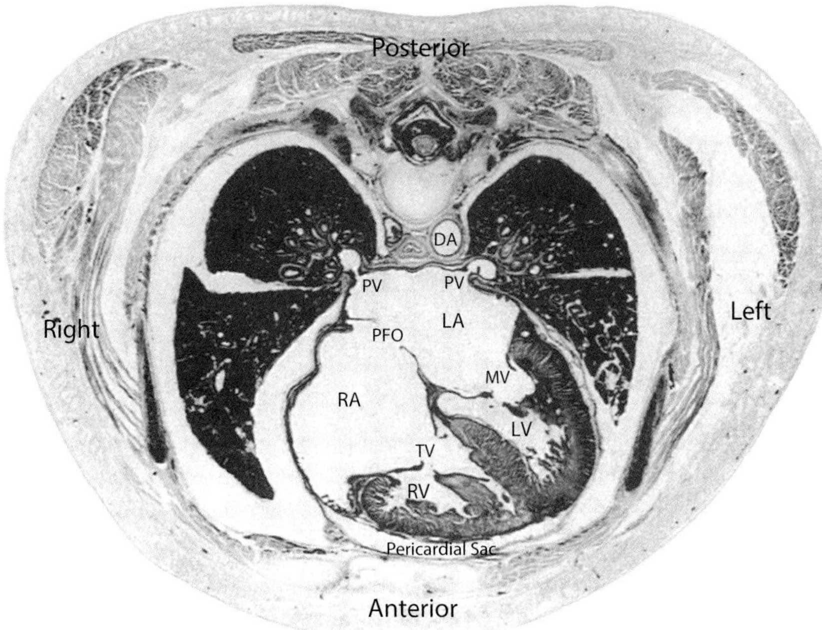

FIGURE 3-3. Transverse section of thorax at level of fourth rib in a newborn infant. Abbreviations: DA, descending aorta; PV, pulmonary vein; PFO, patent foramen ovale; MV, mitral valve, TV, tricuspid valve. (Reproduced with permission from Walmsley R, Monkhouse WS: The heart of newborn child: an anatomical study based upon transverse serial section, *J Anat*. 1988 Aug;159:93–111.)

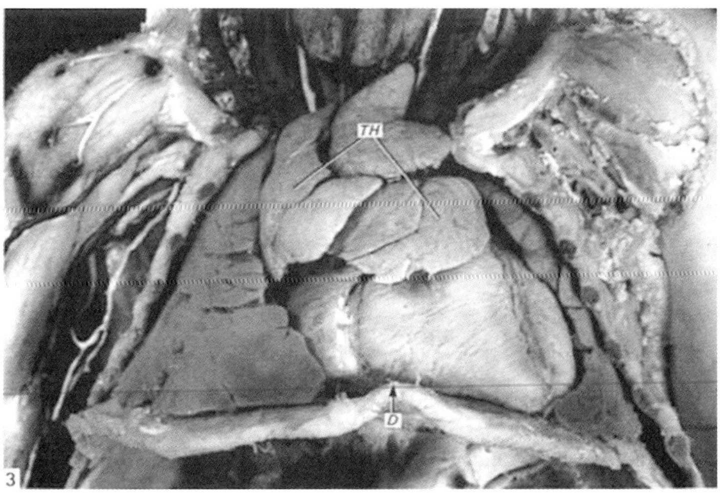

FIGURE 3-4. Thorax of a newborn infant after removal of anterior chest wall. Abbreviations: TH, Thymus; D, Diaphragm. (Reproduced with permission from Walmsley R, Monkhouse WS: The heart of newborn child: an anatomical study based upon transverse serial section, *J Anat*. 1988 Aug;159:93–111.)

heart is situated at the 4th intercostal space at the anterior axillary line. Figure 3-3 shows the relative position of cardiac chambers from a postmortem cross section of a neonatal thorax at the 4th intercostal space.[2] The anterior wall of the right ventricle, the right ventricular outflow, the pulmonary valve, and the initial segment of the main pulmonary are the most anterior, whereas the posterior wall of the left atrium and pulmonary veins are the most posterior structures of the heart, located directly anterior to the descending aorta and esophagus. The ventricles are

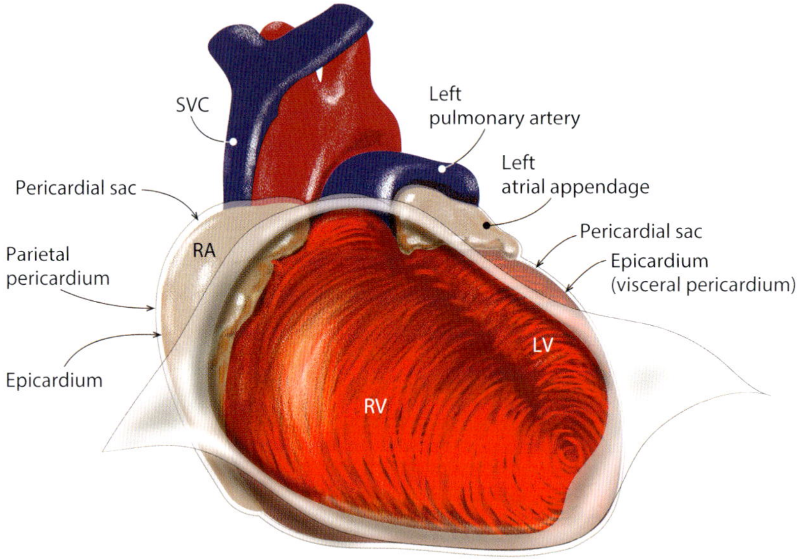

FIGURE 3-5. Diagram of the heart with pericardium split and separated to expose the external appearance of cardiac chambers and great vessels.

inferior and to the left of their corresponding atria. The newborn heart, as is situated in the thoracic cavity at the time of birth, is depicted in Figure 3-4. Newborn infants often have a large thymus which is usually multilobar and covers the upper part of the heart and great vessels.

Differences Between Neonatal and Adult Heart

The neonatal heart has the following characteristics:

- The heart lies more horizontally in the chest at approximately 45° in the frontal plane as opposed to 60° for the adult heart.
- The right ventricular wall has the same thickness as the left ventricular wall. The right ventricular wall thins out gradually during the first month of life.[3]
- The ductus arteriosus and foramen ovale, which are prominent during fetal life, are present at birth.

Upon the opening of the thorax anteriorly, the first structure encountered is the pericardial sac. Pericardium is dense fibrous tissue which encloses the heart and anchors at base to great vessels and inferiorly to the diaphragm (Figure 3-5). It is highly echogenic. The pericardium is separated from the outer layer of heart muscle or epicardium by the pericardial sac containing a small amount of fluid that lubricates and allows for free contraction of the heart. Under pathological conditions, a large amount of fluid under pressure may accumulate in the pericardial sac and may impede cardiac filling (cardiac tamponade).

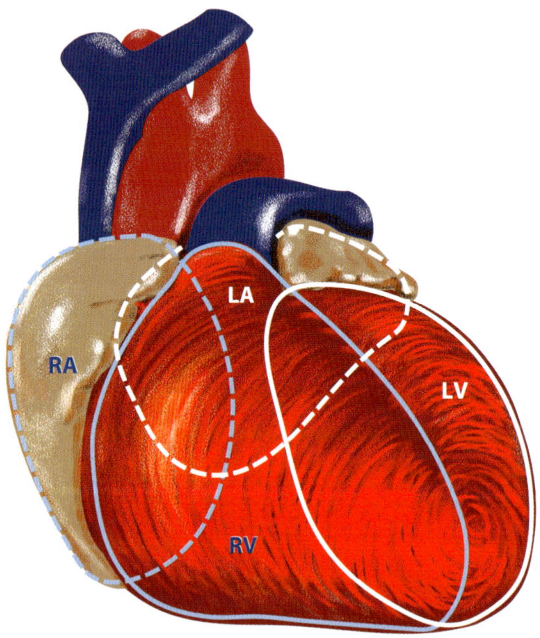

FIGURE 3-6. Diagram of the heart indicating overlapping of cardiac chambers viewed from anteroposterior direction. The right ventricle is the most anterior, whereas the left atrium is the most posterior cardiac chamber.

CARDIAC CHAMBERS, HEART VALVES AND GREAT VESSELS

The right heart chambers are to the same extent anterior as they are to the right of left heart chambers. The extent

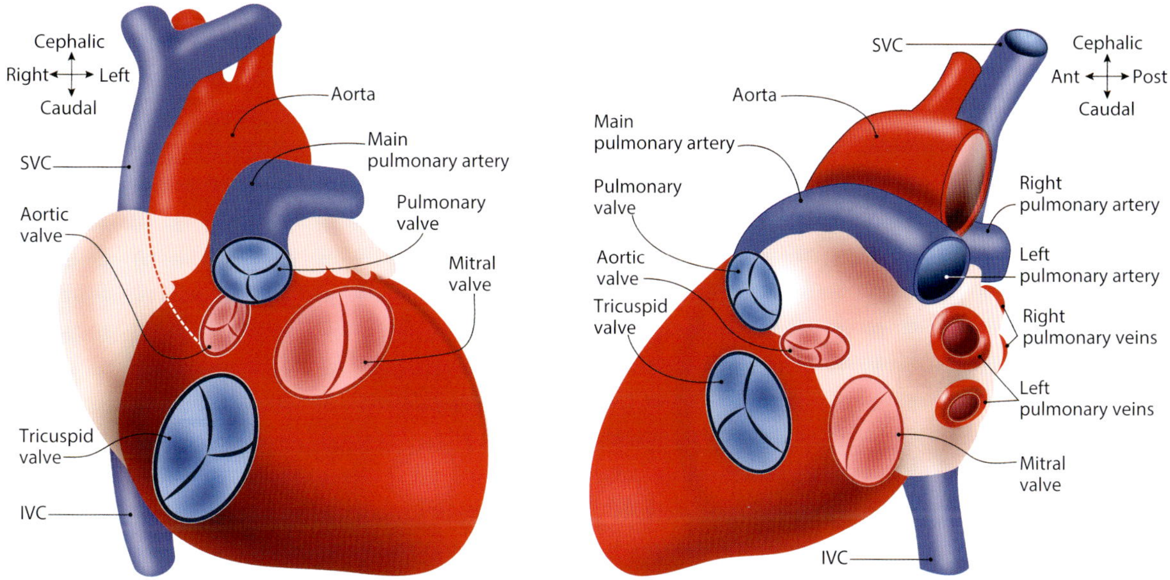

FIGURE 3-7. Schematic representation of location of heart valves. The aortic valve is located in the middle, whereas the mitral valve is the most posterior, the pulmonary valve the most superior and anterior, whereas the tricuspid valve is the most inferior in its location. Abbreviations: Ao, aorta; SVC, superior vena cava; MPA, main pulmonary artery; IVC, inferior vena cava.

of overlap and their relative position is depicted in Figures 3-5 and 3-6. Similarly, the right atrial appendage extends more anteriorly than the left atrial appendage.

Location of the Heart Valves and the Great Vessels

The locations of heart valves are illustrated in frontal and lateral views in Figure 3-7. The pulmonary valve is the most anterior and superior, whereas the tricuspid valve is the most inferior and the mitral valve the most posterior of the cardiac valves. The aortic valve is located in the center.

Imaging Planes of the Heart

In echocardiography, cardiac chambers are imaged from specific acoustic windows through a sector scan. Sector scans do not follow the usual anatomic (coronal, sagittal, and transverse) planes. However, a few approximate these planes and are illustrated here to demonstrate cross-sectional cardiac anatomy. For example, the subcostal coronal planes and the suprasternal coronal posterior plane "crab view" approximate anatomical coronal planes. A complete list of sector scans obtained during neonatal echocardiography is reviewed later in this chapter.

The subcostal coronal anterior plane depicts the heart cut through an anterior frontal plane closest to the anterior chest wall (Figure 3-8). The triangular-shaped right ventricle, right ventricular outflow including crista supraventricularis (a muscle band that separates the upper part of the right ventricle underneath the pulmonary valve), and the initial segment of main pulmonary artery and a small anterior segment of left ventricle are seen in this view. The pulmonary valve, as well as the anterior segment of tricuspid valve, are also seen in this cut.

A subcostal coronal plane at the level of the aortic valve (Figure 3-9) reveals the right atrium, the posterior segment of tricuspid valve, the inflow segment of right ventricle, the aortic valve, the proximal segment of ascending aorta, the anterior segment of the left atrium, and the left atrial appendage, as well as a smooth-walled, ellipsoidal-shaped left ventricle. Only the anterior segment of mitral valve ring is seen in this view.

A posterior subcostal coronal plane (Figure 3-10) depicts the crux of the heart, with septal attachments of the mitral and tricuspid valves, the posterior segment of the interatrial septum, which includes a patent foramen ovale, the posterior segment of the right atrium, the large segment of the left atrium, which often includes left atrial appendage, a small posterior segment of right ventricular inflow, and variable segments of the left ventricle. At this level, the mitral valve, which is the most posterior of heart valves, is well visualized, whereas the tricuspid valve is

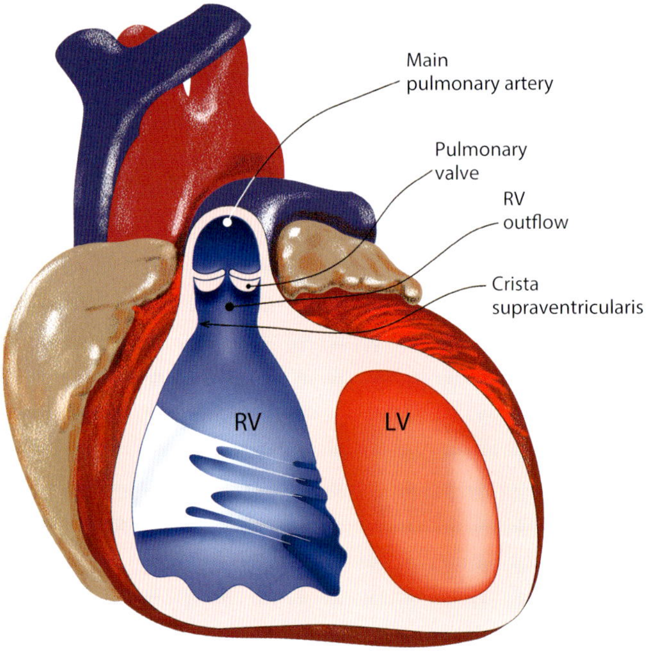

FIGURE 3-8. Diagram of anterior cut through the heart of neonate. Right ventricular outflow, pulmonary valve, and initial segment of main pulmonary artery, which are the most anterior parts of the heart, as well as anterior segment of left ventricle are included in this cut plane. The right atrium, left atrium, and mitral valve are not sectioned because of their posterior location

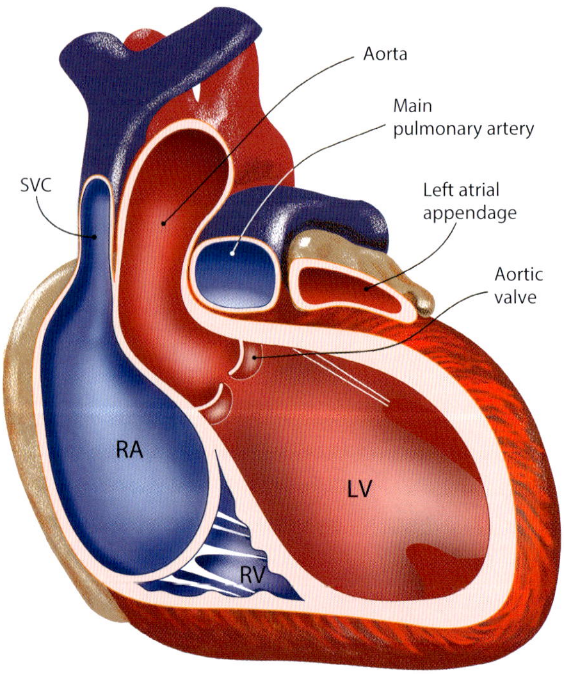

FIGURE 3-9. Diagram of coronal cut at level of aortic valve. Anterior segment of superior vena cava, right atrium, tricuspid valve, inflow segment of right ventricle, left ventricle, aortic valve, initial segment of ascending aorta, small anterior segment of left atrium are sectioned in this plane. Mitral valve is not visualized since it is located posterior to this cut.

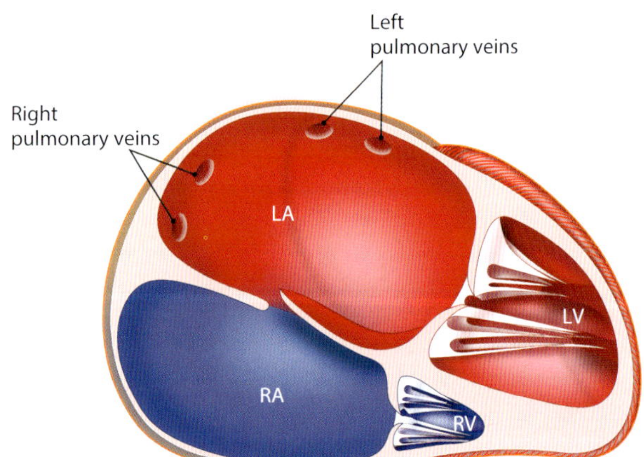

FIGURE 3-10. Diagram of coronal plane through posterior heart chambers. In this cut, the heart is sectioned posterior to the aortic valve and crux of the heart. The attachments of mitral and tricuspid valve, as well as the full length of atrial septum is imaged. Left atrium, mitral valve, left ventricle, and right atrium are well visualized. Posterior segment of tricuspid valve and a small portion of right ventricular inflow are also included in this cut. Abbreviations: RA, right atrium; LA, left atrium; LV,left ventricle, RV, right ventricle.

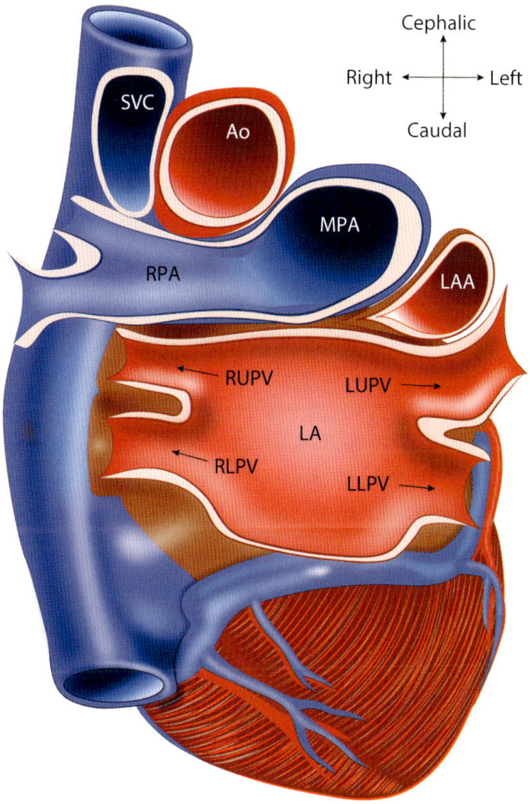

FIGURE 3-11. Diagram of suprasternal coronal posterior cut. Posterior segment of left atrium, pulmonary veins and pulmonary artery and aorta in cross section are delineated in this cut. Abbreviations: LAA, left atrial appendage; MPA, main pulmonary artery; RPA, right pulmonary artery; Ao, aorta; SVC, superior vena cava; RUPV, right upper pulmonary vein; LUPV, left upper pulmonary vein; LA, left atrium; RLPV, right lower pulmonary vein; LLPV, left lower pulmonary vein..

only partially visualized and aortic and pulmonary valves (located anterior to the plane) are not seen.

The suprasternal coronal posterior "crab view" is the most posterior frontal plane obtained from suprasternal window, imaging the posterior wall of the left atrium, pulmonary veins, the left atrial appendage, a cross section of ascending aorta, and the pulmonary artery at its bifurcation (Figure 3-11). Finally, an intact heart displaying the normal posterior structures is shown in (Figure 3-12).

OBTAINING NEONATAL ECHOCARDIOGRAMS

Two-dimensional (2D) echocardiographic cardiac images are fan-shaped, thin slices of the heart obtained from an ultrasound beam transmitted through echocardiographic windows. Standard anatomical planes (coronal, sagittal, and transverse) are used with modifications as necessary, along with planes corresponding to the long and short axes of the heart. During routine echocardiography, one generally obtains 26 tomographic planes from four standard acoustic windows, each plane revealing a 2D image of the heart from a different perspective.[4,5]

Preparing the infant for Echocardiography

Infants should be in an open crib; the upper chest and abdomen are exposed and the hands and feet are gently covered in a wrapping blanket. The infant is placed on the left side at an approximately 30° angle, with the head turned to the left. Electrocardiographic leads are placed away from echocardiographic windows (Figure 3-13). Critically ill neonates under radiant heat warmers and incubators are prepared as much as possible in the same fashion. Leads and sensors covering acoustic windows are displaced to expose unimpeded access to the acoustic windows.

Selection and Manipulation of an Appropriate Probe

The appropriate probe is chosen, as described in Chapter 2. Figure 3-13 depicts the location of echocardiographic windows that are commonly used. The probe is placed with an orientation aimed toward specific cardiac structures of interest, and it is manipulated to obtain the desired sector scans. The probe can be manipulated using several different motions, as shown in Figure and Video 3-14.

Display of 2D images

The orientation mark on the probe indicates the plane of sector scan and the side of the fan-shaped scan that is displayed on the right side of the display screen. Visibility of the structures displayed depends on how they are encountered by the ultrasound beam. Structures perpendicular to the ultrasound beam are effective reflectors and structures parallel to the ultrasound beam are poor reflectors and are less well imaged. For example, in sector scans with the beam parallel to the thin interatrial septum (such as the apical four-chamber view), an echo dropout can occur, indicating a nonexistent atrial septal defect. However, dense structures are highly echogenic and may appear thicker. This can especially be seen for the pericardium, which is a thin but very dense structure, and appears highly echogenic in echocardiographic images.

HOW TO OBTAIN SPECIFIC SECTOR SCANS

The following views are described for a normally located and oriented heart. The apex of the heart is in the left

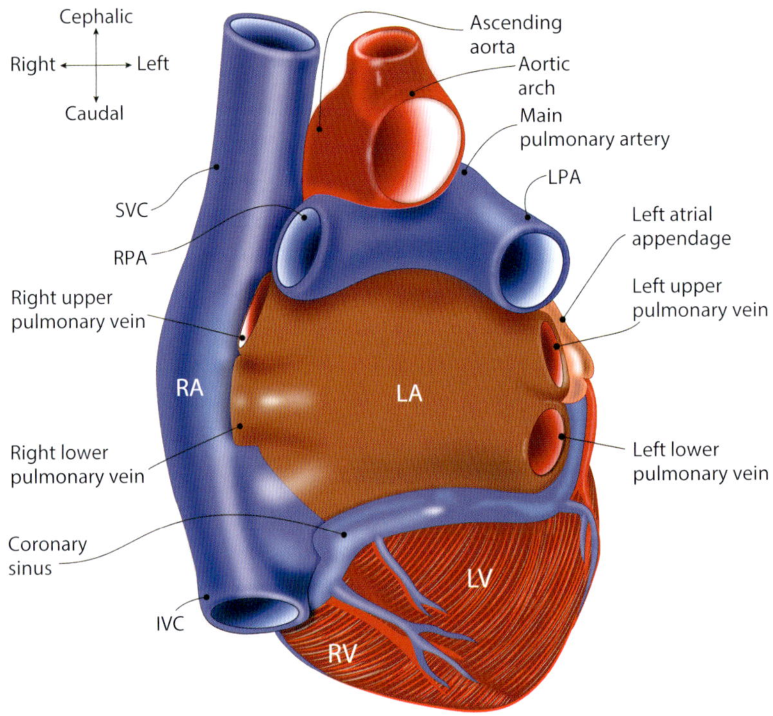

FIGURE 3-12. Diagram of posterior view of an intact heart. Abbreviations: RPA, right pulmonary artery; LPA, left pulmonary artery.

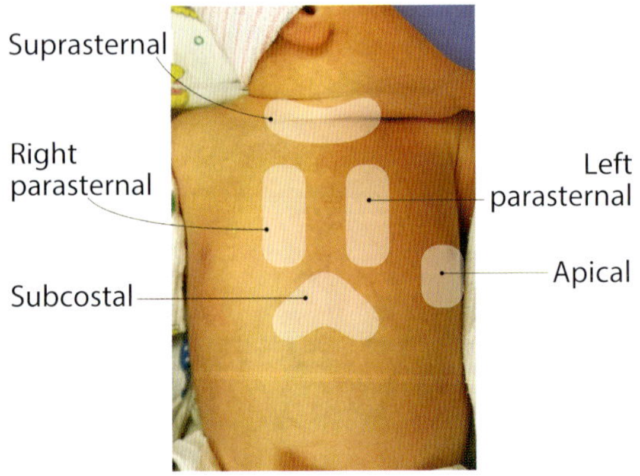

FIGURE 3-13. Location of echocardiographic windows on a newborn chest. Abbreviations: SS, suprasternal; PS, parasternal; AP, apical; SC, subcostal.

chest, and there are normal systemic/pulmonary venous return (the so-called situs solitus) and normally related great vessels. These normal relationships are illustrated in sector scans obtained from the parasternal, apical, subcostal, and suprasternal echocardiographic windows, through a series of Figures and Video clips (Figures and Video clips 3-15 to 3-23).

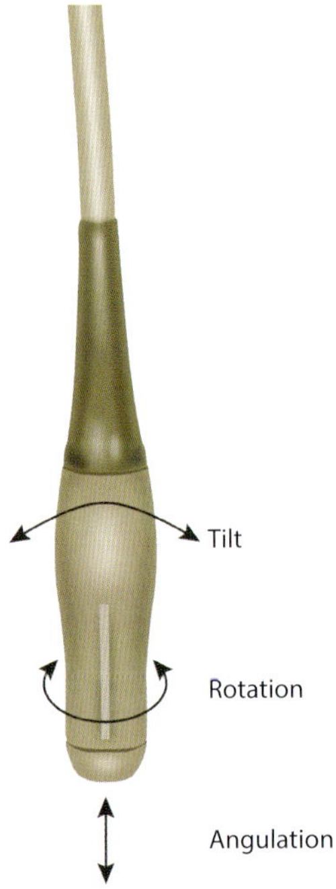

FIGURE and VIDEO 3-14. Transducer position and orientation: transducer orientation may be changed through tilt, rotation, and angulation.

Outline of Sector Scans Obtained from Parasternal Long Axis (FIGURE 3-15)

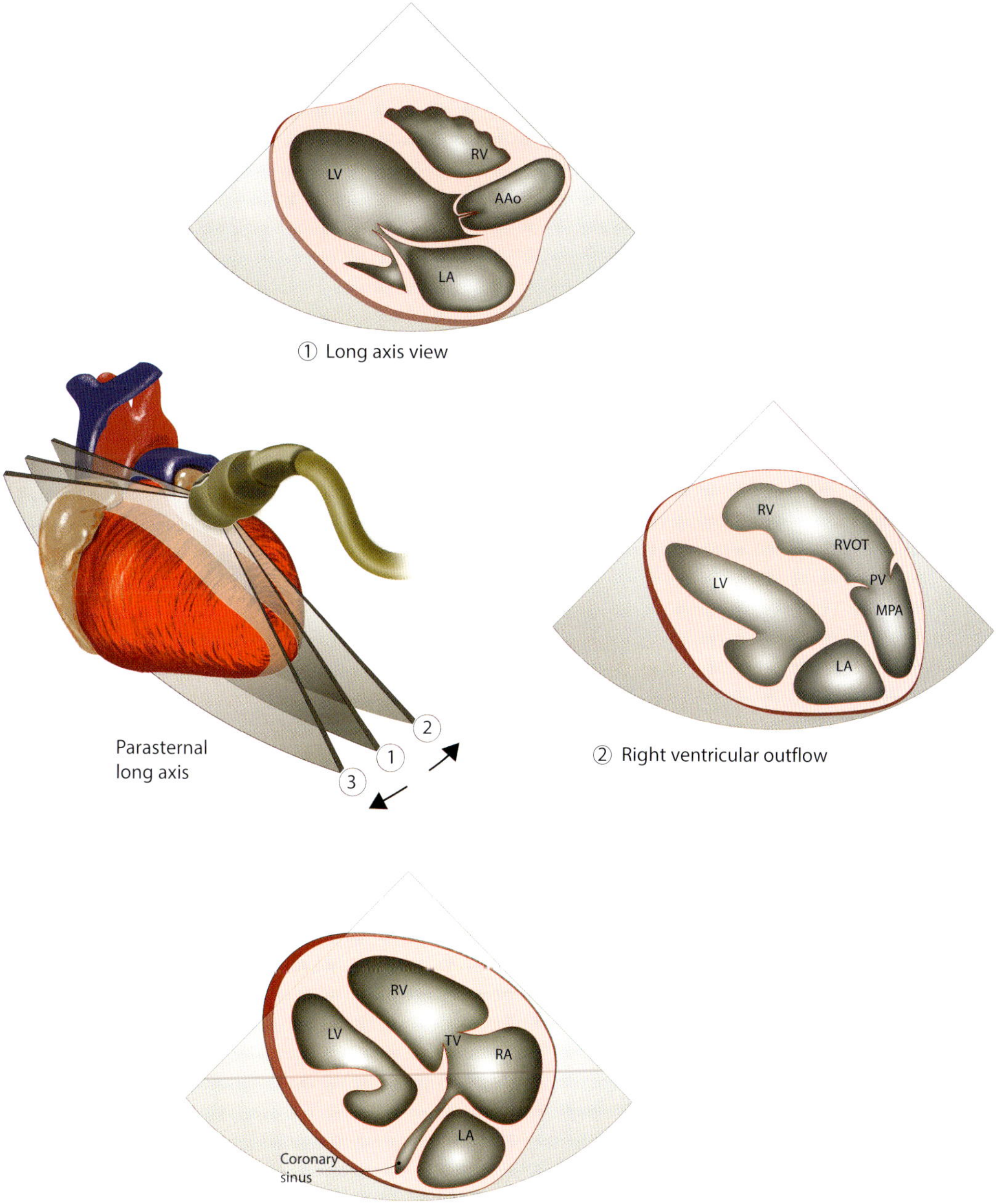

① Long axis view

② Right ventricular outflow

③ Right ventricular inflow

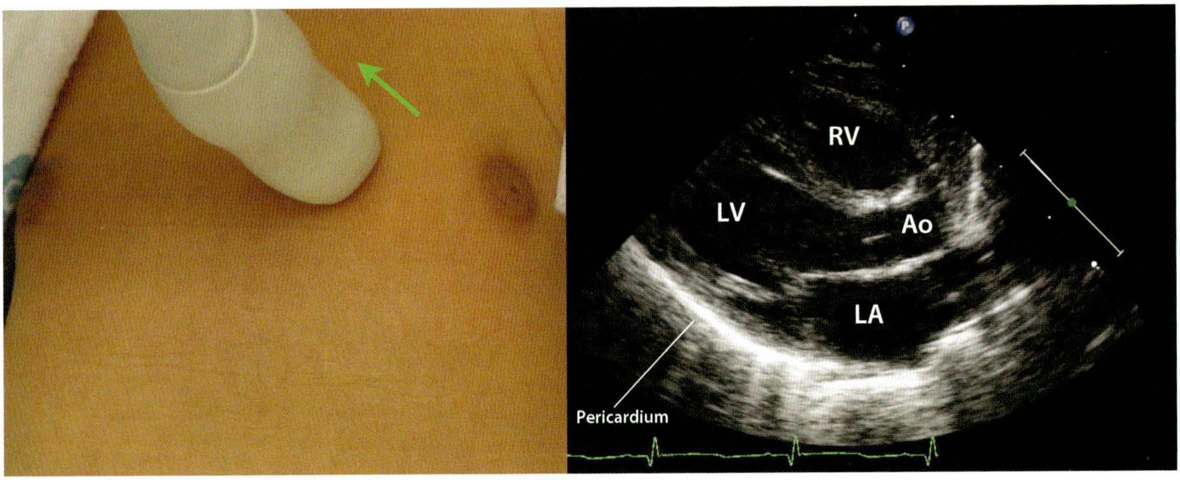

FIGURE and VIDEO 3-15.1. **Parasternal long axis (PLAX).** The transducer is placed perpendicular to the chest, over the parasternal window, with the marker pointing toward the right shoulder. This position is adjusted to obtain a full long-axis view of the heart, as shown in this figure. Since the marker is pointing toward the right shoulder, the apex of the heart, which is in the left chest, is shown on the right. This at first may be confusing to the novice, since on routine chest radiograph, the heart apex is displayed on the left. All long-axis views have the same characteristic. In this view, we will distinguish the anterior portion of the right ventricle (RV), the interventricular septum (IVS), the left ventricle (LV), the aortic valve and the ascending aorta (Ao), and the left atrium (LA). Pericardium, a very dense structure, is highly echogenic and is displayed posterior to the left atrium and ventricle.

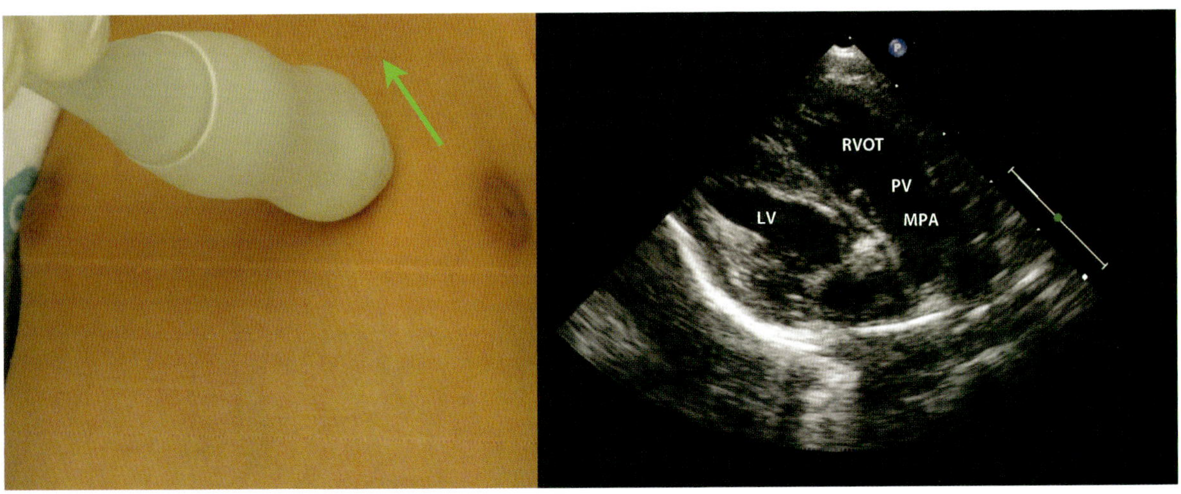

FIGURE and VIDEO 3-15.2. **PLAX right ventricular outflow.** From parasternal long axis (PLAX), a slight clockwise rotation and anterior tilt will bring forward this view. The right ventricular outflow tract (RVOT), pulmonary valve (PV), and main pulmonary artery (MPA) are well visualized.

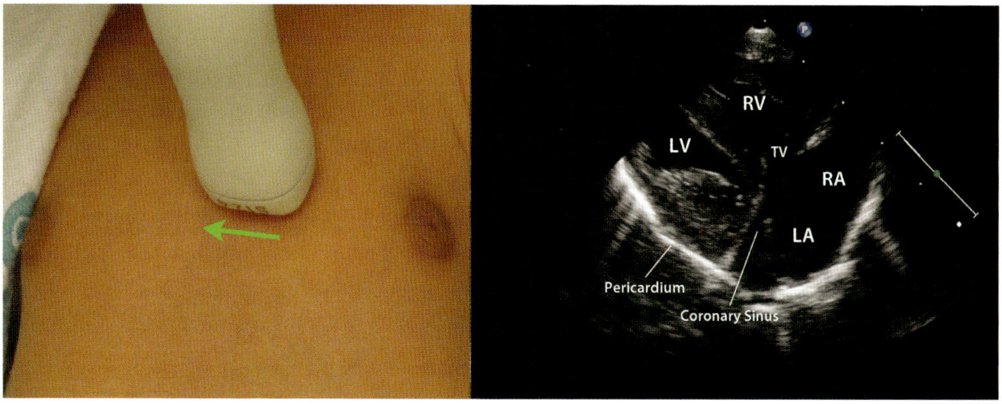

FIGURE and VIDEO 3-15.3. PLAX right ventricular inflow. From the parasternal long axis, a slight rotation counterclockwise and posterior tilt will image this view. The tricuspid valve (TV) and RV inflow portion are visualized. Although the right atrium (RA) and LA are outlined, the interatrial septum is not viewed due to echo dropout. Commonly, the posterior segment of the LV and the mitral valve ring are seen. At times, the coronary sinus extending along the mitral valve ring toward the RA is visualized.

Outline of Sector Scans Obtained from Parasternal Short Axis (FIGURE 3.16)

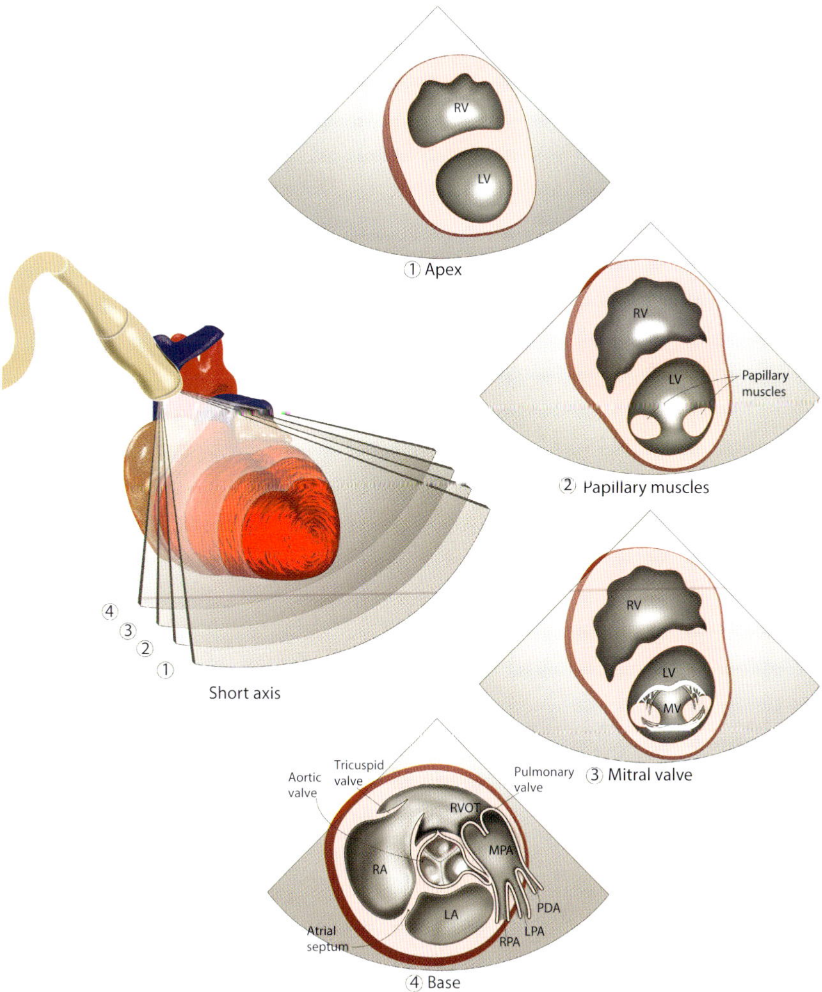

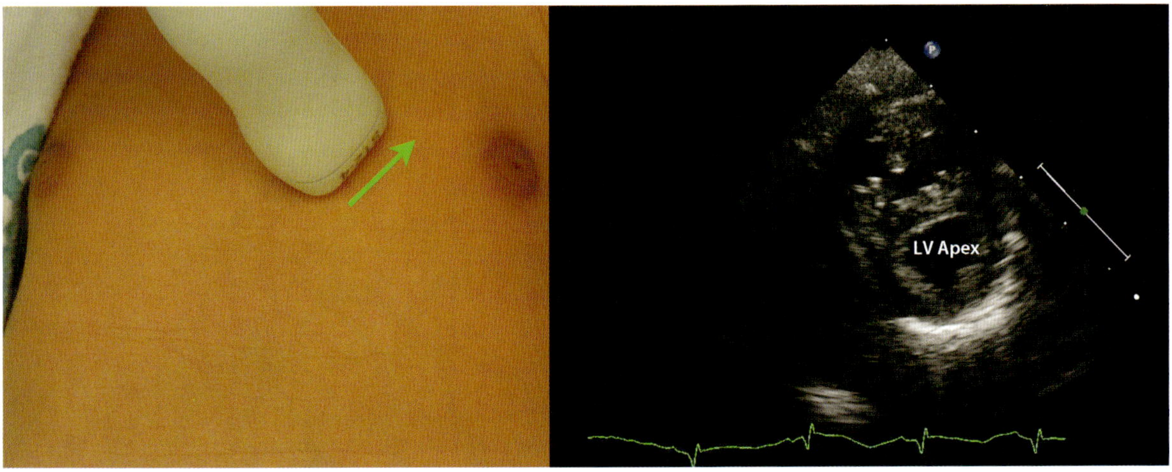

FIGURE and VIDEO 3-16.1. **Parasternal short-axis (PSAX) apical view.** This view is obtained by the clockwise rotation of the transducer for 90° from PLAX. Now the marker will point toward the left shoulder. With the transducer tilted inferiorly and anteriorly, the apical segments of LV and RV are seen.

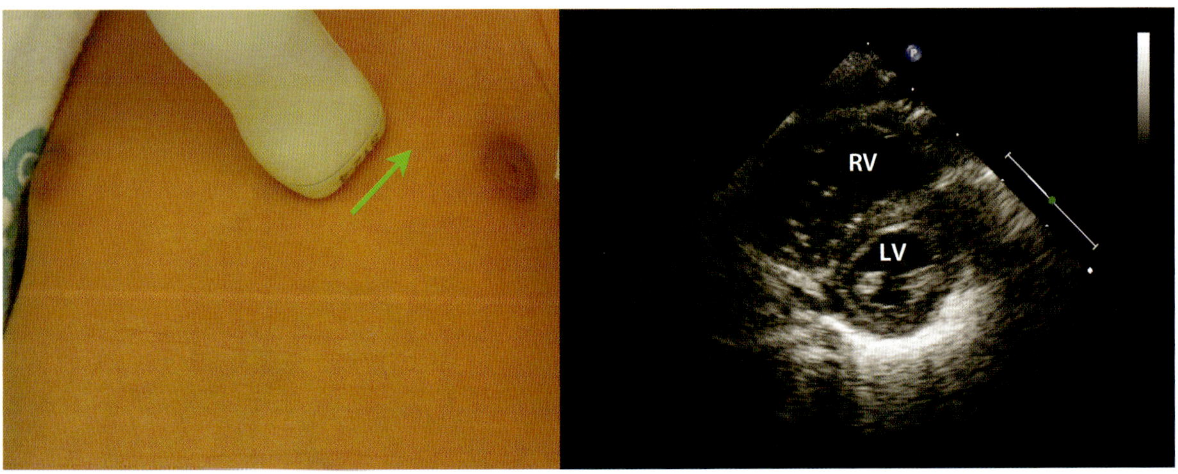

FIGURE and VIDEO 3-16.2. **PSAX at papillary muscle level.** This view Is obtained by further decreasing the angle of the tilt to image the LV through its midsection, which also includes a larger segment of RV that is located anteriorly.

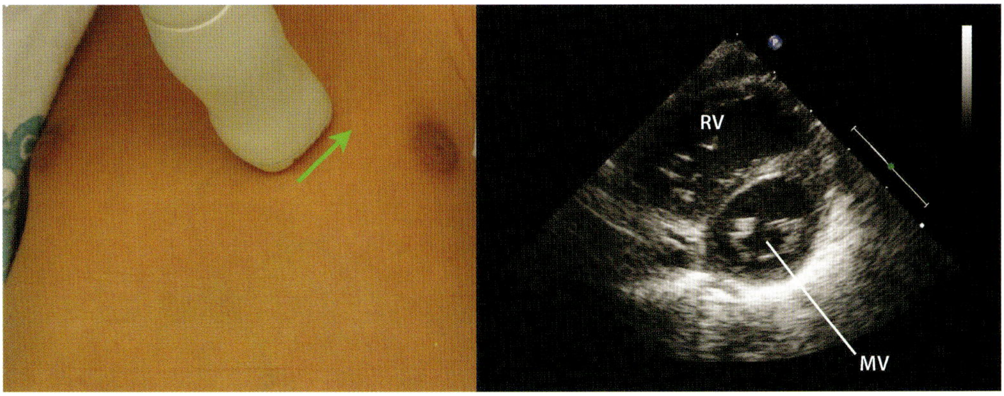

FIGURE and VIDEO 3-16.3. **PSAX at mitral valve level.** This view is obtained by bringing the transducer almost perpendicular to the chest, maintaining the marker pointing toward the left shoulder. This cut will bring in view a cross section of LV at mitral valve (MV) level with the anterior and posterior leaflet of the valve forming the so-called "fish mouth" image. PSAX at MV level can also be used to obtain an M-mode tracing of the LV and anterior portion of the RV.

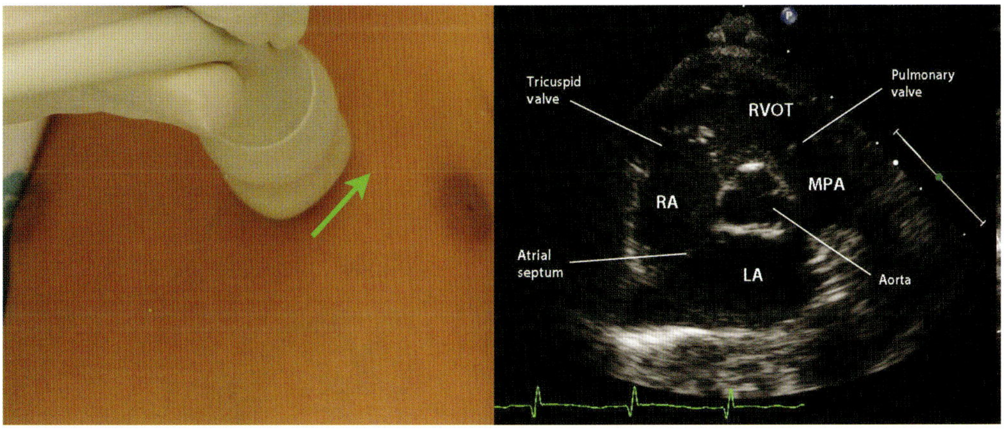

FIGURE 3-16.4. **PSAX at the base of the heart.** This view Is obtained by further tilt of transducer to the right and superiorly from the MV position. This will bring in view the aortic valve and its leaflets in cross section. In this view, the aortic valve is shown in the middle, surrounded by RV outflow (RVOT) anteriorly, the MPA and pulmonary valve (PV) on the left side, the LA inferiorly, and the RA to the right side.

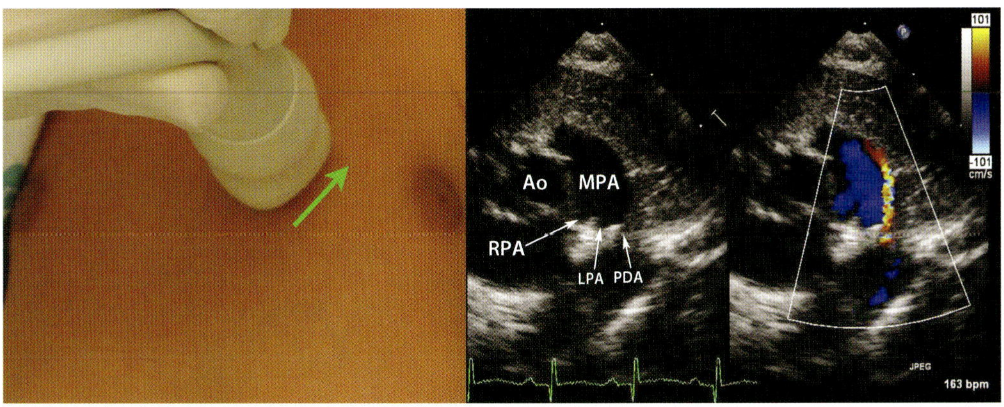

FIGURE and VIDEO 3-16.5. **PSAX at the base with the MPA and its branches.** A further tilt to the right and anteriorly will bring in view the MPA, the origin of the right pulmonary artery (RPA), the left pulmonary artery (LPA), and if present, a patent ductus arteriosus (PDA), the so-called "three-finger sign."

Outline of Sector Scans Obtained from the Apical Window (FIGURE 3-17)

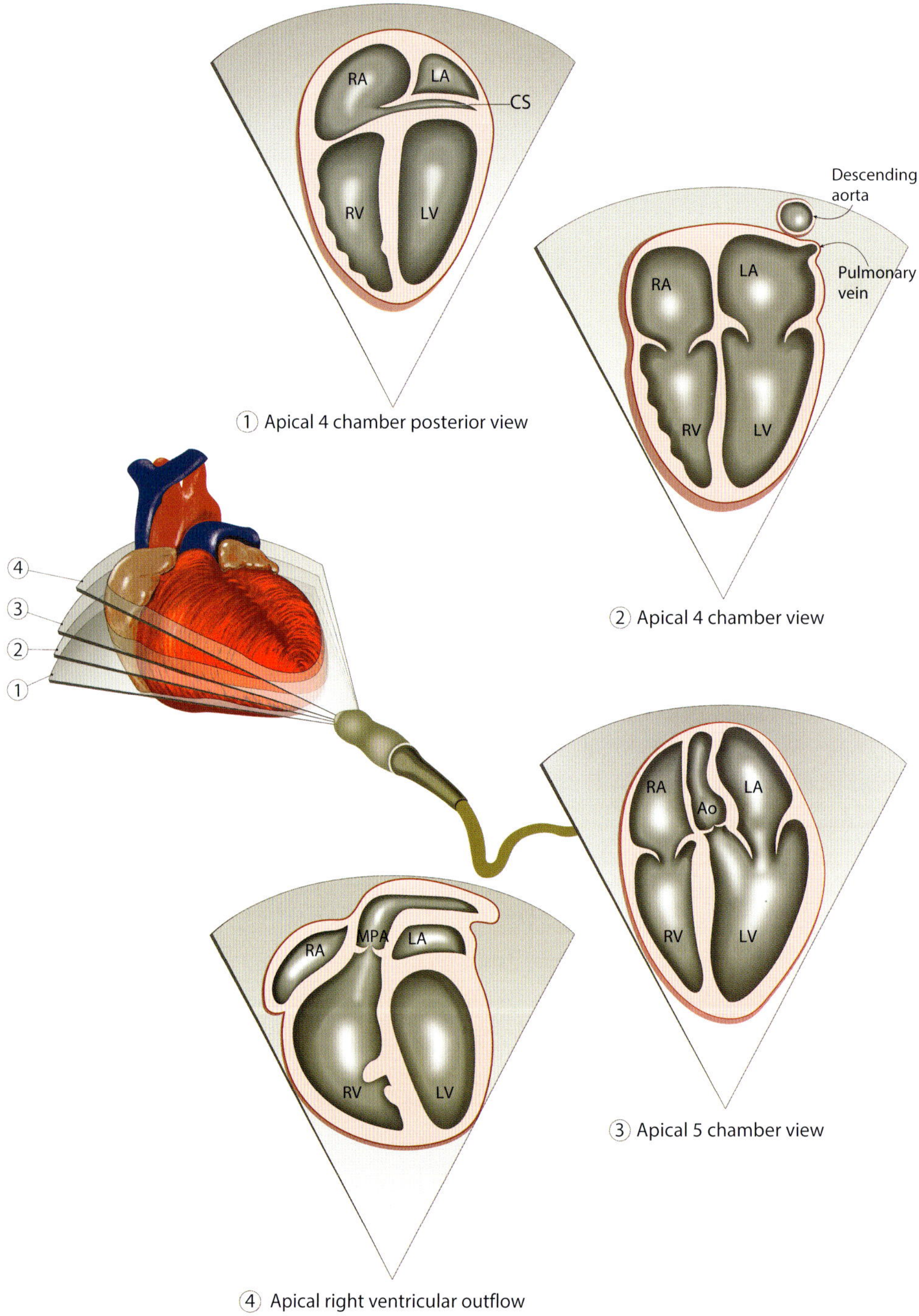

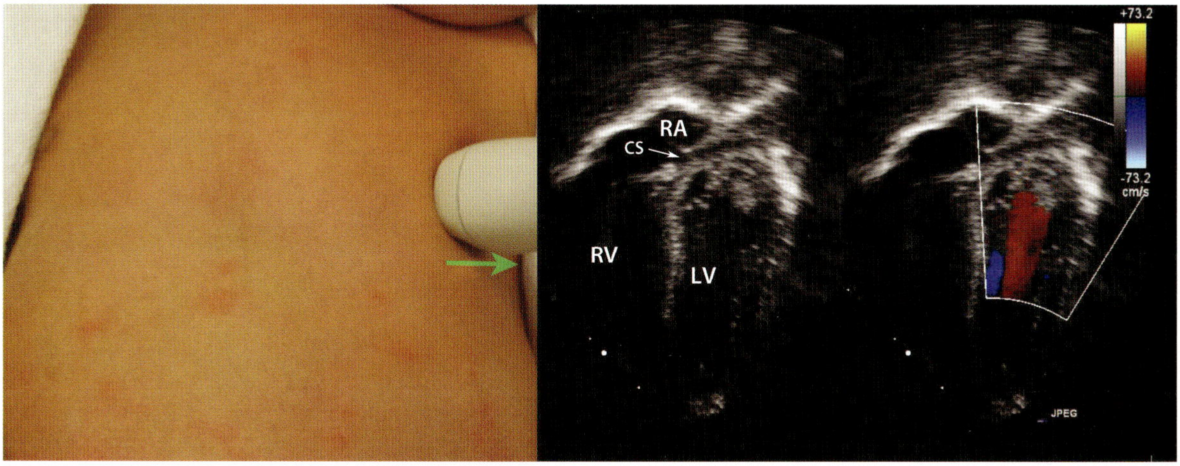

FIGURE and VIDEO 3-17.1. **Apical four-chamber posterior view.** This view is obtained with the marker pointing posteriorly and the plane of the cut going through the transverse section at approximately 5th intercostal space. The sector plane is further adjusted to reveal the posterior view of the chambers. In this view, the posterior aspects of the four cardiac chambers and the two atrioventricular valve rings are detected. Often, the coronary sinus (CS) coursing over the posterior mitral valve ring is noted; it enters the right atrium close to the crux of the heart.

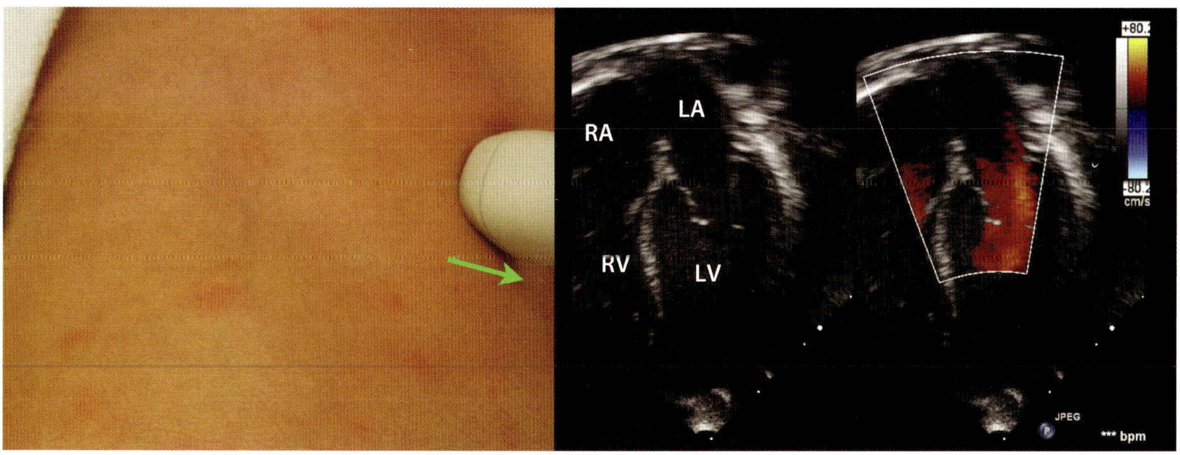

FIGURE and VIDEO 3-17.2. **Apical four-chamber view.** This view Is obtained by a slight superior tilt of the transducer. In this view, LV, RV, RA, and LA are shown In transverse section, whereas atrial septum is only partially visible due to echo dropout. Both MV and TV and their attachments to ventricular septum are clearly defined. Color flow indicates the inflow to the ventricles (red color), and the ventricular outflow is indirectly indicated by the presence of blood flow away from the transducer (blue color).

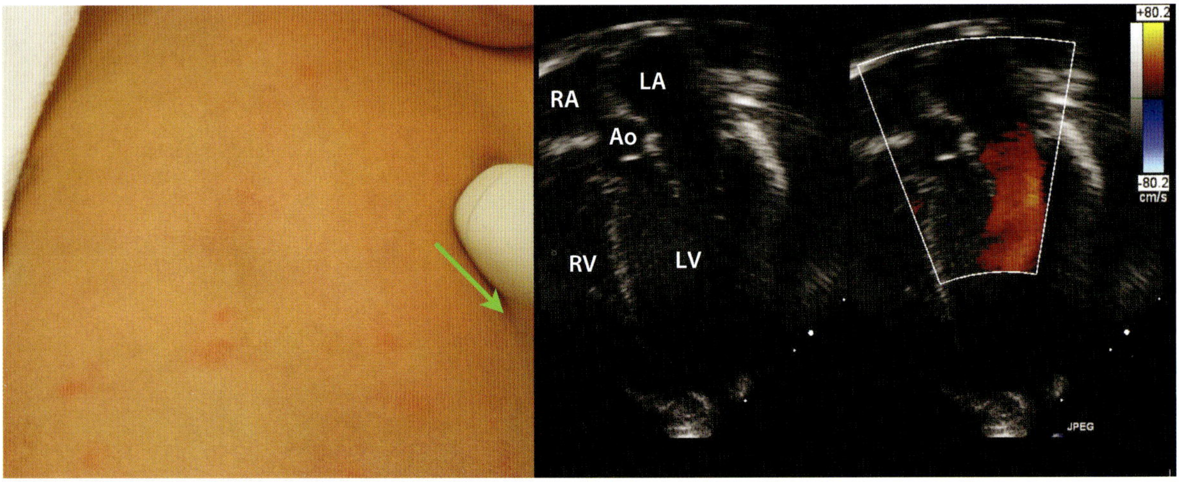

FIGURE and VIDEO 3-17.3. **Apical five-chamber view.** This view Is displayed by a slight clockwise rotation and anterior tilt. In this view, the aortic valve and the proximal segment of ascending aorta (AAo), in addition to the four cardiac chambers (LA, LV, RA, and RV), are brought into view.

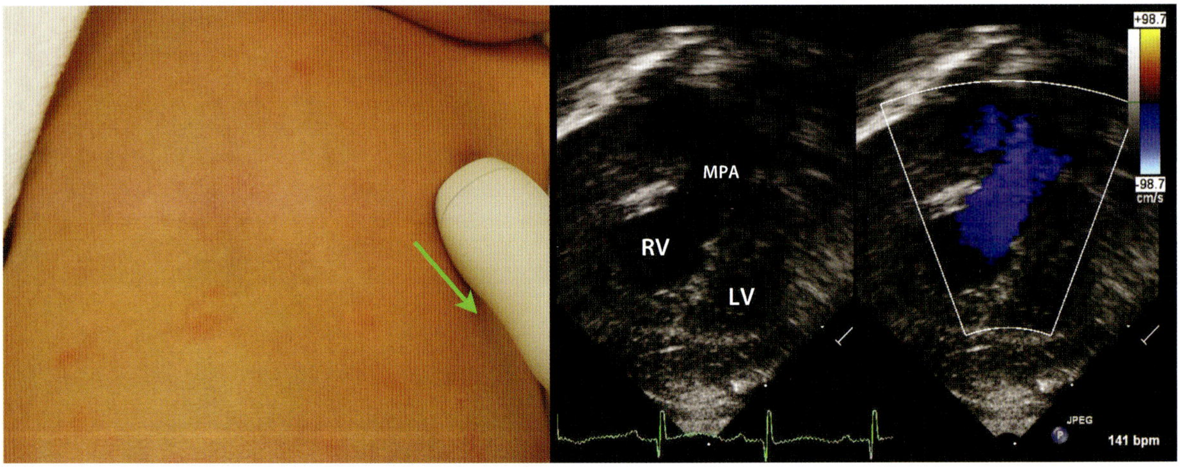

FIGURE and VIDEO 3-17.4. **Apical right ventricular outflow.** This is brought into view by a rightward angulation and further anterior tilt. In this view, left ventricle (LV), right ventricle (RV), pulmonary valve (PV), main pulmonary artery (MPA) can be visualized.

Outline of Sector Scans Obtained from Subcostal Coronal Views (FIGURE 3-18)

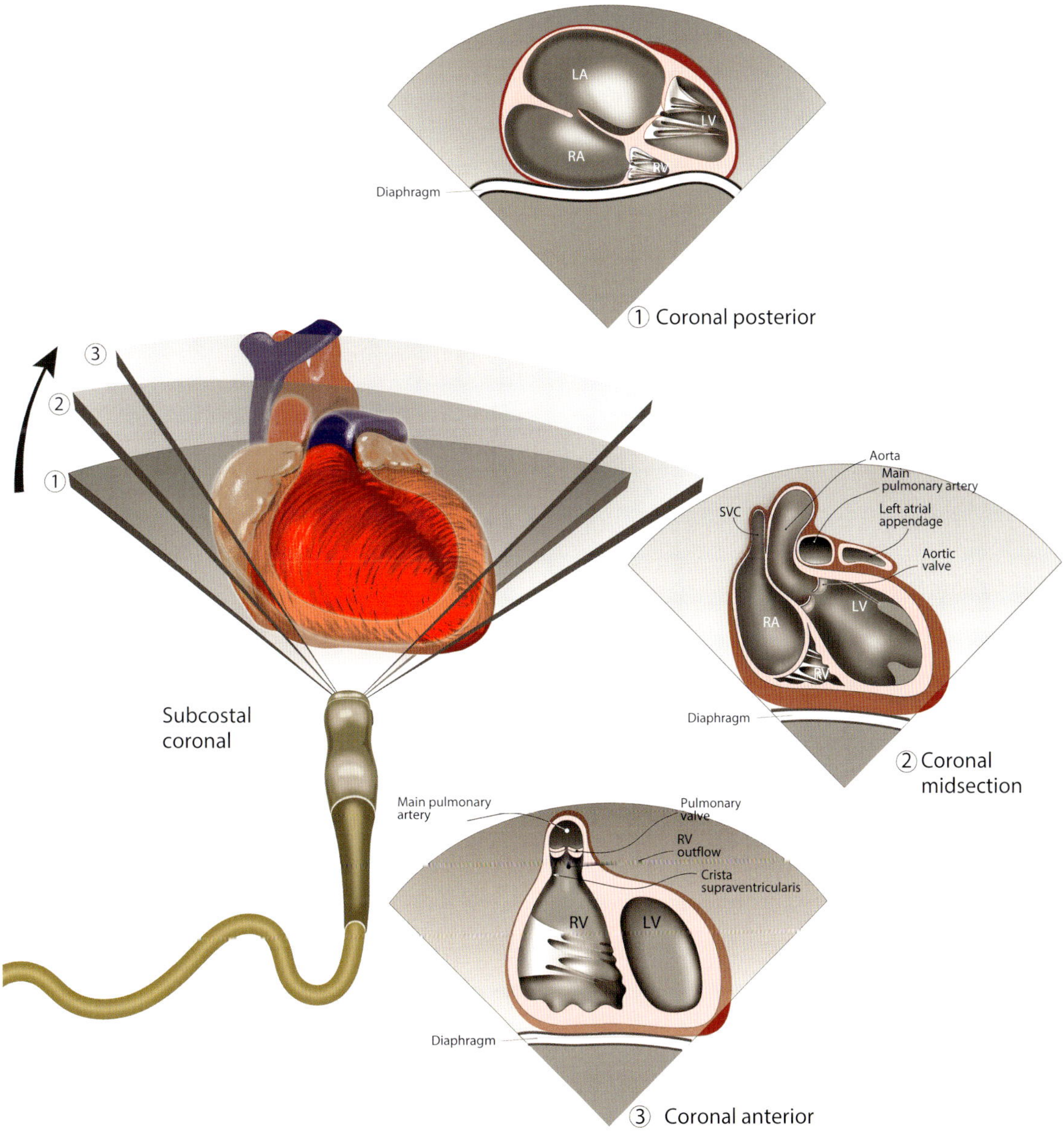

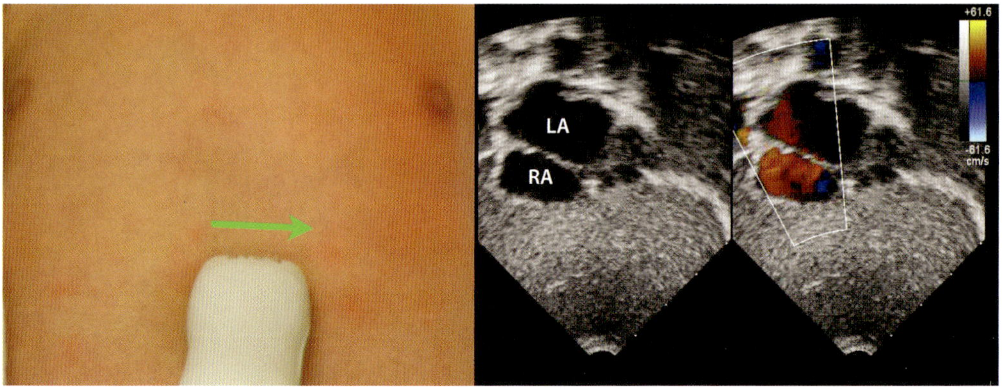

FIGURE and VIDEO 3-18.1. Subcostal coronal posterior. This view is obtained with the marker pointing to the left side of infant and with the transducer tilted posteriorly. In this view, the posterior segment of RA, atrial septum, LA, mitral valve, and posterior segment of left ventricle are visualized. The foramen ovale is usually well-delineated and atrial septum is often seen without echo dropout in this view. Color Doppler often indicates a small left-to-right shunt through the patent foramen ovale.

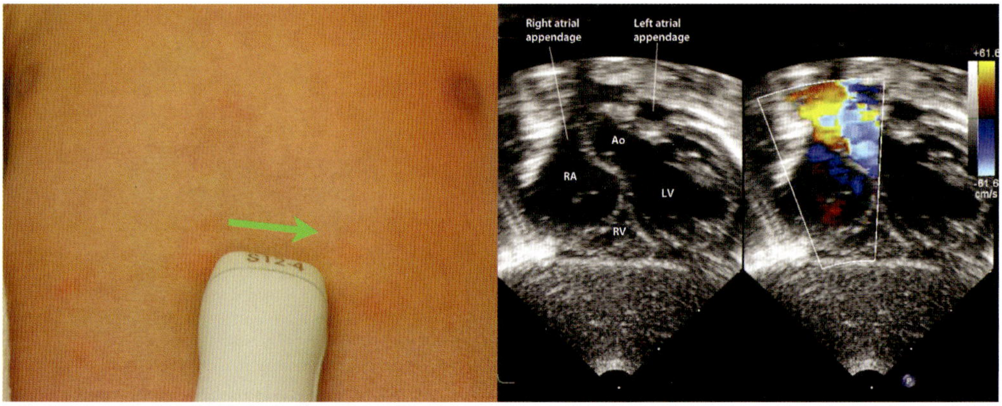

FIGURE and VIDEO 3-18.2. Subcostal coronal midsection. This area is brought in view by a slight anterior tilt. In this view, the RA, the tricuspid valve, the inflow segment of RV, the LV, the aortic valve, the proximal segment of aorta, the anterior segment of LA, and a segment of left atrial appendage are visualized.

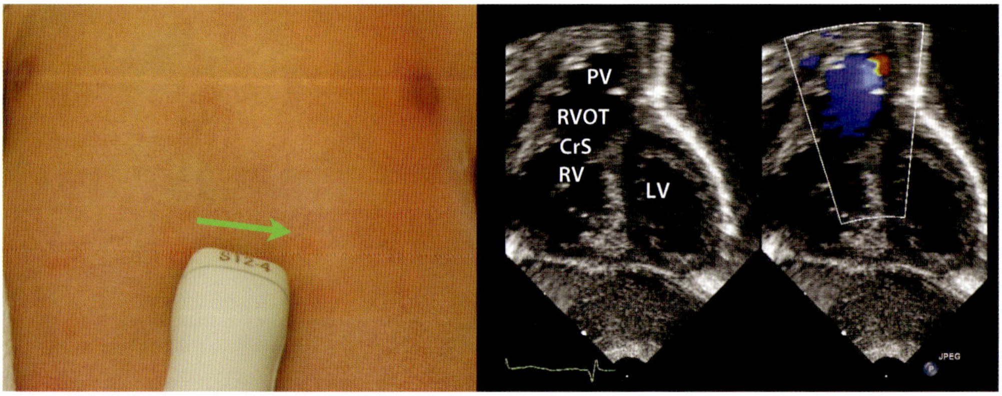

FIGURE and VIDEO 3-18.3. Subcostal coronal anterior. This view is obtained by a further anterior tilt, which displays the anterior segment of the RA, the outflow segment of the RV, the crista supraventricularis (CrS), the main pulmonary artery, and valve, and anterior segment of LV are included in this cut.

Outline of Sector Scan obtained from Subcostal Sagittal Views (FIGURE 3-19)

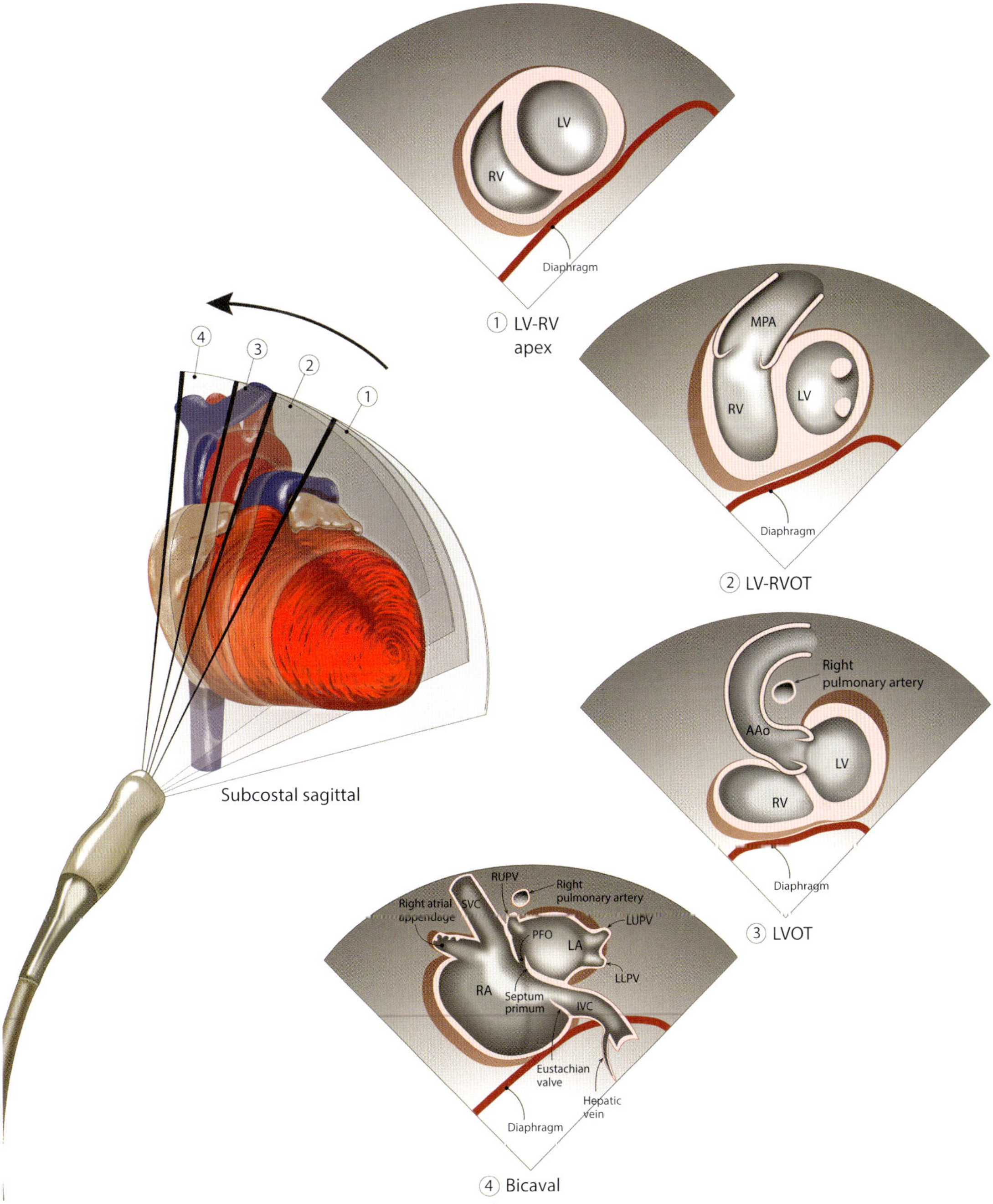

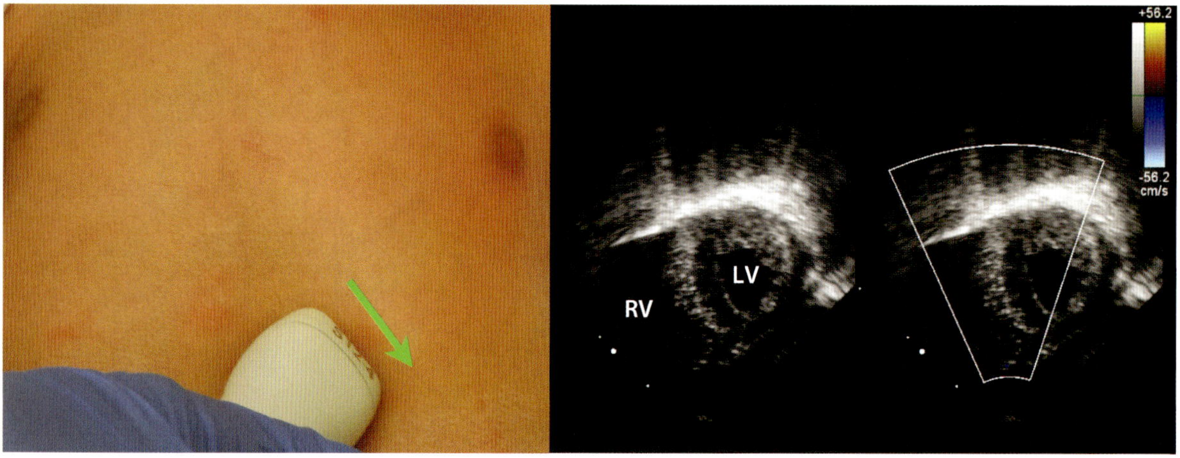

FIGURE and VIDEO 3-19.1. **Subcostal LV-RV apex.** From the subcostal coronal position, 80° of clockwise rotation will point the marker toward the left hip, and a leftward tilt pointing the transducer toward the cardiac apex will display this cut. Some angulation of the transducer toward inferiorly (toward the patient's feet) will bring the heart into the center of the image. The apical sections of the LV, the RV, and the interventricular septum are seen in this view. Since the marker is now pointing posteriorly, the LV is displayed on the left side.

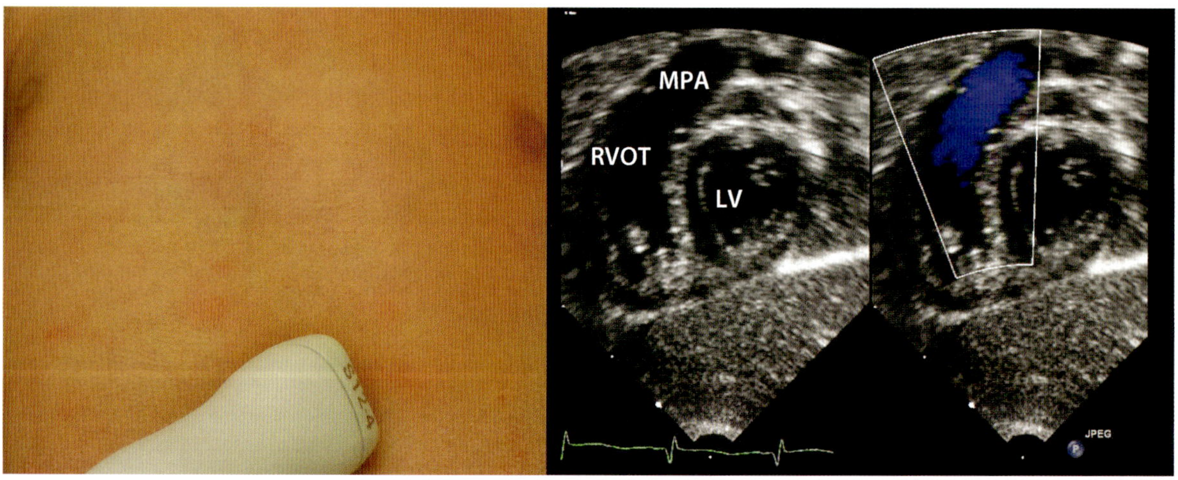

FIGURE and VIDEO 3-19.2. **Subcostal sagittal LV-RVOT.** From the subcostal sagittal apical view, a slight rightward tilt will bring into view the LV in cross section (located posteriorly) and the RV outflow segment (RVOT), the pulmonary valve, and the MPA located anteriorly.

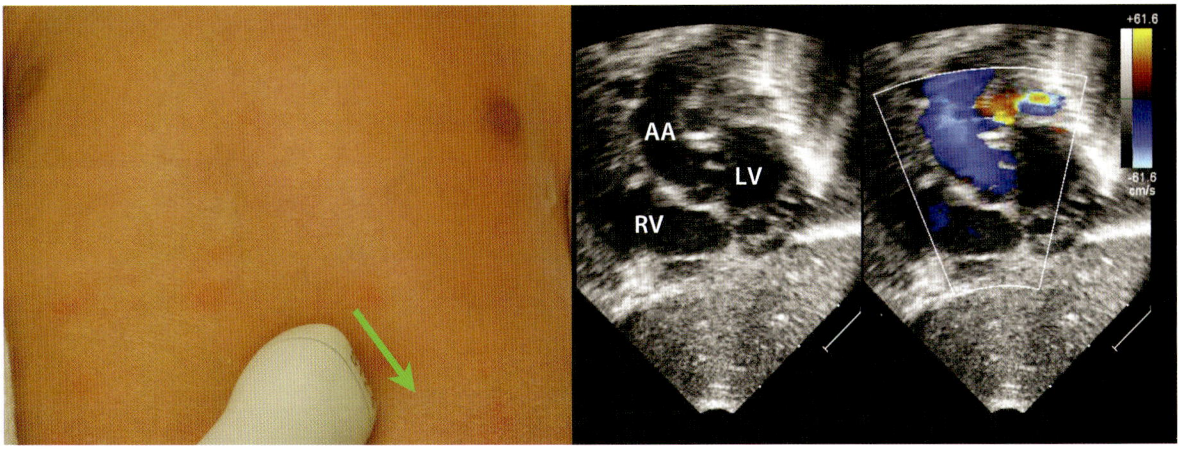

FIGURE and VIDEO 3-19.3. Subcostal sagittal LV-aorta. A further rightward tilt will bring into view the LV, the aortic valve, the ascending aorta (AA), and a small portion of the anterior segment of the RV in cross section.

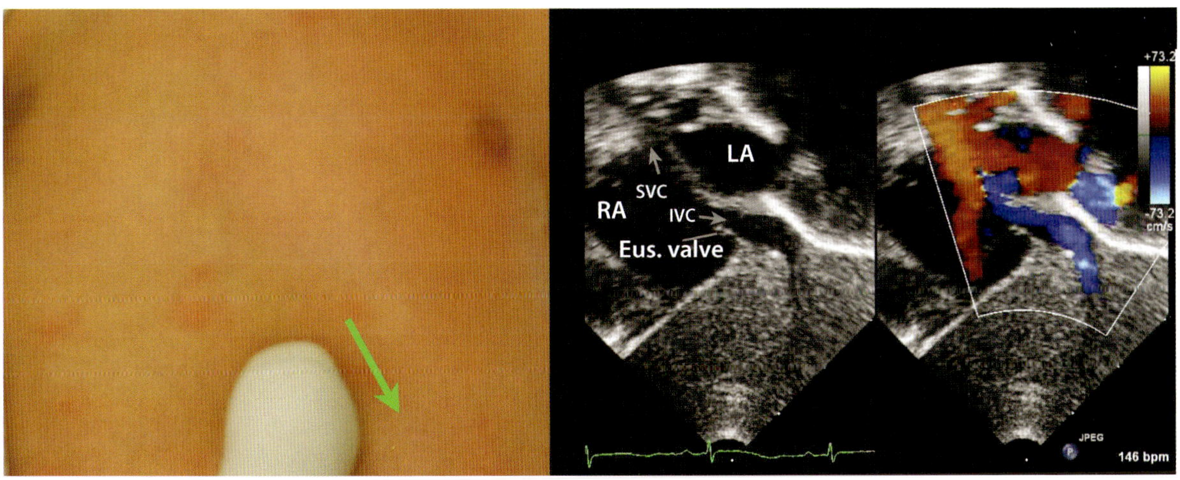

FIGURE and VIDEO 3-19.4. Subcostal sagittal bicaval. A further rightward tilt will image this view. A cut section of the atrial septum extending from the superior vena cava (SVC) to the inferior vena cava (IVC) is visualized. the septum primum is seen overlapping the septum secundum over the opening of the PFO. The LA is located posterior to the RA. The Eustachian valve (Eus. valve) is often noted in neonates anterior to the entrance of the IVC into the RA. The right atrial appendage is viewed in this cut and is located inferior and anteriorly to the opening of the SVC.

Outline of Sector Scans Obtained from Infradiaphramatic Subcostal Views (FIGURE 3-20)

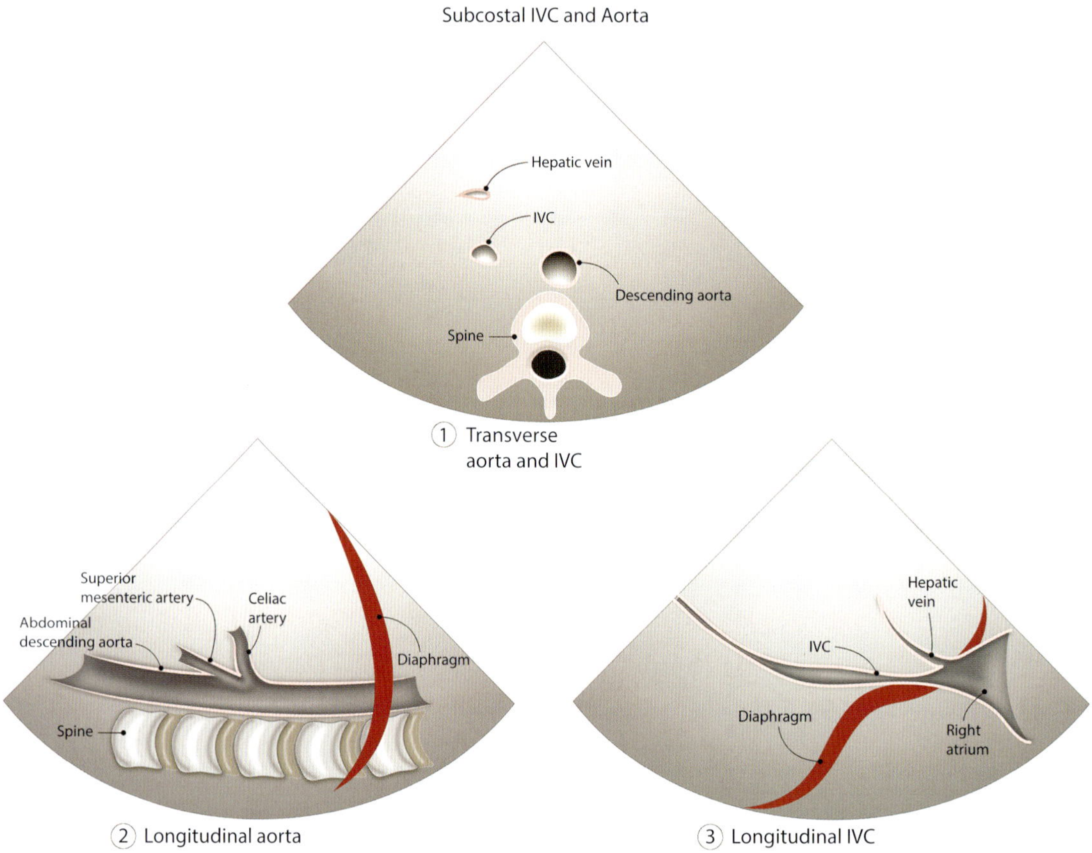

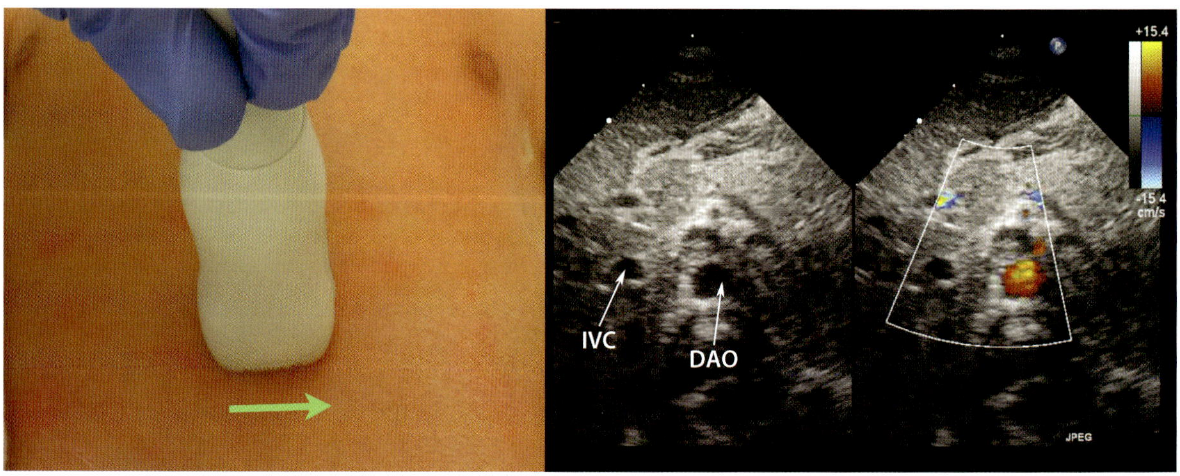

FIGURE 3-20.1. Subcostal cross section of the IVC and the DAo. From the subcostal window, with the transducer perpendicular to the abdominal wall and the marker pointing to the left side, a cross-sectional views of descending aorta (DAo) and inferior vena cava (IVC) are obtained. The IVC is normally located to the patient's right and anterior to the DAo, which overlies the vertebral column. This view confirms a situs solitus position.

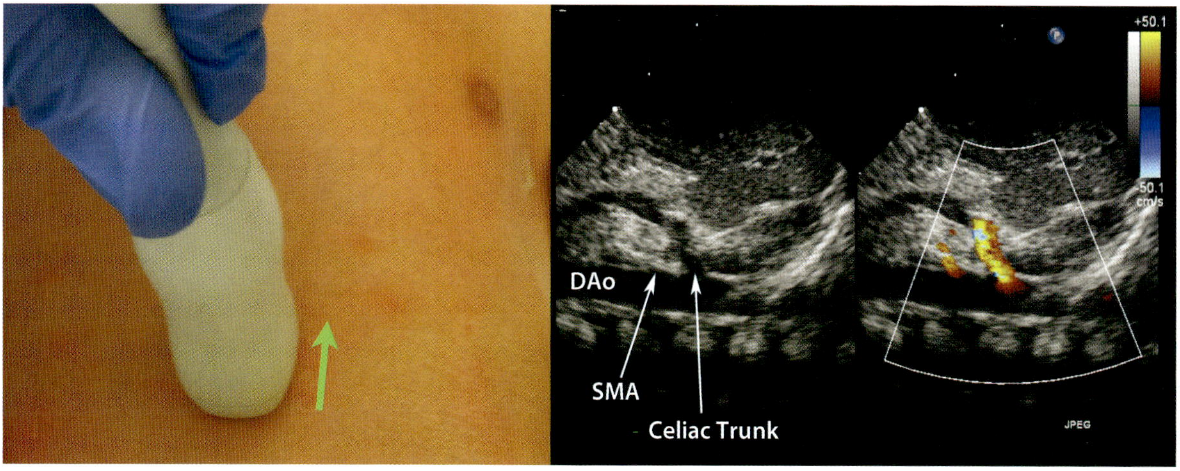

FIGURE and VIDEO 3-20.2. Subcostal sagittal DAo. From a subcostal transverse cut, the transducer is rotated 90° counterclockwise, with the marker pointing toward the head of the neonate. This will result in a sagittal plane that will display the course of the DAo and IVC. A slight tilt to the left from midline position will bring in view the DAo and its major infradiaphragmatic branches as it courses through the diaphragm. Abbreviations: DAo, descending aorta; IVC, inferior vena cava.

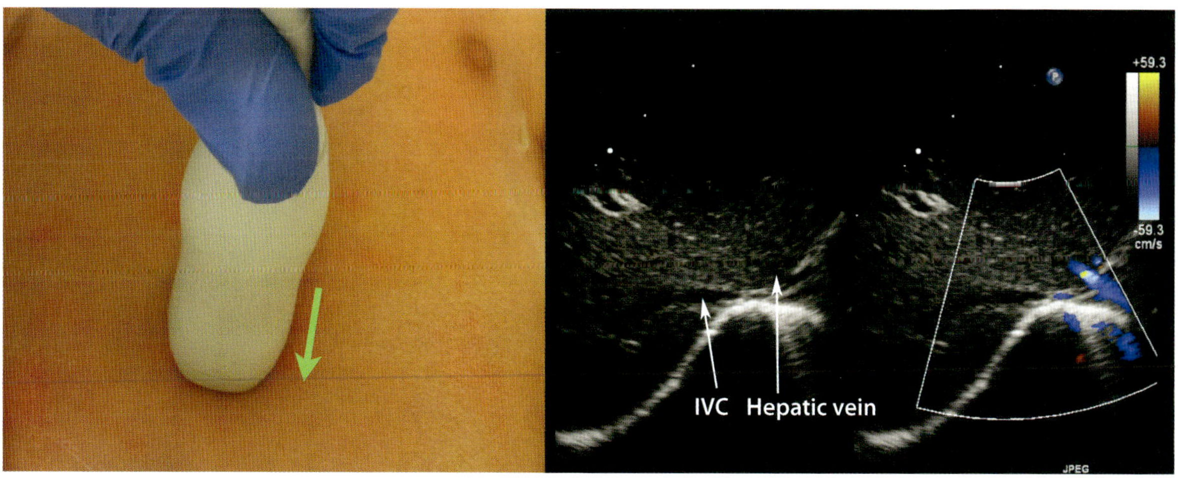

FIGURE and VIDEO 3-20.3. Subcostal sagittal IVC. A slight rightward tilt from midline will bring into view the IVC and hepatic veins, with the IVC entering the RA through the diaphragm.

Outline of Sector Scans Obtained from Suprasternal Window: SVC, Aortic Arch and Ductal Cut (FIGURE 3-21)

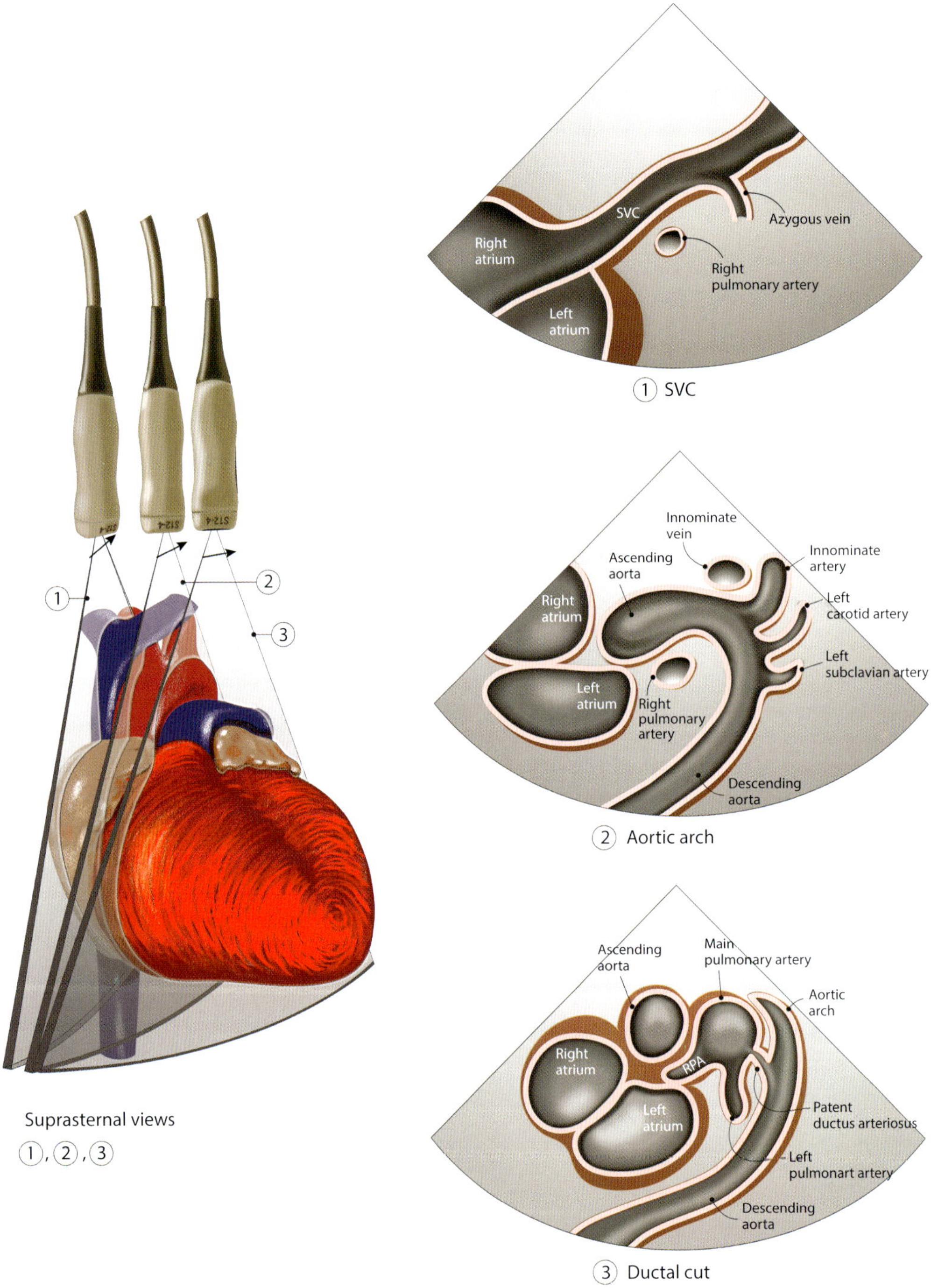

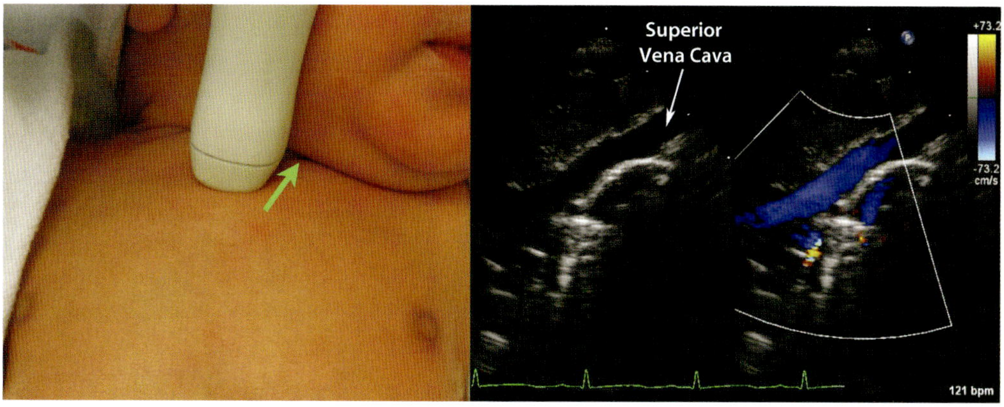

FIGURE and VIDEO 3-21.1. **Suprasternal SVC-RA.** With the marker pointing superiorly and the transducer angled inferiorly toward SVC-RA junction and with slight rightward tilt, the SVC and RA are displayed in anteroposterior orientation. SVC is seen as it enters the RA.

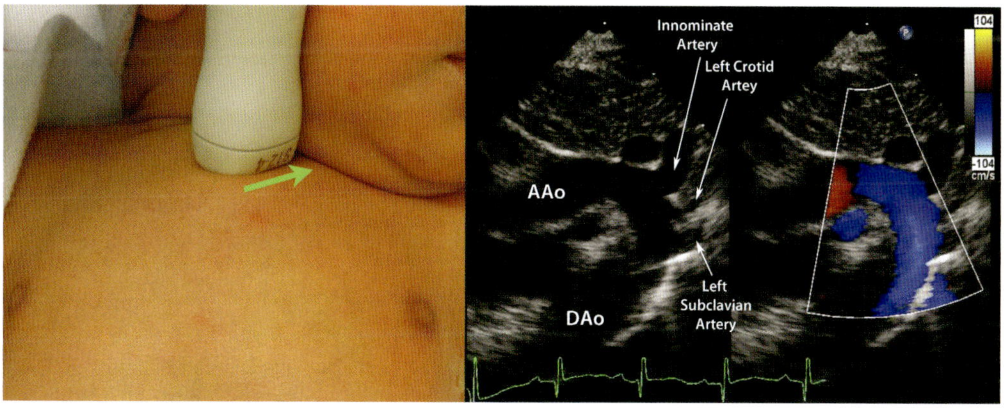

FIGURE and VIDEO 3-21.2. **Suprasternal aortic arch.** The transducer is rotated clockwise to approximately 30° from a straight sagittal plane, and tilted slightly to the left with the plane directed inferiorly, bringing into view the ascending aorta (AAo), the aortic arch and its branches, the descending aorta (DAo), the right pulmonary artery (RPA) in cross section, and a significant segment of the LA.

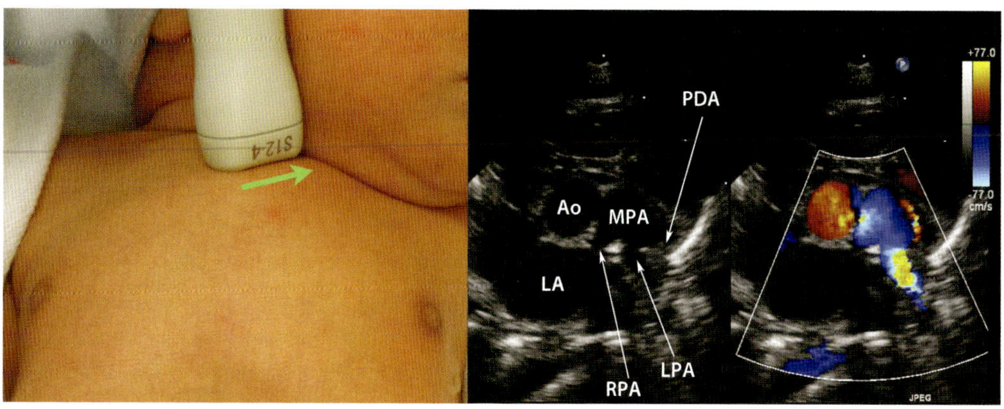

FIGURE and VIDEO 3-21.3. **Suprasternal ductal cut.** Further clockwise rotation of the transducer to approximately 60° from the sagittal plane reveals the main pulmonary artery (MPA) branching into the right pulmonary artery (RPA), the left pulmonary artery (LPA), and the patent ductus arteriosus (PDA, if it remains patent). Variable segments of the LA, the LV, and the AAo may be also be visualized in this view.

Outline of a Sector Scan Obtained from Suprasternal Coronal Posterior View: SVC, Ao, MPA, LA and Pulmonary Veins

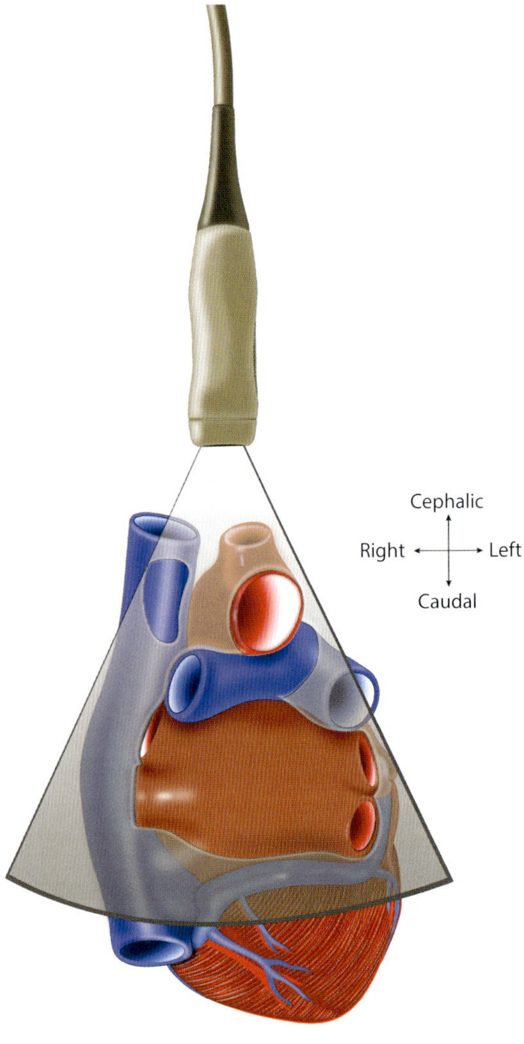

(4) Suprasternal views
(as seen from behind)

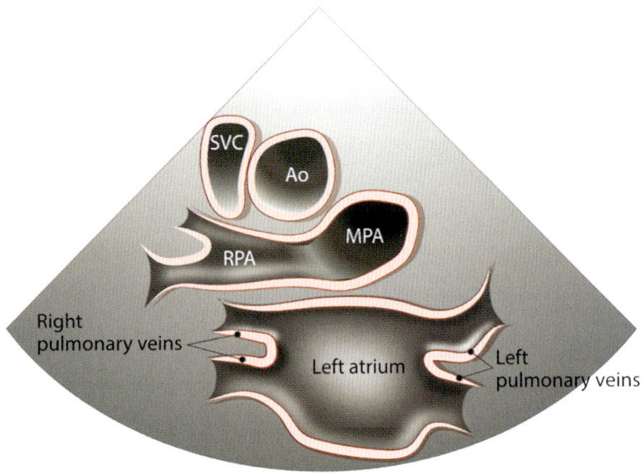

(4) Crab view

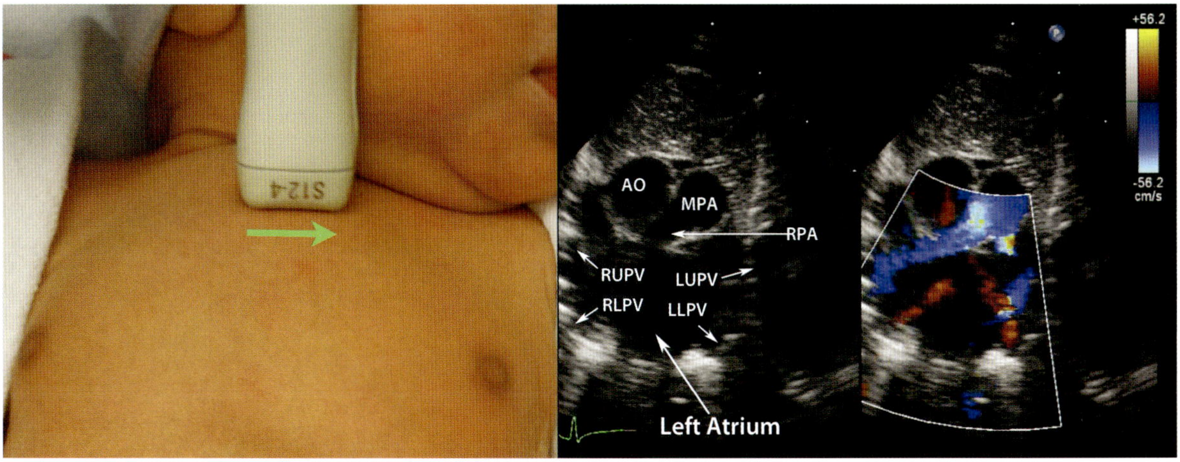

FIGURE and VIDEO 3-22.1. Suprasternal "crab view." With a clockwise rotation of the transducer to 90° from sagittal plane, cutting the heart in a posterior coronal plane, aorta (Ao), main pulmonary artery (MPA), right pulmonary artery (RPA), left atrium (LA), right upper pulmonary vein (RUPV), right lower pulmonary vein (RLPV), left upper pulmonary vein (LUPV), left lower pulmonary vein (LLPV), are visualized in this view.

Outline of Sector Scan from Suprasternal Widow: Innominate Artery, Right Subclavian Artery, and Right Carotid Artery (FIGURE 3-23)

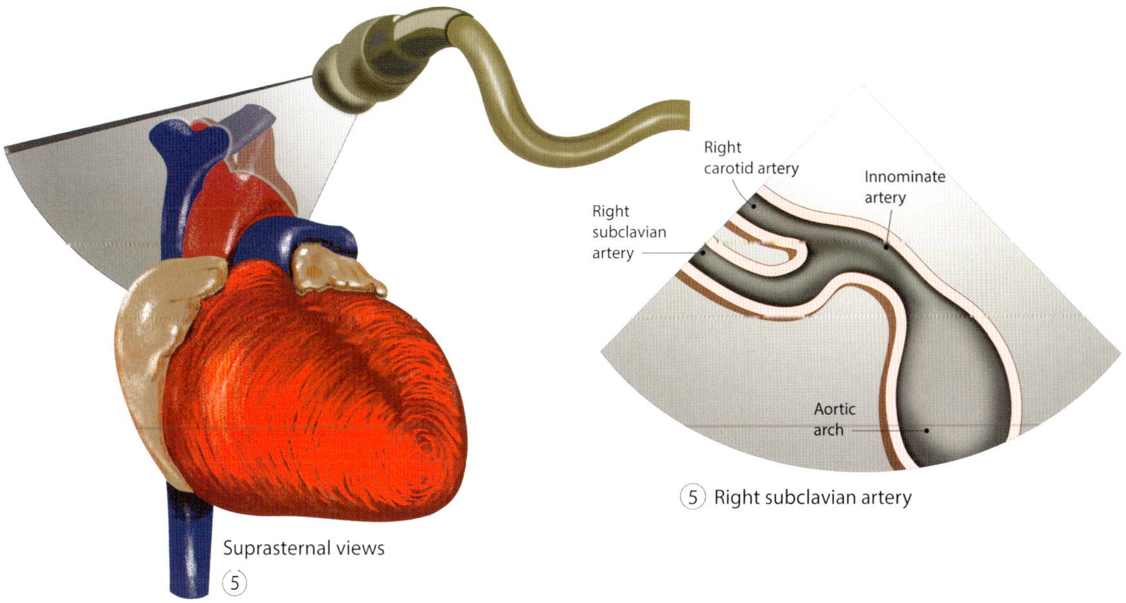

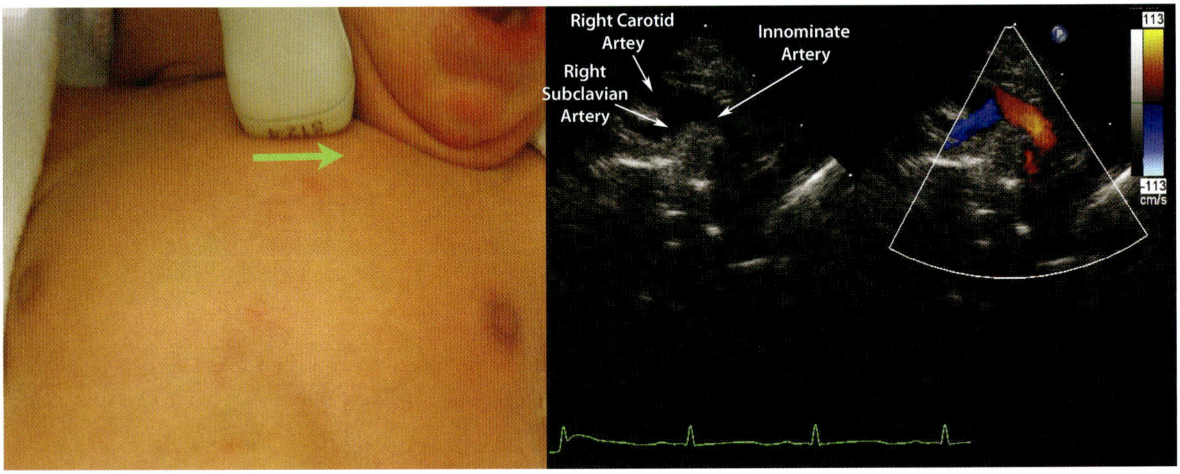

FIGURE and VIDEO 3-23.1. Suprasternal Innominate and right subclavian arteries. The transducer is brought to a vertical position, cutting the thoracic outlet in cross section. Further adjustment will display the innominate artery as it branches into right subclavian and right carotid arteries. Visualization of the right carotid artery coursing toward the right arm confirms the presence of a normal left-sided aortic arch.

In summary, in standard two-dimensional echocardiography, the heart is imaged by a series of thin fan-shaped slices that do not strictly follow the anatomic or cardiac axes of the heart. From each cardiac window, the heart is imaged via multiple planes, with specific aims of looking at certain segments of the heart. Familiarity with these planes and their normal variations will enable the examiner to recognize deviation from normal anatomy, which will then require further detailed study.

REFERENCES

1. Cooper MH, O'Rahilly R. The human heart at seven post-ovulatory weeks. *Acta Anatomica*. 1971;79:280–299.
2. Walmsley RT, Monkhouse WS. The heart of the newborn child: an anatomical study based upon transverse serial sections. *J Anat*. 1988;159:93–111.
3. St. John Sutton MG, Gewitz MH, Shah B, et al. Quantitative assessment of growth and function of cardiac chambers in normal human fetus: a prospective longitudinal study. *Circulation*. 1984;69:645–654.
4. Bulwer EB, Rivero JM. *Echocardiography Pocket Guide: The Transthoracic Examination*. Burlington, MA: Jones and Bartlett Publishers, LLC; 2011.
5. Lai WW, Ko HH. The normal pediatric echocardiogram, Chapter 4. In: *Echocardiography in Pediatric and Congenital Heart Disease*. 2nd ed. Wiley Blackwell; 2016.

CHAPTER 4

Application of Echocardiographic Simulators in Training for Neonatal Echocardiography*

Bijan Siassi, Mahmood Ebrahimi, and Shahab Noori

- INTRODUCTION
- ECHOCOM TRAINING SIMULATOR
- VIRTUAL NEONATAL ECHOCARDIOGRAPHY TRAINING SIMULATOR
- VNETS AS A TRAINING SIMULATOR
- COMPLETE 2D ECHOCARDIOGRAPHY
- COLOR FLOW ECHOCARDIOGRAPHY
- SPECTRAL DOPPLER ECHOCARDIOGRAPHY
- M-MODE ECHOCARDIOGRAPHY
- REFERENCES

INTRODUCTION

Echocardiography is the predominant noninvasive method of assessing cardiac structure and function. Although initially this technique resided exclusively in the domain of the cardiologist, more recently it has been increasingly utilized for point-of-care applications across different specialties.[1] The utility of point-of-care echocardiography has been demonstrated by neonatologists in the neonatal intensive care unit,[2] anesthesiologists during the perioperative period,[3] intensivists in the critical care setting,[4] and emergency medicine physicians in the emergency care setting.[5] The development of more advanced and portable systems has facilitated this change. However, the widespread use of point-of-care echocardiography, especially for neonatal intensive care, has been hampered by the lack of adequately trained non-cardiology specialists and access to patients.

*Videos can be accessed at http://PracticalNeonatalEcho.com.

Training in neonatal point-of-care echocardiography (also known as "targeted" or "functional" echocardiography) is a complex process that requires not only comprehensive theoretical knowledge but also extensive hands-on training to acquire the all-important technical skills. At present, there is no alternative method for achieving technical competence in neonatal echocardiography other than performing studies on actual neonates. However, because of the restricted access to live subjects, particularly neonates, opportunities for practical training are limited. To overcome this obstacle, echocardiography simulators have been developed. Weidenbach et al[6] introduced two-dimensional (2D) echocardiography simulation by the use of real three-dimensional (3D) image volumes, which have been used both for transthoracic and transesophageal echocardiography.[7] In infants and younger children, simulators based on real 3D volumes have been used for training physicians with minimal echocardiography experience with good results. The knowledge of cardiac anatomy as depicted by echocardiography and detection of congenital heart defects is improved, while spatial orientation and hand-eye coordination is enhanced by the use of the simulators.[8–10] However, presently available transthoracic echocardiographic simulators based on real 3D volumes are restricted to 2D echocardiography, which lacks other modalities such as color flow Doppler, spectral Doppler, and M-mode. Furthermore, since image volumes are obtained either from subcostal or apical windows, simulation of echocardiography from parasternal and suprasternal windows may be suboptimal. In general, real transthoracic echocardiographic images obtained in older children and adults are of poor quality and are not suitable for simulation. For these reasons, for transthoracic echocardiography, almost all commercially available simulators obtain their 3D images from other imaging platforms such as MRI and render them to look like echocardiograms. These simulators are used extensively in training intensivists, emergency room physicians, and anesthesiologists, as well as cardiology technologists and trainees.

ECHOCOM TRAINING SIMULATOR

Recently, Weidenbach et al have introduced a training simulator for echocardiography in neonates.[11] Although this simulator includes extensive cases of congenital cardiac defects, along with cases of functional and acquired heart diseases, it only simulates 2D echocardiography for anatomical diagnosis and has the above limitations. In spite of these limitations, it is used by neonatologists for training purposes.

VIRTUAL NEONATAL ECHOCARDIOGRAPHIC TRAINING SIMULATOR (VNETS)

We have developed a simulator with exclusive emphasis on neonates and young infants (Figure and Video 4-1). This system has the capability of simulating real-time scanning from all acoustic windows. It offers the capability of performing 2D imaging, color flow and spectral Doppler, and M-mode modalities. From each infant, four-dimensional (4D) image volumes (3D plus real-time motion) were recorded using Philips IE33 echocardiograph. Up to seven 4D volume datasets were acquired from each infant, and at the same time, 2D video clips of color flow, spectral Doppler, and M-mode were recorded in standard echocardiographic views using five transthoracic echocardiographic acoustic windows (right and left parasternal, apical, subcostal, and suprasternal).

We employed a modified neonatal mannequin, a laptop computer, and an integrated electromagnetic tracking device including a magnetic transmitter and a 6 degrees of freedom (6DOF) sensor incorporated into a dummy transducer for this purpose. Four-dimensional volumes are sliced by invisible cutting planes controlled by roll, pitch, and yaw of the 6DOF sensor incorporated into the dummy transducer, resulting in a continuous real-time display of 2D echocardiographic images, which are shown on the main section of the display window. The location and motion of the cutting planes are duplicated on the fan-shaped cutting planes of the 3D heart displayed on the side section of the display window. A small arrow on the side of the cutting plane indicates the direction of the marker on the transducer (Figure 4-2). The coordinates from 27 specific slices of 3D image volume sets from the five echocardiographic windows are used to initiate the display of video clips of associated color flow Doppler, spectral Doppler, or M-mode, which are recorded and stored at the time of the original 4D volume acquisition.

For each infant, seven 4D DICOM echocardiographic volumes were virtually placed and oriented in their respective five echocardiographic acoustic windows on the doll mannequin. The location of each window is

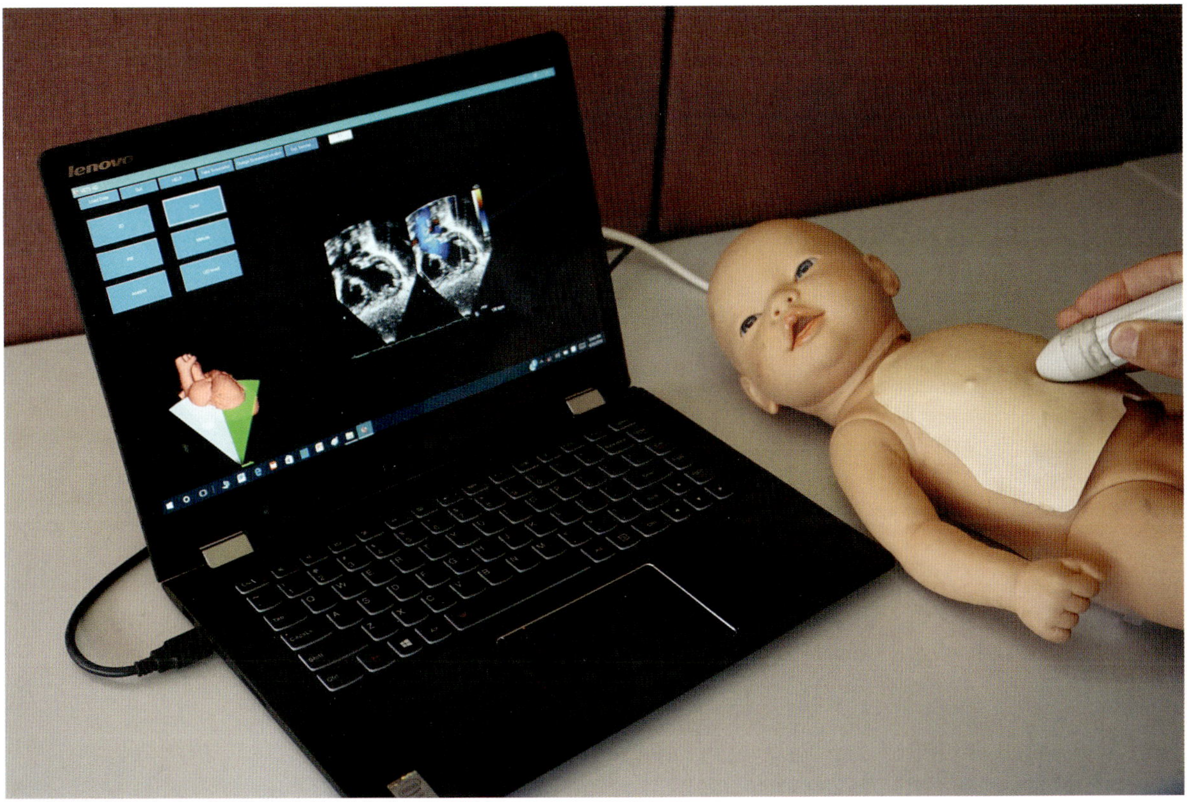

FIGURE and VIDEO 4-1. Virtual Neonatal Echocardiographic Training Simulator (VNETS). Two-dimensional, color flow, Doppler and M-mode are obtained from all cardiac windows and are displayed on the main screen, whereas a fan-shaped cutting plane is shown on the side screen indicating direction of the cut through the 3D image.

specific to each infant according to the variation in the acoustic windows encountered in the clinical setting. The 4D volumes are arranged so that one 4D volume is placed each at the left and right parasternal windows and one at the apex, two at the subcostal window for imaging the heart and abdominal great vessels and two volumes are placed in the suprasternal windows for imaging the heart and the head and neck vessels. The use of multiple volumes allows for the complete range of 2D imaging from each window.

VNETS as a Training Echocardiographic Simulator

Because the simulator was designed for hands-on training purposes, it can simulate actual echocardiography, including image acquisition by the manipulation of the transducer in the standard acoustic windows. All essential echocardiographic modalities can be simulated, including 2D, color and spectral Doppler, and M-mode imaging, along with hemodynamic measurements and report generation (Figure and Video 4-1). The simulator can be used for different levels of training. The beginner and intermediate levels would involve 12 to 17 sector cuts from all cardiac windows and would be appropriate in the training of physicians for point-of-care echocardiography. Pediatric echocardiography technologists and trainees in pediatric cardiology, on the other hand, may be required to master all 27 cuts (Table 4-1). Images for each window can be obtained by paying special attention to the orientation of the cutting planes of the 3D model

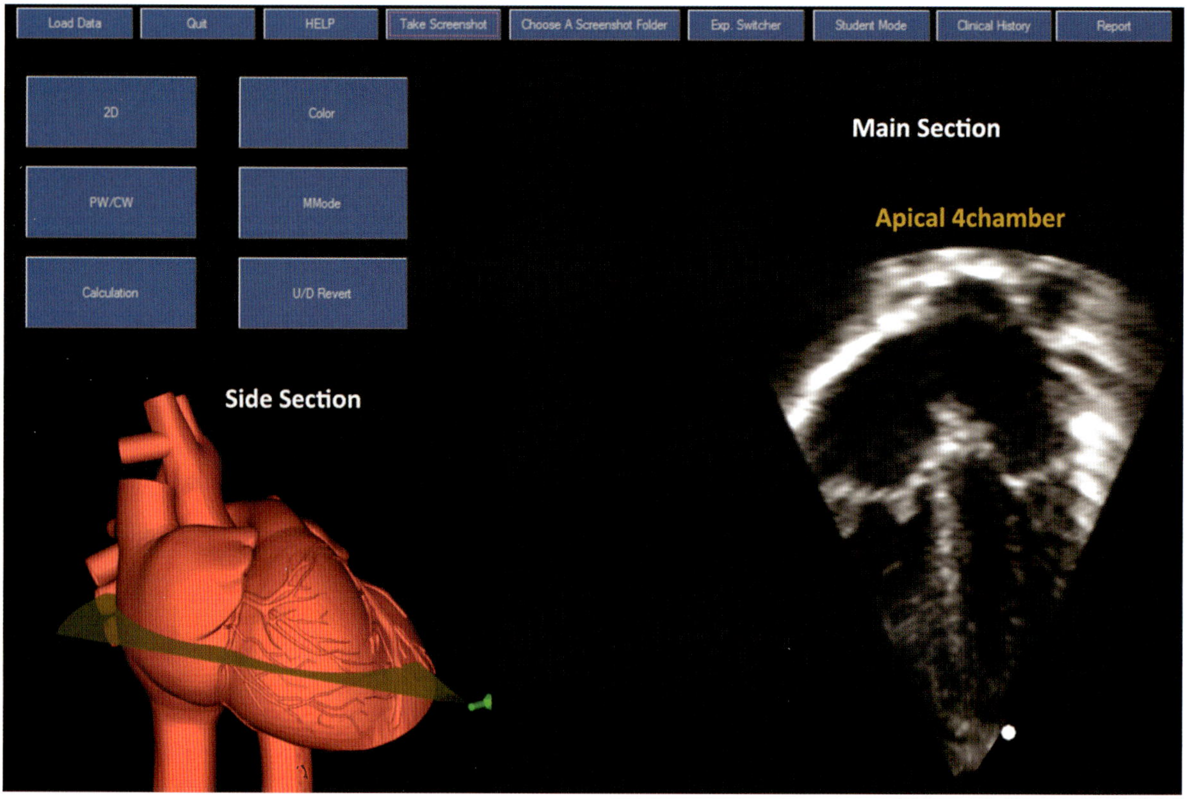

FIGURE 4-2. A 2D echocardiogram obtained from apical window by the slicing of the 4D image volume is displayed on the main screen, and the fan-shaped cutting plane through a 3D heart is demonstrated on the side screen.

of the heart displayed on the side screen, along with the image of 2D echocardiogram on the main screen of the monitor.

Complete 2D Echocardiography

A complete range of echocardiographic images is obtained from the following windows on the mannequin: parasternal window, apical window, subcostal window, right parasternal window, and suprasternal window. Continuous images can be obtained from all windows and optimized for up to 27 standard echocardiographic views. With 2D echocardiography, structural cardiac defects present in congenital heart disease can be detected. Two-dimensional echocardiography can be used for the evaluation of left and right ventricular function. By tracing the endocardial surface of the left ventricle at end-diastole and end-systole from the apical four-chamber view and by using the modified Simpson's algorithm, the user can measure the ejection fraction of the left ventricle (Figure 4-3). Similarly, by measuring the area of right ventricle in end-diastole and end-systole, the user can estimate the right ventricular function. Similarly, measurement of the area of left atrium at end-systole in apical four-chamber view provides a better evaluation of left atrial dimension.

Color Flow Echocardiography

Normal and abnormal color flow Doppler from all standard echocardiographic views can be visualized and investigated. Particular attention is paid to any left-to-right

TABLE 4-1. Suggested Echocardiographic Views at Various Levels of Training

Beginner	Intermediate	Advanced
Parasternal (P) **PL axis (PLAX):** Parasternal long axis **PL RVOT:** Right ventricular outflow (RVOT) **PL RVIN:** Right ventricular inflow **PS Mitral:** Parasternal short axis mitral valve **PS Base:** PS base of the heart	**Parasternal (P)** **PL axis (PLAX):** Parasternal long axis **PL RVOT:** Right ventricular outflow (RVOT) **PL RVIN:** Right ventricular inflow **PS Mitral:** PS mitral valve **PS Base:** PS base of the heart	**Parasternal (P)** **PLAX:** Parasternal long axis **PL RVOT:** Right ventricular outflow (RVOT) **PL RVIN:** Right ventricular inflow **PS Apex:** Parasternal short axis apex **PS Papillary:** PS papillary muscle **PS Mitral:** PS mitral valve **PS Base:** PS base of the heart
Apical (AP) **Ap. 4 Cham:** Apical 4 chamber **Ap. 5 Cham:** Apical 5 chamber	**Apical (AP)** **Ap. 4 Cham:** Apical 4 chamber **Ap. 5 Cham:** Apical 5 chamber **Ap. RVOT:** AP Right ventricular outflow	**Apical (AP)** **Ap. 4 Cham. Post:** Ap. 4 chamber posterior **Ap. 4 Cham:** Apical 4 chamber **Ap. 5 Cham:** Apical 5 chamber **Ap. RVOT:** AP Right ventricular outflow
Subcostal (SC) **SC Cor post:** Subcostal coronal posterior **SC SVC:** Subcostal superior vena cava	**Subcostal (SC)** **SC Cor post:** SC coronal posterior **SC SVC:** SC superior vena cava **SC Sag. Bicaval.** SC sagittal Bicaval **SC Ab. Ao.:** SC abdominal aorta **SC Ab. IVC:** SC inferior vena cava	**Subcostal (SC)** **SC Cor post:** Subcostal coronal posterior **SC SVC:** Subcostal superior vena cava **SC Cor Aorta:** SC coronal aorta **SC cor RVOT:** SC coronal RVOT **SC Sag Apex:** SC sagittal apex **SC Sag. RVOT:** SC sagittal RVOT **SC Sag. Aorta:** SC sagittal Aorta **SC Sag. Bicaval:** SC sagittal Bicaval **SC Ab. Trans.:** SC abdominal transverse **SC Ab. Ao.:** SC abdominal aorta **SC Ab. IVC:** SC abdominal inferior vena cava
Right Parasternal (RP) **RP SVC:** RP superior vena cava **Suprasternal (SS)** **SS Ao arch:** Suprasternal aortic arch **SS Ductal cut:** Suprasternal ductal cut	**Right Parasternal (RP)** **RP SVC:** RP superior vena cava **Suprasternal (SS)** **SS Ao arch:** Suprasternal aortic arch **SS Ductal cut:** Suprasternal ductal cut **SS "Crab view":** SS pulmonary veins	**Right Parasternal (RP)** **RP SVC:** RP superior vena cava **Suprasternal (SS)** **SS Ao arch:** Suprasternal aortic arch **SS Ductal cut:** Suprasternal ductal cut **SS "Crab view":** SS pulmonary veins **SS Innom.:** SS innominate artery

Beginner and intermediate training may be sufficient for physicians involved in point-of-care echocardiography, while advanced training is recommended for physicians and technologists involved in training for pediatric cardiology.

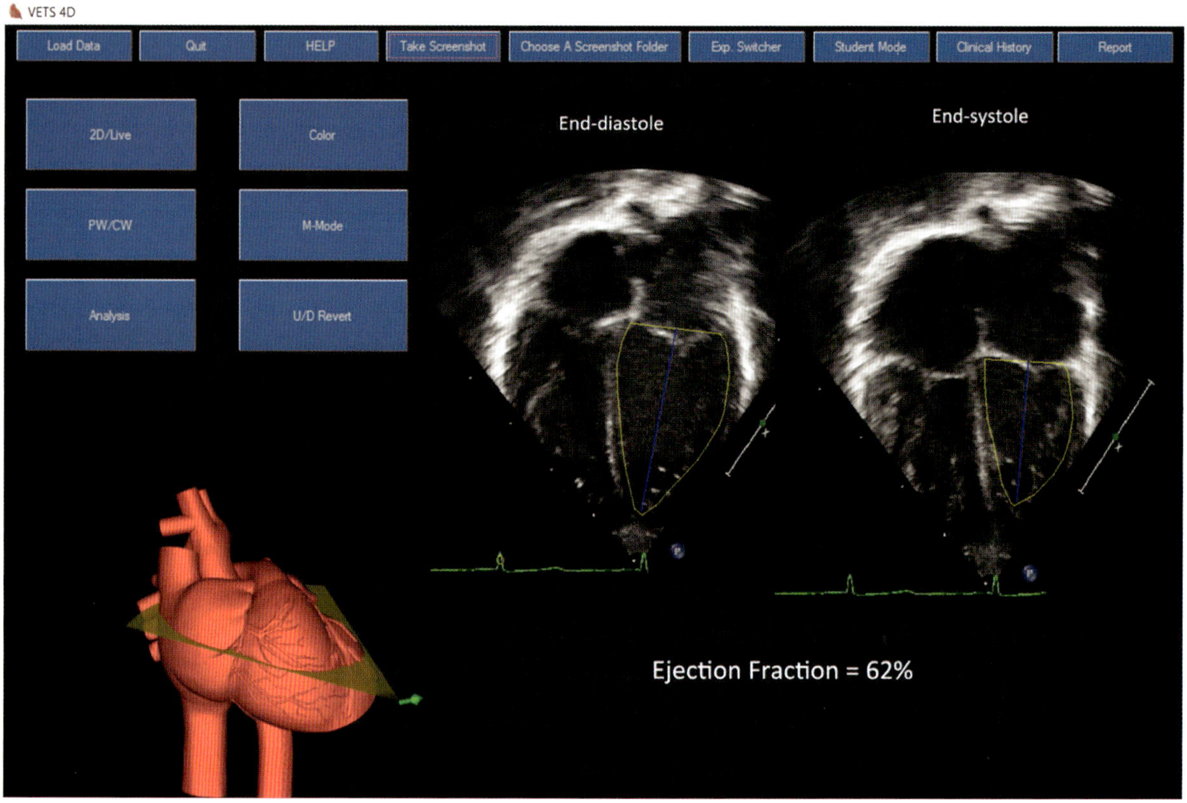

FIGURE 4-3. A four-chamber view obtained from the apical window in end-diastole and end-systole is displayed in the main screen, with the slicing plane on the side screen. The tracing of endocardial planes of the left ventricle in diastole and systole enables the measurement of its ejection fraction. See text for details.

shunting through the atrial/ventricular septa or through a patent ductus arteriosus (Figure 4-4). Regurgitant flows across the mitral, tricuspid, aortic, and pulmonary valves, as well as turbulent flow through stenotic aortic and pulmonary valves, may be evaluated. Careful evaluation of color flow Doppler in addition to the 17 2D echocardiographic images will be sufficient to allow trainees in point-of-care echocardiography to suspect the presence of most congenital cardiac defects (Figure 4-5). Mastery and careful evaluation of 27 2D cuts with color flow Doppler will be sufficient to lead to a detailed diagnosis of most congenital cardiac defects for trainees in pediatric cardiology and pediatric cardiology technologists, provided that appropriate 2D and color flow images were recorded from the index patient for the simulator.

Spectral Doppler Echocardiography

Spectral Doppler can be used to display normal flow profiles through normal vasculature as well as abnormal flow profiles through stenotic or incompetent heart valves, stenotic vessels, or defects in interatrial or interventricular septa. Doppler velocity profiles can be accessed from the apical five-chamber view for aortic flow measurement (Figure 4-6), from the main pulmonary artery for pulmonary flow, and from the subcostal coronal or sagittal bicaval for superior vena cava flow measurement. Similarly, Doppler tracings of the tricuspid flow profiles can be assessed from the apical four-chamber view and from the parasternal long-axis right ventricular inflow view for the inflow and regurgitant flow profile for the assessment of pulmonary arterial pressure. Flow through

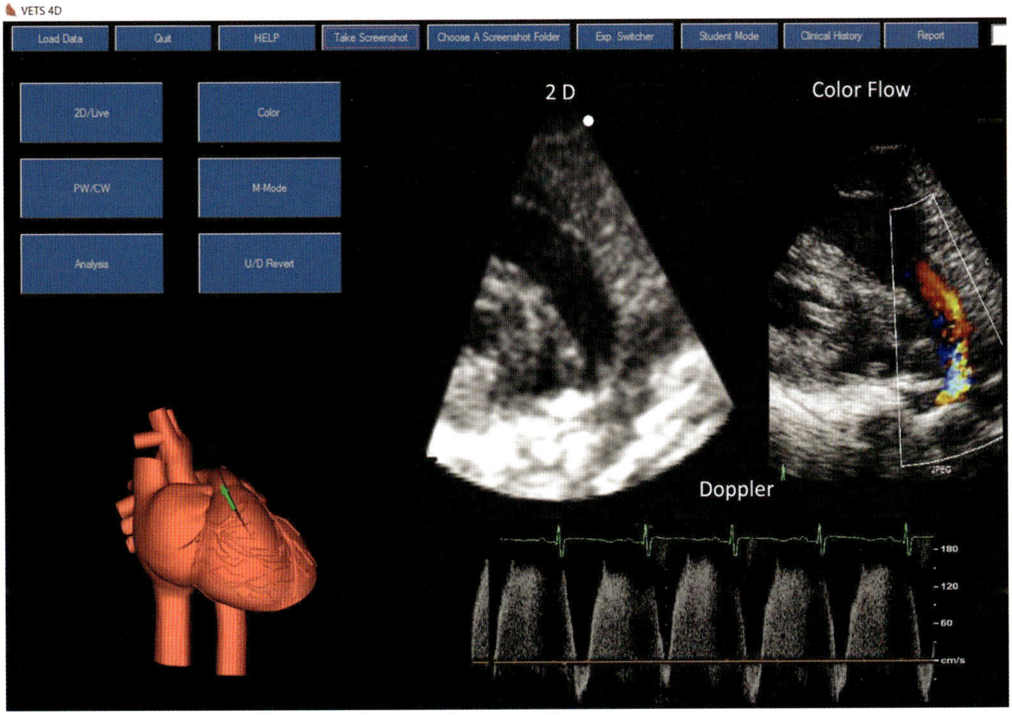

FIGURE 4-4. Slicing plane through parasternal long-axis, right ventricular outflow is displayed on the side screen, while 2D, color flow, and spectral Doppler are displayed on the main screen from a premature neonate with patent ductus arteriosus (PDA). Color flow Doppler confirms presence of PDA with mainly left-to-right shunting. Spectral Doppler indicates the duration and velocity of left-to-right and right-to-left shunts.

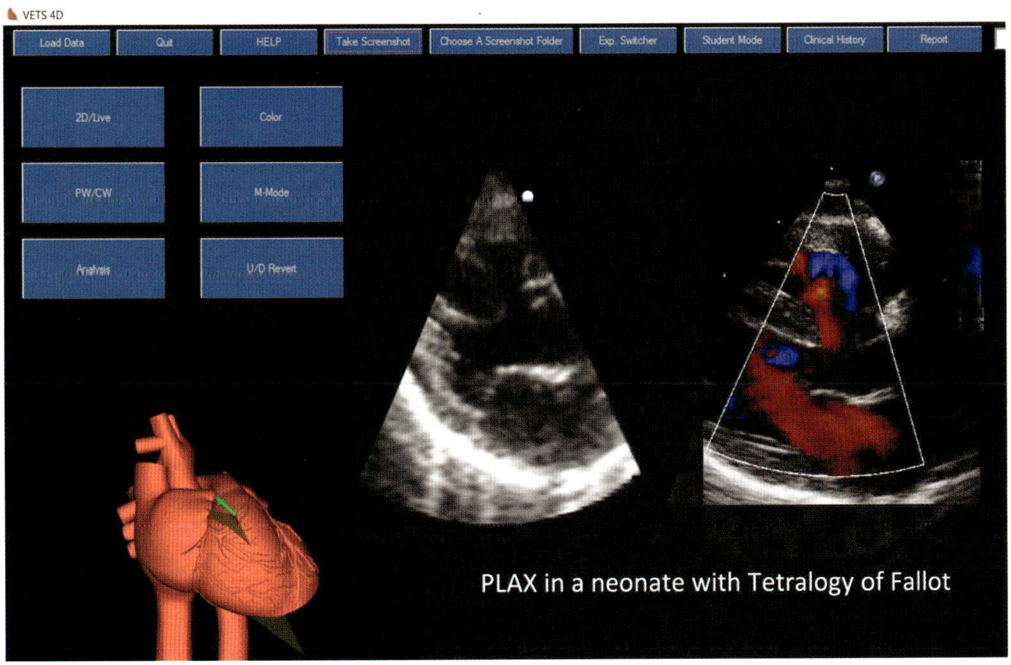

FIGURE 4-5. Slicing plane through the parasternal long axis is displayed on the side screen, while 2D and color flow Doppler are displayed on the main screen from a full-term neonate with tetralogy of Fallot. A 2D echocardiogram indicates the presence of an enlarged aorta overriding a large subaortic ventricular septal defect (VSD). Color flow Doppler displays bidirectional shunting through VSD.

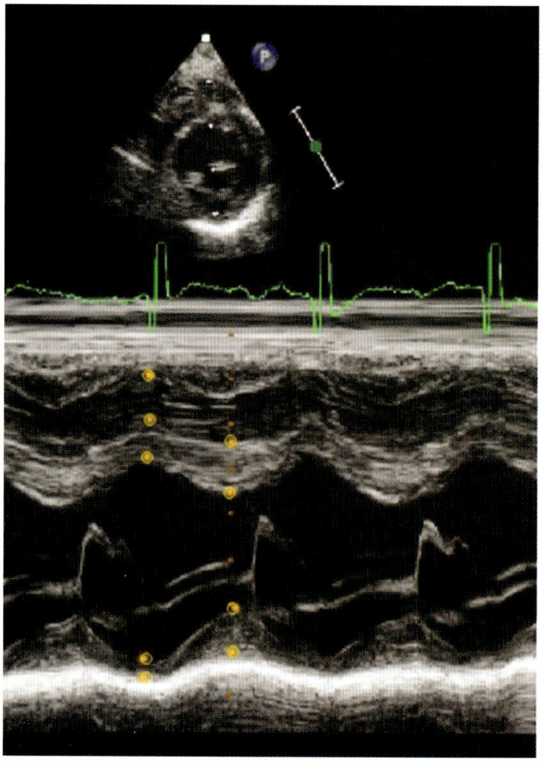

A

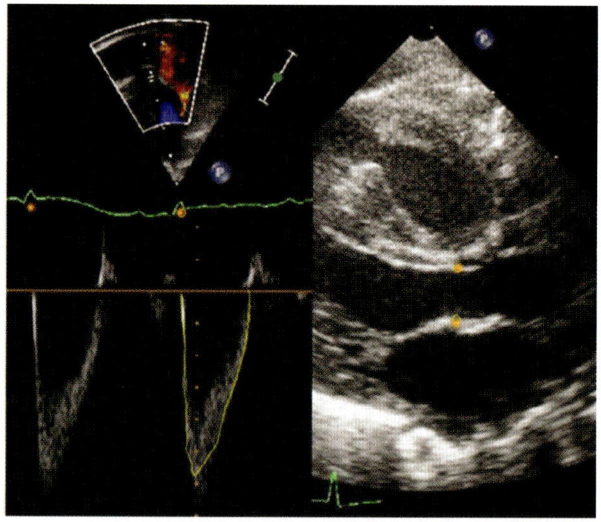

B

FIGURE 4-6. M-mode echocardiography. **Panel A**: M-mode of left ventricle for anatomical and functional measurements. **Panel B**: Aortic blood flow measured from aortic spectral Doppler tracing and aortic diameter. See text for details.

the ductus arteriosus can be assessed from the suprasternal ductal cut or from the parasternal short-axis base or parasternal long-axis outflow for direction of flow and duration of right-to-left and left-to-right shunts through a patent ductus arteriosus. Flow through the foramen ovale may be evaluated from the subcostal coronal posterior or subcostal sagittal bicaval view for its direction and velocity. Finally, other abnormal stenotic or regurgitant flows detected by color Doppler can be further investigated by pulse or continuous-wave Doppler.

M-Mode Echocardiography

M-mode tracings are obtained from the parasternal long-axis or the parasternal short-axis view at the level of the mitral valve leaflets for right and left ventricular sizes, function, and wall thickness, and from parasternal long- and short-axis view at the base of the heart for the measurement of aortic root and left atrial diameters (Figure 4-7). M-mode from other areas of the heart may be obtained as desired.

Case Studies and Report Generation

Although new cases are added to the simulator on an ongoing basis, presently we have stored complete echocardiograms of 25 cases for training purposes. They include normal term and preterm infants as well as neonates with functional or congenital cardiac defects. At various levels of training, the trainee is able to record 2D echocardiography images for evaluation by the instructor. The integrated calculation package allows the trainee to obtain a full range of echocardiographic measurements that are automatically transcribed to the report. For each case, the trainee is able to generate a neonatal echocardiography report describing his or her impression of the case.

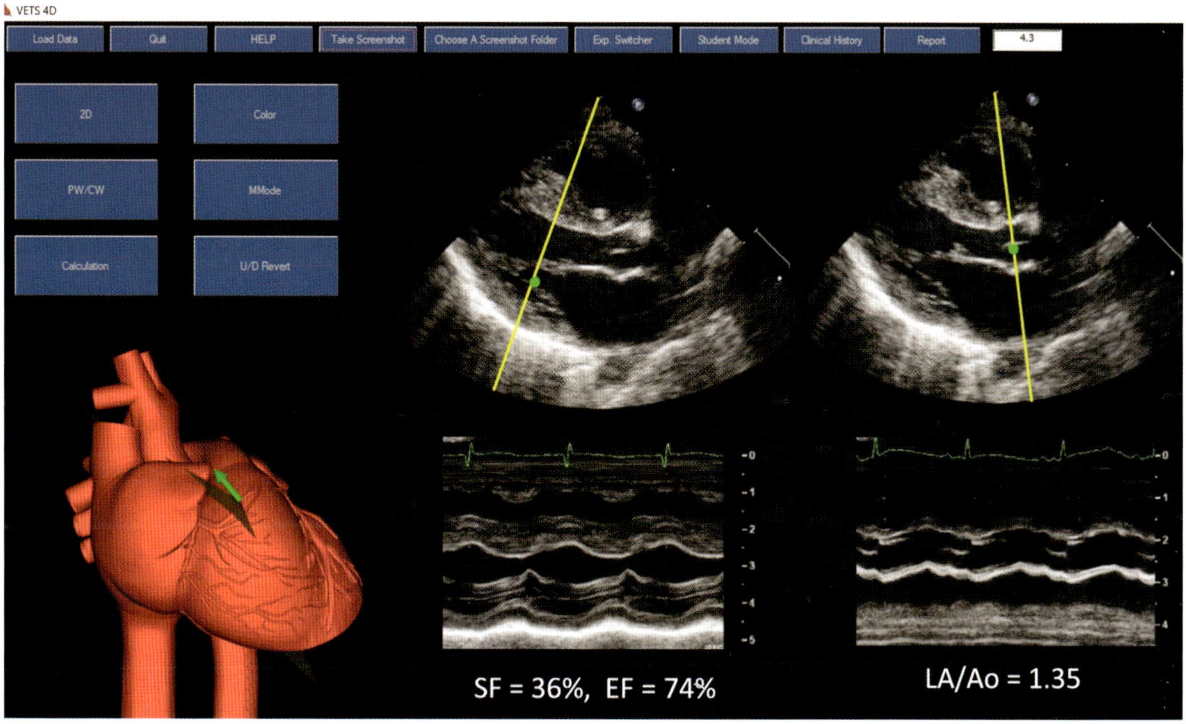

FIGURE 4-7. The slicing plane through the parasternal long axis is displayed on the side screen, while the motion of the M-mode cursor is depicted on the main screen. The M-mode cursor is moved to the tip of mitral valve for the measurement of the shortening fraction and ejection fraction of left ventricle, among other dimensions measured by M-mode. To obtain the aortic root and left atrial dimensions, the user moves the cursor to the base of the heart.

REFERENCES

1. Beaulieu Y. Specific skill set and goals of focused echocardiography for critical care clinicians. *Crit Care Med.* 2007;35:S144–S149.
2. Evans N. Echocardiography in neonatal intensive care units in Australia and New Zealand. *J Paediat Child Health.* 2000;36:169–171.
3. Cowie B. Focused cardiovascular ultrasound performed by anesthesiologists in the perioperative period: Feasible and alters patient management. *J Cardiotborac Vasc Anestb.* 2009;23:450–456.
4. Cholley BP, Vieillard-Baron A, Mebazaa A. Echocardiography in the ICU: Time for widespread use! *Intensive Care Med.* 2006;32:9–10.
5. Mayron R, Gaudio FE, Plummer D, et al. Echocardiography performed by emergency physicians: Impact on diagnosis and therapy. *Ann Emerg Med.* 1988;17:150–154.
6. Weidenbach M, Wick C, Pieper S, et al. Augmented reality simulator in two-dimensional echocardiography. *Comput. Biomed. Res.* 2000;33:11–22.
7. Bose R, Matyal R, Panzica P, et al. Transesophageal echocardiography simulator: A new learning tool. *J Cardiothorac Vasc Anesth.* 2009;23:544–548.
8. Weidenbach M, Razek V, Wild F, et al. Simulation of congenital heart defects: A novel way of training in echocardiography. *Heart.* 2009;95:636–664.
9. Weidenbach M, Wild F, Scheer K, et al. Computer-based training in two-dimensional echocardiography using an echocardiography simulator. *J Am Soc Echocardiogr.* 2005;18:362–366.
10. Shakil O, Mahmood F, Matyal R. Simulation in echocardiography: an ever expanding frontier. *J Cardiothorac Vasc Anesth.* 2012;23:476–485.
11. Weidenbach M, et al. EchoCom-training simulator for echocardiography in neonates. https://www.echocom.de.

CHAPTER 5

M-Mode Echocardiography and 2D Cardiac Measurements*

Merujan Uzunyan and Lindsey Miller

- M-MODE ECHOCARDIOGRAPHY
- USES OF M-MODE ECHOCARDIOGRAPHY
- OBTAINING M-MODE IMAGES
- M-MODE ASSESSMENT OF WALL THICKNESS
- M-MODE ASSESSMENT OF LV SYSTOLIC FUNCTION
  - Fractional Shortening
  - Ejection Fraction
- M-MODE ASSESSMENT OF LV MASS
- M-MODE ASSESSMENT OF PERICARDIAL EFFUSION
- M-MODE ASSESSMENT OF LA SIZE AND OF LA:AO RATIO
- MEASUREMENTS OBTAINED WITH 2D ECHOCARDIOGRAPHY
- MEASUREMENT OF DIAMETER IN ASSESSMENT OF CARDIAC OUTPUT
  - LVOT Diameter Measurement
  - RVOT Diameter Measurement
- SIMPSON'S METHOD FOR LV EJECTION FRACTION
- VISUAL ESTIMATION OF SYSTOLIC FUNCTION BASED ON 2D ECHOCARDIOGRAPHY
- 2D ASSESSMENT OF LV MASS
- 2D ASSESSMENT OF LEFT ATRIAL DIMENSIONS
  - LA Linear Dimensions
  - LA Volume
  - LA Area
- MITRAL AND TRICUSPID VALVE ANNULAR DIMENSIONS
- REFERENCES

This chapter discusses the use of M-mode (movement/motion mode) and its role in neonatal functional echocardiography, as well as common measurements obtained with two-dimensional (2D) imaging.

M-MODE ECHOCARDIOGRAPHY

The original description of M-mode echocardiography in 1953 by Dr. Inge Edler and physicist Hellmuth Hertz marked the beginning of a new noninvasive diagnostic technique. This technique was initially used primarily for the preoperative study of mitral valve stenosis. M-mode is also frequently referred to as an "ice pick view of the heart" for the following reason: Dr. Edler, while pioneering this "new" technology, had realized that a characteristic pattern of echo signals was obtained in patients who displayed mitral stenosis. Determined to find the origin of these signals, he initially performed experiments on calf hearts and later, to verify his observations, he performed ultrasound examinations on dying patients. Upon

*Videos can be accessed at http://PracticalNeonatalEcho.com.

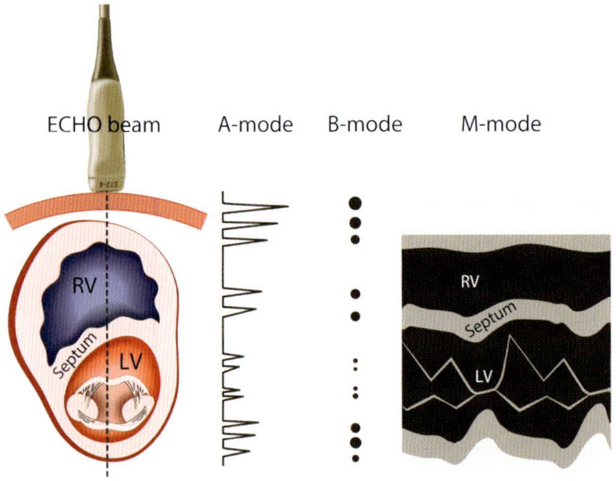

FIGURE 5-1. Schematic drawings showing the 2D parasternal short-axis view of the heart at the level of the mitral valve leaflet tips with corresponding illustrations of A-mode, B-mode, and M-mode assuming single ultrasound beam. Abbreviations: RV, right ventricle; LV, left ventricle.

completion of an examination, he marked the direction of the ultrasonic beam on the patient's chest. After the patient died, he reportedly passed an ice pick through the chest wall in the direction taken by the ultrasonic beam. On postmortem examination, Edler found that the needle had pierced the anterior wall of the right ventricle, had passed through the right ventricular outflow tract, the interventricular septum, and the upper part of the left ventricle, and had entered the left atrium via the mitral valve. Dr. Edler realized that the anterior cusp of the mitral valve was responsible for the echo signal in question.[1]

Another key element in the development of medical ultrasonography was making ultrasound waves visible on the screen. In other words, the returning echoes needed to be displayed in a way that would enable visualization of the cardiac structures. The first display mode was called the amplitude modulated or A-mode display. In A-mode, the presence of a "structure" on the ultrasound beam's path is represented on the screen by a positive deflection (spike) and the strength of the returning signal is represented by its height (amplitude). In intensity modulated display—also known as B-mode (B = brightness)—the signals are converted from spikes to dots. The taller the spikes (the greater the amplitude of the signal), the brighter the dots. This forms the basis of M-mode as well as 2D imaging (Figure 5-1).

Since the cardiac structures are constantly moving, the echo dots from these moving structures will move back and forth along an imaginary vertical line toward and away from the transducer. By electronically sweeping this tracing from left to the right, the "dots" will inscribe the motion pattern of the moving structures (like running an electrocardiogram [ECG] or seismograph paper). In contrast, a fixed (nonmoving) structure will be represented by a straight, horizontal line. Hence, the "M" in M-mode stands for "motion," and the concept is like the ECG. M-mode scans produce a running display of data obtained from the interrogation of a single straight line through a cardiac structure. Imagine a single ultrasound beam piercing the heart to disclose its contents. The ultrasound beam hits all structures in its path, and the ultrasound waves are then reflected. The reflected waves are displayed in B-mode, assigning a brightness value based on their strength and a distance based on time traveled. While 2D echocardiography is essentially a "picture" of the heart, an M-mode echocardiogram is a "diagram" that shows how the positions of its structures change during the cardiac cycle. M-mode recordings allow in-vivo noninvasive measurement of cardiac dimensions and motion patterns of its structures.

M-mode has a higher frequency of sampling than a 2D scan and can therefore give a more detailed analysis of the change in cardiac structures' positions over time. A graph is essentially created on the screen that plots time on the x-axis versus distance from the transducer on the y-axis. This displays motion of a cardiac structure along a single axis in real time. M-mode provides excellent time resolution, since its pulse repetition frequency (PRF, also known as sampling rate; see Chapter 1), which is given in the number of samples obtained in 1 second (usually >1000 cycles per second), is much greater than the heart rate. Therefore, even at a heart rate of 200 beats per minute, 300 pulses of information are acquired for each heartbeat. Assuming a heart rate of 200 beats per minute, there will be 3.33 beats every second, and in a sampling at 1000 cycles per second, there will be 300 looks per heartbeat (1000/3.3=300). Thus, M-mode recordings allow excellent noninvasive measurement of cardiac dimensions and motion patterns. The sweep rate of the M-mode display is analogous to the speed of an ECG paper. This speed varies between 25 mm/s and 100 mm/s and is usually set at 50 mm/s. A series of M-mode recordings may be obtained from the parasternal long-axis view, as illustrated in Figure 5-2.

Currently, 2D imaging, coupled with spectral/color flow Doppler capability, have largely replaced M-mode echocardiography. Noninvasive and bedside diagnostic evaluation of congenital heart defects is accomplished almost entirely with 2D and Doppler echocardiography. M-mode echocardiography, however, does retain a role

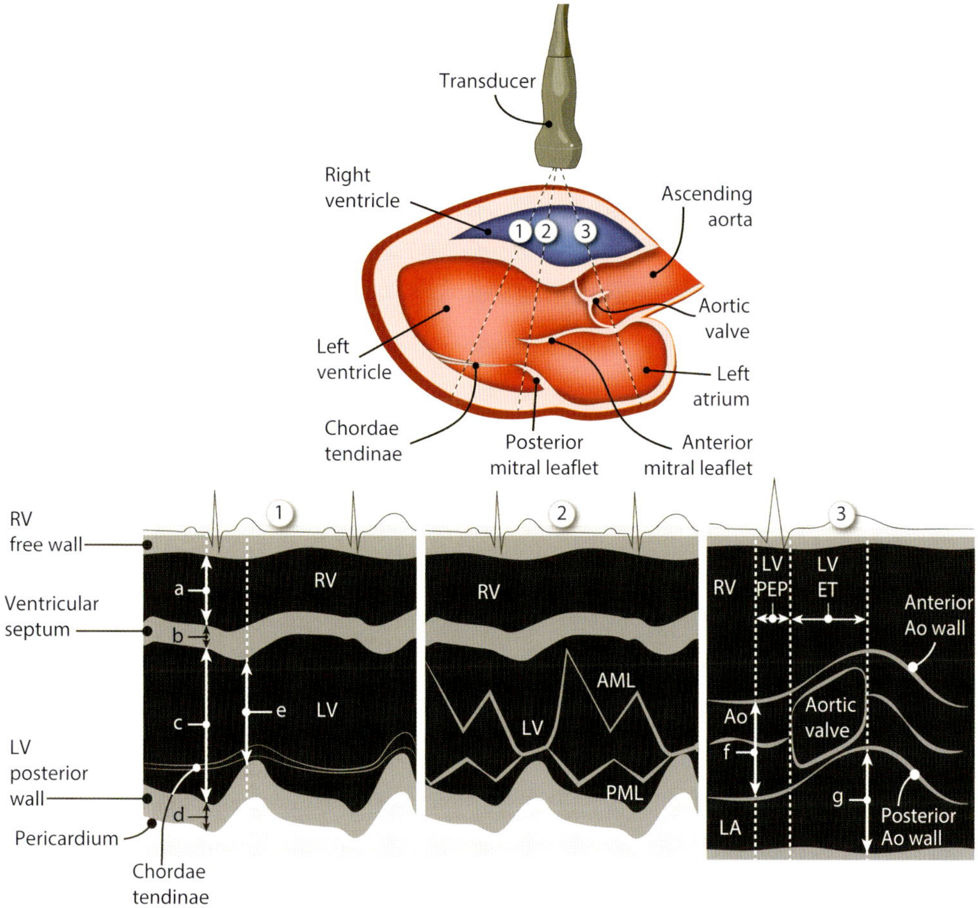

FIGURE 5-2. Schematic drawings showing the 2D parasternal long-axis view of the heart and M-mode tracing at the levels of the papillary muscles (A), the mitral valve tips (B), and the aortic valve (C). Abbreviations: AML, anterior mitral valve; PMV, posterior mitral valve; PEP, pre-ejection period; ET, ejection time; Ao, aorta.

in functional echocardiography and, due to its superior temporal and spatial resolution, is most helpful when used for the timing of rapid cardiac motion and precise linear measurements of cardiac dimensions.

USES OF M-MODE ECHOCARDIOGRAPHY

In our institutions' neonatal intensive care unit (NICU), we routinely perform M-mode scanning for the following measurements:

1. Wall thickness
2. Left ventricular (LV) systolic function
3. LV mass
4. Chamber sizes

OBTAINING M-MODE IMAGES

Since M-mode is a diagram of the heart made over time, it is important for the examiner to have a simultaneous ECG tracing while obtaining echo images. The ECG tracing will help the examiner time the cardiac events that will be recorded by M-mode. This is accomplished easily by connecting the ECHO machine to the patient's bedside cardiac monitor. In certain patients (micropremies) with very delicate skin, ECG lead placement might not be feasible.

Currently, M-mode images are generated from all standard 2D echocardiographic imaging systems. The 2D imaging plane is used to guide the placement of the M-mode ultrasound beam. Therefore, the first step is to obtain a good-quality cross-sectional (2D) image of the

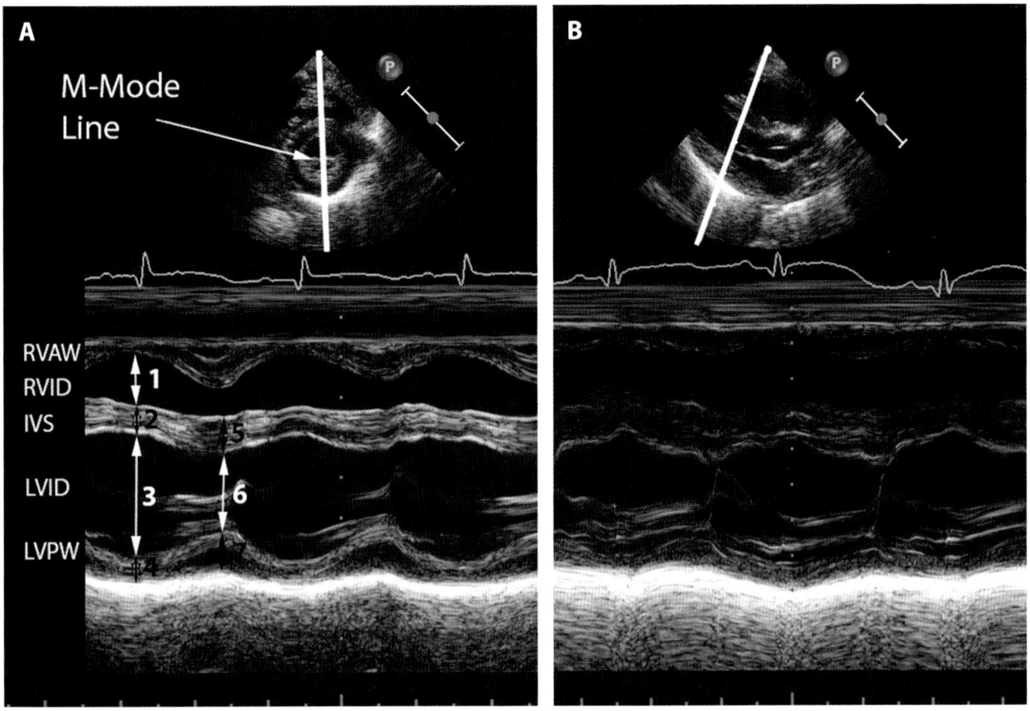

FIGURE 5-3. An M-mode display at the level of the mitral valve leaflet tips is derived from the 2D image obtained at the parasternal short-axis view (A) and long-axis view (B). Arrows 1-4 indicate end-diastolic measurements. Arrows 5-7 indicate end-systolic measurements. Abbreviations: RVAW, right ventricular anterior wall; RVID, right ventricular internal diameter; IVS, interventricular septum; LVID, left ventricular internal diameter; LVPW, left ventricular posterior wall.

heart prior to placing the M-mode beam. It is important to remember that the best resolution is obtained if interrogated structures are perpendicular to the ultrasound beam (see Chapter 1). Most machines are capable of simultaneously displaying a miniaturized version of the 2D image along with the M-mode. In this way, the operator gets to see precisely where the M-mode cursor lies, preventing misplacement of the cursor and consequent misleading images.

The best views for evaluating the left side of the heart are the parasternal views. Both the parasternal long- (LAX) and short-axis (SAX) views can be used to generate M-mode images of the left ventricle (Figure 5-3) and aortic root and left atrium (Figure 5-4). With the SAX view, it is much easier to be certain that the ultrasound beam is perpendicular to the septum and left ventricular posterior wall (LVPW) and, therefore, through the center of the LV cavity. We believe this allows for more accurate and reproducible measurements than the LAX, where the structures can be sectioned tangentially and distort the measurements. Therefore, in our daily practice we prefer to use the parasternal SAX view when performing M-mode evaluation of the LV cavity (Figure 5-5). The two routinely used parasternal SAX views are (1) at the level of the mitral valve tips and (2) at the level of the aortic root. Measurements are made from "leading edge" to "leading edge." The "leading edge" is, by definition, the surface of the structure first encountered by the ultrasound beam.[2]

M-MODE ASSESSMENT OF WALL THICKNESS

Right ventricular (RV) anterior wall, interventricular septum (IVS), and LV posterior wall (LVPW) thicknesses in systole and diastole can be measured using M-mode (Figure 5-5). In the evaluation for hypertrophy, the diastolic measurements must be examined carefully. In the normal newborn, the IVS to LVPW ratio during diastole should be $< 1.3{:}1$; ratios greater than 1.3 are indicative of septal hypertrophy. In the neonate, the presence of myocardial hypertrophy (symmetric and or asymmetric) can be found in several important conditions (Table 5-1).

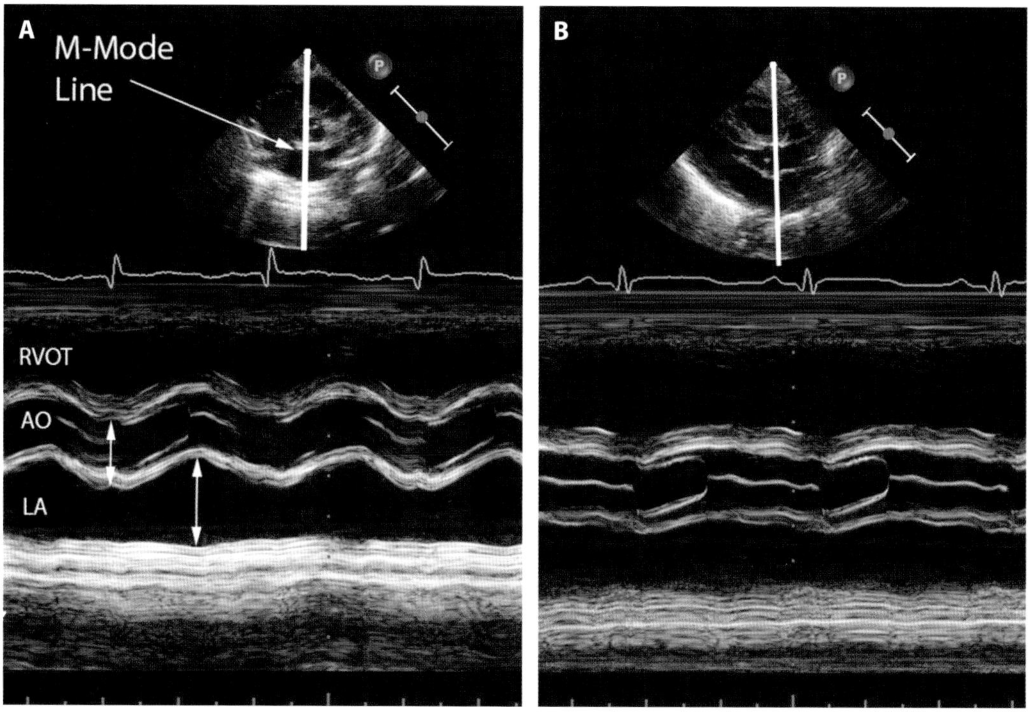

FIGURE 5-4. An M-mode display at the level of the aortic valve is derived from the 2D image obtained at the parasternal short-axis view (A) and long-axis view (B). Arrows indicate aortic root diameter (AO) and left atrial antero-posterior diameter (LA) in end-diastole and end-systole, respectively. Abbreviation: RVOT, right ventricular outflow tract.

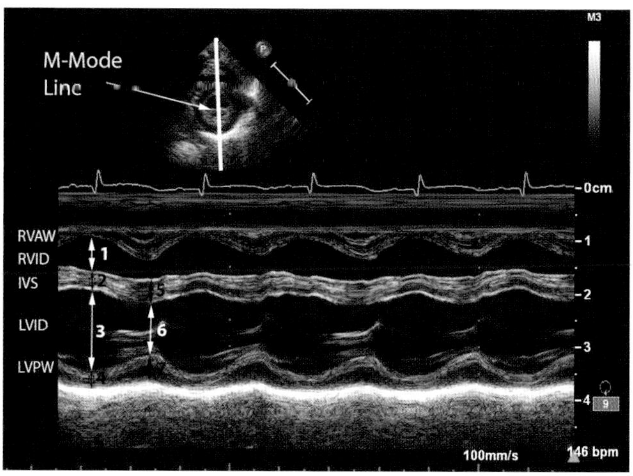

FIGURE 5-5. M-mode tracing obtained from the parasternal short-axis view at the level of the mitral valve leaflet tips. Measurements necessary for the calculation of shortening fraction and ejection fraction. Arrows 1 and 2 indicate LVID in end-diastole and in end-systole, respectively.

TABLE 5-1. Causes of Myocardial Hypertrophy in the Newborn

1. Infants of a diabetic mother
2. Newborns exposed to antenatal or postnatal corticosteroids
3. Genetic syndromes:
   - Noonan's syndrome
   - Leopard syndrome
4. Rare metabolic infiltrative conditions such as Pompe's
5. Familial hypertrophic cardiomyopathy

TABLE 5-2. Definition of End-systole and End-diastole Using Various Markers

	ECG Timed	M-mode Images	Visual Estimation
End Systole	End of T wave	Peak of ventricular wall movement toward the center	Smallest LV internal dimension
End Diastole	Onset of R wave	Maximal posterior excursion of LVPW	Largest LV internal dimension

M-MODE ASSESSMENT OF LV SYSTOLIC FUNCTION

Evaluation of LV systolic function is an essential part of all echocardiographic examinations. Determination of global systolic function is based on changes in ventricular size and volume. LV dimensions are usually measured from 2D guided M-mode echocardiograms at the mitral tips level via the parasternal SAX or LAX views.

First, a parasternal view should be obtained and the M-mode cursor placed through the septal and LV posterior walls just beyond the tip of the mitral leaflets (Figure 5-5). In the resultant M-mode image, measurements should be obtained of the RV internal dimension (RVID), IVS thickness, LV internal dimension (LVID), and LVPW at end-diastole and at end-systole (see Table 5-2 for determination of end-diastole and end-systole). With this information, most machines can generate two numbers that give an objective assessment of LV function: the fractional shortening (FS) and ejection fraction (EF).

Table 5-3 is an example of normal values for M-mode measurements in preterm and normal term neonates in the first week after birth.[3]

TABLE 5-3. M-mode Measurements in Normal Preterm and Term Neonates in the First Week After Birth[4]

	750-1249g	1250-1749g	1750-2249g	2250-2749g	2750-3249g	3250-3749g	3750-4249g	>4250g
LA (cm)	0.72±0.7	0.85±0.10	0.96±0.08	1.03±0.09	1.08±0.10	1.16±0.10	1.2±0.10	1.25±0.07
Ao (cm)	0.63±0.06	0.73±0.06	0.84±0.05	0.89±0.08	0.93±0.06	0.99±0.06	1.03±0.06	1.06±0.08
LA/Ao ratio	1.14±0.11	1.16±0.11	1.14±0.11	1.17±0.10	1.16±0.11	1.17±0.10	1.16±0.09	1.18±0.09
LVIDd (cm)	1.26±0.15	1.33±0.12	1.52±0.15	1.73±0.22	1.79±0.21	1.83±0.20	1.93±0.24	2.12±0.23
LVIDs (cm)	0.85±0.12	0.91±0.10	0.98±0.15	1.15±0.14	1.17±0.15	1.21±0.17	1.25±0.17	1.44±0.16
FS %	33±5	31±4	36±6	34±4	35±4	34±4	35±5	35±5
IVSd (cm)	0.20±0.06	0.26±0.06	0.26±0.06	0.28±0.04	0.29±0.06	0.28±0.05	0.28±0.05	0.30±0.06
IVSs (cm)	0.30±0.10	0.44±0.08	0.44±0.08	0.48±0.07	0.45±0.09	0.46±0.08	0.47±0.07	0.48±0.09

LA = left atrium, Ao = aortic root, LVIDd = left ventricular diameter in diastole, LVIDs = left ventricular diameter in systole, FS = fractional shortening, IVSd = intraventricular septum thickness in diastole, IVSs = intraventricular septum thickness in systole

Limitations

While the M-mode assessment of LV systolic function is easy to learn and perform, it has some drawbacks:

1. M-mode provides information about contractility along a single line. In a patient with regional wall motion abnormalities, such as the newborn with PPHN and paradoxical interventricular septal movement, M-mode measurements can be misleading. In this situation, FS should not be used, and EF should be calculated using a biplane volumetric measurement (Simpson's). See Chapter 8.
2. If the M-mode line is not parallel to the short axis of the LV, the M-mode beam traverses the ventricle in a tangential manner and often misrepresents (overestimates) the true internal dimension.
3. It may be difficult to get clear images when the endocardial surfaces are not well-defined.
4. These measurements are dependent on preload and afterload and thus have the potential to under- or overestimate the true intrinsic contractility of the myocardium.

M-MODE ASSESSMENT OF LV MASS

Although LV mass may be assessed using 2D or 3D echocardiography, M-mode remains the most commonly used method. All modern echocardiography machines automatically generate this value once M-mode measurements are obtained. Myocardial mass is assumed to be equal to the product of the volume and density (specific gravity) of the myocardium. The specific gravity of the myocardium is 1.04-1.05 g/ml. Using wall thickness and LV cavity dimension measurements, the machine software can calculate and report cardiac (LV) mass.

The most commonly used formulas are all variations of the same mathematical principle assuming an ellipsoid geometry. The basic formula could be written as follows:

$$\text{LV mass (g)} = 1.05\,[(\text{LVIDd} + \text{IVSd} + \text{LVPWd})^3 - (\text{LVIDd})^3]$$

All measurements are made at end-diastole (ie, onset of the R wave).

M-MODE ASSESSMENT OF PERICARDIAL EFFUSION

In addition to assessing left ventricular function, chamber sizes, and wall thickness, M-mode can be used to assess for the presence of pericardial effusions. The pericardial space is a potential space and should normally be a single line on M-mode echo. If an effusion is present, an echo-free space will be seen either anterior to the RV or behind (posterior to) the LV posterior wall. However, better assessment of the full extent of pericardial effusions and their hemodynamic consequences is done with 2D plus Doppler echocardiography (see Chapter 10).

M-MODE ASSESSMENT OF LA SIZE AND OF LA:AO RATIO

First obtain a parasternal view and place the M-mode cursor through the root of the aortic valve and precisely at the level of the aortic leaflet tips (Figure 5-5). In order, the anterior wall of the aorta, aortic valve leaflets, the posterior wall of the aorta, the LA cavity, and the posterior wall of left atrium are imaged. The M-mode tracing will show the parallel walls of the aorta moving anteriorly (toward the transducer) in systole and away in diastole. The aortic valve leaflets will be seen separating in systole when the valve is open and assume a box-like appearance, subsequently coming together in diastole as a single line. The left atrium (LA) will be behind the aortic root and will fill during atrial diastole (ventricular systole) and empty in atrial systole (ventricular diastole).

The LA antero-posterior diameter is measured at end-systole using the end of the T wave on the ECG tracing, when the atrium is maximally filled. The aortic root (Ao) is measured at end-diastole from leading edge to leading edge using the start of the QRS on the ECG tracing, right before the aortic valve opens. With these two values, a LA:AO ratio is thus generated.

The concept behind this is that the pulmonary venous return is what fills the LA and this amount of blood must cross the aortic valve. The LA and AO will, therefore, have similar dimensions in a normal heart. In addition, unlike the LA, the aortic valve does not significantly change with changes in preload. An increase in the LA:AO ratio to > 1.5:1.0 has been one of the ultrasound criteria used for the definition of a hemodynamically significant ductus arteriosus in the premature newborn (see Chapter 11).

MEASUREMENTS OBTAINED WITH 2D ECHOCARDIOGRAPHY

In functional echocardiography, the following measurements obtained through 2D imaging are most frequently used in the clinical setting:

LV outflow tract (LVOT) diameter

RV outflow tract (RVOT) diameter

Simpson's method for ejection fraction
LA dimensions
LV mass calculation

■ MEASUREMENT OF DIAMETER IN ASSESSMENT OF CARDIAC OUTPUT

In pediatric cardiology, measurements of the aortic and pulmonary valve annular dimensions carry important diagnostic as well as prognostic information and are routinely used in surgical decision making. In functional echocardiography, left and right ventricular outflow diameters (D) are measured for the calculation of their respective cross-sectional areas (CSA) as per the following formula:

$$CSA(cm^2) = \pi \times (D(cm)/2)^2 = 3.14 \times D^2\,(cm^2)/4$$

and therefore:

$$CSA(cm^2) = D^2(cm)^2 \times 0.785$$

where D is the diameter of LVOT or RVOT.

When CSA is multiplied by the velocity time integral (VTI) of the Doppler flow envelope at the same location (LVOT or RVOT), the stroke volume (SV) is obtained (in milliliters). The calculation of SV indicates how much blood leaves the heart per beat. SV multiplied by heart rate (beats per minute) will yield ventricular output per minute. When the ductus arteriosus is closed, the left ventricular output equals the cardiac output (CO). The following demonstrates the calculations involved:

$$SV\,(ml) = CSA\,(cm^2) \times VTI(cm)$$
$$CO(ml/min) = SV\,(ml) \times heart\,rate(/min)$$

Putting it all together:

$$CO(ml/kg/\,min) = CSA\,(cm^2) \times VTI(cm) \times heart\,rate(/min)/Body\,weight\,(Kg)$$

The CO can also be indexed for body surface area (BSA). In this case the unit would be $ml/m^2/min$.

LVOT Diameter Measurement

With transthoracic 2D echocardiography, the aortic valve annulus can be measured at the parasternal long-axis view. Use of the zoom feature of the ultrasound machine will enlarge the picture and help decrease the margin of error.

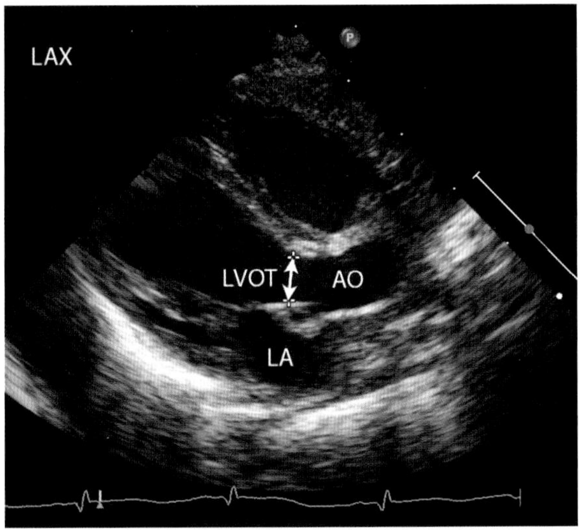

FIGURE 5-6. Two-dimensional image obtained from the parasternal long-axis window at the level of the aortic valve. The arrow indicates the aortic annular diameter made at the hinge points of the aortic valve from inner edge to inner edge. Abbreviations: AO, aorta; LA, left atrium; LAX, long-axis; LVOT, left ventricular outflow tract.

Next, freezing of the zoomed image is performed to obtain a cine loop, which is then scrolled backward and forward to capture a frame in which the aortic valve leaflets are wide open. The measurement for the aortic valve annulus should be made at the hinge points of the aortic valve—for 2D measurements, the preferred technique is from inner edge to inner edge and in mid-systole (Figure 5-6). For the LVOT, the line is drawn from where the anterior (right coronary) aortic cusp meets the ventricular septum to where the posterior (non-coronary) aortic cusp meets the anterior mitral leaflet. This line should be perpendicular to the anterior aortic wall. An alternative location for measurement is at the sino-tubular junction. Wherever the diameter is measured, the pulse wave VTI must be obtained at the same location.

RVOT Diameter Measurement

The diameter of the pulmonary valve annulus (pulmonary artery) is best measured from the parasternal SAX or LAX views using a similar approach to the LVOT measurement (ie, inner edge to inner edge at the hinge points of the pulmonary valve [Figure 5-7]). The outflow diameter will be used by the machine to calculate the CSA, and the VTI from the pulsed Doppler spectral tracing across the

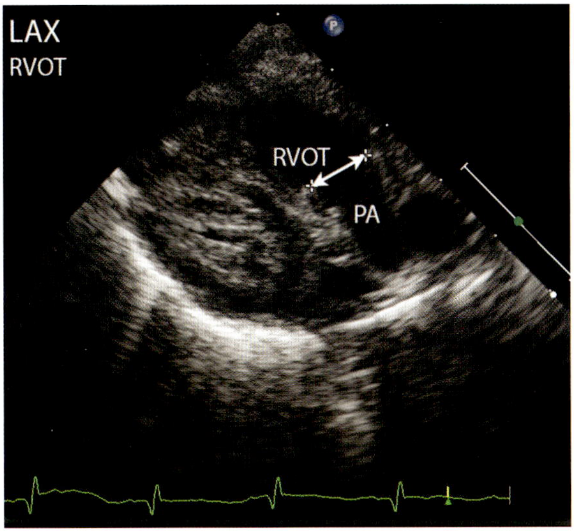

FIGURE 5-7. Two-dimensional image obtained from the parasternal long-axis window at the level of the right ventricular outflow tract (RVOT). The arrow indicates pulmonary annular diameter. Abbreviation: PA, main pulmonary artery.

pulmonary valve will be used to obtain the VTI. Using the CSA and VTI, the output across the RVOT can then be calculated in the same manner as for the LVOT (given above). Remember that the formula for CSA assumes a circular-shaped orifice. It is also obvious that small errors in outflow diameter measurement will lead to large errors in calculated CSA. In determining cardiac output, the eventual error responsible for the variability of the results is almost always due to erroneous measurement of the outflow tract diameter.

For example, assume the following measurements for a given diameter (D):

$$D = 10\,\text{mm CSA} = 78\,\text{mm}^2$$

$$D = 9\,\text{mm CSA} = 64\,\text{mm}^2$$

$$D = 8\,\text{mm CSA} = 50\,\text{mm}^2$$

Between a CSA measurement based on a diameter of 10 vs 8 mm, there is a 56% difference that then will translate into an error of the same magnitude in CO determination if measurement is incorrect. Several measurements should be averaged to minimize this potential source of error.

Obtaining Velocity Time Integral (VTI)

LVOT systolic velocity is best recorded by the apical approach (four chamber with slight cranial angulation to obtain the five chamber) using pulsed wave (PW) Doppler echo and placing the sample volume either immediately above or below the aortic valve. The same could be done by the suprasternal arch view by placing the sample volume in the ascending aorta immediately above the aortic valve. RVOT systolic velocity is obtained with the PW Doppler sample placed at the tips of the pulmonary valve. Once the Doppler tracing is obtained, its contour should be traced to obtain the VTI. The VTI provides information regarding blood flow velocity during systole and is recorded in cm. The VTI is essentially the length of the cylinder of blood ejected on a single heartbeat across the CSA in question. Of note is that this method works only in the presence of laminar flow and is invalidated by the presence of non-laminar flow, as is the case with LVOT or RVOT stenosis.

SIMPSON'S METHOD FOR LV EJECTION FRACTION

LV volume cannot be directly calculated. There is not enough information in one or two 2D echo projections to allow precise and accurate determination of chamber volume. The volumes are thus estimated using mathematical models and assumptions about the shape and symmetry of the LV cavity. The most commonly used 2D method for LV volume measurement is the single or biplane method of disks also known as the Simpson's method. The principle underlying this method is that the total LV volume is calculated from the summation of a stack of elliptical disks. It is based on the idea that the volume of an object can be determined by "cutting" it into thin slices, measuring the volume of each slice, and adding up the volumes of all slices. This principle is applied to the LV by "slicing" it into disks along the long axis.[4]

The apical four-chamber view is routinely used to determine 2D EF. One begins by obtaining a good-quality 2D image, ensuring that the endocardial borders are well visualized. The ECG signal should be simultaneously recorded.

1. Zoom on the LV and freeze the image.
2. Scroll backward and forward to identify a frame at end-diastole. This can be determined by one of the following:
    a. Identifying the frame in which the ventricle appears to have the largest volume
    b. Identifying the frame just before mitral valve closure
    c. Identifying the frame corresponding to the peak of the R wave on the simultaneously recorded ECG tracing

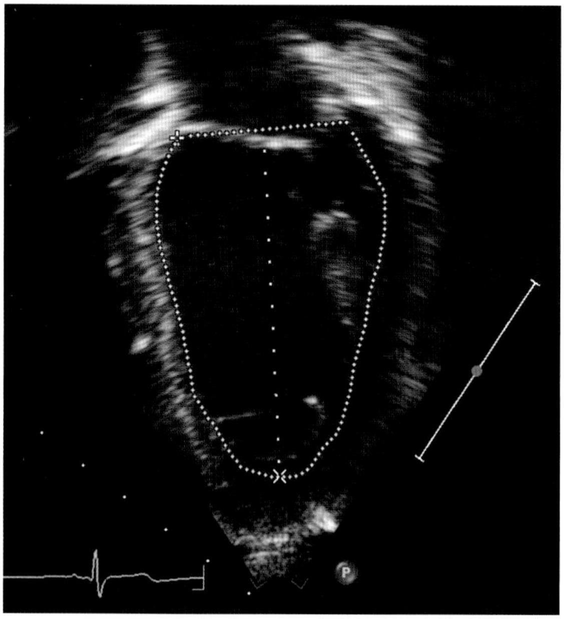

FIGURE 5-8. Tracing of left ventricular endocardial border in end-diastole to be used in Simpson's ejection fraction calculation. Note that the tracing includes the papillary muscles in the volume.

3. Place the cursor on the endocardial border where the anterior mitral valve (MV) leaflet meets the ventricular septum and trace the entire endocardial border of the left ventricle. The papillary muscles are "included" in the LV volume. Therefore, there is no need to trace around the papillary muscles (Figure 5-8).
4. Once this is done, the machine's software calculates the LV end-diastolic volume (LVEDV).
5. Scroll the frozen image again to identify a frame at end-systole. This can be timed by one of the following:
    a. Identifying the frame in which the ventricle appears to have the smallest volume
    b. Identifying the frame just before mitral valve opening
    c. Identifying the frame corresponding to the end of the T wave on the simultaneously recorded ECG
6. Trace the outline of the endocardial border of the LV once again (Figure 5-9).
7. Once this is done, the LV end-systolic volume (LVESV) will be calculated.
8. The machine will then calculate the ejection fraction by using the formula:

$$EF = [(LVEDV - LVESV)/LVEDV] \times 100$$

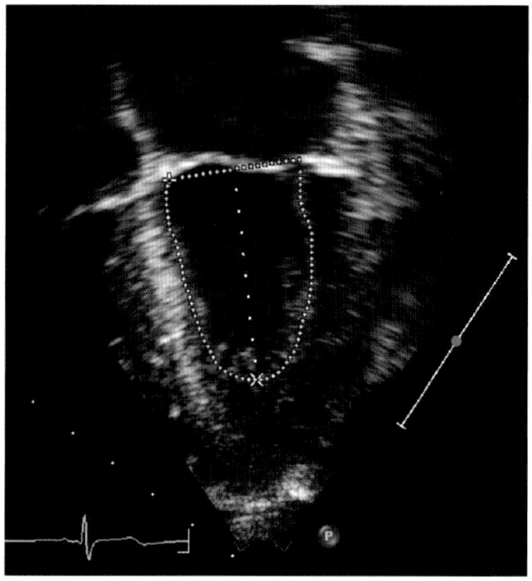

FIGURE 5-9. Tracing of endocardial border in end-systole to be used in Simpson's ejection fraction calculation.

One must be careful to have a true apical four-chamber view and avoid foreshortening of the LV in its long axis. The mitral and tricuspid leaflets and both atria should be visualized very well, without distortion, and the gain settings need to be adjusted to identify the endocardial border. The diastolic and systolic volumes should preferably be measured from the same cardiac cycle.

VISUAL ESTIMATION OF SYSTOLIC FUNCTION BASED ON 2D ECHOCARDIOGRAPHY

Experienced echocardiographers frequently estimate EF without taking measurements by looking at the overall size and contractility as well as the inward movement and thickening of the various segments of the LV walls. This method is obviously very subjective and dependent upon the experience of the operator, yet it has been shown to correlate well with quantitative assessment of the EF.

To give the operator an overall feel about the LV contractility, the parasternal long- and short-axis and four-chamber views are used. One way of doing this is to distinguish three grades of global LV systolic function. This is based on the subjective "eyeballed" radius change of the LV short axis in systole:

Normal (>30% change in radius) **Videos 1 and 2**

Moderate dysfunction (10-30% decrease in radius)

Severe dysfunction (<10% change in radius) **Video 3**

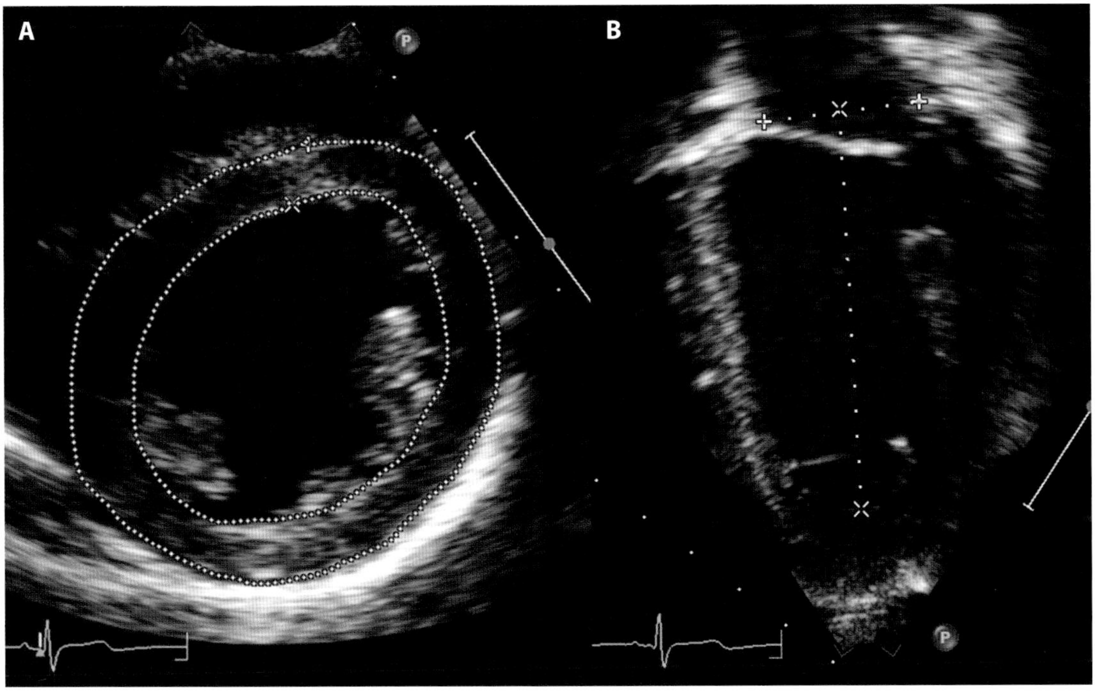

FIGURE 5-10. Calculation of left ventricular mass: tracing of epicardial and endocardial borders at end-diastole from parasternal short-axis view at the papillary muscle level (A) and left ventricular length measurement from plane of mitral valve annulus to the apex from the apical four-chamber view (B).

This approach is obviously prone to inter- and intra-observer variability, and is unreliable for serial evaluation of LV function in the same patient by different operators.

2D ASSESSMENT OF LV MASS

Left ventricular mass from 2D echocardiography is measured from the area-length and truncated ellipsoid method as recommended by the American Society of Echocardiography. It assumes the LV as a prolate ellipsoid. This method requires the parasternal SAX view of the LV at the papillary muscle level and the apical four chambers at end-diastole. It is important to realize that, unlike the LV volume determination (Simpson's method) for EF calculation, the LV mass calculation is based solely on end-diastolic frames. Also, it must again be noted that these measurements are based on mathematical models and geometric assumptions. Nevertheless, studies looking at the correlation between LV mass measured by echocardiography (2D and M-mode) and autopsy have found these assumptions to be reasonable.[5,6]

A discussion of the mathematical details is beyond the scope of this book; however, following is a brief explanation of what this technique entails.

1. Tracing the epicardial border of the heart on parasternal SAX at end diastole
2. Tracing the endocardial border on parasternal SAX at end-diastole
3. Measuring the LV long axis on apical four-chamber view at end-diastole (Figures 5-10 and 5-11)

2D ASSESSMENT OF LEFT ATRIAL DIMENSIONS

Left atrial (LA) size does matter, especially in adult cardiology. The LA size is considered a barometer of LV diastolic burden, and a predictor of adverse cardiovascular outcomes such as atrial fibrillation, congestive heart failure, stroke, and cardiovascular death. It is obvious that its measurement is an important part of an adult echocardiographic examination. The measurements are performed

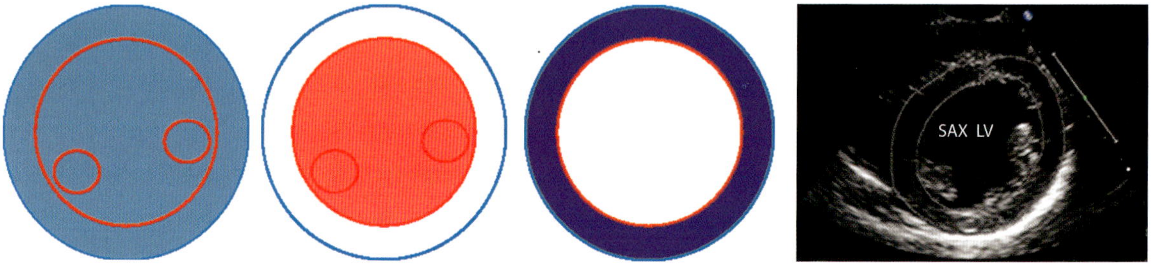

FIGURE 5-11. Left ventricular mass calculations based on 2D imaging method. First, trace the epicardial border (A) to obtain A1 (area in blue color) for the calculation of the total left ventricular volume (wall plus chamber). Next, trace endocardial border (B) to obtain A2 (area in red color) for the calculation of the left ventricular internal cavity volume (chamber only). Finally, subtract A2 from A1 to calculate the area (in purple) representing left ventricular myocardial mass (wall only).

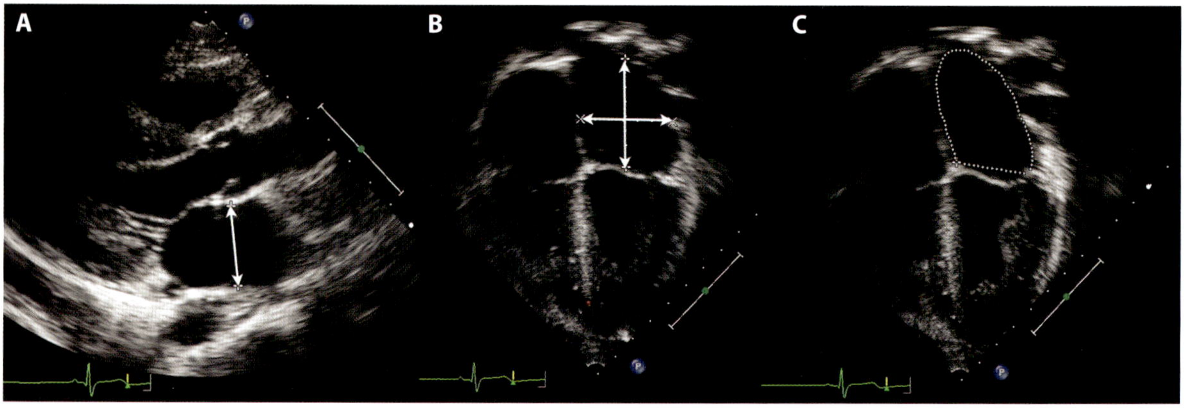

FIGURE 5-12. Two-dimensional measurements of left atrial dimensions: the anteroposterior diameter in a parasternal long-axis view (A), major axis and width in a four-chamber view (B), and planimetered area in a four-chamber view (C). All measurements are taken at ventricular end-systole.

by using M-mode, 2D, and 3D echocardiography. In the context of neonatal echocardiography, LA dimension was historically used for the diagnosis of patent ductus arteriosus (PDA). Currently, LA dimension is used to determine the magnitude of a ductal left-to-right shunt,[7] and as an adjunct to other indices in evaluating hemodynamic significance of a PDA (for details see Chapter 11).

The size of the LA varies during the cardiac cycle. Generally, only the maximum LA size is measured in clinical practice. Maximum LA volume occurs at the end of ventricular systole, just before mitral valve opening. The most common method of LA measurement is the M-mode-based LA anteroposterior diameter as previously described. Two-dimensional measurements do not appear to offer a benefit over M-mode when it comes to everyday bedside decision making.

LA measurements can be performed as linear measure (LA diameters) or surface (LA area), and the machine's software allows for the LA volume calculation.[8] Measurement of LA dimensions is shown in Figure 5-12.

LA Linear Dimensions

LA anteroposterior diameter (D1):

1. Obtain a good-quality parasternal long-axis view where endocardial border is well visualized.
2. Freeze the image.
3. Scroll frames and stop at end-systole (the frame immediately preceding mitral valve opening or end of T wave on ECG).
4. Measure with calipers the distance from the anterior wall to the posterior wall, as shown in Figure 5-12A.

LA perpendicular length (D2) and width (D3):

1. Obtain a good-quality apical four-chamber view where endocardial border is well visualized, and make sure the atria are not foreshortened.
2. Freeze the image.
3. Scroll frames and stop at end-systole (the frame immediately preceding mitral valve opening or end of T wave on ECG).
4. Measure with calipers as shown in the Figures 5-12B.

LA Volume

LA volume will be calculated by the machine's software based on the above-measured linear measurements. There are several mathematical methods for assessing LA volume. They are all based on linear measurements and mathematical manipulations as well as geometrical assumptions. The method illustrated in this chapter is the so-called prolate ellipsoid method (PE) using the following formula with diameters obtained from parasternal LAX and apical four-chamber views (as noted earlier).

LA Area

To measure the LA area:

1. Obtain an apical four-chamber image.
2. Freeze the image.
3. Scroll frames and stop at end-systole.
4. Trace the endocardial border starting from one hinge point of the mitral valve and ending at the opposite hinge point (Figure 5-12C). Exclude the confluence of the pulmonary veins as well as the LA appendage.

MITRAL AND TRICUSPID VALVE ANNULAR DIMENSIONS

The atrioventricular (AV) valve annular dimensions are important in the context of certain complex congenital heart defects. For example, a smaller than normal AV valve is frequently accompanied by a smaller than normal ventricle. In this case, the AV valve dimension is often used in the decision making regarding the feasibility of two-ventricle repair versus single-ventricle palliation. In the context of functional echocardiography, AV valve dimensions can be used:

1. To calculate flow across the given AV valve in a similar fashion as cardiac output determination.

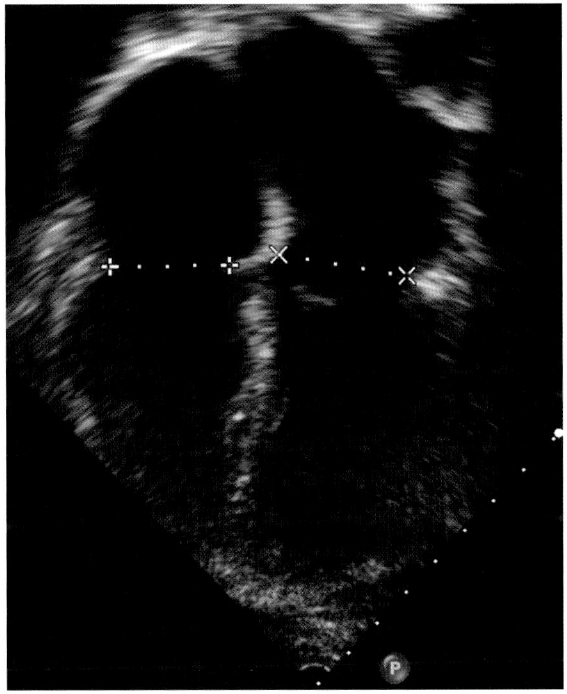

FIGURE 5-13. Two-dimensional image obtained from the apical window showing all four cardiac chambers and measurement of the tricuspid and mitral valve annular diameters.

2. To determine the regurgitant volumes of AV or semilunar valves. This requires a measurement of the flow across the semilunar valve (which includes normal cardiac output plus regurgitant volume), with the regurgitant volume being calculated as follows:

Stroke volume across aortic value − Volume across mitral valve = Aortic regurgitant volume

Stroke volume across mitral value − Stroke volume across aortic valve = Mitral regurgitant volume

The AV valve measurements are taken from the apical four-chamber view in early diastole from the inner septal to the lateral wall margins of the annulus (hinge point to hinge point [Figure 5-13]). These calculations are rarely used in the NICU in an otherwise anatomically normal heart. They could, however, be used as a research tool in the context of shunt volume calculation.

REFERENCES

1. Singh S, Goyal A. The Origin of Echocardiography: A Tribute to Inge Edler. *Tex Heart Inst J*. 2007;34:431–438.
2. Foppa M, Duncan B, Rohde L. Echocardiography-based left ventricular mass estimation. How should we define hypertrophy? *Cardiovascular Ultrasound*. 2005;3:17. doi:10.1186/1476-7120-3-17.
3. Walther FJ, Siassi B, King J, Wu PYK. Echocardiographic Measurements in Normal Preterm and Term Neonates. *Acta Paediatr Scand*. 1986;75:563–568.
4. Mercier JC, DiSessa TG, Jarmakani JM, et al. Two-dimensional echocardiographic assessment of left ventricular volumes and ejection fraction in Children. *Circulation*. 1982;65:5.
5. Devereux RB, Alonso DR, Lutas EM, et al. Echocardiographic assessment of left ventricular hypertrophy: comparison to necropsy findings. *Am J Cardiol*. 1986; 57:450–458.
6. Park SH, Shub C, Nobrega TP, Bailey KR, Seward JB. Two-dimensional echocardiographic calculation of left ventricular mass by the American Society of Echocardiography: correlation with autopsy and M-mode echocardiography. *J Am Soc Echocardiogr*. 1996 March–April;9(2):199–228.
7. Abhayaratna WP, Seward JB, Appleton CP, et al. Left atrial size: physiologic determinants and clinical applications. *J Am Coll Cardiol*. 2006;47:2357–2363.
8. Ujino K, Barnes ME, Cha SS. Two-dimensional echocardiographic methods for assessment of left Atrial volume. *Am J Cardiol*. 2006;98:1185–1188.

CHAPTER 6

Pulsed Wave, Continuous-Wave, and Color Flow Doppler in Assessment of Regurgitant Flow and Measurement of Pressure Gradients*

Merujan Uzunyan and Lindsey Miller

- INTRODUCTION
- DOPPLER PRINCIPLE
- SIMPLIFIED BERNOULLI EQUATION
- DOPPLER DISPLAY MODALITIES
- VALVAR PATHOLOGY
  - Valvar Stenosis/Atresia
  - Valvar Regurgitation/Insufficiency
- DETERMINATION OF PULMONARY ARTERIAL PRESSURE
  - Measurement of the Peak Velocity of Tricuspid Regurgitation
  - Assessment of Direction and Velocity of Blood Flow through a Patent Ductus Arteriosus
  - Measurement of Flow Velocity through a Ventricular Septal Defect
- REFERENCES

INTRODUCTION

This chapter discusses the use of the Doppler principle and the modified Bernoulli equation for the assessment of gradients and regurgitations caused by stenotic or insufficient valves, as well as the evaluation of physiologic or pathologic communications within the circulatory system. These principles are applied to clinical bedside decision making in the context of neonatal functional echocardiography.

An important application of echocardiography is its use in analyzing the direction and velocity of blood flow within the heart and the blood vessels, and the difference in pressure values (pressure gradient) between these chambers. As described in Chapter 1, these measurements are possible thanks to the Doppler principle and the Bernoulli equation. The Doppler principle is used to derive information about velocity of blood flow, and this

*Videos can be accessed at http://PracticalNeonatalEcho.com.

information can then be applied to the Bernoulli equation to extrapolate an estimation of pressure gradients.

■ DOPPLER PRINCIPLE

The Doppler principle states that, to a stationary observer, the original frequency of sound emitted from a source is altered when the source of the sound is moving. The difference in frequency is called the Doppler shift. For echocardiography, the stationary observer is the transducer, emitting the ultrasound waves at a given frequency and receiving the returning ultrasound waves. The red cells within the bloodstream are the moving objects that reflect the incident sound waves and therefore serve as the "source" responsible for producing the Doppler shift. The returning signals will have a higher frequency (positive numerical value) if the red cells are moving toward the transducer, and a lower frequency (negative numerical value) if moving away from the transducer (Figure 6-1).

The Doppler shift (or frequency difference) is calculated using the following formula:

$$\text{Doppler shift (Fd)} = \frac{2 \times \text{Ft} \times \text{V} \times \text{Cos}\,\theta}{\text{C}}$$

where:

Fd = Doppler shift (frequency difference)

2 = Factor used because there are two shifts: one because the wave incident on the moving red blood cells is Doppler shifted and an additional shift because the reflection is from a moving object.

Ft = Frequency of transmitted beam (transducer frequency)

V = Velocity of the blood

Cos θ = Cosine of angle of incidence (insonation) between the ultrasound beam and the blood flow

C = Speed of sound in human tissue (1540 m/sec or m/s)

The importance of the angle of incidence θ becomes obvious when one considers the following:

Cosine of 0° (parallel to beam) is 1.

Cosine of 90° (vertical to beam) is 0.

For any angle between 0° and 90°, the cosine of the angle returns a value <1, which will result in a lower Doppler shift and resultant error, for example:

Cosine of 20° is 0.94 and that means it adds a 6% error.

Cosine of 30° is 0.86 (14% error).

Cosine of 40° is 0.76 (24% error).

Therefore, the greater the angle of incidence, the larger is the error and the more the velocity will be underestimated.

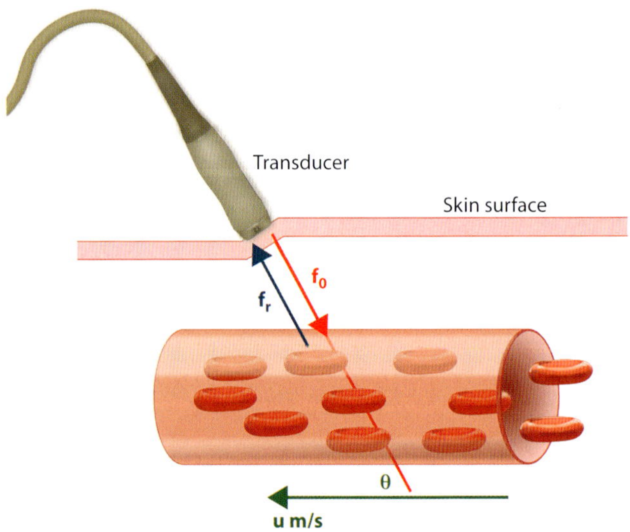

FIGURE 6-1. Doppler shift; fo = transmitted frequency, fr = reflected frequency, V = velocity of red blood cells, Θ = Doppler angle.

Once the Doppler shift is measured, the Doppler formula can be rearranged to solve for velocity:

$$\text{Velocity} = \frac{C \times \text{Doppler shift}}{2 \times \text{Ft} \times \text{Cos}\theta}$$

All modern echocardiography systems offer the technology to perform Doppler evaluation of moving structures, such as blood. Several different Doppler modalities are available (as described below). With this technology, the following information can be obtained:

1. If there is blood flow (sound, color flow, and spectral Doppler)
2. The direction of blood flow (color flow and spectral Doppler)
3. The magnitude of blood flow velocity (color flow Doppler for a qualitative visual assessment, spectral Doppler for a quantitative estimation of velocity)

SIMPLIFIED BERNOULLI EQUATION

Once velocity of flow is determined, the modified Bernoulli formula is applied to calculate a pressure difference (gradient or drop) by relating velocity to pressure. Bernoulli's principle states: "As the velocity of a fluid increases, the pressure exerted by that fluid decreases." Higher velocities are therefore associated with a greater pressure drop, resulting in a larger pressure gradient. According to the simplified Bernoulli equation, velocity can be related to change in pressure by the following formula:

$$\Delta P = 4V^2$$

where ΔP is the pressure gradient and V is flow velocity.

DOPPLER DISPLAY MODALITIES

The Doppler-measured flow values can be displayed by the ultrasound machine as a graph of *time* on the x-axis versus *velocity* (meters/second) on the y-axis; this method of display is commonly known as **spectral Doppler**. By convention, positive values are represented above the baseline and negative values are represented below the baseline. The two spectral Doppler modes are **pulsed wave (PW)** and **continuous-wave (CW)**. PW Doppler offers the advantage of being able to evaluate a Doppler velocity at any point on the two-dimensional (2D) echocardiographic image. However, this requires range gating, in which the selected area of interest (also known as a sample volume) is localized a specific distance from the transducer, as calculated from the transmit/receive time of an emitted pulse of sound (assumed speed of sound 1540 m/s). Only the signals from the selected area are evaluated for Doppler shifts. This dependence on awaiting the return of the range-gated signals results in an upper velocity limit for PW Doppler that depends on the echocardiography system, the depth of the selected area of interest, and the frequency of the transducer (lower-frequency transducers can detect higher velocities). On the other hand, CW Doppler is not range-gated. Therefore, CW can be aimed in a direction but not at any pinpoint location in that direction. CW Doppler detects velocities all the way along its path and does not have an upper limit to detectable velocities. The highest velocity along that path produces the highest velocity on the spectral tracing.

Color flow Doppler presents a visual map of mean Doppler velocities, shown as colors, superimposed upon a concurrently obtained 2D image. The color represents moving blood within the heart or a vascular structure. With color flow Doppler, assignment of color to velocities is usually based upon direction (red toward transducer and blue away from it) and magnitude (different color hues, with higher velocities shown as lighter saturations). This type of Doppler is extremely useful for obtaining a comprehensive, global picture of blood flow within the heart or a vascular structure. It is particularly useful for overall assessment of valvar pathology and intracardiac shunts, and plays an invaluable role in directing spectral Doppler evaluation.

It is important to remember that the ultrasound machine is not capable of directly detecting or measuring pressures and velocities; direct noninvasive measurement of pressure in any cardiac chamber is not possible. *Therefore, what is ultimately determined by echocardiography is not an absolute pressure value, but a pressure difference (gradient or drop).* The presence of gradients and regurgitation caused by stenotic or insufficient valves, as well as physiologic or pathologic communications within the circulatory system, allows the observer to extrapolate values of pressures. Stenotic or regurgitant valves, as well as intra- or extracardiac shunts, create pressure gradients that in turn are responsible for the velocity changes detected by Doppler. By properly analyzing the Doppler information, one can gain important hemodynamic as well as structural information.

VALVAR PATHOLOGY

Diseases of the cardiac valves can produce total absence of flow across the valve (atresia) or varying degrees of narrowing (stenosis), backflow (regurgitation/insufficiency), or a combination of stenosis/regurgitation. Doppler echocardiography is used to interrogate the valves and obtain a numerical value for flow velocity in m/s. Then, by using the simplified Bernoulli equation, the echocardiography machine translates this velocity into a pressure difference (gradient).

The best views to interrogate each valve are as follows:

- Mitral valve: Apical four chamber, left parasternal long axis
- Aortic valve: Apical four chamber, subcostal sagittal and coronal, suprasternal
- Tricuspid valve: Apical four chamber, left parasternal long axis, parasternal right ventricular inflow, left parasternal short axis at aortic valve level
- Pulmonic valve: Parasternal long and short axis, subcostal sagittal and coronal

Valvar Stenosis/Atresia

Valvar stenosis/atresia and their evaluation will not be extensively discussed, since the detection of these conditions in a neonate should prompt a pediatric cardiology consultation. However, given below are brief discussions of the various type of valvar pathologies.

Mitral Valve and Tricuspid Valve Stenosis/Atresia

Mitral and tricuspid valve stenosis can be found as isolated conditions in an otherwise anatomically normal heart, but they are extremely rare conditions. In contrast, both mitral and tricuspid valve atresia (atresia being defined as complete lack of patency with no flow across the valve plane) are always associated with other significant cardiac anomalies.

Aortic and Pulmonic Valve Stenosis/Atresia

Aortic and pulmonic valve atresia are, for practical purposes, always associated with other cardiac malformations. In contrast, mild to moderate pulmonic stenosis—in the absence of any other associated cardiac anomaly—is the most common isolated valvar disease in the neonate, and its presence or absence must be considered when right ventricular pressure (RVP) is determined with the TR jet.

The most common aortic valve abnormality found in newborn patients is a bicuspid aortic valve. However, most bicuspid aortic valves are neither stenotic nor regurgitant, and might not become hemodynamically significant until later in life. Isolated aortic valve stenosis due to an abnormal aortic valve (which can be tricuspid, bicuspid, or unicuspid) can be found in the neonate, though it is an uncommon. When encountered, the clinical severity depends upon the degree of aortic valve stenosis—from mild (patients are asymptomatic and present only with a murmur) to critical (patients are dependent upon a patent ductus arteriosus for survival).

The severity of semilunar valve stenosis is based upon:

1. The Doppler-derived numerical value of the flow velocity (in m/s) across the valve
2. The same value (flow velocity) translated into a pressure gradient expressed in mmHg, using the simplified Bernoulli equation ($4 \times \text{Velocity}^2$)

Detection of these anomalies should prompt a pediatric cardiology referral, as the grading of severity of such an anomaly is beyond the scope of neonatal functional echocardiography.[1] A classic example is the severe malformation "critical aortic stenosis" (mentioned above), in which the forward flow through the aortic valve is so limited that ductal closure is incompatible with life. Invariably this condition is associated with severe left ventricular dysfunction, making the ventricle unable to generate enough pressure to create high-velocity flow across the valve. Therefore, one cannot always rely on the pressure gradient to present a complete picture of disease severity.

Practical Tips

In bedside clinical application of echocardiography, one needs experience to identify reliably an abnormal valve with 2D imaging. Turbulent flow across a valve noted by color Doppler is an excellent clue to such an abnormality, and it can be easily confirmed by PW and/or CW Doppler measurement of the abnormal (high) flow velocity (Figure and Video 6-2; Figures 6-3 and 6-4). In fact, color Doppler screening of all valves, followed by spectral (PW and CW) Doppler interrogation of any potential areas of flow turbulence, should be standard practice to obtain rapid, practical, and clinically relevant information about valvar pathology. Conversely, the absence of turbulent flow by color Doppler, when used with appropriate Nyquist levels (see Chapter 1), effectively eliminates the possibility of semilunar valve stenosis (**Videos 3 and 4**).

One important caveat regarding high-velocity flow detected by CW Doppler is that this Doppler modality is not range-gated, as previously discussed. Therefore, aortic stenosis (AS) can be confused with mitral regurgitation (MR), since both are high-velocity flows away from the transducer and their paths can overlap when the operator is using the apical window. Remember that mitral regurgitation will produce a high velocity due to the pressure gradient between left ventricle and left atrium, which translates into a pressure gradient reflecting systemic blood pressure. However, such a high gradient would be

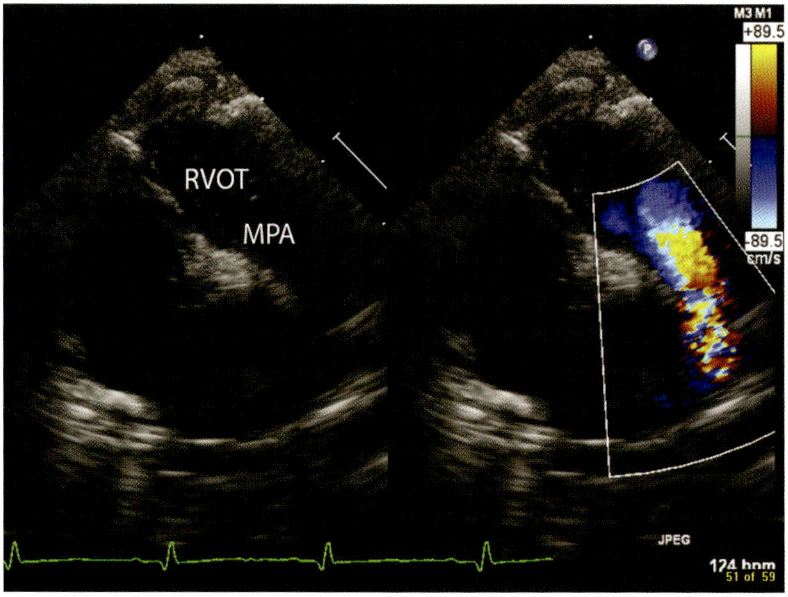

FIGURE and VIDEO 6-2. Parasternal long-axis view with leftward angulation of the transducer to display the right ventricular outflow tract (RVOT), with simultaneous 2D imaging and color flow Doppler displayed in the color compare mode. The image on the right demonstrates aliasing by color Doppler at the pulmonary valve level. Abbreviation: MPA, main pulmonary artery.

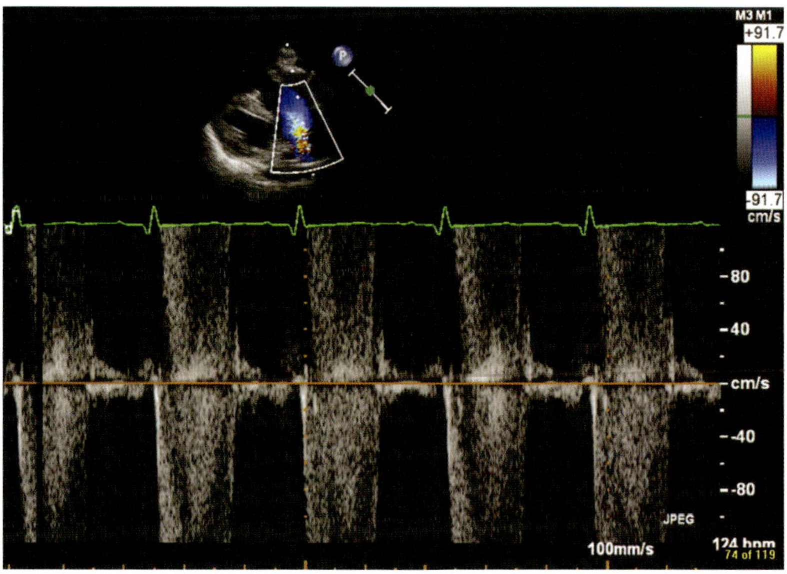

FIGURE 6-3. Pulsed wave Doppler spectral recording from the same patient depicted in Figure 6-2. The image is obtained from the parasternal long-axis RVOT view with PW sample volume placed immediately above the pulmonic valve, demonstrating aliasing.

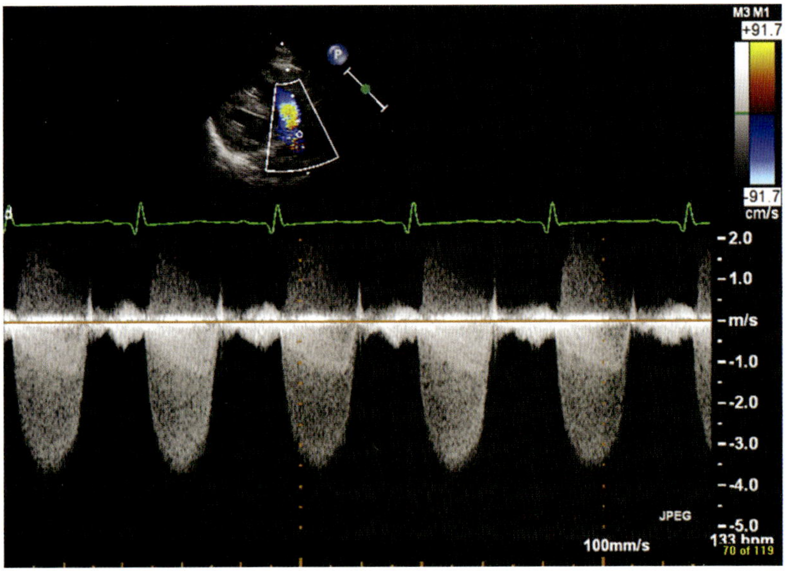

FIGURE 6-4. Continuous-wave Doppler spectral recording from the same patient depicted in Figures 6-2 and 6-3 showing a full envelope (spade-shaped) spectral Doppler tracing consistent with moderate pulmonary valve stenosis. The measured velocity is approximately 3.5 m/s, or about 49 mm Hg as calculated by the simplified Bernoulli equation.

unusual in the newborn with aortic valve stenosis and, if detected, would be indicative severely and obviously abnormal aortic valve morphology. Another example of the potential error caused by range ambiguity is coarctation of the aorta, which can be confused with left pulmonary artery stenosis (and vice versa) from a suprasternal view. These issues can be avoided by a careful and precise color Doppler directed interrogation of each structure in question.

Correlation of Doppler-derived Pressures to Cardiac Catheterization Values

A well-validated fact is the lack of correlation of the Doppler-derived pressure drop across the semilunar valves with those measured during cardiac catheterization (with the Doppler-derived values being higher). The main reason for this discrepancy is that the Doppler-derived pressure gradient represents the *maximal* instantaneous gradient; it is simply the pressure difference between two chambers at a given instant. On the other hand, the pressure difference measured during cardiac catheterization is typically reported as the peak-to-peak gradient and measures the difference between the peak pressures in the same two chambers, and in general, these pressures simply do not occur simultaneously. In addition, patients are sedated for catheterization and thus a lowering of pressures is observed.

Valvar Regurgitation/Insufficiency

It is important to understand that the following discussion of valvar regurgitation/insufficiency assumes otherwise normal cardiac anatomy. It is also critical to understand that the volume of blood regurgitating across a valve is not the same as the velocity of the regurgitant jet. For example, a high regurgitant jet velocity does not imply a large amount of regurgitation. Instead, it merely indicates there is a large pressure gradient between the two chambers being evaluated.

Mitral and Tricuspid Regurgitation

Assuming an anatomically normal heart, mitral regurgitation (MR) and tricuspid regurgitation (TR) in the context of myocardial depression (perinatal asphyxia, sepsis, etc.) are common. This myocardial depression-related mild to moderate MR and TR are most likely due to myocardial/papillary muscle dysfunction with anatomically normal valves (Figure and Video 6-5).[2]

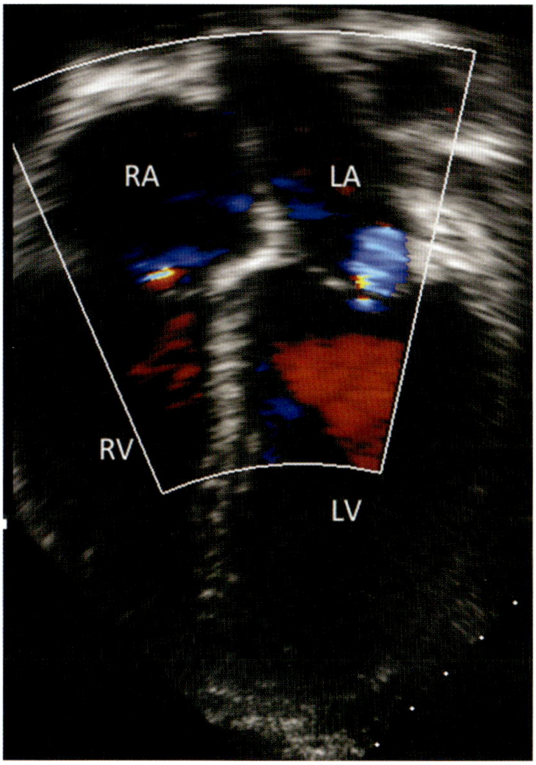

FIGURE and VIDEO 6-5. 2D color Doppler image of the heart obtained from the apical four-chamber view showing mild tricuspid and mitral regurgitation.

Grading of regurgitation across valves is a complicated process that involves multiple ultrasound modalities/views and an experienced echocardiographer. A simplified bedside estimation of valvar regurgitation can be attempted by subjective assessment of the amount of regurgitant volume on the color Doppler (Figure and Video 6-6).

It is recommended that one first traces the area regurgitant jet, then traces the atria, to obtain a ratio of regurgitant jet area:left atrial area. The corresponding ratios represent good estimates of severity: 1+ (15%), 2+ (25%), 3+ (35%), and 4+ (60%). However, it is important to remember that regurgitant jets are three-dimensional (3D) structures, often asymmetric, and therefore they might not be adequately represented with just one specific 2D view. This underlines the importance of assessing any regurgitant jet with multiple echocardiographic windows and views.

Aortic and Pulmonic Regurgitation

Trace pulmonary regurgitation with an anatomically normal pulmonary valve is also a common occurrence in the neonate. Aortic regurgitation of any quantity implies an anatomic abnormality with the valve itself (eg, bicuspid aortic valve, truncal valve in the presence of truncus arteriosus, tetralogy of Fallot).[3] A simplified bedside qualitative estimation of semilunar valve regurgitation can be attempted by subjective assessment of the amount of regurgitant volume by color Doppler (Figure and Video 6-7).

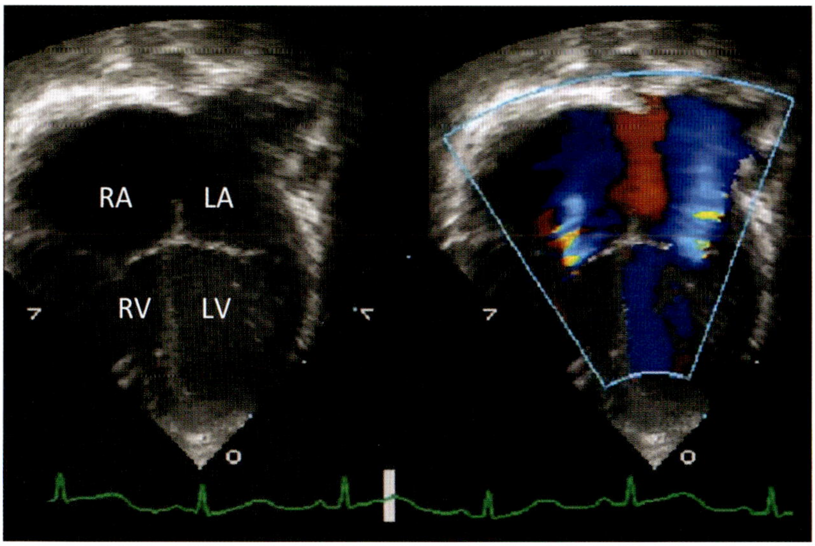

FIGURE and VIDEO 6-6. Two-dimensional color Doppler image of the heart obtained from the apical four-chamber view showing severe tricuspid and mitral regurgitation.

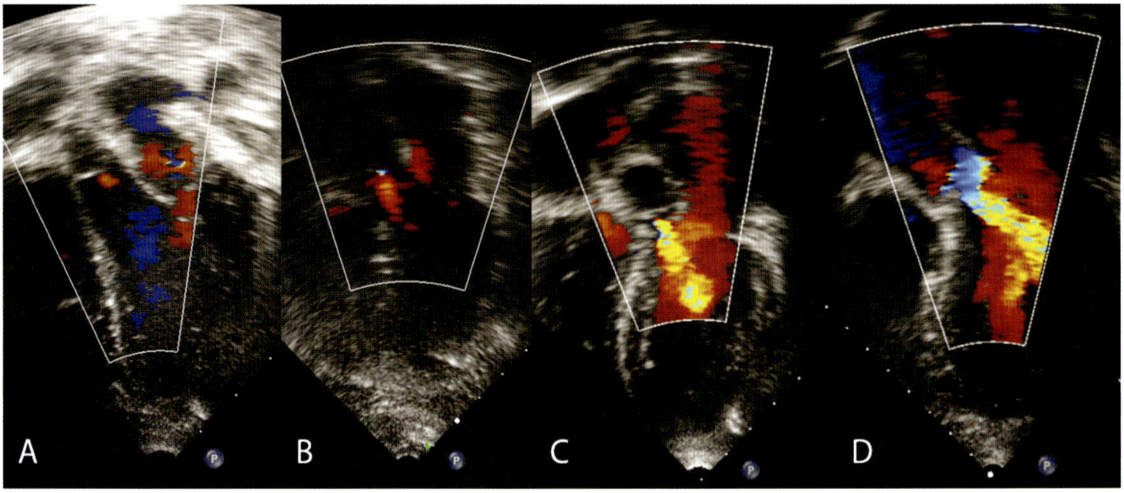

FIGURE and VIDEO 6-7. Two-dimensional color Doppler images obtained from the apical five-chamber window showing trace (A), mild (B), moderate (C), and severe (D) aortic regurgitation.

DETERMINATION OF PULMONARY ARTERIAL PRESSURE

Of great interest to neonatologists is the noninvasive estimation of pulmonary artery (PA) pressures. Pulmonary artery systolic pressure (PASP) can be obtained by three different methods:

1. Measurement of the peak velocity of tricuspid regurgitation
2. Doppler interrogation of the direction and velocity of flow through a patent ductus arteriosus (PDA), when a PDA is present
3. Doppler interrogation of the direction and velocity of flow through a ventricular septal defect (VSD), when a VSD is present

As will be discussed in Chapter 12, obtaining a PASP pressure by these methods, along with other complementary findings on 2D echocardiography (short-axis left ventricular cavity shape and interventricular septal morphology and motion), will assist the clinician in making informed clinical decisions.

Measurement of the Peak Velocity of Tricuspid Regurgitation

Continuous-wave Doppler is the most common method to determine the peak tricuspid regurgitation jet velocity (V), which estimates the pressure difference (gradient) between the right ventricle (RV) and the right atrium (RA) using the simplified Bernoulli equation. RV systolic pressure can be determined by adding the mean RA pressure (directly measured, or estimated at 0-5 mm Hg) to the pressure gradient between the RV and RA. In the absence of pulmonary valve stenosis or right ventricular outflow obstruction, PASP is considered equal to RV systolic pressure, as determined by the following equation:

$$\text{PASP} = 4\text{V}^2 + \text{RA pressure}$$

The steps to estimate PASP are as follows:

1. Normal cardiac anatomy must be established.
2. Sufficient TR must exist for interrogation. The absence of TR precludes pressure assessment via this method.
3. Obtain a good-quality 2D image.
4. The following sector cuts are best for imaging:
   a. Apical four-chamber (Figure 6-8)
   b. Parasternal long-axis RV inflow (Figure 6-9)
5. Color compare mode (side-by-side display of simultaneous color flow Doppler and 2D imaging) is best to visually detect flow problems.
6. Interrogate with color Doppler to "see" if there is TR and determine its direction and shape, as well as estimate its amount.
7. Use spectral Doppler to measure flow velocity. Pinpoint the problem with PW Doppler, and if aliasing occurs, utilize CW Doppler to measure the highest possible velocity.

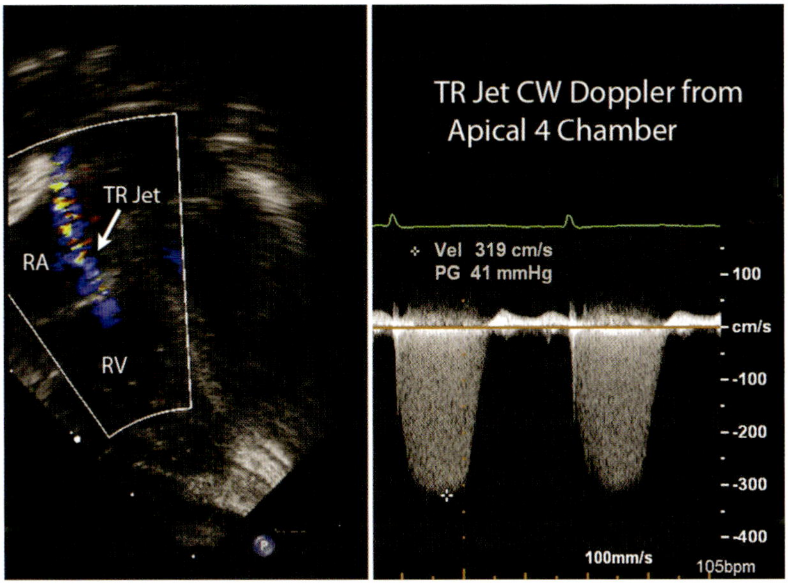

FIGURE 6-8. On the left is a 2D color Doppler image obtained from the apical four-chamber window demonstrating tricuspid regurgitation (TR). The right image is a continuous-wave (CW) Doppler spectral recording of the velocity of the TR jet. Abbreviations: RA, right atrium; RV, right ventricle.

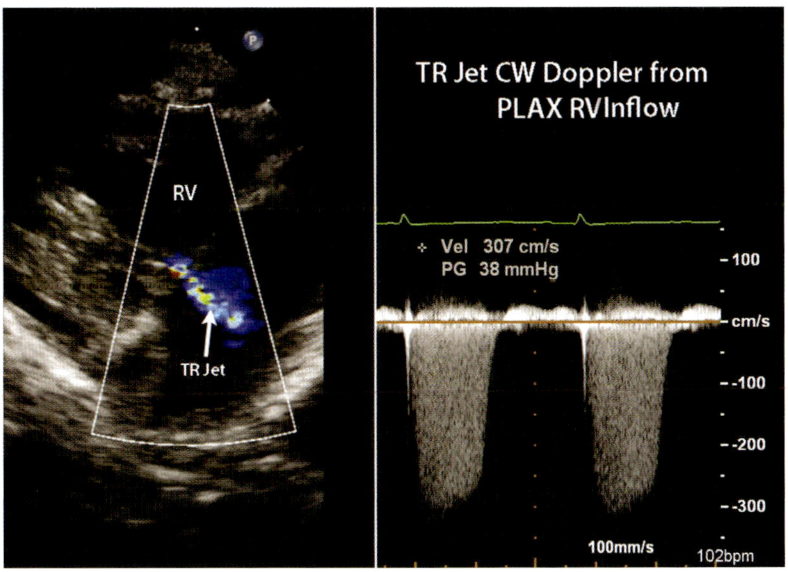

FIGURE 6-9. On the left is a 2D color Doppler image obtained from the parasternal long-axis (PLAX) window right ventricle (RV) inflow view demonstrating tricuspid regurgitation (TR). The right image is a continuous-wave (CW) Doppler spectral recording of the velocity of the TR jet.

8. Ensure proper Doppler alignment (as close to parallel to the TR jet as possible). Minimize underestimation by keeping the angle of insonation (alignment) under 20°.
9. Obtain an excellent high-intensity Doppler signal with full "spade-shaped" Doppler envelope with clearly visualized peak.
10. Ensure absence of RV outflow tract obstruction by using color Doppler screening followed by PW and CW Doppler confirmation.
11. Obtain the highest velocity from multiple echo windows.
12. Use the highest velocity rather than averaging several readings.
13. Determine accurate estimate of RA pressure (since exact measurements of RA pressure can only be obtained by invasive methods; in the newborn, one can assume a value between 5 and 10 mm Hg based upon ventilation status and other associated pathology).
14. Do not confuse severity of TR (how much blood is regurgitating) with the numerical value of the TR jet as determined by Doppler. A higher velocity does not signify more regurgitation; rather, it signifies a higher-pressure gradient between RV and RA and therefore higher RV pressure.

Using this method, several investigators have demonstrated an adequate correlation between the Doppler estimates of RV pressure and direct measurements from right-heart catheterization.[4]

Assessment of Direction and Velocity of Blood Flow through a Patent Ductus Arteriosus

The flow pattern and velocity across the PDA can be analyzed to gain important hemodynamic information regarding PA pressure values.[5] The windows used are as follows:

- Parasternal short and long axis
- High parasternal (the ductal cut)
- Suprasternal window (arch view)

Doppler interrogation of the direction and velocity of ductal blood flow can reveal either an unrestrictive large PDA or a restrictive small PDA.

Large Unrestrictive PDA

A large PDA does not allow the establishment of a significant pressure gradient between the aorta and pulmonary artery. Instead, systemic and pulmonary artery pressures will be equalized and the shunting pattern will be based on the relationship between pulmonary (PVR) and systemic (SVR) vascular resistance:

1. Pure right-to-left flow indicates that PVR is higher than SVR. This can be seen in severe pulmonary hypertension.
2. Bidirectional flow occurs when the aortic and pulmonary pressures are approximately equal. Flow is right to left in systole and left to right during diastole (Figure 6-10).
3. Pure left-to-right flow occurs once PVR drops and aortic pressure is higher than pulmonary artery pressure.

Small Restrictive PDA

A restrictive PDA allows establishment of a discernible pressure gradient between the aorta and pulmonary artery. Shunting across a restrictive duct is often exclusively left to right, generally at high velocity. With a higher flow velocity, the actual PA pressure determination may be irrelevant, since the PA pressure and PVR are likely low (Figures 6-11 and 6-12).

Theoretically, PASP should be calculated by measuring the pressure gradient using the simplified Bernoulli equation. The calculated gradient is then added to or subtracted from the systemic systolic blood pressure to estimate PASP when ductal flow is right to left and left to right, respectively. However, this method of estimation of PASP has not been adequately validated. Therefore, when interrogating ductal flow, do not rely simply upon the absolute numerical value, but focus rather on flow patterns and trends over time to gain valuable clinical information.

Refer to Chapter 11 for further details about how to obtain and interpret ductal Doppler flow patterns and hemodynamics.

Measurement of Flow Velocity through a Ventricular Septal Defect

The flow pattern and velocity across the VSD can be analyzed in a similar way to a PDA.[6] The best views for this evaluation are as follows:

- Parasternal long axis
- Parasternal short axis at aortic valve level
- Parasternal short axis at the level of papillary muscle or apex if the VSD is muscular

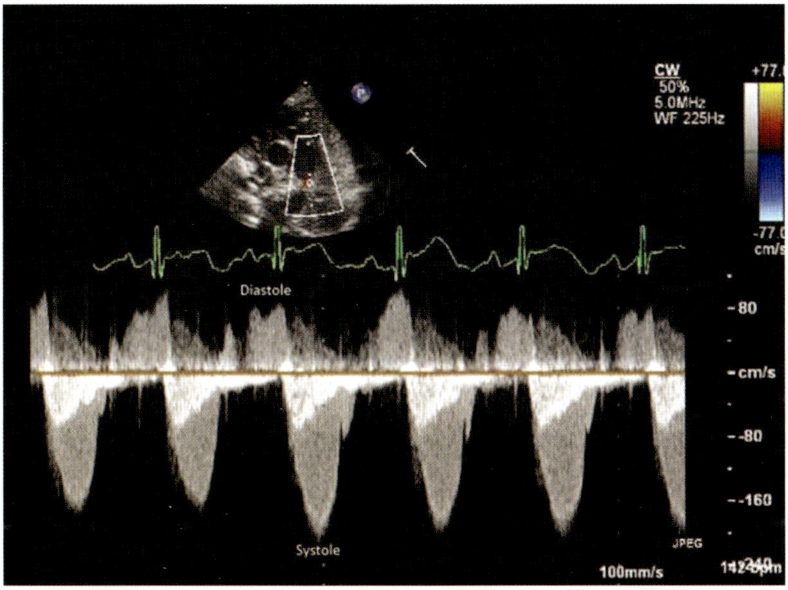

FIGURE 6-10. Pulsed wave Doppler obtained from parasternal short axis at aortic valve level through MPA demonstrating left-to-right shunt during diastole and right-to-left shunt during systole through a patent ductus arteriosus.

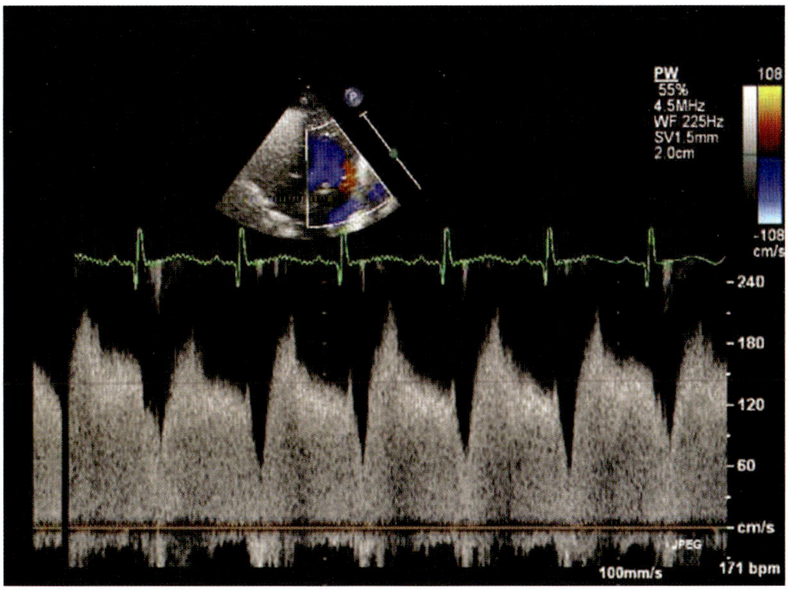

FIGURE 6-11. Pulsed wave Doppler obtained from parasternal short axis at aortic level through MPA demonstrating left-to-right shunt throughout cardiac cycle.

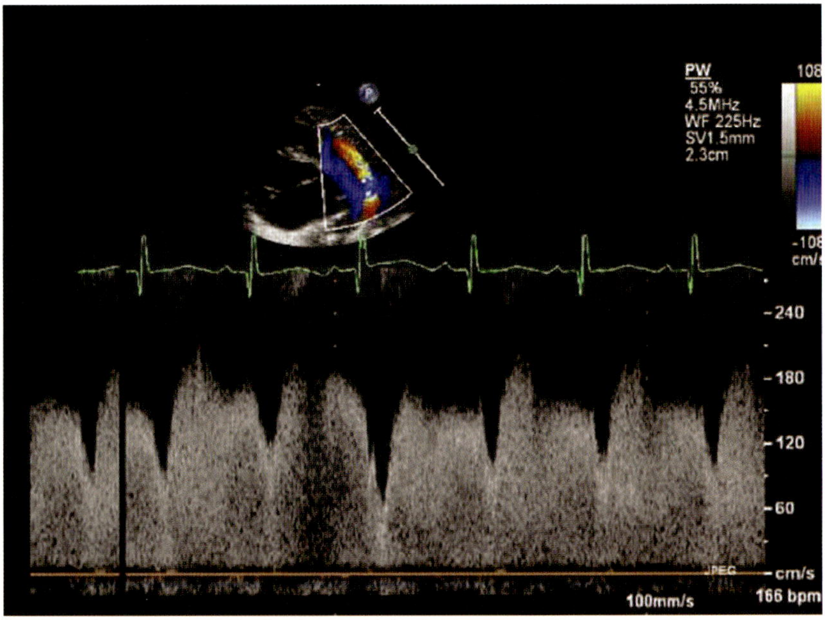

FIGURE 6-12. Pulsed wave Doppler obtained from parasternal long-axis right ventricular outflow view demonstrating continuous left-to-right shunt throughout cardiac cycle. Peak flow velocity of 2m/sec is indicative of a constricted patent ductus arteriosus.

Interpretation of flow pattern across the VSD depends upon the size of the defect.

Large VSD

A "large" VSD is defined as a defect close to or equal to the diameter of the aortic valve annulus. When present, left and right ventricular pressures equalize and the shunting pattern depends upon the PVR/SVR relationship. Physiologic possibilities include the following:

1. Low-velocity bidirectional shunting, as is often seen in the newborn (first hours to several days of life)
2. A pure right-to-left shunt, which is unusual unless the VSD is present in the context of complex cardiac malformations, or severe persistent pulmonary hypertension
3. A pure left-to-right shunt once PVR has decreased to the usual low postnatal levels (Figures 6-13 and 6-14)

Whenever there is a large interventricular communication (large perimembranous VSD, endocardial cushion defect, tetralogy of Fallot, etc.), the ventricular pressures are, by definition, equalized and shunting pattern will be dependent on the PVR/SVR relationship.

Restrictive VSD

A small or so-called "restrictive" VSD is a defect that will produce a pressure gradient between the two ventricles by its small size (Figures 6-15 and 6-16). Theoretically, by measuring the flow velocity and applying the simplified Bernoulli equation, one would expect to be able to derive the RV pressure, but it is important to keep in mind that studies have shown that VSD-derived pressure values might not always closely match those obtained with catheterization, and therefore these derived pressures are approximations. Nonetheless, it is safe to say that a left-to-right peak velocity of a VSD greater than 4 m/s almost always indicates a normal pulmonary artery pressure in the infant, and a velocity less than 3 m/s might indicate elevated pulmonary artery pressure (in the absence of right ventricular outflow obstruction). The gestational and chronological ages of the baby, and the systemic blood pressure at that time, are also important factors to consider when evaluating the VSD jet.

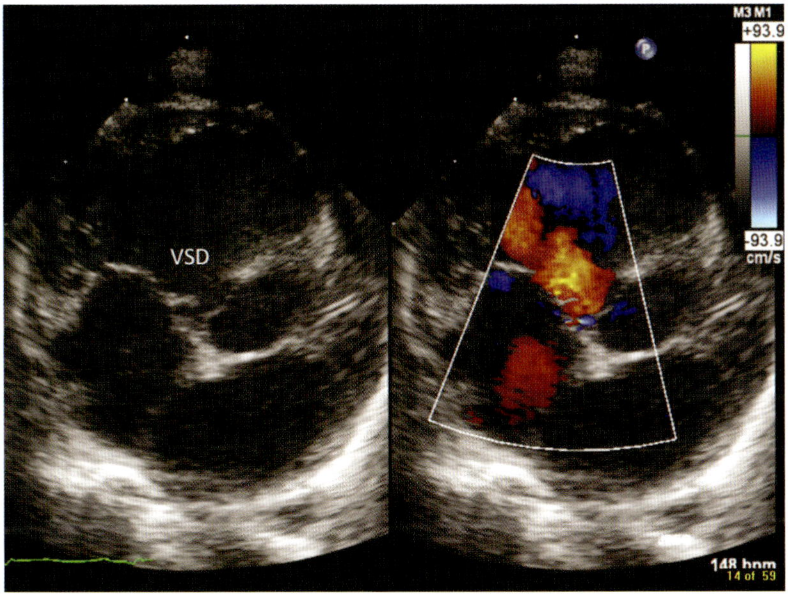

FIGURE 6-13. Two-dimensional color Doppler image obtained from the parasternal short-axis window at the aortic valve level in the color compare mode showing a large ventricular septal defect with a left-to-right shunt. The lack of aliasing is an indication of the low velocity of the flow across the defect.

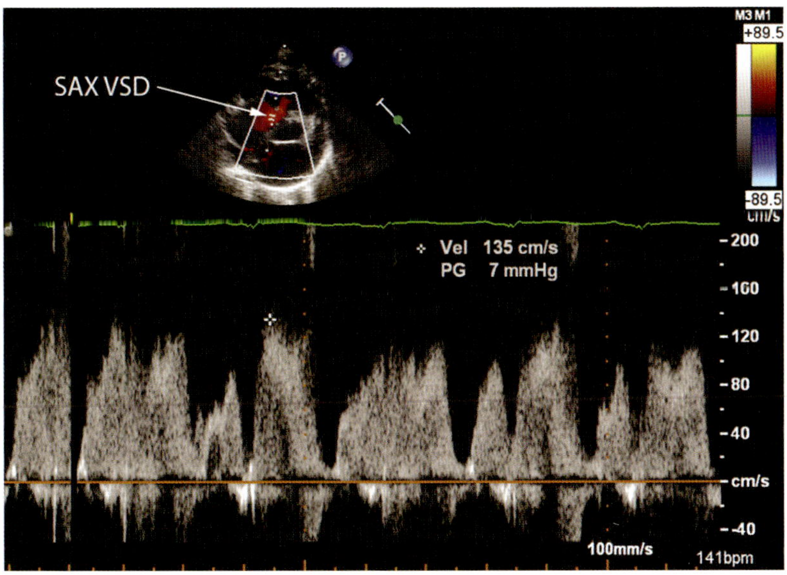

FIGURE 6-14. Two-dimensional image obtained from the parasternal short-axis (SAX) view at the level of the aortic valve. A spectral pulse wave recording of the direction and velocity of the flow across the ventricular septal defect (VSD) is derived. Since the flow is red (toward the transducer) in color mode and above the baseline in spectral mode, the shunt is left to right.

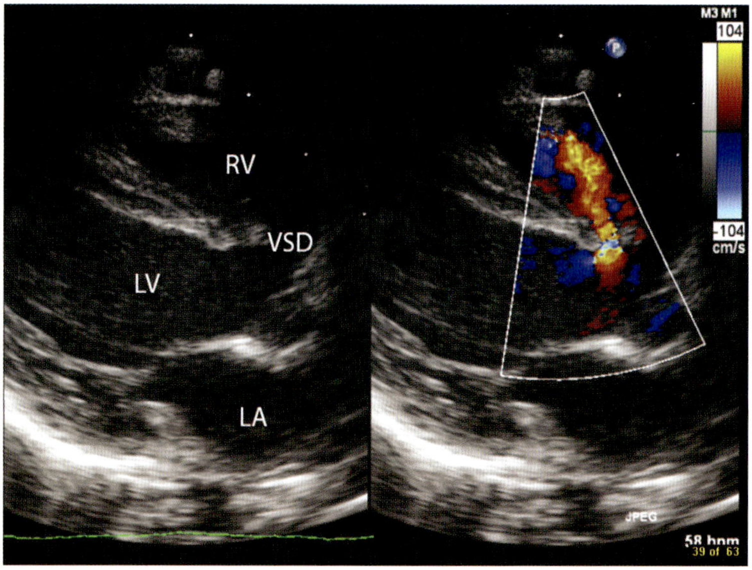

FIGURE 6-15. Two-dimensional color Doppler image obtained from the parasternal long-axis view and displayed in the color compare mode. Note the red color indicating flow toward the transducer and hence left to right. In addition, the aliasing suggests a high flow velocity, signifying a restrictive VSD. Abbreviations: LA, left atrium; LV, left ventricle; RV, right ventricle; VSD, ventricular septal defect.

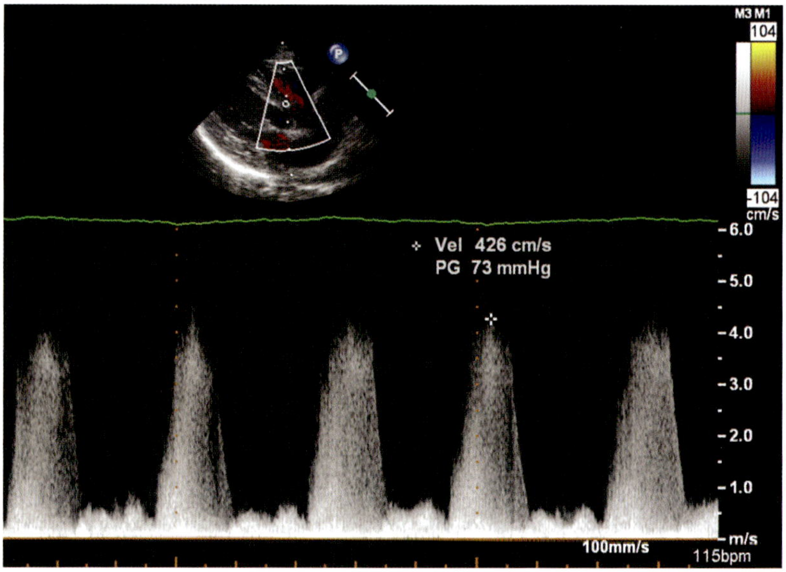

FIGURE 6-16. From the 2D color Doppler image in Figure 6-15, a continuous-wave Doppler spectral tracing is obtained. The Doppler flow is above the baseline, indicating a left-to-right shunt, and high velocity, indicating a restrictive VSD. The calculated Doppler gradient between the two ventricles is 73 mm Hg.

REFERENCES

1. Mertens L, Seri I, Marek J, et al. Targeted Neonatal Echocardiography in the Neonatal Intensive Care Unit: Practice Guidelines and Recommendations for Training. *J Am Soc Echocardiogr*. 2011;24:1057–1078.
2. Lancellotti P, Moura L, Pierard LA, et al. European Association of Echocardiography recommendations for the assessment of valvular regurgitation. Part 2: mitral and tricuspid regurgitation (native valve disease). *Euro J of Echo*. 2010;11:307–332.
3. Lancellotti P, Moura L, Pierard LA, et al. European Association of Echocardiography recommendations for the assessment of valvular regurgitation. Part 1: aortic and pulmonary regurgitation (native valve disease). *Euro J of Echo*. 2010;11:223–244.
4. Skinner JR, Stuart AGS, O'Sullivan J, Heads A, Boys RK, Hunter S. Validation of right heart pressure determination by Doppler in infants with tricuspid regurgitation. *Arch Dis Child*. 1993; 69:216–220.
5. Musewe NN, Poppe D, Smallhorn JF, et al. Doppler echocardiographic measurement of pulmonary artery pressure from ductal Doppler velocities in the newborn. *J Am Coll Cardiol*. 1990;15:446–456.
6. Houston AB, Lim MK, Doig WB, Reid JM, Coleman EN. Doppler assessment of intraventricular pressure drops in patients with ventricular septal defects. *BMJ*. 1988;60:50–56.

CHAPTER 7

Application of Pulsed Wave and Continuous-Wave Doppler in the Assessment and Measurement of Cardiac and Systemic Blood Flow*

Shahab Noori

- INTRODUCTION
- LEFT VENTRICULAR OUTPUT
- RIGHT VENTRICULAR OUTPUT
- SUPERIOR VENA CAVA FLOW
- MITRAL AND TRICUSPID FLOW DOPPLER
- REGIONAL AND ORGAN BLOOD FLOW
  - Cerebral Blood Flow
    - Middle Cerebral Artery
    - Anterior Cerebral Artery
- SUPERIOR MESENTERIC ARTERY
- RENAL ARTERY
- REFERENCES

INTRODUCTION

The measurement of blood flow through any vascular structure using ultrasound requires two basic pieces of information: the velocity of blood flow and the cross-sectional area of the vessel. The velocity of blood flow can be measured using spectral Doppler. As pulsed wave (PW) Doppler allows for measurement of velocity at a specific point in the vessel (ie, range resolution), it is the preferred mode of spectral Doppler. When measuring the velocity, the echocardiographer must take care to use an angle of insonation as parallel as possible to the direction of flow. If the ultrasound beam is intercepting the blood flow at an angle, the velocity will be underestimated (see Chapter 6). In clinical practice, an angle of less than 20° is generally considered acceptable, as the effect on velocity is negligible. An angle greater than 20° will require angle correction, which often produces inconsistent results. Another important point in measuring the velocity is that, in the presence of a turbulent flow, the measured velocity by PW Doppler cannot be used to estimate the flow because of

*Videos can be accessed at http://PracticalNeonatalEcho.com.

aliasing that occurs with higher velocities (see Chapters 1 and 4). Therefore, the operator should assess the flow by color Doppler first to ensure that the flow is laminar before attempting to obtain the velocity by PW Doppler.

In the measurement of the cross section of the vessel, it is assumed that the vessel is cylindrical in shape and therefore the vessel cross section is a circle. By measuring the diameter of the vessel, one can calculate the area using the following formula:

$$\pi D^2/4$$

where π is the constant 3.14 and D is the diameter of the vessel.

Blood flow can be calculated using either of these two formulas:

$$\text{Blood flow} = \text{Velocity time integral} \times \text{Cross} - \text{sectional area} \times \text{Heart rate}$$
$$\text{Blood flow} = \text{Mean velocity} \times \text{Cross} - \text{sectional area} \times 60$$

Velocity time integral (VTI) is the area under the curve of the Doppler envelope for each cardiac cycle. Mean velocity is the time-averaged velocity over the entire cardiac cycle (see below).

Important: The assumption that the vessel in cross section is circular is thought to be acceptable for clinical use of flow estimation in the arterial system. However, for the venous system (such as the superior vena cava, due to collapsibility of the veins), this assumption is more problematic. This will be discussed below.

In this chapter, estimation of left and right ventricular output and superior vena cava flow will be discussed. This will be followed by a brief description of mitral and tricuspid flow Doppler. Use of mitral and tricuspid flow Doppler in the assessment of diastolic function will be discussed in Chapter 8. Finally, the assessment of organ blood flow using Doppler flow indices will be reviewed.

LEFT VENTRICULAR OUTPUT

When the ductus arteriosus is closed, left ventricular output (LVO) represents systemic blood flow. Conversely, in the presence of a patent ductus arteriosus (PDA), the systemic blood flow can be over- or underestimated by LVO, depending upon whether the shunt through the PDA is predominantly left to right (overestimate) or right to left (underestimate). While there are different techniques (eg, thermodilution and magnetic resonance imaging) available to estimate cardiac output, echocardiography is the only noninvasive bedside modality that can be used clinically. Recent reports suggest that electrical velocimetry, which is based on thoracic bioimpedance, has the potential for noninvasive and continuous cardiac output monitoring.[1–3] As for echocardiography, given the percentage error of up to 30%, except for the extreme values, the absolute LVO should be used with caution in assessing the systemic blood flow. Rather, serial measurements used to assess changes in LVO would be a more reliable indicator of the hemodynamics status.

The normal value of LVO varies in different studies, with mean values ranging from 100 ml/kg/min to as high as 300 ml/kg/min.[4–15] There are several reasons for this apparent discrepancy in the literature. The timing of measurement appears to be of significant importance. Immediately after birth, LVO is relatively low and then increases as the pulmonary vascular resistance drops and the left-to-right shunt through the PDA increases.[8,15] Subsequently, the LVO decreases with the closure of ductus arteriosus[8,15] and remains stable or mildly increases during the first year.[6,10,13] Moreover, there is more variability in estimated LVO in preterm infants, especially during the early postnatal period.[9,12] Another reason for variability of LVO is the variation in methodology. This is especially true for the measurement of aortic diameter: the measured diameter is smallest when the aortic annulus is measured at the valve hinge points and progressively increases when ascending aorta and sinus of Valsalva are used. Furthermore, the potential to overestimate the aortic diameter is greater when M-mode rather than two-dimensional (2D) ultrasound is used. For practical purposes, mean LVO is considered to be about 200 ml/kg/min with a range of 150–300 ml/kg/min.[4–15]

Technique

A. Measurement of Velocity

Position. The patient should be placed in a supine or a slight left lateral decubitus position.

Transducer. A high-frequency (10–12 MHz) probe is preferable to maximize spatial resolution. However, in some cases (eg, in larger infants or when a subcostal approach is used), a lower-frequency probe can be used for better penetration (see details on transducer frequency in Chapters 1 and 2).

View. The apical five-chamber view is usually the best way to ensure a good angle of insonation (<20°) (Figure and Video 7-1). Alternatively, the suprasternal view can be used, especially if flow from the ascending aorta is assessed. When significant lung disease such as air leak

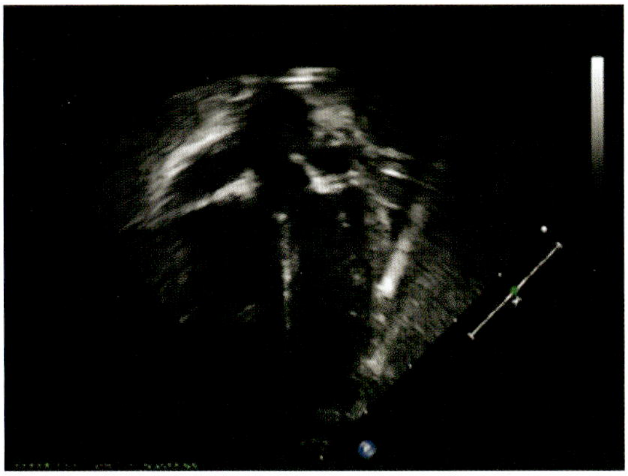

FIGURE and VIDEO 7-1. Apical five-chamber view of the heart is often used for Doppler interrogation of left ventricular outflow tract and aortic valve. With practice, the angle of insonation can be reduced to close to 0°.

or fibrosis is present, the apical and suprasternal acoustic windows might not be available. In such cases, the subcostal view can be helpful, although the angle of insonation across the aortic valve might not be optimal.

Procedure. For the apical view, place the transducer slightly lateral to the left midclavicular line at the level of 6th or 7th intercostal space (also see the standard views in Chapter 3). The transducer's marker should be pointing toward the patient's left. Once a 2D image of the left ventricular outflow tract is obtained, place the PW Doppler cursor at the level of aortic valve to obtain the velocity profile (Figure 7-2). Next, trace the spectral Doppler envelope to determine the VTI (Figure 7-2). It is preferable to use the machine's analysis system by designating each measurement appropriately (eg, aorta VTI); this will save time because the machine's software package will perform the necessary calculations. Depending upon the echocardiography system, the heart rate might be automatically acquired through the EKG recording obtained via the bedside monitor, or by manual placement of the leads. Otherwise, the heart rate can be calculated by measuring the time between identical points on the EKG or flow Doppler envelope (RR interval on most echo system).

B. Measurement of Aortic Valve Diameter

Position. The patient should be placed in a supine position.

Transducer. A high-frequency (10-12 MHz) probe is preferable to maximize spatial resolution. However,

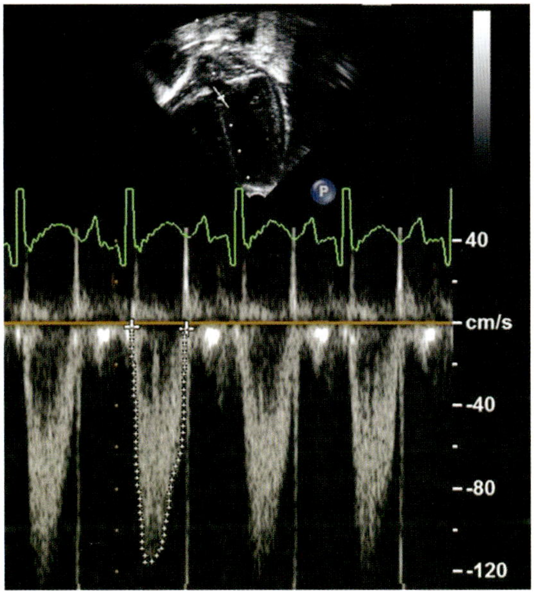

FIGURE 7-2. PW Doppler at the level of aortic valve obtained from apical five-chamber view. Tracing the Doppler envelope yields the velocity time integral (VTI).

in some cases (eg, in larger infants or when a subcostal approach is used) a lower-frequency probe can be used for better penetration (see details on transducer frequency in Chapters 1 and 2).

View. The parasternal long-axis view is the preferred approach for measuring the aortic valve diameter (Figure and Video 7-3).

Procedure. Place the transducer slightly medial to the left midclavicular line at the level of the 4th or 5th intercostal

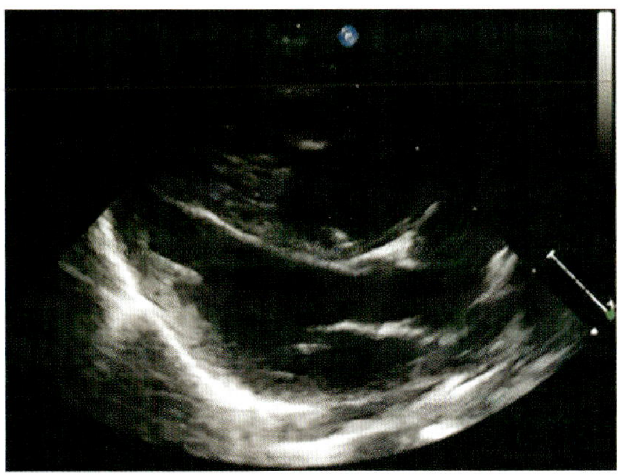

FIGURE and VIDEO 7-3. The parasternal long-axis view is the preferred approach to measuring the aortic diameter.

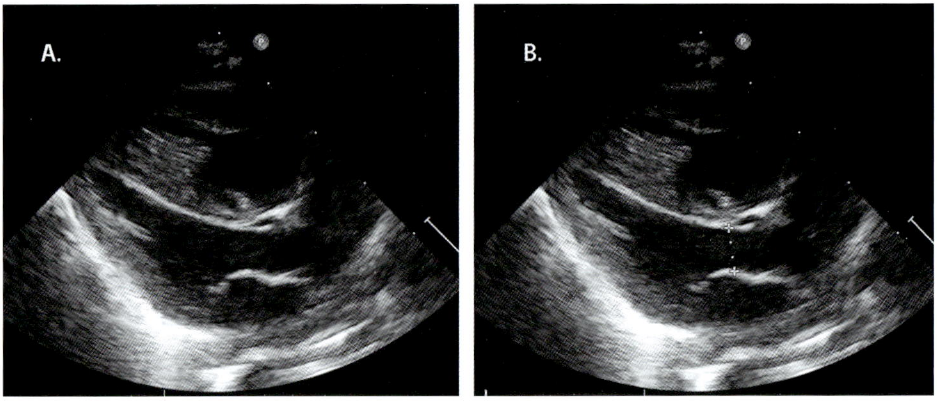

FIGURE 7-4. 2D image of the aortic valve obtained from parasternal long-axis view (**A** and **B**). The diameter used for calculation of left ventricular output is measured between the two visible valve hinges in systole (**B**).

space (also see the standard views in Chapter 3). The transducer's marker should be pointing toward the patient's right shoulder. As the valve structure is less distensible with a change in volume or pressure, measurement of the diameter at the valve is preferable (Figure 7-4). Care must be taken to obtain a standard long-axis view of the heart in order to have the echo reflection of aortic valve cusps (during diastole) in the center. This will ensure that the measured distance is the true valve diameter. The diameter is measured when the valve is open in systole. Alternatively, for the calculation of the surface area, the diameter at the ascending aorta (distal to the sinuses of Valsalva) can be used. This is easier to measure but might be less reliable for serial measurements if there is a significant change in cardiac output. Regardless of whether the valve or ascending aorta is used, it is more important that the diameter and Doppler measurements are performed in the same location.

RIGHT VENTRICULAR OUTPUT

As mentioned above, in the presence of a PDA, LVO does not represent systemic blood flow. This poses a significant limitation on utility of LVO measurements during the transitional period when a PDA is common. In such circumstances, estimation of right ventricular output (RVO) can be useful in the assessment of systemic flow. In the absence of significant flow through the patent foramen ovale (PFO), blood returning to the right side of the heart and flowing through the pulmonary artery should be equal to the systemic output. Although PFO is a common finding during the transition, usually the flow is not significant. However, it is important to note that in general, the estimated RVO (when measured noninvasively) is higher than LVO.[9,11,13,15,16] This is in contradistinction to the fact that the circulation of the neonate is in series, thus LVO and RVO should be equal. The likely reasons for this apparent discrepancy are the difficulty in visualizing the pulmonary valve hinge points (producing an error in measurement of the diameter) and the presence of a PFO. The difference between LVO and RVO in most studies is about 20-50 ml/kg/min,[9,15,16] but some authors reported a difference as high as 120-130 ml/kg/min.[11,13] In addition, the difference appears to be greater in preterm infants. Therefore, similar to LVO, serial measurements would be a more reliable indicator of a patient's hemodynamics status than a single RVO measurement.

Technique

A. Measurement of Velocity

Position. The patient should be placed in a supine position.

Transducer. Same as for LVO measurement.

View. Pulmonary artery flow velocity can be assessed from the modified apical (Figure and Video 7-5), modified parasternal long-axis (Figure and Video 7-6), parasternal short-axis (Figure and Video 7-7), and subcostal views. When significant lung disease exists (such as an air leak or fibrosis) that renders other views impossible, the subcostal view might be the only option.

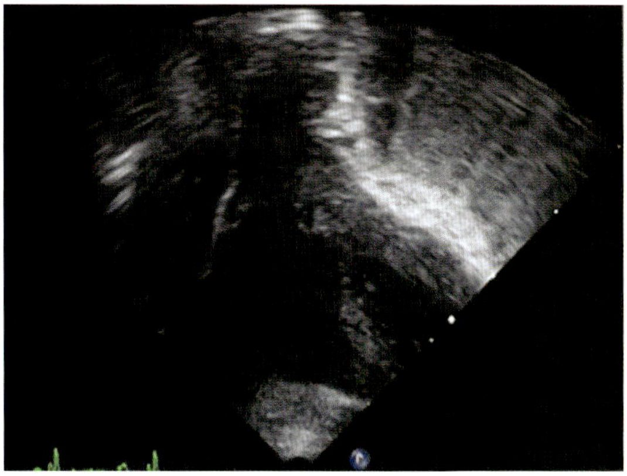

FIGURE and VIDEO 7-5. Pulmonary artery flow velocity can be assessed from different views. This video clip shows visualization of the pulmonary artery from the modified apical view. As both aortic and pulmonary flow can be assessed from the apical view, this view is preferable for hemodynamic assessment. The close temporal proximity of acquisition of the two flow Doppler tracings from this view along with minimal disturbance of the patient can be advantageous compared to assessment of aortic and pulmonary flow from separate echo windows and views.

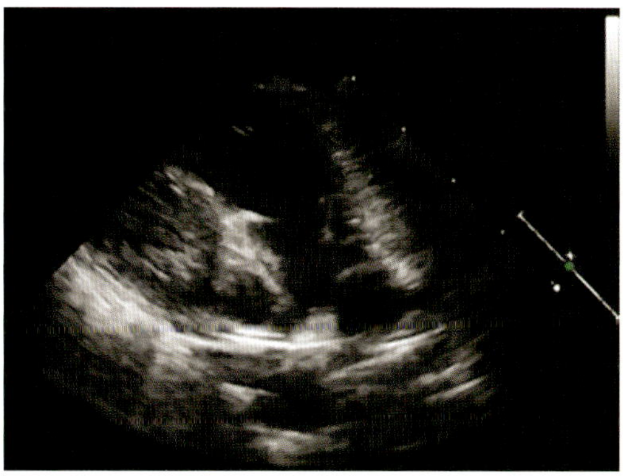

FIGURE and VIDEO 7-6. Modified parasternal long-axis view, with the transducer rotated clockwise and tilted anteriorly. Both pulmonary artery diameter and flow velocity can be measured.

Procedure. When the apical view is used to acquire a Doppler tracing at the aortic valve, the view can be modified to acquire pulmonary flow Doppler tracing as well. In this approach, after obtaining the aortic Doppler tracing, slide the transducer horizontally toward the midline by 1-2 cm, rotate it clockwise slightly, and tilt it anteriorly to visualize the right ventricular outflow tract, pulmonary valve, and pulmonary artery. The Doppler cursor is placed at the pulmonary valve and a Doppler tracing is obtained (Figure 7-8).

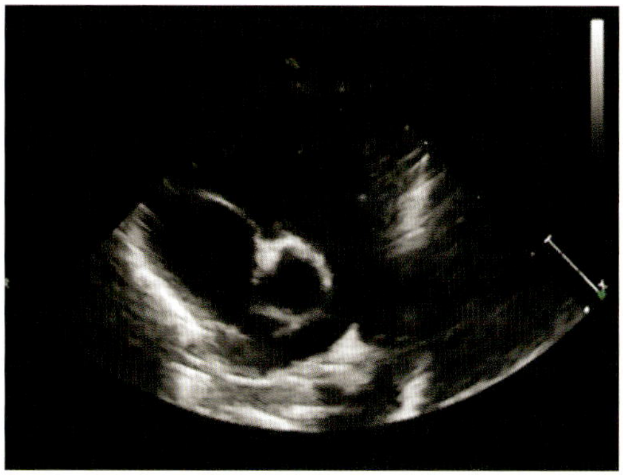

FIGURE and VIDEO 7-7. Pulmonary artery flow velocity can be measured from the standard parasternal short-axis view.

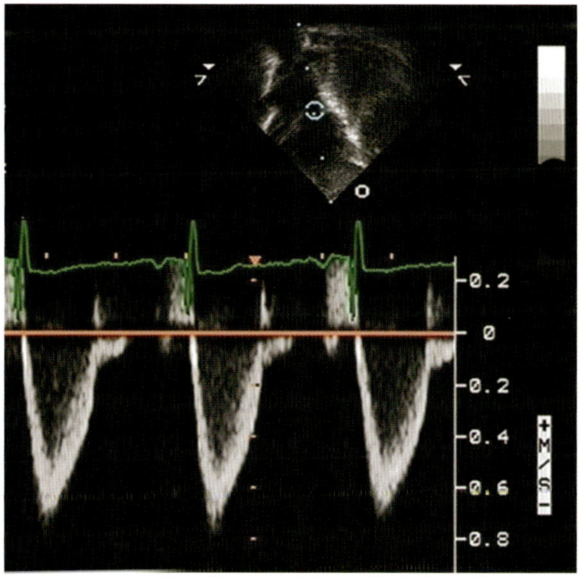

FIGURE 7-8. PW Doppler at the level of pulmonary valve obtained from the subcostal view.

For the modified parasternal long-axis view, place the transducer slightly medial to the left mid clavicular line at the level of the 4th intercostal space (also see the standard views in Chapter 3). The transducer's marker should be pointing toward the right shoulder. This should reveal standard long axis of the heart. Rotating the probe slightly clockwise and tilting it anteriorly will yield the pulmonary valve and artery. Place the PW Doppler cursor at the level of pulmonary valve to obtain the velocity profile. Tracing the spectral Doppler envelope and determining the heart rate are performed in the same manner as for LVO measurement (see above).

B. Measurement of Diameter

Position. The patient should be placed in a supine position.

Transducer. Same as for LVO measurement.

View. All the above four views can be used to measure the diameter. The preferred method is the parasternal long-axis view.

Procedure. The view and the procedure are the same as the ones used for measuring the velocity. The pulmonary valve annulus should be measured during systole. However, since the plane of pulmonary valve attachment is parallel to the transthoracic ultrasound beam, the cusps attachments are poorly visualized in all the views (Figure 7-9). This makes estimation of valve diameter less reliable compared to the aortic valve. Alternatively, the main pulmonary artery (pulmonary trunk) diameter distal to the sinus of Valsalva can be measured (Figure 7-10). However, using this diameter to calculate the RVO often overestimates the actual output. In addition, the repeatability of this measurement is worse than that of pulmonary valve.[16]

SUPERIOR VENA CAVA FLOW

As mentioned above, application of LVO and RVO in assessing systemic flow can be limited by the presence of a significant PDA and PFO, respectively. Kluckow and Evans proposed SVC flow measurement as a surrogate for cerebral and systemic blood flow.[17] There are several advantages of SVC flow over ventricular output. SVC flow measurement is not affected by a PDA or PFO. As regional blood flow, in general, and cerebral blood flow, in particular, is of more interest than the entire systemic cardiac output during the early postnatal transition, SVC flow measurement is advantageous. However, SVC flow measurement also has its own set of limitations. Given the collapsibility of the vein, the assumption of a circular cross section (as used for an artery) is not valid. The contribution of brain blood flow to SVC flow in the preterm infant is unknown. Nevertheless, SVC flow, when used in conjunction with other indicators of systemic flow or in a research setting, can be useful. Table 7-1 shows the range of normal SVC flows in preterm and full-term infants.[11,17,18] In the very preterm infant, SVC flow <30–45 mL/kg/min is considered low during the first postnatal day and the low SVC flow is associated with increased risk for development of intraventricular hemorrhage and poor neurodevelopmental outcome.[19–22]

Technique

A. Measurement of Velocity

Position. The patient should be placed in a supine position.

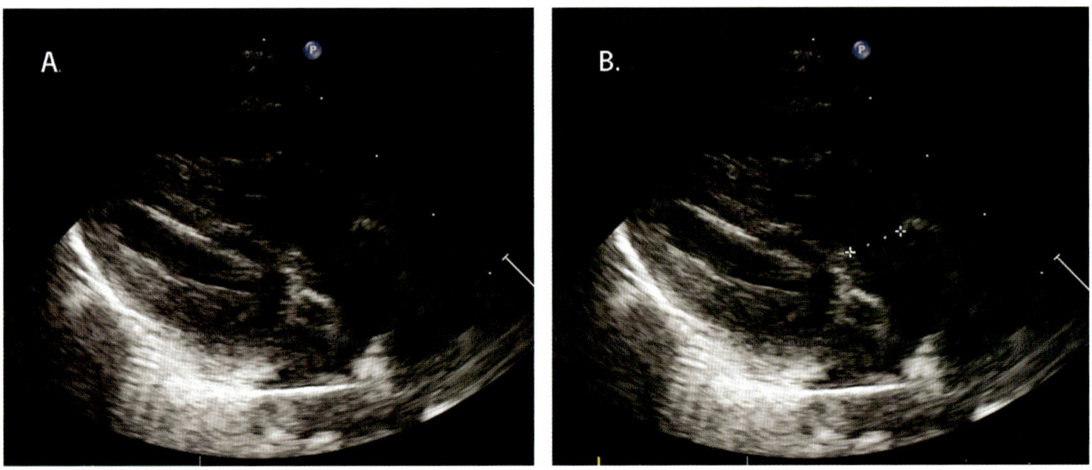

FIGURE 7-9. Two-dimensional image of pulmonary valve obtained from modified parasternal long-axis view (**A** and **B**). The diameter used for calculation of right ventricular output is measured between the two visible valve hinge points in systole (**B**).

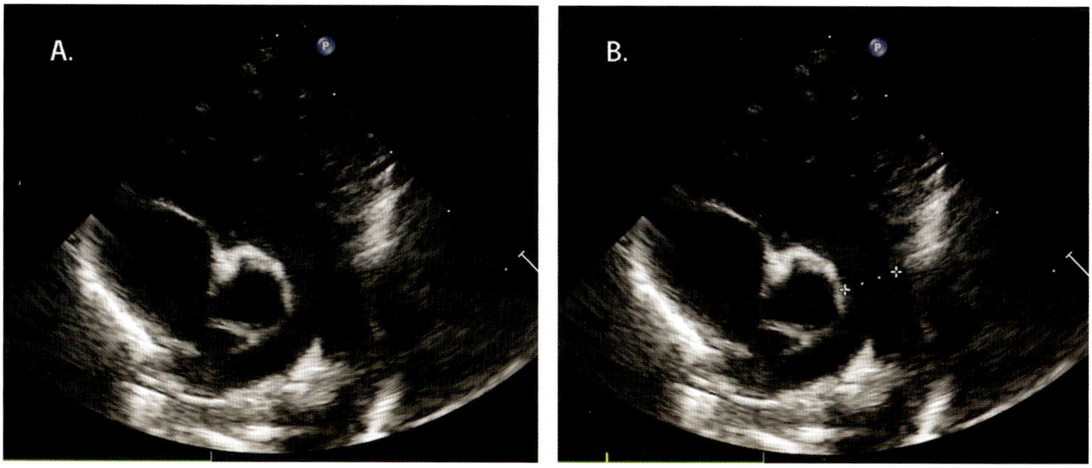

FIGURE 7-10. Measurement of the diameter of pulmonary trunk from parasternal short axis (**A** and **B**). For the purpose of calculation of right ventricular output, pulmonary trunk diameter distal to the sinus of Valsalva (**B**) can be measured as an alternative to pulmonary valve diameter.

TABLE 7-1. Range of SVC Flow in Preterm Infants During the Transition

Authors		n	VTI	max D	min D	Flow
	5 hr					
Kluckow & Evans[17]		25	9.7 (6.3–13.0)	3.0 (2.1–4.5)	2.4 (1.6–3.5)	**62 (30–140)**
Groves et al[11]		80	10.0 (5.5–12.2)			**90 (41–132)**
	12 hr					
Kluckow & Evans[17]		25	9.3 (5.4–15.5)	3.4 (2.0–4.1)	2.6 (1.6–3.6)	**75 (34–117)**
Groves et al[11]		80	9.0 (5.0–15.4)			**101 (40–183)**
Holberton et al[18]		165				**114 (82, 150)[a]**
	24 hr					
Kluckow & Evans[17]		24	11.0 (4.3–17.6)	3.5 (2.4–4.3)	2.5 (1.6–3.3)	**82 (42–150)**
Groves et al[11]		80	11.0 (7.6–16.6)			**112 (64–193)**
	48 hr					
Kluckow & Evans[17]		21	10.6 (5.7–17.2)	3.5 (2.4–4.3)	2.5 (1.6–3.3)	**86 (46–140)**
Groves et al[11]		80	12.6 (8.0–17.3)			**113 (82–179)**

Data are presented as median (range) except where indicated by "a" in which case it is presented as median (interquartile).
Abbreviations: max D, maximum diameter; min D, minimum diameter; SVC, superior vena cava; VTI, velocity time integral
Data from references 11, 17 and 18.

Transducer. Same as for LVO measurement.

View. Subcostal (Figure and Video 7-11)

Procedure. Place the transducer on the abdomen between the xiphoid process and the umbilicus (also see the standard views in Chapter 3). With the marker pointing toward the patient's left, gently tilt the transducer posteriorly. After visualization of the right atrium in 2D, the SVC can be identified using color Doppler. Place the PW Doppler cursor in the SVC as it joins the right atrium to obtain the velocity profile. Identify the typical triphasic flow pattern (Figure 7-12). Tracing the flow Doppler envelope and determining the heart rate is done in the same manner as for LVO (see above). It is important to trace at least 3-5 cardiac cycles to capture the variation in Doppler envelopes, which at times can be quite significant, as shown in Figure 7-13. Simultaneous acquisition of the

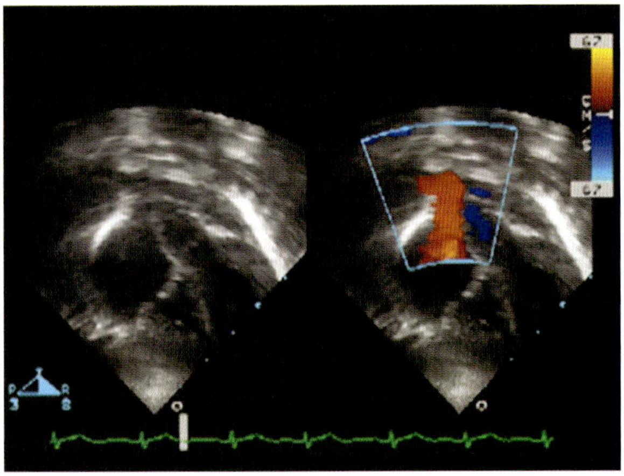

FIGURE and VIDEO 7-11. Subcostal coronal view can be used to measure superior vena cava flow velocity.

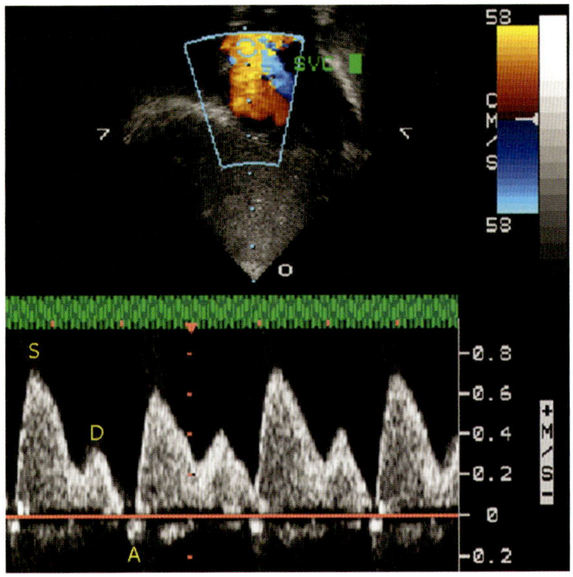

FIGURE 7-12. Typical triphasic Doppler flow pattern of superior vena cava obtained from subcostal view. S and D waveforms are forward flow and represent systole and early diastole, respectively. The waveform A is reversed flow and represents atrial contraction.

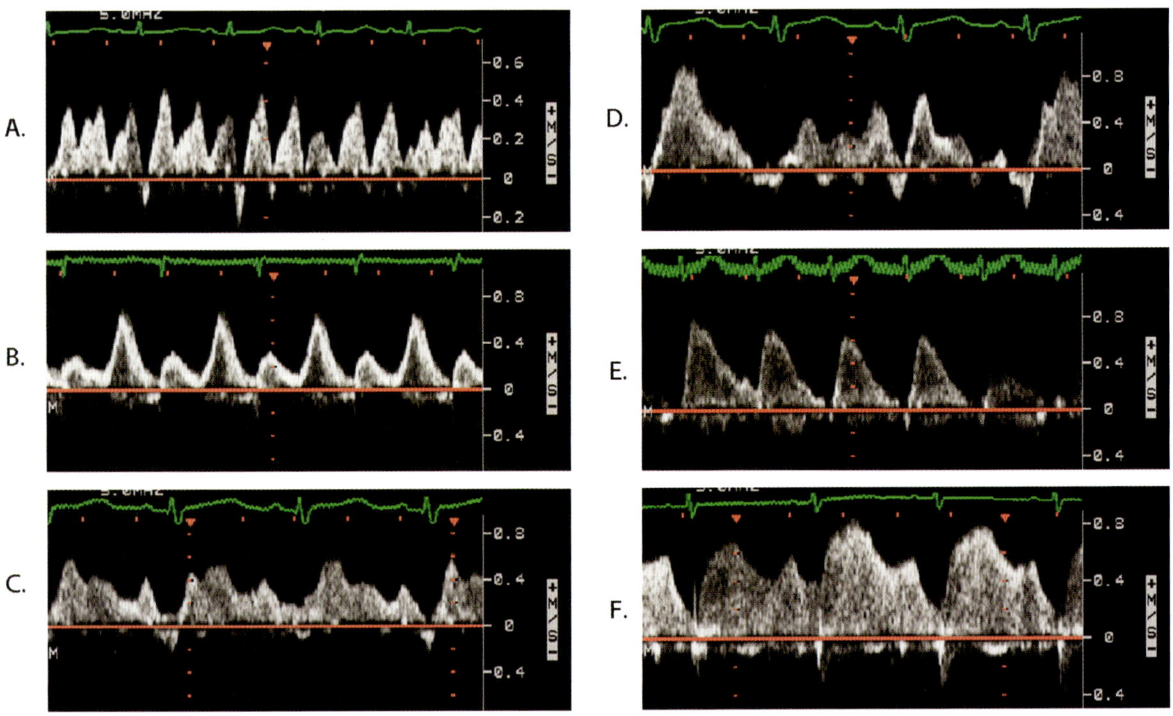

FIGURE 7-13. Examples of variation in superior vena cava flow patterns (**A**-**F**). Simultaneous acquisition of the EKG tracing helps in identifying the cardiac cycle, when determination of the start and end of cycle based on flow pattern is not feasible.

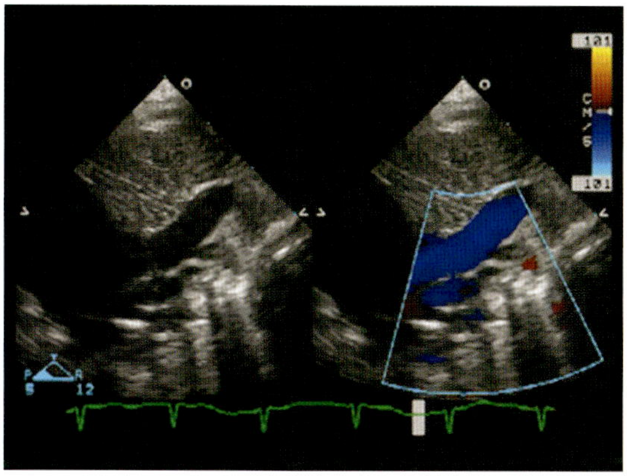

FIGURE and VIDEO 7-14. Superior vena cava diameter can be measured from high parasternal view.

EKG tracing helps in identifying the cardiac cycle when the determination of the cardiac cycle by flow pattern is not feasible (Figure 7-13D).

B. Measurement of Diameter

Position. The patient should be placed in a supine position.

Transducer. Same as for LVO measurement

View. SVC diameter can be measured in modified suprasternal or parasternal long-axis view (Figure and Video 7-14).

Procedure. In suprasternal view, first the brachiocephalic (innominate) vein is identified by counterclockwise rotation, and moving the transducer downward using color Doppler, the vein can be traced as it drains to SVC and right atrium (also see the standard views in Chapter 3). The diameter can be measured using 2D or M-mode. Due to significant diameter change over the cardiac cycle, for flow measurement, the average of maximum and minimum diameter is used. The change in diameter over the cardiac cycle is better visualized by the M-mode than 2D. However, placing the M-mode line perpendicular to the SVC can be challenging. An oblique section of SVC by the M-mode leads to overestimation of cross-sectional area and hence overestimation of SVC flow. Therefore, the 2D measurement of diameter is generally preferable (Figure 7-15).

MITRAL AND TRICUSPID FLOW DOPPLER

Estimation of blood flow through mitral and tricuspid valves is inaccurate due to the inability of measuring

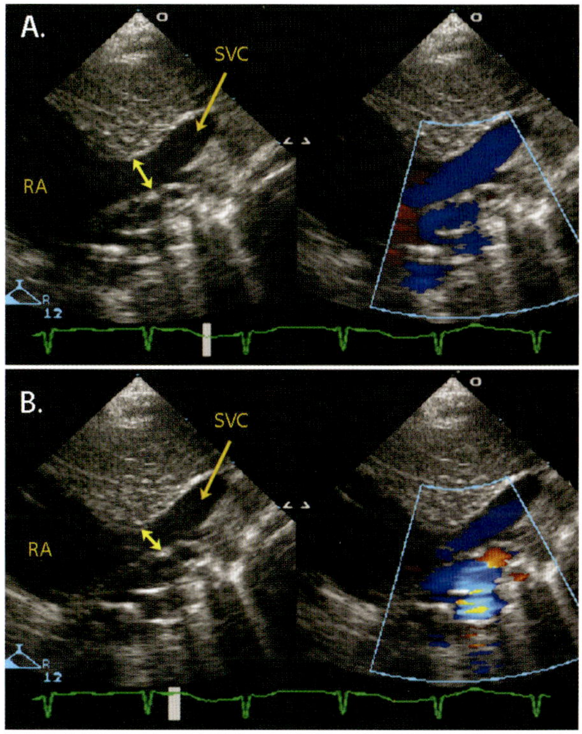

FIGURE 7-15. Two-dimensional and color Doppler images of superior vena cava (SVC) obtained from high parasternal long-axis view (**A** and **B**). Measurement of SVC diameter is shown by the double arrow. The average of maximum (**A**) and minimum (**B**) diameters is used for calculation of SVC flow. Abbreviation: RA, right atrium.

accurately the surface area of the valves. PW Doppler is used to evaluate the flow pattern rather than the flow. The characteristics of flow pattern can be useful for assessment of diastolic function, which is discussed in detail in Chapter 8.

Technique

Measurement of Velocity

Position. The patient should be placed in a supine or slight left lateral decubitus position.

Transducer. Same as for LVO measurement

View. While atrioventricular valves can be interrogated from subcostal and parasternal views, the apical four-chamber is the preferred view (Figure and Video 7-16).

Procedure. For the apical view, place the transducer slightly lateral to the left midclavicular line at the level

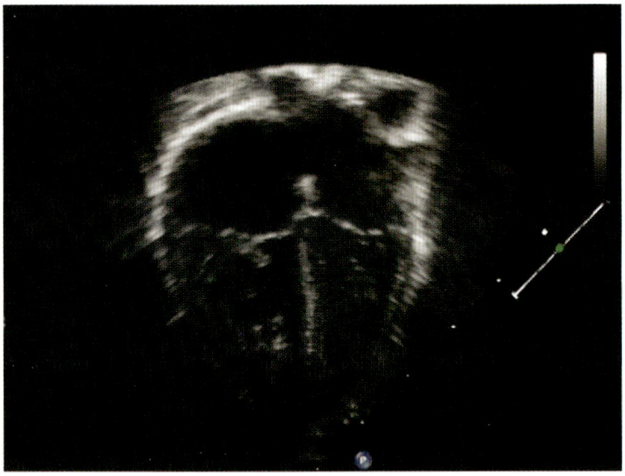

FIGURE and VIDEO 7-16. Apical four-chamber view can be used for assessment of mitral and tricuspid valves.

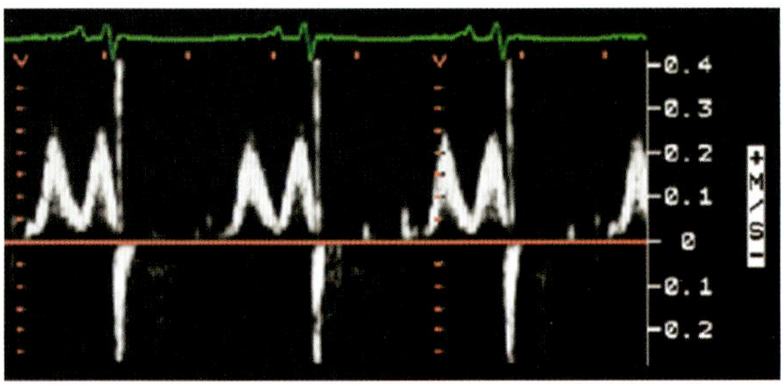

FIGURE 7-17. The M-shaped flow Doppler typical of mitral and tricuspid valve.

of 6th or 7th intercostal space (also see the standard views in Chapter 3). The transducer's marker should be pointing toward the patient's left. Place the PW Doppler cursor at the level of mitral or tricuspid valve tip to obtain the velocity profile. The Doppler envelope is typically biphasic similar to the letter "M" (Figure 7-17; see details in Chapter 8).

REGIONAL AND ORGAN BLOOD FLOW

Regional and organ blood flow can be assessed by Doppler. However, due to the size of the smaller arteries supplying the individual organs, most commercially available ultrasound systems cannot accurately measure the vessel diameters; therefore, quantification of blood flow is generally inaccurate. Despite this limitation, there is still a wealth of information contained within the Doppler envelope. Doppler-derived blood flow *indices* (rather than blood flow) can be utilized (Figure 7-18). For example, changes in stroke volume are primarily reflected by changes in systolic flow velocity. Conversely, change in vascular resistance of the organ primarily affects the diastolic flow velocity. Mean blood flow velocity (MV) and velocity time integral (VTI, area under the curve) are affected by blood flow; these measurements can be used as a surrogate for blood flow. In both cases, it is assumed that the diameter of the vessel is constant and does not change with time. While this assumption is not necessarily true, in several studies MV and VTI have been shown to have a good correlation with invasive measure of blood flow.[23–25] MV appears to be a better index of blood flow than VTI, since it is not affected by the changes in the heart rate.

Pulsatility and resistance indices are designed to overcome the limitation of not being able to measure the diameter of an artery and, to a certain extent, the variability in the angle of insonation. While there is a good correlation between these indices and blood flow, they are best used as indicators of resistance, rather than flow.[23–25]

Cerebral Blood Flow

The brain blood supply comes from the internal carotid and vertebral arteries. The confluence of the paired vertebral arteries gives rise to the basilar artery, which, together with the left and right internal carotid arteries, forms the circle of Willis at the base of the brain (Figure 7-19). It is important to note that there are significant variations in vessel caliber of the circle of Willis.

In general, the main intracranial arteries can be evaluated with relative ease in the neonatal population. In addition to the standard approaches, the open fontanelle provides additional windows to evaluate the intracranial arteries. While basilar, posterior cerebral, and ophthalmic arteries and the circle of Willis have all been evaluated, the middle (MCA) and anterior cerebral artery (ACA) are the most commonly assessed intracranial arteries in the neonatal population.

Middle Cerebral Artery

Each internal carotid artery terminates by dividing into an MCA and ACA. The MCA travels laterally and enters the Sylvian fissure. The course of MCA makes it ideal for Doppler assessment, as the angle of insonation from the temporal region of the head can be 0°. It is the largest branch of internal carotid artery and supplies the basal ganglia and the frontal, parietal, and temporal lobes. The

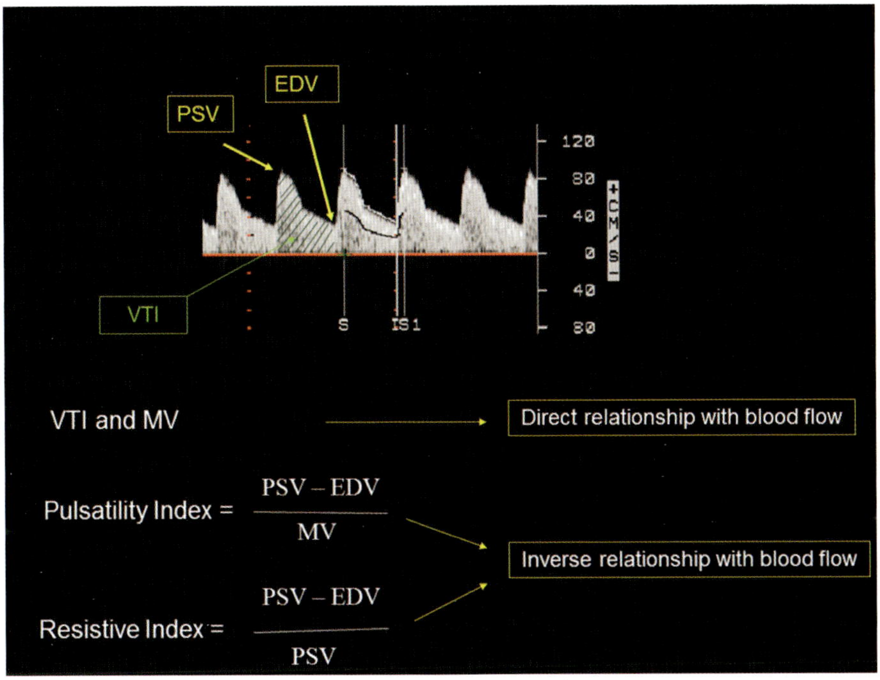

FIGURE 7-18. Doppler tracing of an artery (in this example of the middle cerebral artery), velocity-derived Doppler indices and their relationship with blood flow. Velocity time integral (VTI) and mean velocity (MV) have a direct relationship with blood flow, and pulsatility index and resistance index have inverse relationship with blood flow. Abbreviations: PSV, peak systolic velocity; EDV, end-diastolic velocity; MV, mean velocity.

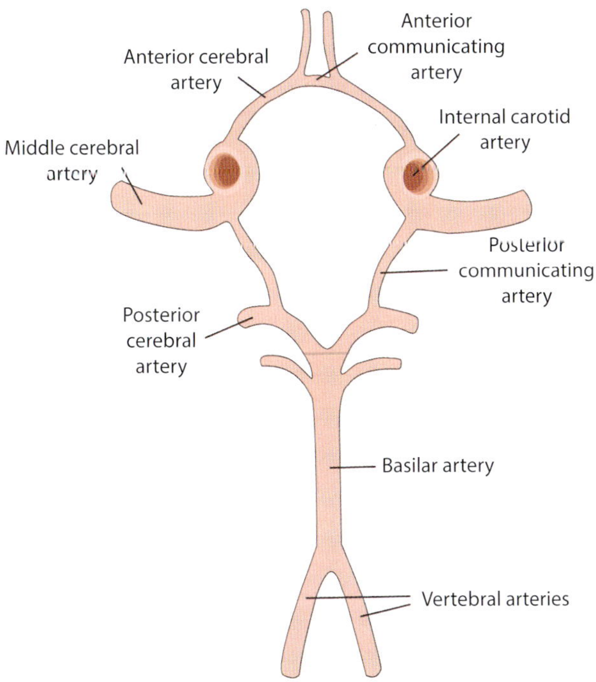

FIGURE 7-19. Brain blood supply.

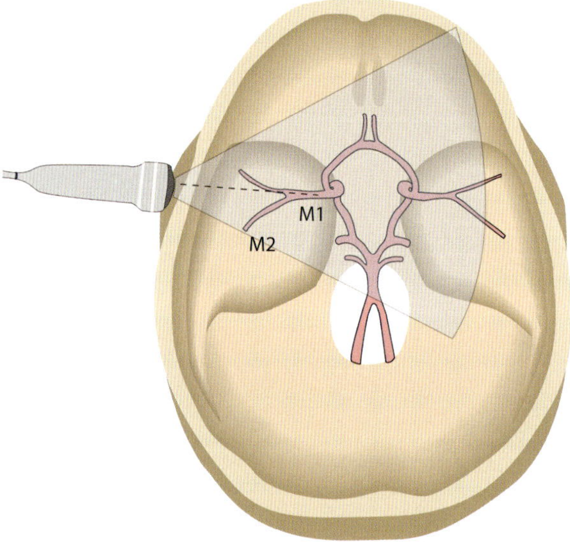

FIGURE 7-20. Schematic drawing depicting position of the transducer and placement of PW Doppler cursor in the proximal (M1) portion of the middle cerebral artery to obtain the velocity profile.

TABLE 7-2. Middle and Anterior Cerebral Arteries Doppler-derived Indices in Term Infants During the First Five Postnatal Days of Life

	Day 1	Day 3	Day 5
MCA			
PSV (cm/s)	45.4 ± 9.3	53.5 ± 11.0	56.9 ± 8.6
EDV (cm/s)	16.5 ± 5.6	21.5 ± 7.9	21.2 ± 5.6
MV (cm/s)	27.8 ± 6.6	34.0 ± 10.0	34.9 ± 6.4
RI	0.63 ± 0.09	0.60 ± 0.08	0.62 ± 0.07
ACA			
PSV (cm/s)	29.1 ± 7.2	31.2 ± 7.4	32.6 ± 7.1
EDV (cm/s)	11.3 ± 2.7	13.0 ± 3.9	13.7 ± 3.8
MV (cm/s)	18.6 ± 3.7	19.7 ± 5.0	21.0 ± 4.6
RI	0.59 ± 0.09	0.57 ± 0.08	0.57 ± 0.08

ACA = Anterior cerebral artery; EDV= End diastolic velocity; MCA = Middle cerebral artery; MV = Mean velocity; PSV = Peak systolic velocity; RI = Resistance index

Data from Ozek E, Köroğlu TF, Karakoç F, et al. Transcranial Doppler assessment of cerebral blood flow velocity in term newborns, *Eur J Pediatr*. 1995 Jan;154(1):60–63.

MCA has been divided into two segments: the proximal segment M1 and the distal segment M2 (Figure 7-20). For the purpose of cerebral blood flow (CBF) assessment, Doppler measurement of the M1 portion is preferable.

MCA Doppler flow indices depend upon the gestational age and chronological age.[26–29] The flow velocities are higher in more mature neonates and increase with chronological age. As CBF is affected by a host of factors including blood pressure, cardiac output, carbon dioxide, oxygen, hematocrit, and metabolism, one must take into account the changes in these factors when interpreting Doppler indices. An example of a population-based range of MCA Doppler values for different gestational and chronological ages is shown in Tables 7-2 and 7-3).[26,29]

Technique

Assessment of Flow Pattern and Measurement of Velocity

Position. Ideally, the patient should be placed in a supine position with the head in midline. However, to minimize disturbance of the patient, any position would be acceptable as long as access to the temporal region is possible.

Transducer. A transducer designed for vascular ultrasonography is ideal; however, any transducer used for cardiac ultrasonography, eg, an 8-MHz or 12-MHz phased-array sector transducer, would be sufficient.

View. Temporal region of the head.

Procedure. Place the transducer superior and parallel to the zygomatic arch with the probe marker directed anteriorly (Figure 7-21). Set the field of view to 5–10 cm. Using color Doppler, tilt or slide the probe gently to identify the circle of Willis at the base of the brain (Figure and Video 7-22). The MCA will be seen coming directly toward the probe and therefore the flow will be seen as red. It is important to set the color scale low (eg, 10–20 cm/s) if low cerebral blood flow is suspected; otherwise, it can be difficult to visualize the vascular structure by color Doppler. Conversely, if aliasing is present, one needs to set the color scale high to prevent aliasing, especially if one intends to measure the size of the vessel. However, as mentioned earlier, due to small vessel size, the diameters of the cranial arteries are not routinely measured. The sampling gate should be set to the smallest size due to the small diameter of the MCA.

Place the PW Doppler cursor in the proximal (M1) portion of the MCA to obtain the velocity profile (Figure 7-18).

TABLE 7-3. Middle Cerebral Artery Doppler-derived Indices in Preterm Infants During the First Month of Postnatal Life

	MCA-PSV (cm/sec)			MCA-EDV (cm/sec)			MCA-RI			MCA-MV (cm/sec)			MCA-PI		
	10th	50th	90th	10th	50th	90th	10th	50th	90th	10th	50th	90th	10th	50th	90th
GA ≤ 28 wk															
Day															
1	16.40	21.00	32.50	5.00	6.00	7.00	0.70	0.75	0.78	8.20	12.00	18.90	1.09	1.37	1.58
3	27.00	33.75	37.90	7.00	8.75	12.00	0.67	0.70	0.79	12.10	19.00	23.80	1.16	1.31	1.55
7	34.30	39.75	47.80	7.00	8.75	18.60	0.67	0.74	0.81	18.00	23.00	37.80	1.05	1.31	1.72
14	37.20	45.00	52.90	8.00	10.00	17.70	0.66	0.76	0.79	18.10	25.50	31.80	1.09	1.42	1.92
21	40.00	48.00	58.70	7.20	11.00	14.00	0.70	0.79	0.82	12.30	26.00	31.90	1.19	1.56	1.92
28	47.70	58.50	75.40	11.00	13.50	18.60	0.74	0.76	0.82	22.60	31.00	37.50	1.23	1.46	1.90
GA = 29-30 wk															
Day															
1	22.80	21.n	32.60	5.00	7.17	9.60	0.64	0.73	0.81	12.00	14.17	20.60	1.18	1.27	1.68
3	30.80	35.33	43.40	5.80	9.25	14.20	0.66	0.74	0.81	15.40	21.67	32.20	1.04	1.30	1.64
7	33.00	43.50	54.60	6.00	9.33	17.80	0.65	0.77	0.84	15.80	20.17	37.60	1.03	1.51	1.80
14	37.00	49.D7	60.40	8.00	11.17	14.60	0.71	0.77	0.83	20.40	27.83	30.80	1.11	1.47	1.75
21	48.00	55.83	60.80	7.00	11.33	18.20	0.70	0.78	0.84	24.80	29.00	35.00	1.22	1.47	1.81
28	44.40	57.50	67.80	7.40	12.33	19.60	0.70	0.79	0.84	21.80	31.83	42.00	1.16	1.44	1.76
GA = 31-32 wk															
Day															
1	24.70	28.75	35.60	4.70	8.00	11.00	0.68	0.73	0.85	12.70	15.50	21.60	1.12	1.28	1.95
3	30.70	38.50	44.90	7.00	10.00	12.30	0.70	0.75	0.78	16.40	20.00	27.00	1.08	1.31	1.47
7	38.40	44.50	49.20	6.00	10.00	15.60	0.64	0.77	0.83	19.50	23.50	32.50	0.91	1.44	1.73
14	46.20	51.50	56.30	6.00	11.50	14.60	0.72	0.77	0.84	17.80	27.00	31.30	1.22	1.46	1.77
21	47.70	54.50	62.30	6.00	12.50	17.00	0.73	0.78	0.86	19.90	30.00	36.00	1.09	1.43	1.88
28	52.10	64.00	81.40	8.00	13.00	22.00	0.68	0.79	0.85	26.40	33.50	48.30	1.00	1.46	1.74
GA > 32 wk															
Day															
1	23.40	31.83	39.60	4.20	8.00	13.00	0.67	0.74	0.84	12.20	18.17	25.60	1.03	1.35	1.68
3	33.20	38.00	47.80	7.00	10.00	12.80	0.70	0.75	0.79	17.00	20.83	28.00	1.20	1.39	1.60
7	40.00	46.00	55.60	8.20	12.00	17.40	0.68	0.73	0.81	18.60	26.00	35.60	1.10	1.35	1.55
14	47.20	55.00	59.00	7.20	12.00	17.00	0.70	0.77	0.83	20.00	30.83	40.20	1.15	1.35	1.94
21	54.20	62.17	66.00	10.00	13.25	18.80	0.70	0.75	0.82	28.20	35.25	42.60	1.10	1.32	1.75
28	61.40	71.17	86.00	12.00	18.83	25.00	0.69	0.74	0.85	33.00	42.00	51.60	1.03	1.29	1.71

EDV = End diastolic velocity; GA = gestational age; MCA = Middle cerebral artery; MV = Mean velocity; PI = Pulsatility index; PSV = Peak systolic velocity; RI = Resistance index
Reproduced with permission from Romagnoli C, Giannantonio C, De Carolis MP, et al. Neonatal color Doppler US study: normal values of cerebral blood flow velocities in preterm infants in the first month of life. Ultrasound. *Med Biol*. 2006 Mar;32(3):321–331.

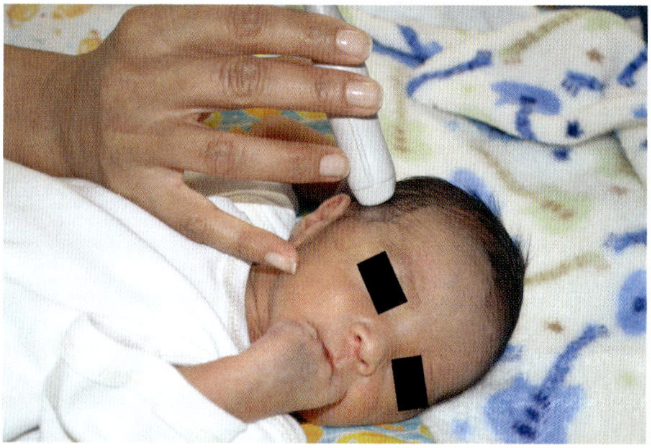

FIGURE 7-21. Transducer position for assessing middle cerebral artery. Place the transducer superior and parallel to the zygomatic arch with the probe marker directed anteriorly.

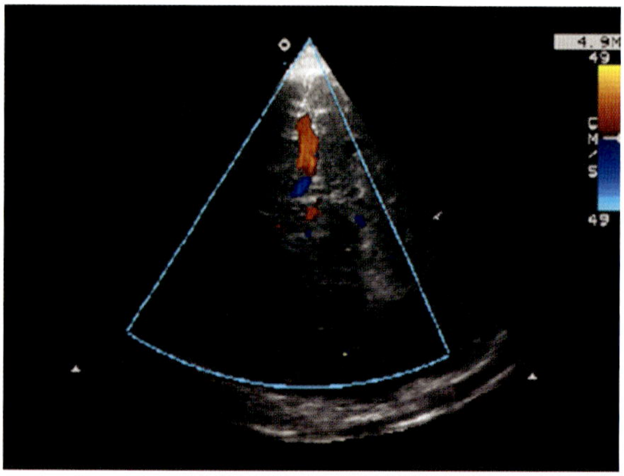

FIGURE and VIDEO 7-22. Color Doppler imaging of the circle of Willis from temporal view. The large artery flowing toward the probe (red) is the middle cerebral artery.

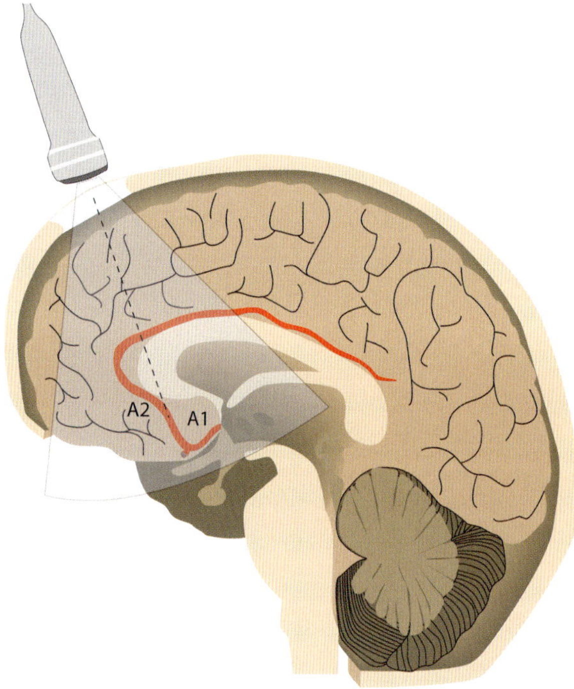

FIGURE 7-23. Schematic drawing depicting the position of the transducer and the placement of PW Doppler cursor in the distal (A2) portion of the anterior cerebral artery in order to obtain the velocity profile.

Anterior Cerebral Artery

After branching off the internal carotid artery, the ACA runs slightly medially and anteriorly and connects with the contralateral ACA via the anterior communicating artery. Thereafter, the ACA runs in the longitudinal fissure and curves around the genu of the corpus callosum. The ACA has been divided into two segments: the proximal or pre-communicating segment A1 and the distal or post-communicating segment A2 (Figure 7-23). The distal portion (A2) is preferable for assessing the flow profile and velocity, as it runs a straighter course. The ACA supplies the basal ganglia and the frontal and parietal lobes of the brain.

As mentioned earlier, CBF is affected by many factors, and therefore defining normative values for a given population need to take into consideration factors such as gestational and chronological age. An example of a population-based range of ACA Doppler values for different gestational and chronological ages is shown in Table 7-4.[29]

Technique

Assessment of Flow Pattern and Measurement of Velocity

Position. Ideally, the patient should be placed in a supine position with the head in midline position. However, to minimize disturbance of the patient, any position would be acceptable as long as access to the temporal region and anterior fontanelle is possible.

Transducer. Same as MCA (see above).

View. In general, the anterior fontanelle is the preferable approach because A2 is best visualized in this view. However, the temporal approach is acceptable if access to the

TABLE 7-4. Anterior Cerebral Artery Doppler-derived Indices in Preterm Infants During the First Month of Postnatal Life

	ACA-PSV (cm/sec)			ACA-EDV (cm/sec)			ACA-RI			ACA-MV (cm/sec)			ACA-PI		
	10th	50th	90th	10th	50th	90th	10th	50th	90th	10th	50th	90th	10th	50th	90th
GA ≤ 28 wk															
Day															
1	13.20	16.00	21.70	5.00	4.50	3.10	0.68	0.74	0.82	7.10	10.00	12.80	1.27	1.13	1.74
3	17.30	25.00	33.90	9.90	8.00	4.00	0.64	0.71	0.80	9.10	15.25	20.00	1.18	0.99	1.71
7	23.30	32.75	41.70	8.80	6.00	4.10	0.73	0.79	0.86	12.20	18.00	21.00	1.38	1.19	1.71
14	24.30	36.75	45.60	13.60	8.00	5.10	0.70	0.77	0.81	10.50	19.75	25.60	1.46	1.12	1.79
21	30.20	38.50	42.90	10.00	8.00	6.10	0.71	0.76	0.82	10.00	20.00	25.70	1.37	1.18	1.92
28	35.20	45.50	48.00	11.90	8.75	6.10	0.74	0.80	0.86	18.10	23.50	28.00	1.54	1.28	1.91
GA = 29-30 wk															
Day															
1	17.40	18.83	26.00	7.00	4.33	3.40	0.68	0.71	0.85	7.00	10.83	16.60	1.31	0.95	1.64
3	24.20	27.83	37.60	12.20	8.00	4.40	0.67	0.75	0.82	12.60	16.33	24.60	1.28	1.03	1.62
7	28.00	37.17	47.20	11.60	8.00	4.40	0.64	0.74	0.85	13.00	18.25	24.20	1.36	1.04	1.75
14	27.40	41.25	47.60	12.00	9.17	5.40	0.71	0.75	0.85	15.40	21.17	25.20	1.34	1.24	1.86
21	37.20	44.25	51.60	13.80	9.50	5.80	0.70	0.78	0.85	17.20	24.00	30.60	1.49	1.18	1.77
28	36.40	47.67	61.60	19.20	11.67	6.40	0.67	0.74	0.86	21.00	28.17	36.00	1.51	1.03	1.98
GA = 31-32 wk															
Day															
1	17.00	21.50	29.30	7.00	5.00	3.00	0.72	0.76	0.86	9.70	12.00	16.00	1.39	1.08	1.67
3	24.10	30.00	35.30	10.00	7.50	4.70	0.70	0.74	0.80	11.70	16.00	20.00	1.33	1.12	1.90
7	30.00	35.00	39.80	10.30	8.00	4.00	0.69	0.74	0.85	14.40	19.00	22.30	1.28	1.11	1.64
14	35.40	40.00	45.30	13.50	9.50	4.70	0.66	0.76	0.87	14.40	21.00	26.50	1.38	1.08	1.95
21	37.70	45.00	56.70	14.30	9.75	5.70	0.68	0.78	0.85	15.80	23.50	32.60	1.36	1.12	1.89
28	39.70	51.50	70.30	15.00	11.50	8.00	0.74	0.78	0.85	20.10	28.50	36.30	1.57	1.18	1.84
GA > 32 wk															
Day															
1	16.00	22.33	28.80	9.80	6.00	3.00	0.70	0.75	0.85	7.20	12.83	19.80	1.39	1.04	1.80
3	27.00	32.00	37.80	10.80	8.00	6.00	0.67	0.75	0.81	15.00	18.00	21.00	1.30	1.06	1.56
7	30.40	37.17	41.60	12.00	8.17	6.00	0.70	0.75	0.83	14.20	19.83	25.00	1.29	1.11	1.73
14	35.20	40.00	45.00	12.80	8.83	5.20	0.69	0.74	0.81	15.00	21.83	26.80	1.31	1.10	1.65
21	38.00	45.00	54.00	13.80	9.83	6.00	0.69	0.76	0.83	15.20	24.83	28.00	1.35	1.17	1.83
28	44.40	55.83	65.80	18.00	12.00	8.00	0.69	0.78	0.84	20.40	31.00	42.00	1.39	1.09	1.73

EDV = End diastolic velocity; GA = gestational age; ACA = Anterior cerebral artery; MV = Mean velocity; PI = Pulsatility index; PSV = Peak systolic velocity; RI = Resistance index
Reproduced with permission from Romagnoli C, Giannantonio C, De Carolis MP, et al. Neonatal color Doppler US study: normal values of cerebral blood flow velocities in preterm infants in the first month of life, Ultrasound. *Med Biol*. 2006 Mar;32(3):321–331.

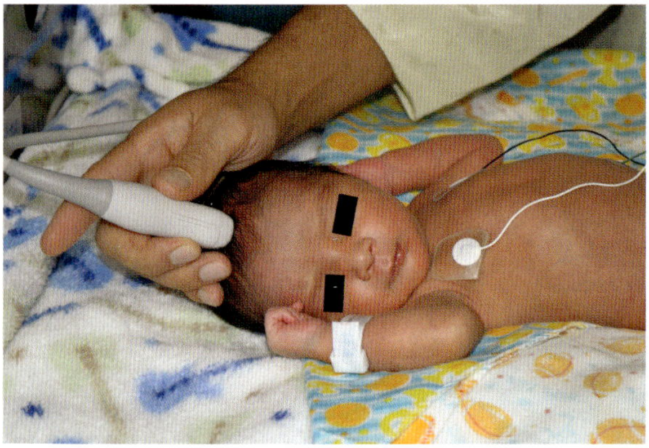

FIGURE 7-24. Transducer position for assessing anterior cerebral artery. Place the transducer on the anterior fontanelle in the midline, with the probe marker directed anteriorly.

anterior fontanelle is not possible or assessment of the A1 portion is desired.

Procedure. Place the transducer on the anterior fontanelle in the midline with the probe marker directed anteriorly (Figures 7-23 and 7-24). Set the field of view to 5-10 cm. Using 2D imaging, identify brain structure in sagittal view. Using the color box, tilt or slide the probe gently to identify the color flow of the ACA curving upward and coming toward the probe. Again, it is important to set the color scale low (eg, 10-20 cm/s) if low cerebral blood flow is suspected; otherwise, with a high color scale, visualization of vascular structure become very difficult. The sampling gate should be set to the smallest size due to the small diameter of the ACA. Place the PW Doppler cursor in the distal (A2) portion of the ACA in order to obtain the velocity profile (Figure 7-23). As for the temporal approach, the procedure is similar to Doppler interrogation of MCA except that, after the circle of Willis and MCA is identified, the probe is tilted slightly anteriorly to visualize the proximal portion of ACA (A1).

SUPERIOR MESENTERIC ARTERY

The celiac trunk and superior mesenteric artery (SMA) are the first arteries arising from the abdominal aorta. The celiac trunk branches off the anterior aspect of the abdominal aorta just below the diaphragm, and the SMA branches off a few millimeters below the celiac trunk. The SMA supplies nearly the entire small intestine (except for the superior portion of duodenum) and a good portion of the large intestine (the cecum, ascending and first half of transverse colon). Unlike the celiac trunk, which has a flow pattern typical of a low-resistance circulation (high forward flow during diastole), the flow pattern in SMA varies significantly and depends on feeding status. In a fasting state, the flow pattern is that of a high-resistance vascular bed with a low or absent diastolic flow. Conversely, the postprandial pattern is consistent with a low-resistance vascular bed with a high forward diastolic flow. However, in preterm infants the difference in fasting and postprandial flow patterns can be small. Furthermore, in the case of the right hepatic artery arising from the SMA rather than from the celiac trunk (a normal anatomic variation), the SMA flow pattern mimics that of the celiac trunk, even in the fasting state.

SMA Doppler flow changes with gestational and chronological age, but there can be significant variability.[30] The published data on normative values for SMA Doppler also varies.[30-34] An example of a population-based range of SMA Doppler values for different gestational and chronological ages is shown in Table 7-5.[34]

Technique

Assessment of Flow Pattern and Measurement of Velocity

Position. The patient should be placed in a supine position.

Transducer. In general, a lower frequency (in the range of 5-8 MHz) is preferable.

View. Abdominal.

Procedure. Place the transducer just below the xiphoid process and slightly left of the midline with the probe marker directed superiorly (Figure 7-25). Using 2D imaging, identify the abdominal aorta in a sagittal plane. Using color Doppler, identify the celiac trunk flow directed more or less straight toward the probe and the SMA flow also directed toward the probe but at an angle (Figure and Video 7-26). Remember to adjust the color scale low enough to visualize the low flow and high enough to prevent aliasing. Slide and tilt the probe sideways to decrease the angle of insonation. The sampling gate should be set to the smallest size due to the small diameter of the SMA. Place the PW Doppler cursor in the SMA, taking care to avoid interrogation of the celiac trunk, which can occur because of the close proximity of the two arteries and respiratory movement.

TABLE 7-5. Superior Mesentric Artery Doppler-derived Indices in Preterm and Term Infants During the First Postnatal Day of Life

	Day of Life	25–28 wk	29–32 wk	33–36 wk	37–41 wk
PSV (cm/s)	1	26±6	35±6	40±8	75±14
	3	31±5	50±11	59±9	86±14
	7	38±5	56±12	63±8	90±13
	14	43±8	64±11	71±9	
	21	55±9	66±11	75±10	
	28	62±8	75±9	88±12	
EDV (cm/s)	1	6±2	9±2	10±3	15±4
	3	8±2	10±2	13±4	20±7
	7	8±2	12±4	14±3	25±11
	14	10±4	12±3	15±4	
	21	12±4	15±4	16±6	
	28	13±4	17±4	21±9	
MV (cm/s)	1	12±4	19±4	19±6	35±11
	3	17±5	22±6	27±6	36±8
	7	17±5	24±5	31±7	38±9
	14	19±5	27±6	32±8	
	21	28±9	32±6	33±11	
	28	29±7	34±8	38±17	
RI	1	0.78±0.06	0.73±0.05	0.75±0.05	0.80±0.02
	3	0.74±0.07	0.79±0.04	0.78±0.06	0.77±0.05
	7	0.79±0.05	0.78±0.05	0.78±0.03	0.74±0.10
	14	0.76±0.05	0.80±0.04	0.79±0.04	
	21	0.80±0.05	0.77±0.06	0.78±0.05	
	28	0.80±0.05	0.78±0.05	0.79±0.07	
PI	1	1.76±0.58	1.41±0.37	1.67±0.47	1.78±0.35
	3	1.57±0.93	1.83±0.45	1.77±0.46	1.89±0.37
	7	1.84±0.56	1.85±0.49	1.69±0.32	1.82±0.50
	14	1.73±0.35	1.94±0.48	1.69±0.32	
	21	1.71±0.58	1.69±0.58	1.80±0.49	
	28	1.79±0.50	1.82±0.53	1.97±0.65	

EDV = End diastolic velocity; MV = Mean velocity; PI = Pulsatility index; PSV = Peak systolic velocity; RI = Resistance index
Reproduced with permission from Papacci P, Giannantonio C, Cota F, et al. Neonatal colour Doppler ultrasound study: normal values of abdominal blood flow velocities in the neonate during the first month of life. *Pediatr Radiol*. 2009 Apr;39(4):328–35.

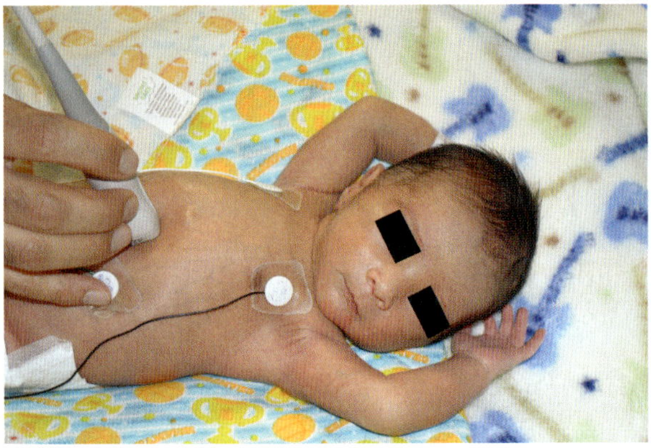

FIGURE 7-25. Transducer position for assessing the superior mesenteric artery. Place the transducer just below the xiphoid process and slightly left of the midline, with the probe marker directed superiorly.

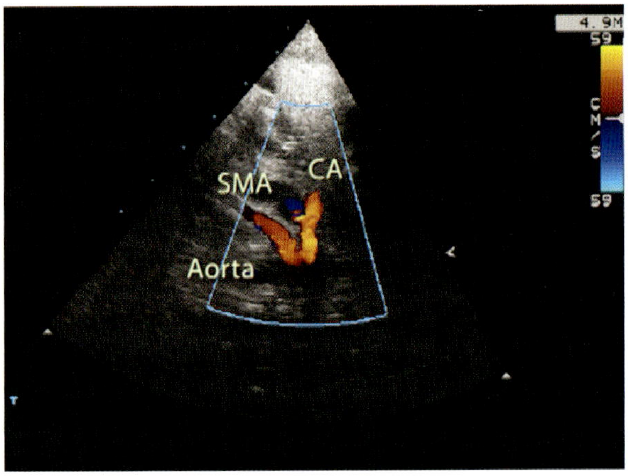

FIGURE and VIDEO 7-26. Color Doppler imaging of the celiac (CA) and superior mesenteric artery (SMA).

TABLE 7-6. The Range of Average Value for Common Renal Doppler Indices Reported in Different Studies

	PSV (cm/s)	EDV (cm/s)	MV (cm/s)	RI	PI
Preterm	22–53	5–7	19–22	0.75–0.87	1.51–1.79
Term	27–69	2–16	12–29	0.70–0.88	1.49–1.67

EDV = End diastolic velocity; MV = Mean velocity; PI = Pulsatility index; PSV = Peak systolic velocity; RI = Resistance index
Based on references 35–41.

RENAL ARTERY

The renal arteries branch off the abdominal aorta at almost a right angle at the level of the first to second lumbar vertebrae. At the level of the renal hilum, each renal artery divides into anterior and posterior branches. For the purpose of hemodynamic assessment, the renal artery should be evaluated before branching occurs.

Renal artery Doppler indices are affected by common conditions such as hypotension and PDA, and by frequently used medications such as dopamine and indomethacin. The Doppler indices also change with gestational and chronological ages. The average values for Doppler indices vary in different studies. Table 7-6 shows the average value ranges based on several publications.[35–41]

Technique

Assessment of Flow Pattern and Measurement of Velocity

Position. In a supine position, the proximal segment can be visualized. In slight lateral decubitus, the kidney and mid-distal segments can be visualized.

Transducer. In general, a lower frequency (in the range of 5-8 MHz) is preferable.

View. Mid-abdominal for visualizing the origin of the renal arteries, and flank approach to visualize the kidneys and mid to distal renal artery segments.

Procedure. For the purpose of hemodynamic assessment and evaluating the flow pattern in normal kidneys, the flank approach is adequate. Place the transducer on the flank a few centimeters above the level of umbilicus with the probe marker directed superiorly (Figure 7-27). Using 2D imaging, identify the kidney in its long axis. Using color Doppler, identify blood flow from the aorta to the renal hilum directed more or less straight toward the probe (Figure and Video 7-28). Slide and tilt the probe gently to decrease the angle of insonation. The sampling gate should be set to the smallest size due to the small diameter of the artery. Place the PW Doppler cursor in the renal artery prior to the point in which it branches in the renal hilum. Visualization of renal arteries can be limited due to excessive bowel gas.

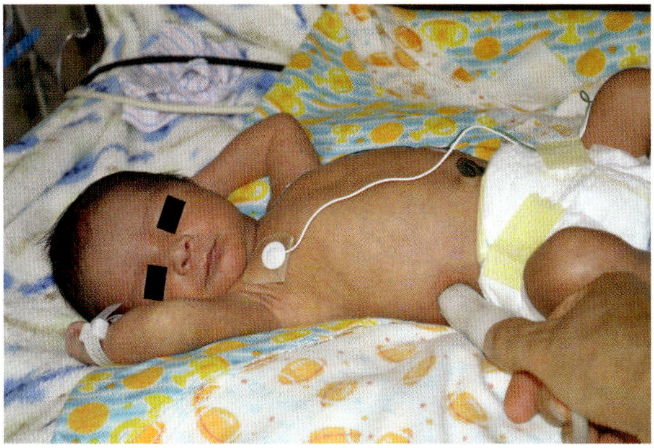

FIGURE 7-27. Transducer position for assessing renal artery. Place the transducer on the flank a few centimeters above the level of umbilicus, with the probe marker directed superiorly.

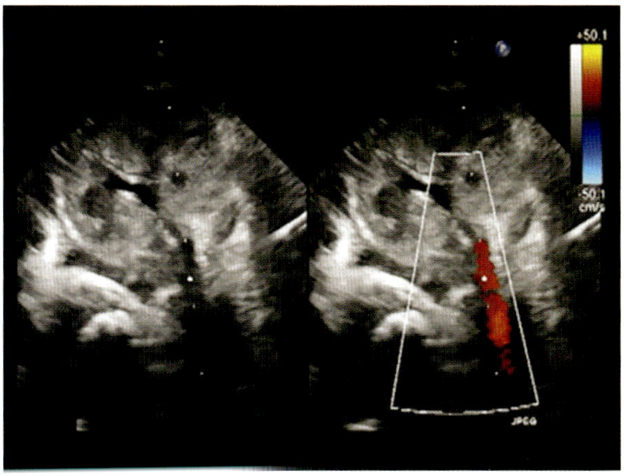

FIGURE and VIDEO 7-28. Color compare mode showing the renal artery.

REFERENCES

1. Noori S, Drabu B, Soleymani S, Seri I. Continuous noninvasive cardiac output measurements in the neonate by electrical velocimetry: a comparison with echocardiography. *Arch Dis Child Fetal Neonatal Ed.* 2012. doi:10.1136/archdischild-2011-301090.
2. Torigoe T, Sato S, Nagayama Y, Sato T, Yamazaki H. Influence of patent ductus arteriosus and ventilators on electrical velocimetry for measuring cardiac output in very-low/low birth weight infants. *J Perinatol.* 2015;35:485–489.
3. Trinkmann F, Berger M, Doesch C, et al. Comparison of electrical velocimetry and cardiac magnetic resonance imaging for the non-invasive determination of cardiac output. *J Clin Monit Comput.* 2016;30:399–408.
4. Alverson DC, Eldridge MW, Johnson JD, Aldrich M, Angelus P, Berman W Jr. Noninvasive measurement of cardiac output in healthy preterm and term newborn infants. *Am J Perinatol.* 1984;1:148–151.
5. Walther FJ, Siassi B, Ramadan NA, Ananda AK, Wu PY. Pulsed Doppler determinations of cardiac output in neonates: normal standards for clinical use. *Pediatrics.* 1985;76:829–833.
6. Alverson DC, Aldrich M, Angelus P, Backstrom C, Werner S. Longitudinal trends in left ventricular cardiac output in healthy infants in the first year of life. *J Ultrasound Med.* 1987;6:519–524.
7. Mandelbaum VH, Alverson DC, Kirchgessner A, Linderkamp O. Postnatal changes in cardiac output and haemorrheology in normal neonates born at full term. *Arch. Dis. Child.* 1991;66:391–394.
8. Agata Y, Hiraishi S, Oguchi K, et al. Changes in left ventricular output from fetal to early neonatal life. *J. Pediatr.* 119:441–445.
9. Evans N, Kluckow M. Early determinants of right and left ventricular output in ventilated preterm infants. *Arch Dis Child Fetal Neonatal Ed.* 1996;74:F88–F94.
10. Schmitz L, Stiller B, Pees C, Koch H, Xanthopoulos A, Lange P. Doppler-derived parameters of diastolic left ventricular function in preterm infants with a birth weight <1500 g: reference values and differences to term infants. *Early Hum Dev.* 2004;76:101–114.
11. Groves AM, Kuschel CA, Knight DB, Skinner JR. Does retrograde diastolic flow in the descending aorta signify impaired systemic perfusion in preterm infants? *Pediatr Res.* 2008;63:89–94.
12. Sehgal A, Mak W, Dunn M, et al. Haemodynamic changes after delivery room surfactant administration to very low birth weight infants. *Arch Dis Child Fetal Neonatal Ed.* 2010;95:F345–F351
13. Sloot SC, de Waal KA, van der Lee JH, van Kaam AH. Central blood flow measurements in stable preterm infants after the transitional period. *Arch. Dis. Child. Fetal Neonatal Ed.* 2010;95:F369–F372.
14. Noori S, Drabu B, McCoy M, Sekar K. Non-invasive measurement of local tissue perfusion and its correlation with hemodynamic indices during the early postnatal period in term neonates. *J Perinatol.* 2011;31:785–788.
15. Noori S, Wlodaver A, Gottipati V, McCoy M, Schultz D, Escobedo M. Transitional changes in cardiac and cerebral hemodynamics in term neonates at birth. *J. Pediatr.* 2012;160:943–948.
16. Tsai-Goodman B, Martin RP, Marlow N, Skinner JR. The repeatability of echocardiographic determination of right ventricular output in the newborn. *Cardiol Young.* 2001;11:188–194.

17. Kluckow M, Evans N. Superior vena cava flow in newborn infants: a novel marker of systemic blood flow. *Arch Dis Child Fetal Neonatal Ed*. 2000;82:F182–F187.

18. Holberton JR, Drew SM, Mori R, König K. The diagnostic value of a single measurement of superior vena cava flow in the first 24 h of life in very preterm infants. *Eur J Pediatr*. 2012. doi:10.1007/s00431-012-1755-z.

19. Kluckow M, Evans N. Low superior vena cava flow and intraventricular haemorrhage in preterm infants. *Arch Dis Child Fetal Neonatal Ed*. 2000;82:F188–F194.

20. Hunt RW, Evans N, Rieger I, Kluckow M. Low superior vena cava flow and neurodevelopment at 3 years in very preterm infants. *J Pediatr*. 2004;145:588–592.

21. Osborn DA, Evans N, Kluckow M, Bowen JR, Rieger I. Low superior vena cava flow and effect of inotropes on neurodevelopment to 3 years in preterm infants. *Pediatrics*. 2007;120:372–380.

22. Paradisis M, Evans N, Kluckow M, Osborn D. Randomized trial of milrinone versus placebo for prevention of low systemic blood flow in very preterm infants. *J. Pediatr*. 2009;154:189–195.

23. Hansen NB, Stonestreet BS, Rosenkrantz TS, Oh W. Validity of Doppler measurements of anterior cerebral artery blood flow velocity: correlation with brain blood flow in piglets. *Pediatrics*. 1983;72:526–531.

24. Greisen G, Johansen K, Ellison PH, Fredriksen PS, Mali J, Friis-Hansen B. Cerebral blood flow in the newborn infant: comparison of Doppler ultrasound and 133xenon clearance. *J Pediatr*. 1984;104:411–418.

25. Raju TN. Cerebral Doppler studies in the fetus and newborn infant. *J. Pediatr*. 1991;119:165–174.

26. Ozek E, Köroğlu TF, Karakoç F, et al. Transcranial Doppler assessment of cerebral blood flow velocity in term newborns. *Eur J Pediatr*. 1995;154:60–63.

27. Pezzati M, Dani C, Biadaioli R, et al. Early postnatal doppler assessment of cerebral blood flow velocity in healthy preterm and term infants. *Dev Med Child Neurol*. 2002;44:745–752.

28. Evans N, Kluckow M, Simmons M, Osborn D. Which to measure, systemic or organ blood flow? Middle cerebral artery and superior vena cava flow in very preterm infants. *Arch Dis Child Fetal Neonatal Ed*. 2002;87:F181–184s.

29. Romagnoli C, Giannantonio C, De Carolis MP, Gallini F, Zecca E, Papacci P. Neonatal color Doppler US study: normal values of cerebral blood flow velocities in preterm infants in the first month of life. *Ultrasound Med Biol*. 2006;32:321–331.

30. Havranek T, Miladinovic B, Wadhawan R, Carver JD. Factors that affect the postnatal increase in superior mesenteric artery blood flow velocity in very low birth weight preterm infants. *J Perinat Med*. 2012;40:565–570.

31. Leidig E. Pulsed Doppler ultrasound blood flow measurements in the superior mesenteric artery of the newborn. *Pediatr Radiol*. 1989;19:169–172.

32. Van Bel F, Van Zwieten PH, Guit GL, Schipper J. Superior mesenteric artery blood flow velocity and estimated volume flow: duplex Doppler US study of preterm and term neonates. *Radiology*. 1990;174:165–169.

33. Martinussen M, Brubakk AM, Vik T, Yao AC. Mesenteric blood flow velocity and its relation to transitional circulatory adaptation in appropriate for gestational age preterm infants. *Pediatr Res*. 1996;39:275–280.

34. Papacci P, Giannantonio C, Cota F, et al. Neonatal colour Doppler ultrasound study: normal values of abdominal blood flow velocities in the neonate during the first month of life. *Pediatr Radiol*. 2009;39:328–335.

35. Bömelburg T, Jorch G. Investigations of renal artery blood flow velocity in preterm and term neonates by pulsed Doppler ultrasonography. *Eur J Pediatr*. 1988;147:283–287.

36. Agata Y, Hiraishi S, Misawa H, et al. Regional blood flow distribution and left ventricular output during early neonatal life: a quantitative ultrasonographic assessment. *Pediatr Res*. 1994;36:805–810.

37. Cleary GM, Higgins ST, Merton DA, Cullen JA, Gottlieb RP, Baumgart S. Developmental changes in renal artery blood flow velocity during the first three weeks of life in preterm neonates. *J Pediatr*. 1996;129:251–257.

38. Pezzati M, Danesi G, Pozzessere A, Cosenza EB, Rubaltelli FF. Renal blood flow velocity in preterm and term neonates during the fourth day of life: changes in relation to gestational age and birth weight. *Biol Neonate*. 1998;73:19–23.

39. Andriani G, Persico A, Tursini S, Ballone E, Cirotti D, Lelli Chiesa P. The renal-resistive index from the last 3 months of pregnancy to 6 months old. *BJU Int*. 2001;87:562–564.

40. Yildirim H, Gungor S, Cihangiroglu MM, Aygun AD. Doppler studies in normal kidneys of preterm and term neonates: changes in relation to gestational age and birth weight. *J Ultrasound Med*. 2005;24:623–627.

41. Ilves P, Lintrop M, Talvik I, Muug K, Asser K, Veinla M. Developmental changes in cerebral and visceral blood flow velocity in healthy neonates and infants. *J Ultrasound Med*. 2008;27:199–207.

CHAPTER 8

Assessment of Systolic, Diastolic, and Global Cardiac Function*

Shahab Noori

- INTRODUCTION
- SYSTOLIC FUNCTION
  - Shortening Fraction
  - Ejection Fraction
    - Linear Left Ventricular Minor-axis Dimensions
    - Modified Simpson's Biplane Method
  - Velocity of Circumferential Fiber Shortening
  - Stress-Velocity Index
  - Wall Stress
- DIASTOLIC FUNCTION
  - Mitral and Tricuspid Flow Doppler
  - Tissue Doppler
  - Pulmonary Vein Doppler
- GLOBAL MYOCARDIAL FUNCTION
  - Myocardial Performance Index

INTRODUCTION

In the previous chapter, methods of estimation of cardiac output and organ blood flow indices were discussed. These are essential components of the echocardiographic assessment of adequacy of cardiovascular function. The current chapter focuses upon the noninvasive assessment of systolic and diastolic cardiac function.

SYSTOLIC FUNCTION

Shortening Fraction

Assessment of systolic function is a basic component of functional echocardiography. Shortening fraction (SF), also known as fractional shortening, is the most commonly used index of left ventricular systolic function in children. This index reflects the degree of myocardial fiber shortening during systole. As the loading condition affects the initial myocardial fiber length (preload effect) and the degree of shortening (afterload effect), this index of cardiac systolic function is considered to be load-dependent. Therefore, changes in loading condition impact the myocardial contractility as assessed by SF without necessarily a change in the inherent myocardial function. In addition, the most commonly used method to measure SF has significant limitations (see below). Nevertheless, SF provides the clinician with a simple and quick way to assess myocardial systolic function. Assessment of SF is generally performed with M-mode echocardiography (see also Chapter 5).

*Videos can be accessed at http://PracticalNeonatalEcho.com.

The normal value of SF for all gestational and postnatal ages is considered to be in range between 27% and 42%. In hemodynamically stable preterm infants ≤30 weeks' gestation, average SF was 34%±5% (range 23–48%) in the first 3 postnatal days and 38%±6% (range 25–51%) from 4–14 days after birth.[1]

Technique

Position. The patient should be placed in a supine position.

Transducer. For better resolution, a high-frequency (10–12 MHz) probe is preferable.

View. Optimal visualization of the left ventricle (LV) can be achieved using standard parasternal short- or long-axis views. In neonates it is preferable to use a parasternal short-axis view.

Procedure. Using the parasternal short-axis view, obtain a cross section of the LV at the level of the papillary muscles or the tip of mitral valve leaflet (Figure 8-1). The latter is preferred in neonates. Care should be taken to obtain a two-dimensional (2D) image of the cross section of the LV in such a way as to have mitral valve closure as a horizontal line. Next, place the M-mode line to be perpendicular to the septum, the above-mentioned horizontal line, and the posterior wall, with about equal distance between the two papillary muscles. Initiating the M-mode setting on the ultrasound machine will yield the motion of the various structures along the M-mode line.

Measurement. It is customary to start by measuring the right ventricle internal diameter in diastole followed in sequence by measuring the ventricular septal thickness, LV internal diameter (LVIDD), and posterior wall thickness in diastole. Subsequently, in systole the septal thickness, LV internal diameter (LVIDS), and posterior wall thickness are measured. Normal data for the above measurements varies for different gestational ages and weights.[2–4] For the purpose of estimating SF, only LVIDD and LVIDS are needed. The echo system will automatically calculate SF, provided the above measurements are assigned using the analysis package of the system. SF is calculated as [(LVIDD−LVIDS)/LVIDD]×100. The above measurements can also be performed using 2D images. However, M-mode has better temporal resolution and is preferable in the neonatal population.[5]

Limitations

The main limitation of SF in estimating contractility and systolic function is generalizability of relative linear

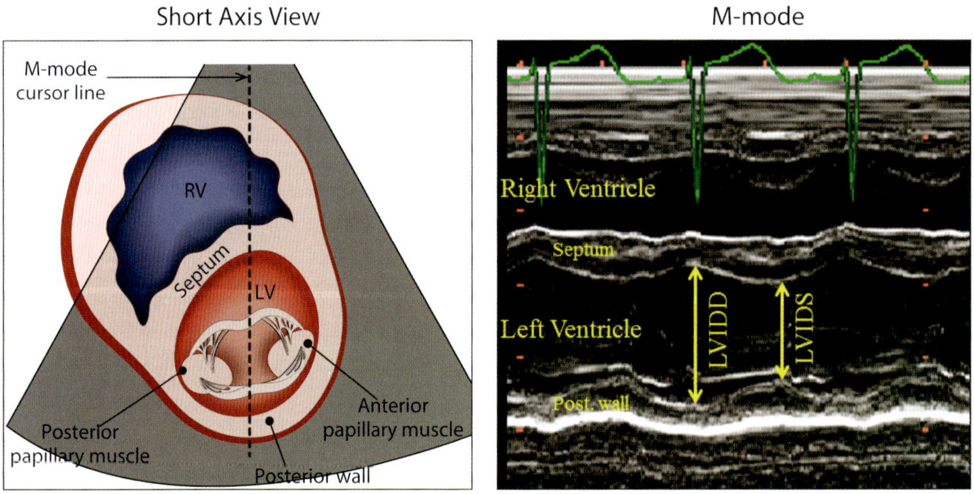

FIGURE 8-1. A schematic drawing of the short-axis view of the heart at the level of mitral valve tip. The dotted line on the drawing depicts where the M-mode cursor line is placed. The motion of various structures along this dotted line is displayed in the M-mode tracing. For the purpose of measuring the shortening fraction, an M-mode tracing of the short-axis view of the heart at the level of papillary muscles or tip of the mitral valve is obtained. In neonates, it is preferable to obtain M-mode at the level of the tips of mitral valve. Left ventricular internal diameter in diastole (LVIDD) and systole (LVIDS) are measured as shown.

movement of the two points along the M-mode cursor (the endocardial borders of the ventricular septum and the LV posterior wall) to the entire LV myocardium. While in normal myocardium this is not an issue, in pathological conditions, where accurate estimate of systolic function is even more important, SF may not reflect the overall contractile function of the LV. In the presence of myocardial dysfunction, different parts of the myocardium can have different degrees of fiber shortening. For example, the LV might have greater shortening in the lateral direction compared to the anteroposterior direction. In such a case, the SF (which measures shortening in anteroposterior direction) would underestimate overall LV systolic function (Figures and Videos 8-2 to Figure 8-4). In the case of elevated pulmonary artery pressure, the septal wall may be flattened or bowed into the LV, or the motion might be paradoxical (Figure and Video 8-5). Similarly, the septal and posterior wall motion might be dyskinetic in dilated cardiomyopathy, rendering SF much less useful as a measure of myocardial function (Figure and Video 8-6). In such cases, measuring changes in area can be more useful than SF. To measure fractional change in area, a 2D cross section of the LV at the level of the tips of the mitral valve is obtained using parasternal short-axis view (similar to SF measurement). Fractional area change is calculated using the formula [(LVAD−LVAS)/LVAD]×100, where LVAD and LVAS are LV area (traced by planimetry) at the end of diastole and systole, respectively. There are limited data on the normal ranges in neonates; in adults, a value > 36% is considered normal.[6] Alternatively, volumetric changes (ejection fraction) can be used when septal motion is abnormal, as will be discussed below. Another limitation of SF is load dependency; however, most echocardiographic indices of systolic function share this limitation.

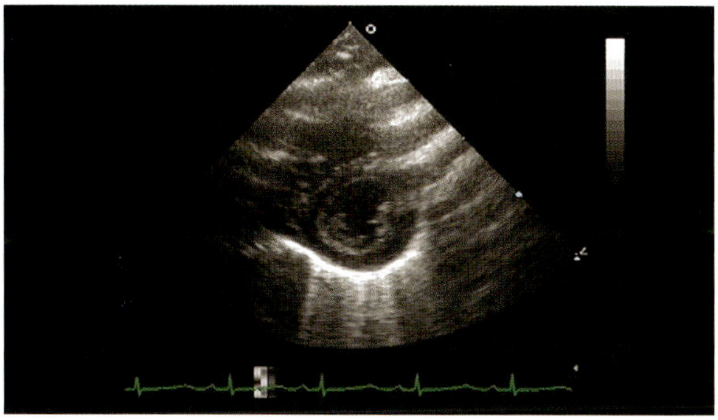

FIGURE and VIDEO 8-2. Short-axis view of the left ventricle in an extremely preterm infant. In the video, note the greater change in left ventricular diameter in the lateral direction compared to the anteroposterior direction. (Also see Figures 8-3 and 8-4.)

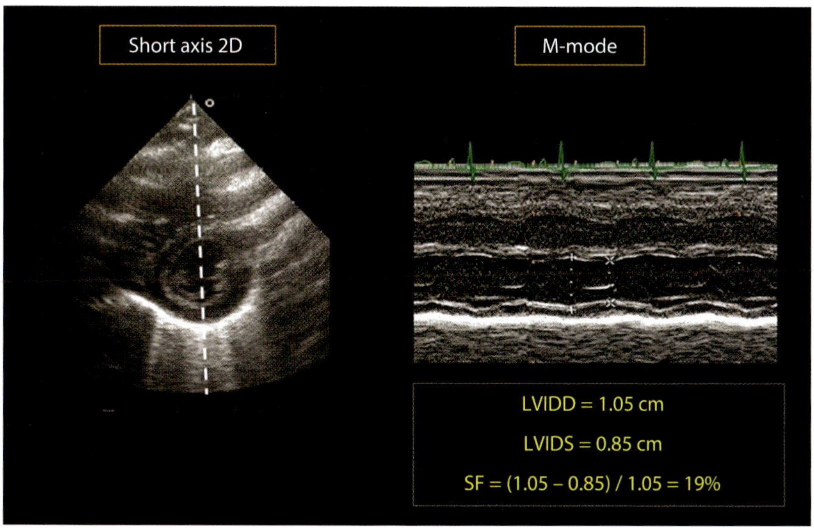

FIGURE 8-3. On the left, a short-axis view of the left ventricle at the level of the tip of the mitral valve is shown. Note the dotted line representing the thin section of the heart where the M-mode tracing is obtained. On the right, the M-mode tracing with the measurements of left ventricular internal diameter in diastole (LVIDD) and systole (LVIDS) is displayed. Using these measurements, the shortening fraction (SF) is 19%.

Ejection Fraction

Ejection fraction (EF) is another measure of the LV systolic function. This index is an estimate of the proportion of LV volume that is ejected during each cardiac cycle. There are several ways to estimate EF. Two echocardiographic methods that can be used to calculate EF include (1) methods based upon linear LV M-mode minor-axis dimensions and (2) modified Simpson's biplane. The area-length, or bullet, method is another way to estimate EF.[7] This method is more laborious, as it involves measurements in both minor and major axis and is not further discussed.

Linear Left Ventricular Minor-axis Dimensions

This method is essentially the same as the method of measuring SF. The parasternal short axis view of heart and M-mode are used to measure LVIDD and LVIDS. EF is calculated by $[(LVIDD^3 - LVIDS^3)/LVIDD^3] \times 100$, and the normal value ranges from 56% to 78%. Given the fact that one is cubing the same diameter used in the calculation of SF, the limitations of this index are also the same as those for SF mentioned above. Therefore, this method of calculation of EF is not useful when the same conditions exist that interfere with the utility of SF (discussed above).

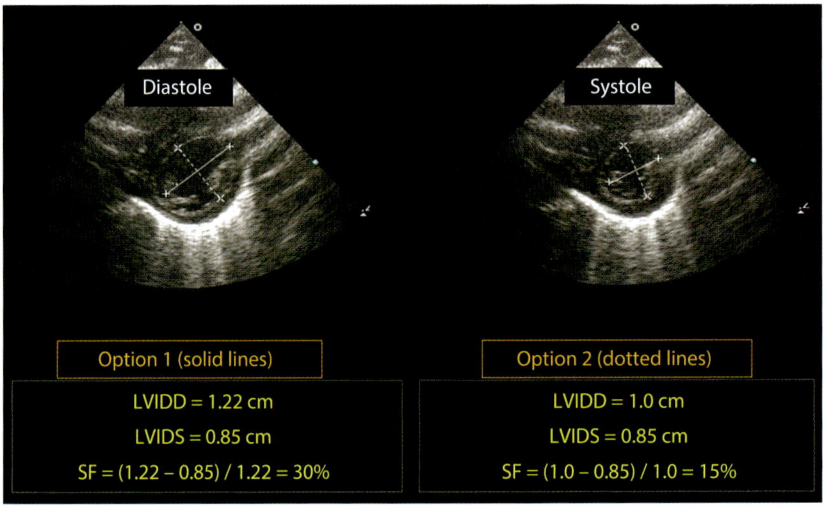

FIGURE 8-4. Two-dimensional views of the left ventricle in diastole (left) and systole (right). Shortening fraction (SF) is calculated based on 2D measurements of left ventricular internal diameter in diastole (LVIDD) and systole (LVIDS) in two different orientations (the solid and dotted lines). Limitation of SF in estimating systolic function is evident in this example, as using different orientations yield very different results.

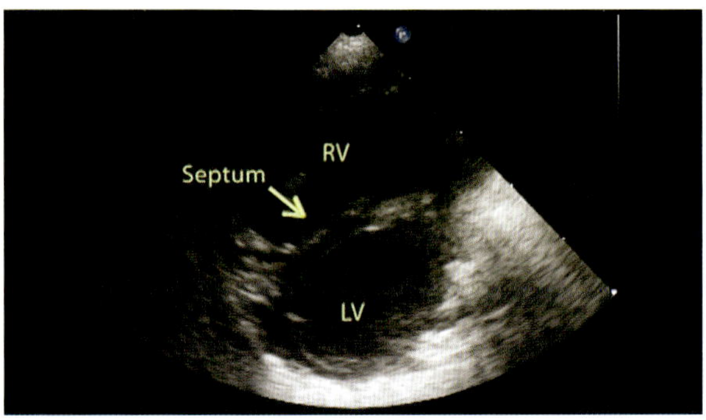

FIGURE and VIDEO 8-5. Short-axis view of the left ventricle in an infant with pulmonary hypertension. In the video, note the dilated right ventricle (RV) and flattening of the septum (arrow). Abbreviation: LV, left ventricle.

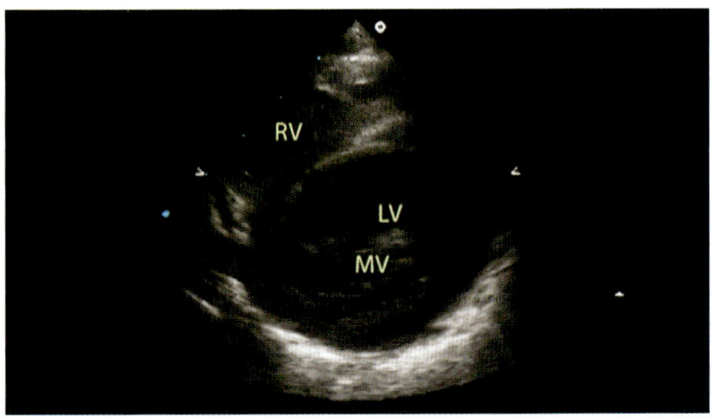

FIGURE and VIDEO 8-6. Short-axis view of the left ventricle in an infant with dilated cardiomyopathy. In the video, note dyskinetic motion of interventricular septum and left ventricular (LV) free wall motion. Abbreviations: MV, mitral valve; RV, right ventricle.

Modified Simpson's Biplane Method

Technique

Position. The patient should be placed in a supine or in a slight left lateral decubitus position.

Transducer. For better resolution, a high frequency (10–12 MHz) probe is preferable

View. Optimal visualization of the LV for this purpose can be achieved using an apical four- or two-chamber views (Figure and Video 8-7).

Procedure. Using the apical view, obtain a longitudinal section of the LV through the mitral valve. Adjust the image gains and contrast (compression) so that there is good endocardial border definition and discrimination between the blood/tissue interface. Care should be taken to obtain a 2D image where the endocardial border is clearly visible. In addition, one must be aware of potential of foreshortening the LV.

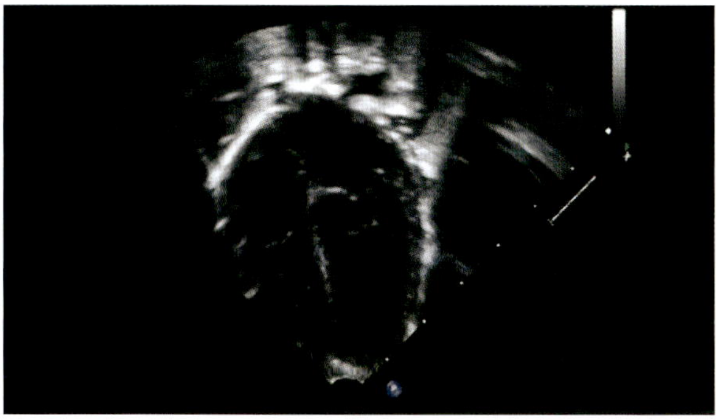

FIGURE and VIDEO 8-7. Apical four-chamber view of the heart.

Measurement. First, the endocardium and mitral valve plane are traced during diastole, and then the longitudinal axis is determined by measuring the distance from the apex to the midpoint of mitral valve plane (Figure 8-8). The mitral valve plane is determined by a line connecting the lateral and medial hinge points. The echocardiography machine built-in software calculates the volume based on the assumption that the LV is cone shaped and consists of a series of discs. The calculated volume is the end-diastolic volume (EDV). The same process is then repeated at end-systole to determine the end-systolic volume (ESV). The EF (expressed as a percentage) is calculated as [(EDV−ESV)/EDV]×100, with a normal value being 56–78%. This method can also be used to estimate stroke volume (EDV-ESV) and ventricular output ([EDV−ESV]×heart rate). Of note, when one is tracing the blood-endocardium interface, it is customary to include the papillary muscles in the blood pool. Newer echocardiography systems have the autotrace capability.

Limitations

The main limitation of the modified Simpson's method in estimating EF is the difficulty in obtaining high-quality images with adequate enough resolution to visualize clearly the endocardial border. The procedure requires slightly more time to perform than SF, which is another shortcoming of the method. Finally, load dependency is another limitation of this method.

Velocity of Circumferential Fiber Shortening

Velocity of circumferential fiber shortening (VCF) is another measure of contractility and systolic function. Like SF, VCF is also load-dependent, but it is thought to be less preload-dependent and less sensitive to abnormal

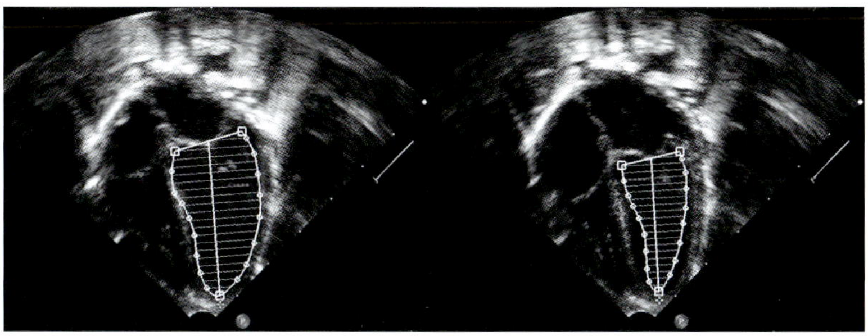

FIGURE 8-8. An example of measurement of ejection fraction (EF) using the modified Simpson method. Some echocardiography system can autotrace the endocardium as in this example. The end-diastolic volume (EDV) and end-systolic volume (ESV) are 6 and 2 ml, respectively. Using [(EDV−ESV)/EDV]×100, the EF is 67%.

septal motion. VCF is significantly affected by changes in heart rate; as such, it is often corrected for heart rate (VCF_C). This measure of contractility is not currently part of routine assessment of cardiac function. However, as discussed below, one needs to calculate VCF_C in order to assess the stress-velocity index, a load-independent index of contractility.

Technique

Position. The patient should be placed in a supine position.

Transducer. For better resolution, a high-frequency (10–12 MHz) probe is preferable

View. To measure VCF, two views of the heart are needed. The first view can be a parasternal short-axis (preferable) or standard parasternal long-axis. This is the same view used for measuring SF. The second view is apical five-chamber.

Procedure. The first step of the procedure is the same as the one used for measuring SF (see above). In this step, the relative motion of interventricular septum and posterior wall are assessed by M-mode. The second step involves Doppler interrogation of the aortic flow at the valve level from the apical five-chamber view. After obtaining a four-chamber apical view of the heart, turn the transducer slightly counterclockwise and anteriorly to visualize the LV outflow track and proximal part of ascending aorta. Take care to obtain an upright 2D image of heart. Next, place the Doppler gate at the aortic valve level. Activating the PW-Doppler button will produce the spectral Doppler envelope of aortic flow velocity. From this tracing, the LV ejection time (LVET) can be calculated using the duration of aortic flow. Alternatively, LVET can be calculated from the duration of aortic valve opening using M-mode tracing of aortic valve in parasternal long-axis view.

Measurement. The first step in measuring VCF is the same as for SF. In this step, LVIDD and LVIDS are measured. Next, LVET can be measured using the duration of the aortic flow spectral Doppler envelope obtained in apical five-chamber view (discussed above). Care must be taken to ensure that the heart rate is similar during the M-mode and Doppler image acquisitions. Alternatively, using the M-mode at the level of aortic valve in parasternal long-axis view, LVET can be calculated as the time span from opening to closure of aortic valve. The echo system will automatically calculate VCF, provided the above measurements are assigned using analysis package of the system. VCF is calculated as [(LVIDD−LVIDS)/LVIDD]/LVET. However, VCF is affected by changes in heart rate (because LVET is heart rate-dependent). Therefore, VCF is often corrected for heart rate to yield VCF_C. To calculate the VCF_C, the duration of the cardiac cycle (R-R interval) is measured. This can be obtained from the M-mode image used for measurement of LVIDD and LVIDS; in this view, two identical points from either the electrocardiogram (ECG) or the M-mode tracing can be used to measure the R-R interval. Alternatively, the spectral Doppler tracing of the aortic valve can be used (provided the heart rate is similar to the M-mode); the time span between two identical points on the ECG or from the start of one Doppler envelope to the next is used to derive the R-R value. Once the R-R interval is obtained, the echocardiography machine software calculates the VCF_C using the following formula: $VCF_C = VCF \times \sqrt{RR}$. The normal VCF_C is 1.28±0.22 circ/s in full-term neonates and 1.08±0.14 circ/s in the older pediatric population.[8] In hemodynamically stable preterm infants, we have found an average VCF_C to be 1.22±0.26 circ/s (range 0.78–1.77) in the first 3 postnatal days and 1.45±0.27 circ/s (range 0.89–2.21) from 4–14 days after birth.[1]

Limitations

In general, the limitations of VCF_C are similar to SF except that it is less sensitive to abnormal geometry of the ventricle (see above).

Stress-Velocity Index, Part 1

The stress-velocity index is a measure of myocardial contractility that is largely load-independent. In other words, the stress-velocity index represents true contractile function of the myocardium, whereas SF and VCF_C represent systolic function of the myocardium for a given preload and afterload. Both load-dependent and load-independent measures of contractility provide important and clinically relevant information. SF and VCF_C provide information on the myocardial systolic function with the current loading conditions. Conversely, in the case of the stress-velocity index, one can gain insight into the myocardial contractility capability relative to the normal heart, independent of any loading conditions. The stress-velocity index is defined as the relationship between VCF_C and wall stress (WS). Prior to any further discussion of the index, it is important to first describe the derivation of WS, which is given in the subsequent section.

Wall Stress

Wall stress (WS) is a measure of afterload; afterload is the force that the LV has to overcome to pump blood out of the ventricle into the aorta during systole. This force can be estimated, as it exerts its effect per unit area in the direction of apex-base (meridional) or in the direction of minor axis (circumferential). Because meridional WS is easier to estimate and correlates well with circumferential WS, meridional WS is more commonly used. In this book, all further comments and discussions on WS are made with reference to meridional WS.

While the concept of preload in terms of end-diastolic volume is relatively easy to grasp, afterload can be more difficult. Indeed, afterload is often confused with systemic vascular resistance (SVR). While related, WS and SVR are two different indices of cardiovascular function. SVR is resistance to flow generated by characteristics of vasculature, vascular tone, and viscosity of the blood, and according to Ohm's law, $SVR=\Delta P/Q$, where ΔP is the pressure gradient (Mean blood pressure – Central venous pressure) and Q is the cardiac output. On the other hand, WS depends on the LV cavity pressure and diameter and LV wall thickness, according to the law of Laplace. The law of Laplace states that surface tension (ie, WS) is directly related to LV cavity pressure and diameter and inversely related to wall thickness. Because the pressure, diameter, and wall thickness change during the cardiac cycle, WS also varies during the cardiac cycle. The best indicator of afterload as a limiting factor for myocardial contractility is the end-systolic WS. While LV cavity diameter and wall thickness can be measured noninvasively by echocardiography, end-systolic ventricular pressure can only be measured invasively. Tracing the arterial pressure waveform may be helpful, as the arterial pressure at the time of the dicrotic notch on the pressure waveform corresponds to the ventricular pressure at the end of systole. However, this type of tracing, which can be obtained noninvasively, is cumbersome to perform routinely. Fortunately, several investigators have shown that the mean arterial blood pressure correlates well with end-systolic ventricular pressure. Because this value is much easier to measure, it can be used for the calculation of end-systolic WS.[9]

Technique

Position. The patient should be placed in a supine position.

Transducer. For better resolution, a high-frequency (10–12 MHz) probe is preferable.

View. To measure wall stress, the parasternal short axis view is used.

Procedure. The procedure is the same as the one used for measuring SF (see above).

Measurement. The LVIDS and posterior wall thickness in systole (PWS) are measured using M-mode tracing image. Blood pressure at the time of M-mode tracing acquisition is recorded (as discussed above, mean blood pressure is an adequate surrogate for end-systolic ventricular pressure). The echo system will automatically calculate the WS, provided the above measurements are assigned using analysis package of the system. WS is calculated as $(0.334\ P\times LVIDS) / (PWS\ [1+(PWS/LVIDS)])$. The normal WS is 30.2 ± 8.7 g/cm^2 in full-term neonates and 37.3 ± 8.8 g/cm^2 in the older pediatric population.[8] In hemodynamically stable preterm infants, we have found an average WS to be 28.4 ± 12.3 g/cm^2 (range 8.2–86.6) in the first 3 postnatal days and 20.1 ± 8 g/cm^2 (range 7.4–43.6) from 4–14 days after birth.[1]

Limitations

Inaccuracy in estimating LVIDS due to septal motion abnormalities can affect the accuracy of WS.

Stress-Velocity, Part 2

Now that VCF_C and WS have been defined, the discussion on the stress-velocity index can continue. When one plots the VCF_C obtained for any given WS value, the graph that is produced is known as the stress-velocity index. There is an inverse relationship between the two parameters, such that the graph that is produced is negative and linear: the higher the wall stress, the lower the VCF_C (Figure 8-9). However, in neonates the y-intercept of this regression line is higher and the slope is steeper than in older children. In other words, the myocardium functions at a higher baseline contractile state and is more sensitive to increase in afterload than older children. Some studies have found an even higher y-intercept and steeper line in preterm compared to full-term neonates,[10,11] while others found no such a difference.[12]

The stress-velocity index is usually presented as a z-score. Z-score is based upon population normative data, with one z-score equivalent to one standard deviation. Normal contractility is considered to be with ±2 standard deviations; therefore, normal is considered a z-score of ± 2, with $>+2$ and <-2 representing a hyperdynamic state and poor contractility, respectively. For a given

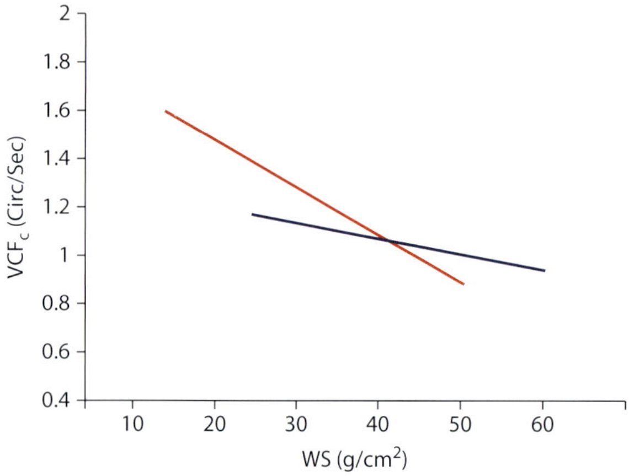

FIGURE 8-9. The blue line represents the normal inverse relationship that exists between the heart rate-corrected velocity of circumferential shortening (VCF_C, myocardial contractility) and the wall stress (WS, afterload) in children. In neonates, the y-intercept of the regression line (red) is higher and the slope is steeper than in older children. In other words, the myocardium functions at a higher baseline contractile state and with an increase in afterload the contractility of immature myocardium decreases more than that of the mature heart of older children. (Modified with permission from Rowland DG and Gutgesell HP. Noninvasive assessment of myocardial contractility, preload, and afterload in healthy newborn infants. *Am J Cardiol*. 1995;75(12):818–821.)

end-systolic WS, the z-score is estimated as follows: [VCF_C (actual)$-VCF_C$(calc)] /SD, where VCF_C (actual) is the measured heart rate-corrected velocity of circumferential fiber shortening, VCF_C(calc) is the calculated VCF_C based on measured WS and the normal relationship between VCF_C and WS (based upon a normal population), and SD is the standard deviation of VCF_C of the normal population. Based upon normative data in full-term neonates,[8] VCF_C(calc) is calculated as -0.020 mWS + 1.88. Standard deviation (SD) of VCF_C in normal population is 0.22. For example, if measured VCF_C and WS are 0.91 circ/s and 10 g/cm^2, respectively, the VCF_C(calc) is $(-0.020\times10)+$ 1.88 or 1.68 circ/s. The z-score would be [0.91–1.68]/0.22 or – 3.5. In this example the contractility is reduced (3.5 SD below the mean for normal population). In hemodynamically stable preterm infants, VCF_C (calc) can be calculated using -0.0123 mWS + 1.58, with SD 0.23 for the transitional period (first 3 days) and -0.0241 mWS +1.93 with SD 0.27 for postnatal day 4–14.[1]

DIASTOLIC FUNCTION

Assessment of diastolic function is important and useful for the diagnosis and management of patients with cardiovascular compromise. This might be even more important in the neonatal population, as the immature myocardium in preterm and full-term infants is known to have reduced diastolic function due to poor compliance. However, challenges in finding appropriate echocardiographic methods and the lack of specificity of the currently available echocardiographic indices have often resulted in complete omission of evaluation of diastolic function during routine echocardiography.

The two main components of diastole are ventricular relaxation and compliance. Ventricular relaxation is an active, complex, energy-dependent process. In adults, relaxation abnormalities occur early in disease states, resulting in poor filling in early diastole and relative increase in filling with atrial contraction. Ventricular relaxation can be assessed by peak negative change in LV pressure over time ($-dP/dt$), and also by the time constant of relaxation (τ), which is generally measured invasively by cardiac catheterization. On the other hand, ventricular compliance is passive and defined as change in volume over change in pressure. As mentioned earlier, the immature neonatal myocardium has inherently poorly compliance. Further decrease in compliance can be caused by myocardial stiffness, increased pericardial constraint (eg, pericardial effusion), and increase intraventricular volume. Other factors that can affect diastole include systolic function, left atrial pressure, and intrathoracic pressure.

For the analysis of diastolic function, it is useful to divide diastole into four phases: (1) *isovolumetric relaxation,* which depends on systolic function and relaxation; (2) *early rapid filling,* which depends upon both ventricular relaxation and compliance; (3) *diastasis,* which depends upon heart rate and ventricular compliance, and (4) *atrial contraction,* which represents atrial contraction (corresponding to the P-wave on the ECG) and depends on both atrial function and ventricular compliance.

The gold standard methods for assessment of diastolic function are the time constant of relaxation (τ) and the pressure-volume curve (compliance). However, both these methods require cardiac catheterization and as such are too invasive for clinical use in the neonatal and infant population. Nevertheless, echocardiographic methods are available for the general noninvasive assessment of diastolic function.

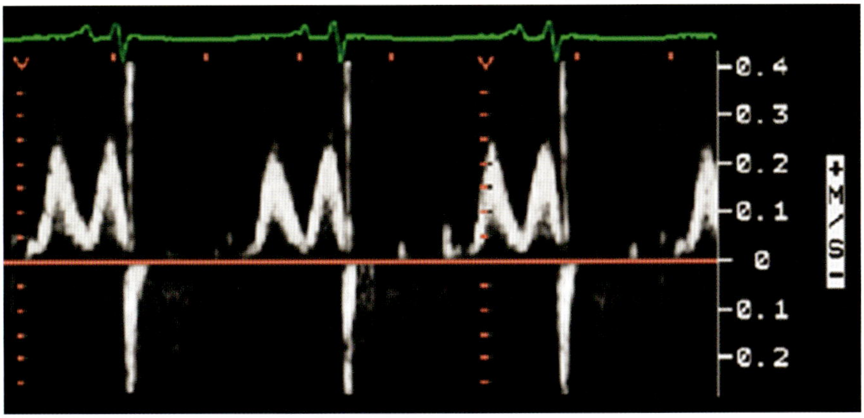

FIGURE 8-10. The M-shaped flow Doppler typical of the mitral and tricuspid valves. In the waveform, the first peak is the E wave and is due to early passive filling, and the second peak is the A wave and is caused by atrial contraction.

In this chapter, the more commonly used echocardiographic methods for evaluation of diastolic function will be discussed: mitral and tricuspid flow Doppler, tissue Doppler, and pulmonary vein Doppler. Left atrial area (volume) is used in older children and adults to assess diastolic function.[7,13] However, due to lack of data in the neonates, it is not discussed in this book. Finally, the myocardial performance index will be reviewed as a measure of combined systolic and diastolic function. For evaluation of preload, refer to Chapter 10.

Mitral and Tricuspid Flow Doppler

Flow across the mitral and tricuspid valves are the most commonly used measures of diastolic function. However, indices based on atrioventricular valve flow Doppler have poor sensitivity and specificity. The spectral Doppler tracing across the atrioventricular valves is M-shaped (Figure 8-10) and has two flow waveforms: early passive filling (E) and atrial contraction (A). The E and A flow patterns depend not only on ventricular diastolic function but also on other factors such as the age, preload, atrial function, heart rate, and atrioventricular valve function. With a high heart rate, the two waveforms may merge. Early stages of relaxation abnormalities result in a reduction in E flow and an increase in A flow. On the other hand, poor compliance results in an increase in atrial pressure and therefore an increase in flow in E rather than A phase. In adults, early diastolic dysfunction is marked by relaxation abnormality, resulting in a reversal of the E/A ratio (E<A).[14] With worsening diastolic function, compliance is also affected, which leads to increase in left atrial pressure and an increase in E. This results in the reversal of the E/A ratio back to normal. The normalization of E/A ratio despite worsening diastolic function is termed **pseudonormalization of E/A**.

Technique

Position. The patient should be placed in a supine position.

Transducer. For better spatial resolution, a high -frequency (10–12 MHz) probe is generally preferable. However, to obtain an optimal spectral Doppler tracing, a lower frequency (5–8 MHz) transducer might be necessary.

View. Apical four-chamber view.

Procedure. Once the four-chamber view of the heart is obtained, we need to pay attention to the atrioventricular valve, noting for any abnormality in echogenicity, leaflet attachment, and valve plane (tricuspid lower than mitral). Next, place the color Doppler box over the mitral and tricuspid valve to document any regurgitation or turbulence suggestive of insufficiency and stenosis, respectively. Place the pulsed wave Doppler gate just below the valve plane and press the PW Doppler button to obtain first mitral and then tricuspid flow Doppler.

Measurement. The most commonly used measurements are peak E and A velocities. These velocities and their ration (E/A) are different in preterm and term infants and change with chronological age.[15–17] In older children, E/A ratio is greater than 1. As mentioned above, due to immaturity of myocardium, the newborn heart is less compliant than that of older children. This results in less ventricular filling during the early phase (E) as compared to older children. As such, in neonates, especially preterm infants, the E/A ratio is less than 1. Table 8-1 shows the normative data for the E, A, and E/A ratios in preterm and term subjects during the neonatal period and infancy. The peak flow velocity is increased in case of an increase in blood flow through the valve (eg, increased preload or regurgitation) or if the valve is stenotic. While increases in preload can raise the E velocity, the velocity often does not exceed 1.2 m/s. When peak E velocity is greater than 1.5 m/s, valvular stenosis should be suspected.

Other useful information that can be obtained from flow Doppler is the E wave deceleration time. With worsening diastolic function as the compliance deteriorates, the duration of deceleration time is reduced.

Limitations

The main limitation of the atrioventricular Doppler indices is lack of specificity. As mentioned earlier, the flow pattern across the atrioventricular valves and the resultant Doppler indices are not only affected by ventricular relaxation and compliance but also altered by other variables, including the loading condition. In addition, with progression of ventricular diastolic function from mild to moderate severity, the increase in atrial pressure results in changes in E and A waveform back to a normal pattern, which, as mentioned, is a condition called pseudonormalization.

Tissue Doppler

Tissue Doppler is a relatively newer method of diastolic function evaluation. In this method, Doppler is used to assess myocardial velocity, which in diastole is primarily reflective of myocardial relaxation. Compared to atrioventricular flow Doppler indices, tissue Doppler indices are less sensitive to loading condition. Tissue Doppler has both systolic (S') and diastolic (E' and A') components. E' and A' represent early and late diastolic phase, respectively, corresponding to the E and A waves of atrioventricular valve inflow. Low E' velocity and high E/E' ratio are indicative of diastolic dysfunction.[13,14] In adults, a mitral E'$<$10 cm/s or E/E' $>$13 in the presence of other positive signs are considered to be indicative of diastolic dysfunction.[13] Similar E/E' cut off has been reported to be useful in children with congenital heart defect after surgery as an index of diastolic function, especially in predicting high atrial pressure.[18,19]

Technique

Position. The patient should be placed in a supine position.

Transducer. For better spatial resolution, a high-frequency (10–12 MHz) probe is generally preferable. However, to obtain an optimal spectral Doppler tracing, a lower-frequency (5–8 MHz) transducer might be necessary.

View. Apical four-chamber view.

Procedure. Once the four-chamber view of the heart is obtained, place the Doppler gate at the lateral mitral annulus and activate the tissue Doppler module on the echocardiography machine. This will yield the typical tissue velocity Doppler profile (Figure 8-11). Given the relatively low values for myocardial velocity (much lower than the atrioventricular valve inflow), the Doppler scale should be lowered to facilitate better visualization and therefore more accurate measurement of velocities (most echocardiography machines have preprogrammed settings for tissue Doppler imaging). It is also very important to obtain an upright image of a four-chamber view and align the ultrasound beam parallel to the wall. Otherwise, the velocity is underestimated. Tissue Doppler tracing can also be obtained from the septal and tricuspid annuli.

Measurement. For purposes of diastolic function, the maximum velocity of E' and A' is measured. The maximum S' velocity can be used as a measure of systolic function. Normal values for preterm and term infants are shown in Table 8-2.[20–22]

Limitations

The main limitation of tissue Doppler is the extrapolation of regional motion as a predictor of global diastolic function. In addition, load independence of E' has recently been questioned, as it can be affected with acute changes in preload.

TABLE 8-1 Normative Data for E, A and E/A Ratio in Preterm and Term Subjects During Neonatal Period and Infancy

	Age	n	E (cm/s)	A (cm/s)	E/A	Authors
Preterm						
	Early Postnatal					
<1000 g	13 ± 10 days	34	32.7 ± 12.3	36.9 ± 10		Schmitz et al.[17]
1000–1499 g	12 ± 9 days	29	38.5 ± 11.4	43.6 ± 11.9		Schmitz et al.[17]
26–32 wk	14 ± 4 days	18	31 ± 9	33 ± 7	0.93 ± 0.19	Harada et al.[12,15,24]
32–36 wk	≤4 days	15	40.1 ± 5.6	43.2 ± 6	0.93 ± 0.03	Kozak-Barany et al.[16]
	Later					
<1000 g	132 ± 33 days	22	82 ± 14.5	66.5 ± 24.5		Schmitz et al.[17]
1000–1499 g	138 ± 70 days	25	79 ± 10.9	75.1 ± 10.7		Schmitz et al.[17]
26–32 wk	94 ± 17 days	18	78 ± 14	61 ± 12	1.29 ± 0.18	Harada et al.[12,15,24]
32–36 wk	30 days	15	61.5 ± 5.2	56.9 ± 4.8	1.08 ± 0.04	Kozak-Barany et al.
Term						
	Early Postnatal					
	≤5 days	19	46.9 ± 5.2	44.3 ± 5.7	1.06 ± 0.05	Kozak-Barany et al.
	7 ± 1 days	13	58 ± 8	49 ± 10	1.21 ± 0.21	Harada et al.[12,15,24]
	15 ± 14 days	74	56.2 ± 16.4	50.8 ± 13.9		Schmitz et al.[17]
	Later					
	30 days	19	62.8 ± 6.1	56.9 ± 5.4	1.11 ± 0.05	Kozak-Barany et al.
	135 ± 36 days	28	86.2 ± 10.5	70.6 ± 13.1		Schmitz et al.[17]

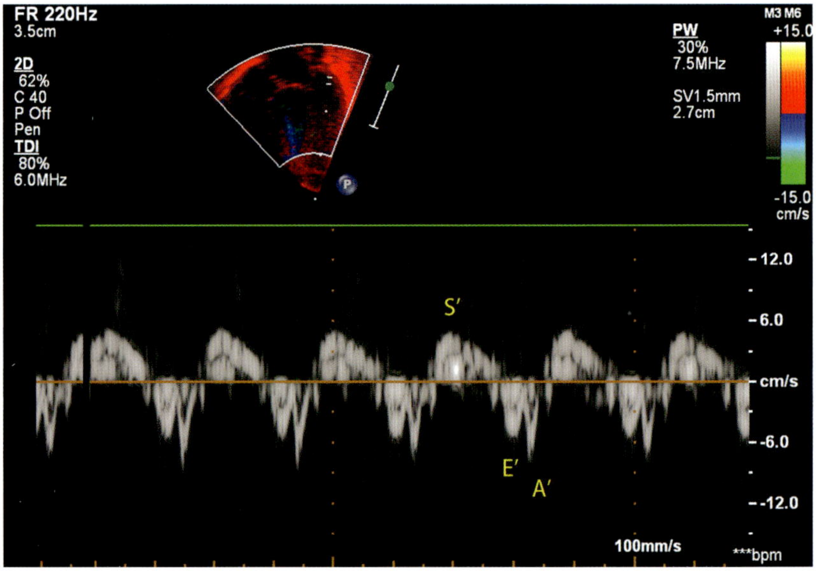

FIGURE 8-11. Tissue Doppler of lateral mitral valve annulus in a 7-day-old extremely low-birth-weight infant. S' represents left ventricular (LV) systole and E' and A' correspond to the early and late phases of LV diastole.

Pulmonary Vein Doppler

Evaluation of pulmonary vein spectral Doppler can provide valuable information about diastolic function in older children and adults. Unfortunately, little is known about the normal pattern in neonates[23–25] and about the utility of pulmonary vein Doppler in the assessment of diastolic function in this population.[5] Furthermore, this method of diastolic evaluation is load-dependent, and as such it can be affected by PDA and significant PFO flow.

The pulmonary vein Doppler tracing is similar to that of the superior vena cava (SVC). It consists of 3 waveforms: S, D, and A (Figure 8-12). "S" stands for systole, and the waveform represents forward flow as a result of movement of valve plane toward the apex during systole. "D" stands for diastole, and the waveform is the result of forward flow with the opening of mitral valve during early diastole (corresponding to the E wave of mitral valve inflow). The 'A' stands for atrium and the waveform represents reversal of flow as a result of atrial contraction during late diastole (corresponding to the A wave of mitral valve inflow). In fetal life and the early postnatal period, the flow is biphasic and consists of S and D waves only and on occasion when the heart rate is too high S and D can merge. In addition, the flow might be continuous in the first few postnatal days. In one study, by one week after birth the flow had changed from continuous to intermittent with a brief period of zero flow after the D wave, and at 1 month the flow became triphasic to include an A wave.[25] Other than the flow pattern, the peak velocity is also different in newborn than older children. In first few hours, the S and D velocity can be > 80 cm/s and in the ensuing hours and days the velocities decrease to an average of about 50 cm/s. By one week to one month, the velocities have decreased to about 40 cm/s with a slightly higher S velocity compared to D velocity in normal term infants.

In newborns, the S and D peak velocities are either about the same or the S is slightly less than D. After the first week, the S peak velocity could be slightly higher than D. In older children and adults, the normal flow pattern is characterized by S≥D. As mentioned earlier, the impact of diastolic dysfunction on pulmonary vein Doppler in the neonatal population has not been adequately studied. In older children and adults, with diastolic dysfunction, initially the S wave exceeds the D wave. Then, as left atrial pressure increases, D will be greater than S. In addition, high velocity or increased duration of the A waveform reflects an increase in left atrial pressure which (in the absence of mitral valve disease) generally signifies decreased LV compliance. In adults, pulmonary vein

TABLE 8-2 Normal Values of Tissue Doppler Velocities E′ and A′ in Preterm and Term Infants

		Mitral			Septal			Tricuspid			
	Age	n	E′ (cm/s)	A′ (cm/s)	n	E′ (cm/s)	A′ (cm/s)	n	E′ (cm/s)	A′ (cm/s)	Authors
Preterm											
	Early Postnatal										
23–26 wk	7 days	85	4 (4–5)	7 (5–8)	88	4 (3–5)	6 (5–7)	81	5 (4–6)	9 (8–10)	Di Maria et al.[22]
27–29 wk	7 days	80	5 (4–7)	6 (5–8)	85	4 (4–5)	6 (5–7)	75	6 (5–7)	9 (8–10)	Di Maria et al.[22]
30–33 wk	7 days	21	5 (5–6)	5 (4–7)	22	4 (3–5)	6 (5–7)	21	5.5 (5–7)	8 (7–9)	Di Maria et al.[22]
34.3 ± 1.5	3.8 ± 2.1 days	20	7.6 ± 1.2	7.3 ± 1.3	20	5.7 ± 0.7	6.2 ± 0.7	20	6.2 ± 1.3	9.4 ± 1.1	Ciccone et al.[22]
	Later										
23–26 wk	36 weeks PMA	76	7 (6–9)	8 (6–10)	75	6 (5–7)	8 (6–9)	61	9 (7–11)	11 (9–13)	Di Maria et al.[22]
27–29 wk	36 weeks PMA	66	7 (6–9)	9 (7–11)	68	6 (5–7)	8 (7–10)	56	9 (7–11)	11 (9–13)	Di Maria et al.[22]
30-33 wk	36 weeks PMA	23	8 (6–10)	7 (6–9)	21	6 (6–7)	7 (6–7)	13	7 (5–8)	9 (8–11)	Di Maria et al.[22]
Term											
	Early Postnatal										
	<1 day	130	7.5 ± 1.5	6.2 ± 1.4	130	5.0 ± 1.0	4.9 ± 1.0	130	7.5 ± 1.4	9.2±1.6	Mori et al.[20]
	3.9 ± 2 days	135	7.7 ± 1.5	6.5 ± 1.2	135	5.4 ± 0.9	5.2 ± 0.9	135	7.5 ± 1.3	9.2±1.5	Mori et al.[20]
	3.8 ± 2.1 days	33	7.9 ± 1.2	7.3 ± 1.3	33	5.8 ± 0.7	5.9 ± 1.0	33	7.9 ± 1.1	9.5±1.5	Ciccone et al.[21]

Values are median (interquartile) or mean ± SD

A duration exceeding mitral A duration is suggestive of increased LV end-diastolic pressure.[26]

Technique

Position. Patient should be placed supine.

Transducer. For better spatial resolution, a high frequency (10–12 MHz) probe is generally preferable. However, to obtain an optimal spectral Doppler tracing, a lower frequency (5–8 MHz) transducer might be necessary.

View. Apical four-chamber view.

Procedure. In the standard four-chamber view of the heart, identify the upper pulmonary veins. The right upper pulmonary vein is often easier to visualize and interrogate with Doppler, and the angle of insonation is nearly parallel to the direction of blood flow in this vessel (Figure and Video 8-13). Next, the Doppler sample volume is placed in the pulmonary vein just before it enters the left atrium, and PW Doppler mode is activated on the echocardiography machine. As the flow velocity in the pulmonary vein is lower than in the pulmonary artery, it is important to ensure that the velocity scale is adjusted accordingly to display an optimal spectral Doppler envelope. Furthermore, care should be taken to avoid inadvertent sampling of SVC flow, due to its proximity to right upper pulmonary vein. This is more likely to occur with a suboptimal apical view.

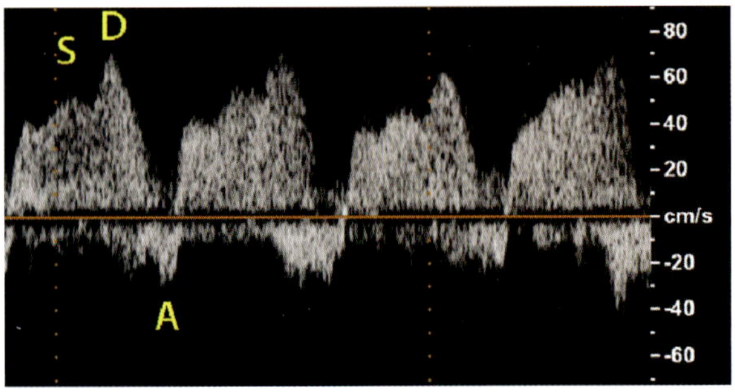

FIGURE 8-12. Right upper pulmonary vein Doppler in a 24-hour old term infant. Note the S, D and A waveforms. Similar to the superior vena cava, the Doppler flow pattern can be quite variable. In this case, the forward flow appears to be triphasic.

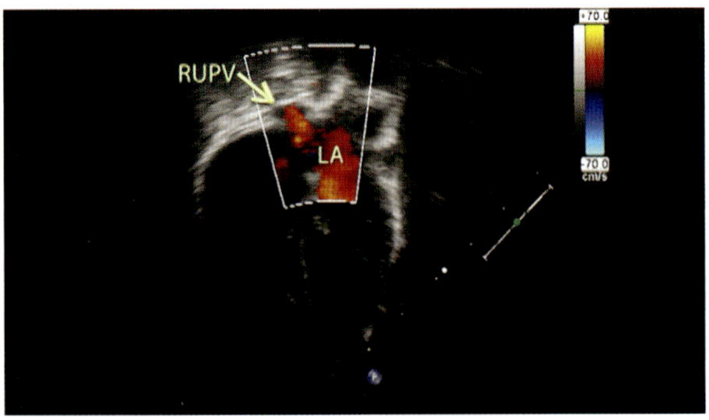

FIGURE and VIDEO 8-13. Color Doppler of the standard four-chamber view of the heart. Note the right upper pulmonary veins (RUPV, arrow). Abbreviation: LA, left atrium.

Measurement. For purposes of diastolic function, the maximum velocity of S and D is measured. In addition, the maximum velocity and duration of the A wave should be measured. Similar to SVC flow, pulmonary vein flow is affected by respiration; therefore, when measuring S, D and A velocities, use an average of 3–5 cardiac cycles.

Limitations

The main limitation of pulmonary vein Doppler in assessment of diastolic function is its load dependency. Although rare, when present, pulmonary vein stenosis affects the spectral Doppler tracing, and therefore in such cases pulmonary vein Doppler cannot be used for assessment of diastolic function. In addition, mitral valve dysfunction (especially mitral regurgitation) can also affect the pulmonary vein flow pattern. However, other than asphyxiated neonates, mitral valve dysfunction is uncommon in the absence of congenital heart disease.

GLOBAL MYOCARDIAL FUNCTION

Myocardial Performance Index

The myocardial performance index (MPI), also known as the Tei index, is a measure of global myocardial function, ie, combined systolic and diastolic function.[27] The index has a good correlation with accepted indices of LV performance as measured by cardiac catheterization.[28] In the last decade, this index has been increasingly used in the assessment of cardiac function and as a predictive tool in preterm and full-term neonates. For example, MPI appears to be a more sensitive marker of deterioration of cardiac function after PDA ligation than conventional indices.[29] Persistently elevated MPI after birth may help identify preterm infants at risk for bronchopulmonary dysplasia.[30] In addition, abnormal MPI can be used as a marker of right ventricular dysfunction in neonates with pulmonary hypertension.[31] MPI is inversely related to myocardial performance: the higher the numerical value of MPI, the worse the cardiac function. MPI is a quick and easy way to assess cardiac function. However, similar to most other indices of cardiac function, it is affected by changes in loading condition.[32,33]

Technique

Position. The patient should be placed in a supine position.

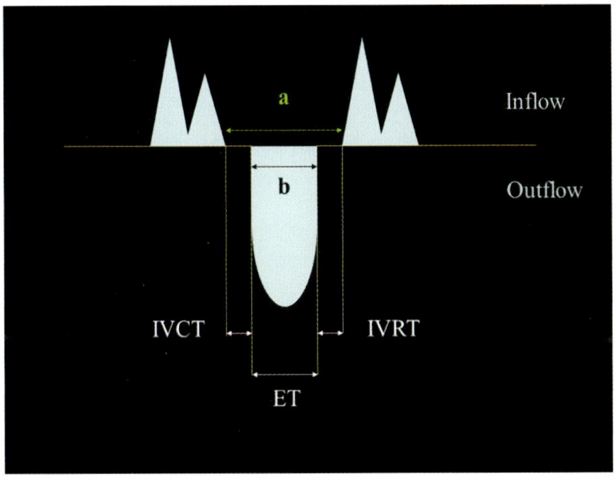

FIGURE 8-14. A schematic drawing of inflow and outflow pulsed wave Doppler depicting isovolumetric contraction (IVCT) and relaxation time (IVRT) and the ejection time (ET). We can assign "a" to the time span between the end of one inflow Doppler to the beginning of the next one and "b" to the ET. Myocardial performance index (MPI) is calculated as (a-b)/b. See Figures 8-15 and 8-16.

Transducer. For better spatial resolution, a high-frequency (10–12 MHz) probe is generally preferable. However, to obtain an optimal spectral Doppler tracing, a lower-frequency (5–8 MHz) transducer might be necessary.

View. Standard and modified apical four- and five-chamber views.

Procedure. The MPI can be obtained for either the right or left ventricle. It is a simple ratio that is calculated from isovolumetric contraction time (IVCT), relaxation time (IVRT), and ejection time (ET) (Figure 8-14). There are two methods to obtain these measurements: through the Doppler assessment of flows through the atrioventricular/semilunar valves, or through use of tissue Doppler measurements of the mitral/tricuspid valve annulus. The author prefers Doppler assessment of flow across the atrioventricular and semilunar valves. With this method, the procedure is the same whether acquiring Doppler flows through the right or left side of the heart. For the left side, aortic flow Doppler is obtained followed by a mitral valve flow tracing (Figure 8-15). For the right side, pulmonary and tricuspid valve Doppler tracings can similarly be acquired. Care must be taken to minimally disturb the patient, as a change in heart rate between inflow and outflow Doppler image acquisitions will affect the measured time periods. Therefore, it is imperative that the heart rate at the

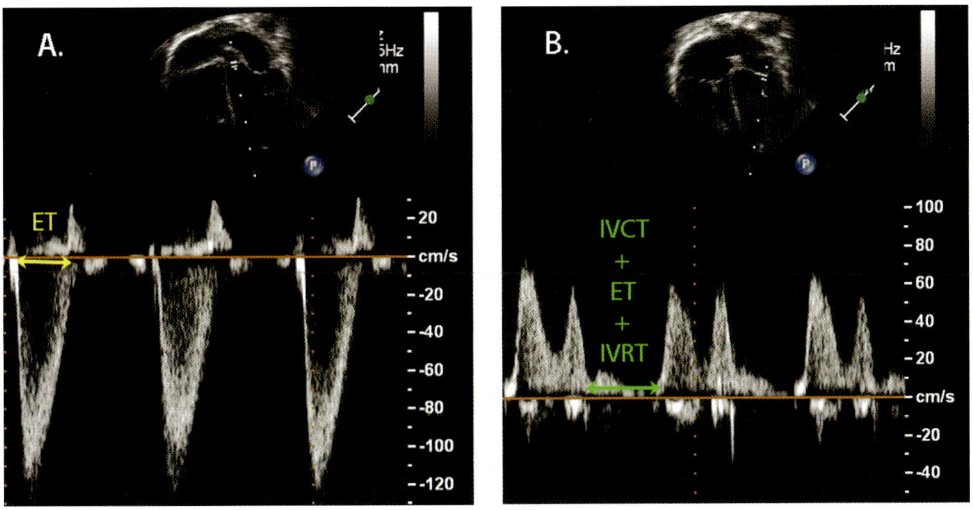

FIGURE 8-15. Measurement of left ventricular myocardial performance index (MPI) using separate Doppler tracings of aorta and mitral flow. A. Measurement of ejection time (ET). **B.** Measurement of time span between the end of one mitral valve flow Doppler to the beginning of the next one; this time span encompasses isovolumetric contraction (IVCT) and relaxation times (IVRT) as well as ET. If we assign "a" to this time period and "b" to ET, then (a-b)/b would yield the MPI. In this example, "a" or IVCT+ET+IVRT was 0.240 second and "b" or ET was 0.187 second. MPI was calculated to be 0.28.

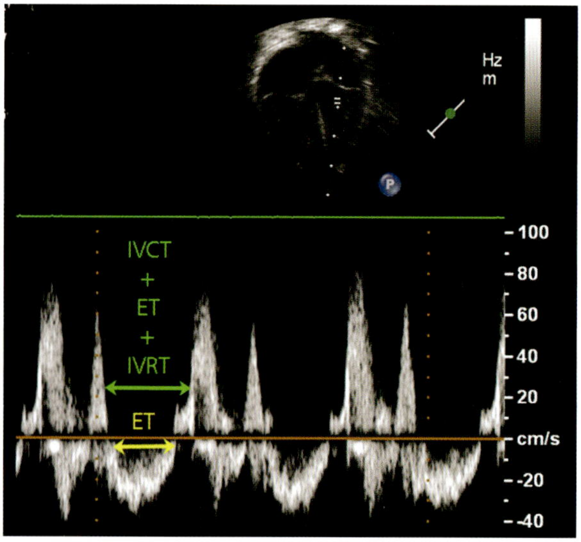

FIGURE 8-16. Measurement of left ventricular MPI using single Doppler tracing of combined aorta and mitral flow in the same patient and time as in Figure 8-8. In this method, the sampling gate is placed between the mitral and outflow tract to capture both the inflow and outflow Doppler tracings. In this example, "a" or IVCT+ET+IVRT was 0.246 second and "b" or ET was 0.190 second. MPI was calculated to be 0.29.

time of inflow and outflow Doppler tracing be the same. Alternatively, the Doppler gate can be placed between the inflow and outflow to capture both tracings at the same time (Figure 8-16). However, while this technique solves the problem of discrepancy in heart rate, additional error can be introduced, as the Doppler tracing might not be clearly visible (this is particularly true for the right heart).

Measurement. For the left side of the heart, the LV ejection time is recorded by measuring the duration of aortic flow. For the purpose of the MPI calculation, this time period is referred to as **b**. Next, the mitral valve spectral Doppler tracing is obtained, and the time span between the end of one mitral Doppler envelope to the beginning of the following envelope is measured. This time period is here referred to as **a**, and includes IVCT, ET (**b**), and IVRT. Therefore, the calculation of **a** − **b** will yield the combined time periods of IVCT and IVRT. MPI can then be calculated as follows:

$$\mathbf{MPI} = (\mathbf{a} - \mathbf{b})/\mathbf{b}$$

Again, one must ensure that the heart rates at the time of acquisition of inflow (**b**) and outflow (**a**) Doppler recordings are about the same. The same process can be repeated for the right side of the heart, using inter-tricuspid valve and pulmonary flow durations. Normal left and right MPI in infants are 0.33±0.08 and 0.29±0.09, respectively.[34] The reported MPI in preterm and term neonates and during infancy are similar. In hemodynamically stable preterm infants, we have found the average left and right MPI to be 0.29±0.10 (range 0.04–0.57) and 0.31±0.14 (range 0.06–0.86), respectively, in the first 3 postnatal days. On days 4–14 after birth, left and right MPI were 0.34±0.13 (range 0.11–0.66) and 0.31±0.16 (range 0.07–0.95), respectively.[1]

Limitations

The main limitation of MPI is its load dependency, and the fact that it is an indicator of global systolic function and does not separate the systolic from diastolic components. Therefore, when an abnormal MPI is obtained, other methods must be utilized to determine whether systolic or diastolic function (or both) are abnormal.

REFERENCES

1. Noori S., Wu T-W, Seri I. pH Effects on Cardiac Function and Systemic Vascular Resistance in Preterm Infants. *J. Pediatr*. 2012; doi:10.1016/j.jpeds.2012.10.021.
2. Kampmann C, Wiethoff CM, Wenzel A et al. Normal values of M mode echocardiographic measurements of more than 2000 healthy infants and children in central Europe. *Heart*. 2003;83:667–672.
3. Zecca E, Romagnoli C, Vento G, De Carolis MP, De Rosa G, Tortorolo G. Left ventricle dimensions in preterm infants during the first month of life. *Eur. J. Pediatr*. 2001;160:227–230.
4. Güzeltaş A, Eroğlu AG. Reference values for echocardiographic measurements of healthy newborns. *Cardiol Young*. 2012;22:152–157.
5. Mertens L, Seri I, Marek J et al. Targeted Neonatal Echocardiography in the Neonatal Intensive Care Unit: practice guidelines and recommendations for training. Writing Group of the American Society of Echocardiography (ASE) in collaboration with the European Association of Echocardiography (EAE) and the Association for European Pediatric Cardiologists (AEPC). *J Am Soc Echocardiogr*. 2011;24:1057–1078.
6. Urbanowicz JH, Shaaban MJ, Cohen NH, et al. Comparison of transesophageal echocardiographic and scintigraphic estimates of left ventricular end-diastolic volume index and ejection fraction in patients following coronary artery bypass grafting. *Anesthesiology*. 1990;72:607–612.

7. Lopez L, Colan SD, Frommelt PC, et al. Recommendations for quantification methods during the performance of a pediatric echocardiogram: a report from the Pediatric Measurements Writing Group of the American Society of Echocardiography Pediatric and Congenital Heart Disease Council. *J Am Soc Echocardiogr*. 2010;23:465–495–577.
8. Rowland DG, Gutgesell HP. Noninvasive assessment of myocardial contractility, preload, and afterload in healthy newborn infants. *Am J Cardiol*. 1995;75:818–821.
9. Rowland DG, Gutgesell HP. Use of mean arterial pressure for noninvasive determination of left ventricular end-systolic wall stress in infants and children. *Am. J. Cardiol.* 1994;74:98–99.
10. Igarashi H, Shiraishi H, Endoh H, Yanagisawa M. Left ventricular contractile state in preterm infants: relation between wall stress and velocity of circumferential fiber shortening. *Am. Heart J.* 1994;127:1336–1340.
11. Barlow AJ,Ward C, Webber SA, Sinclair BG, Potts JE, Sandor GGS. Myocardial contractility in premature neonates with and without patent ductus arteriosus. *Pediatr Cardiol.* 2004;25:102–107.
12. Harada K, Takahashi Y, Toyono M, Orino T, Takada G. Peak systolic stress-rate-corrected mean velocity of fiber shortening in preterm and fullterm infants. *Tohoku J Exp Med.* 1998;184:13–20.
13. Nagueh SF, Smiseth OA, Appleton CP, et al. Recommendations for the Evaluation of Left Ventricular Diastolic Function by Echocardiography: An Update from the American Society of Echocardiography and the European Association of Cardiovascular Imaging. *J Am Soc Echocardiogr.* 2016;29:277–314.
14. Khouri SJ, Maly GT, Suh DD, Walsh TE. A practical approach to the echocardiographic evaluation of diastolic function. *J Am Soc Echocardiogr*. 2004;17:290–297.
15. Harada K, Takahashi Y, Tamura M, Orino T, Takada G. Serial echocardiographic and Doppler evaluation of left ventricular systolic performance and diastolic filling in premature infants. *Early Hum Dev*. 1999;54:169–180.
16. Kozák-Bárány A, Jokinen E, Saraste M, Tuominen J, Välimäki I. Development of left ventricular systolic and diastolic function in preterm infants during the first month of life: a prospective follow-up study. *J Pediatr.* 2001;139:539–545.
17. Schmitz L, Stiller B, Pees C, Koch H, Xanthopoulos A, Lange P. Doppler-derived parameters of diastolic left ventricular function in preterm infants with a birth weight <1500 g: reference values and differences to term infants. *Early Hum Dev*. 2004;76;101–114.
18. Larrazet F, Bouabdallah K, Le Bret E, Vouhé P, Veyrat C, Laborde F. Tissue Doppler echocardiographic and color M-mode estimation of left atrial pressure in infants. *Pediatr Crit Care Med*. 2005;6:448–453.
19. Figueras-Coll M, Sanchez-de-Toledo J, Gran F, Abella R, Perez-Hoyos S, Rosés F. Echocardiography in the Assessment of Left Atrial Pressure After Pediatric Heart Surgery: A Comparison Study with Measurements Obtained from Left Atrial Catheter. *World J Pediatr Congenit Heart Surg*. 2015;6:438–442.
20. Mori K, Nakagawa R, Nii M, et al. Pulsed wave Doppler tissue echocardiography assessment of the long axis function of the right and left ventricles during the early neonatal period. *Heart*. 2004;90:175–180.
21. Ciccone MM, Scicchitano P, Zito A, et al. Different functional cardiac characteristics observed in term/preterm neonates by echocardiography and tissue doppler imaging. *Early Hum Dev*. 2011;87:555–558.
22. Di Maria MV, Younoszai AK, Sontag MK, et al. Maturational Changes in Diastolic Longitudinal Myocardial Velocity in Preterm Infants. *J Am Soc Echocardiogr*. 2015;28:1045–1052.
23. Agata Y, Hiraishi S, Oguchi K, et al. Changes in pulmonary venous flow pattern during early neonatal life. *Br Heart J*. 1994;71:182–186.
24. Harada K, Takahashi Y, Shiota T, Tamura M, Takada G. Changes in transmitral and pulmonary venous flow patterns in the first day of life. *J Clin Ultrasound*. 1995;23:399–405.
25. Hong YM, Choi JY. Pulmonary venous flow from fetal to neonatal period. *Early Hum Dev*. 2000;57:95–103.
26. Rossvoll O, Hatle LK. Pulmonary venous flow velocities recorded by transthoracic Doppler ultrasound: relation to left ventricular diastolic pressures. *J Am Coll Cardiol*. 1993;21:1687–1696.
27. Tei C, Ling LH, Hodge DO, et al. New index of combined systolic and diastolic myocardial performance: a simple and reproducible measure of cardiac function–a study in normals and dilated cardiomyopathy. *J Cardiol*. 1995;26:357–366.
28. Tei C, Nishimura RA, Seward JB, Tajik AJ. Noninvasive Doppler-derived myocardial performance index: correlation with simultaneous measurements of cardiac catheterization measurements. *J Am Soc Echocardiogr*. 1997;10:169–178.
29. Noori S, Friedlich P, Seri I, Wong P. Changes in myocardial function and hemodynamics after ligation of the ductus arteriosus in preterm infants. *J Pediatr*. 2007;150:597–602.
30. Czernik C, Rhode S, Metze B, Schmalisch G, Bührer C. Persistently elevated right ventricular index of myocardial performance in preterm infants with incipient bronchopulmonary dysplasia. *PLoS ONE*. 2012;7:e38352.

31. Patel N, Mills JF, Cheung MMH. Use of the myocardial performance index to assess right ventricular function in infants with pulmonary hypertension. *Pediatr Cardiol.* 2009;30:133–137.

32. Lavine SJ. Effect of heart rate and preload on index of myocardial performance in the normal and abnormal left ventricle. *J Am Soc Echocardiogr*. 2005;18:133–141.

33. Lavine SJ. Index of myocardial performance is afterload dependent in the normal and abnormal left ventricle. *J Am Soc Echocardiogr*. 2005;18:342–350.

34. Eidem BW, McMahon CJ, Cohen RR, et al. Impact of cardiac growth on Doppler tissue imaging velocities: a study in healthy children. *J Am Soc Echocardiogr*. 2004;17:212–221.

CHAPTER 9

Shunts Through a Patent Foramen Ovale*

Bijan Siassi

- INTRODUCTION
- ANATOMY AND PHYSIOLOGY OF THE FORAMEN OVALE
  - Developmental Anatomy
  - Eustachian Valve
  - Interatrial Pressure Differences during the Normal Transitional Circulation
- ECHOCARDIOGRAPHY OF ATRIAL SEPTUM
  - Two-Dimensional Echocardiography of the Foramen Ovale
  - Color Flow and Pulsed Doppler Evaluation of Shunts through the PFO
- ATRIAL SHUNTS DURING TRANSITIONAL CIRCULATION
  - Left-to-Right Shunting through PFO in Healthy Full-Term Neonates
  - Left-to-Right Shunting through a PFO in Healthy Preterm Neonates
  - Left-to-Right Shunting through a PFO in Premature Neonates with a Patent Ductus Arteriosus or Systemic to Pulmonary Collaterals
- ESTIMATION OF LEFT-TO-RIGHT SHUNT VOLUME
  - Pulmonary to Systemic Flow Ratios
  - Diameter of Color Flow Doppler
- RIGHT-TO-LEFT SHUNT THROUGH FORAMEN OVALE
  - Detection of Right-to-Left Atrial Shunting
  - Transient Right-to-Left Atrial Shunt Secondary to Crying, Valsalva Maneuver, and Deep Inspiration
  - Cyanosis Secondary to Persistent Prominent Eustachian Valve
  - Right-to-Left Atrial Shunt in PPHN, RV Dysfunction, or Severe Lung Disease
- INTERATRIAL SHUNTS IN NEONATES WITH CONGENITAL HEART DEFECTS
- REFERENCES

INTRODUCTION

A patent foramen ovale, patent ductus arteriosus, and patent ductus venosus are the three vital fetal channels that ensure a normal fetal circulation. Right-to-left shunting through the foramen ovale significantly contributes to the output of the left ventricle, which functions in parallel with the right ventricle to ensure normal fetal cardiac output. This chapter focuses on the important role of the patent foramen ovale in the fetus, and its function and impact in postnatal life. Of note, this chapter will not address other types of atrial defects producing interatrial shunting in neonates with congenital heart disease. This topic will be addressed in Chapter 15.

*Videos can be accessed at http://PracticalNeonatalEcho.com.

ANATOMY AND PHYSIOLOGY OF THE FORAMEN OVALE

Developmental Anatomy of the Foramen Ovale

During early cardiac morphogenesis in the fetus, the first portion of the atrial septum that develops is known as the **septum primum**. The septum primum arises from the roof of the common atrium, and begins to divide it into the left and the right atria. Beginning from the fifth week of gestation, the septum primum develops and grows toward the endocardial cushions.[1] The progressively diminishing space between the growing septum primum and the endocardial cushions is known as the **ostium primum**. Prior to complete closure of the ostium primum, enlarging perforations occur in the upper portion of the septum primum. At the same time, to the right of the septum primum, a second atrial septum, the **septum secundum**, develops and extends, overlapping the margins of the septum primum. The slit-like gap between the septum primum and the septum secundum is known as the **foramen ovale** (Figure 9-1). The portion of the septum primum that covers the foramen ovale bulges into the left atrium during fetal life, allowing a large right-to-left shunt. This portion of atrial septum is known as the **flap valve**. The opening of foramen ovale is the same size as the inferior vena cava at 9 weeks' gestation, and it is reduced to 40% to 55% at birth.[2] A small patent foramen ovale (PFO) can remain patent throughout postnatal and adult life, with an incidence of approximately 27% of cases noted in an autopsy series of 965 patients (of all age groups) with normal hearts.[3] In most such cases, the PFO is clinically silent, but it can serve as a significant source of paradoxical embolism in later adult life.[4]

Eustachian Valve

The Eustachian valve[5] is a remnant of the right valve of the sinus venosus. It functions principally as the valve of the inferior vena cava (IVC), dividing the flow of the IVC into two streams: (1) a stream that is derived mainly from ductus venosus flow, carrying a relatively higher oxygen content from the umbilical vein, is directed into left atrium; (2) the other stream will join superior vena cava (SVC) flow and will be directed into the right ventricle. After birth, with elimination of umbilical circulation and closure of the ductus venosus, any right-to-left shunt through the PFO that is facilitated by the Eustachian valve will cause systemic arterial desaturation and cyanosis.[6]

Interatrial Pressure Differences during the Normal Transitional Circulation

Right atrial pressure is higher than left atrial pressure during fetal circulation, resulting in a large right-to-left shunt through the PFO. Atrial pressures include the following wave forms: **a-wave**, generated during atrial systole; **c-wave,** generated during the closure of tricuspid valve; and **v-wave,** generated during rapid filling of the atrium during ventricular systole. Usually the a-wave is the highest of the three in the right atrial pressure tracing, whereas the v-wave is dominant in the left atrial pressure tracing. These pressure waveforms are higher in the right atrium during fetal life. However, following birth in

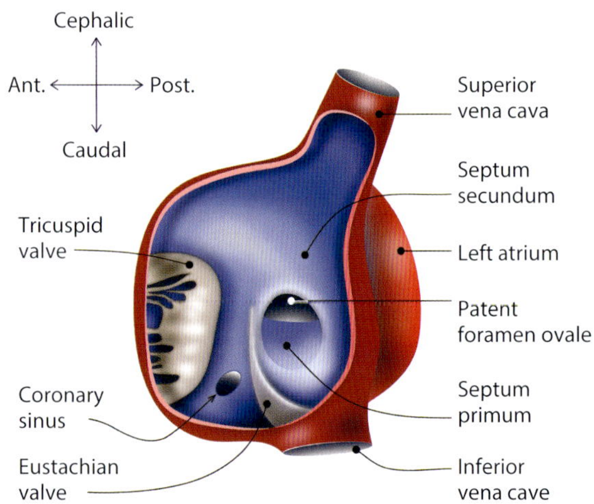

FIGURE 9-1. Diagram of foramen ovale and Eustachian valve as depicted in bicaval sagittal cut of echocardiogram.

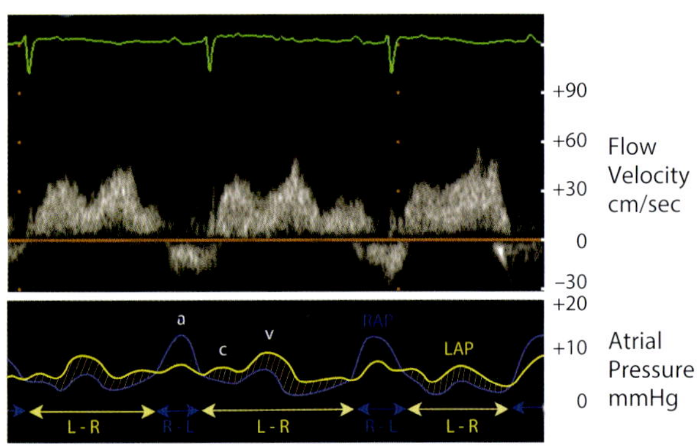

FIGURE 9-2. Directioal Doppler of blood flow across a patent foramen ovale, and corresponding atrial pressure wave forms. Abbreviations: R-L, right to left; L-R, left to right; RAP, right atrial pressure; LAP, left atrial pressure; a, a-wave, c, c-wave; v, v-wave of atrial pressure.

normal neonates, with the rapid decrease in right atrial blood inflow and increase in left atrial blood flow, except for a brief period during atrial systole, left atrial pressure exceeds right atrial pressure, resulting in a left-to-right atrial shunt (Figure 9-2).

■ ECHOCARDIOGRAPHY OF THE ATRIAL SEPTUM

Two-dimensional Echocardiography of the Foramen Ovale

Subcostal coronal posterior (Figure and Video 9-3) and subcostal sagittal bicaval (Figure and Video 9-4) are the best sector scans to evaluate interatrial septal anatomy (Chapter 3). The presence and dimensions of the PFO can often be delineated from these views. Overlapping of the flap valve of the septum primum and the septum secundum is best seen in a sagittal bicaval cut, whereas the gap between the two septa is best imaged by a coronal cut. Thus, the measurement of a PFO from a single cross-sectional cut, as an indication of significance of a left-to-right shunt, is often misleading, especially when it is not highlighted by the presence of color flow. Bulging of the atrial septum into the right or left atrium gives a good indication of pressure differential between the two atria. In other sector scans, such as the parasternal long-axis (Figure and Video 9-5), apical four-chamber (Figure and Video 9-6) and parasternal short axis, the atrial septum is not fully imaged (although parts of it are included in the cross-sectional scan) due to echo dropout, since the plane of the atrial septum is parallel or has an acute angle with the plane of the ultrasound beam.

Color Flow and Pulsed Doppler Evaluation of Shunts through the PFO

Pulsed and color flow Doppler are essential for demonstrating shunts through a PFO or atrial septal defect. In contrast to the imaging of the atrial septum, which is best visualized when the ultrasound beam is oriented perpendicular to the structure, the direction of blood flow should be *parallel* to the ultrasound beam to obtain an optimal Doppler flow measurement. For the parasternal long-axis and apical four-chamber views, the atrial septum is parallel or forms an acute angle with the ultrasound beam, resulting in echo dropout, but atrial shunt flow directed toward the tricuspid valve might also be directed either parallel or at an acute angle with the ultrasound beam, resulting in a good visualization of atrial shunt flow (Figures and Videos 9-5 and 9-6). In a subcostal imaging of the atrial septum, atrial shunt flow is often either parallel or at an acute angle with the ultrasound beam, enabling adequate color and directional Doppler flow recording. However, one complicating factor is the constant presence of SVC flow, which has the same velocity and direction as PFO flow, and can therefore mask small atrial left-to-right shunts. It is often necessary to advance color flow recordings frame by frame to distinguish small PFO flows (Figure and Video 9-7).

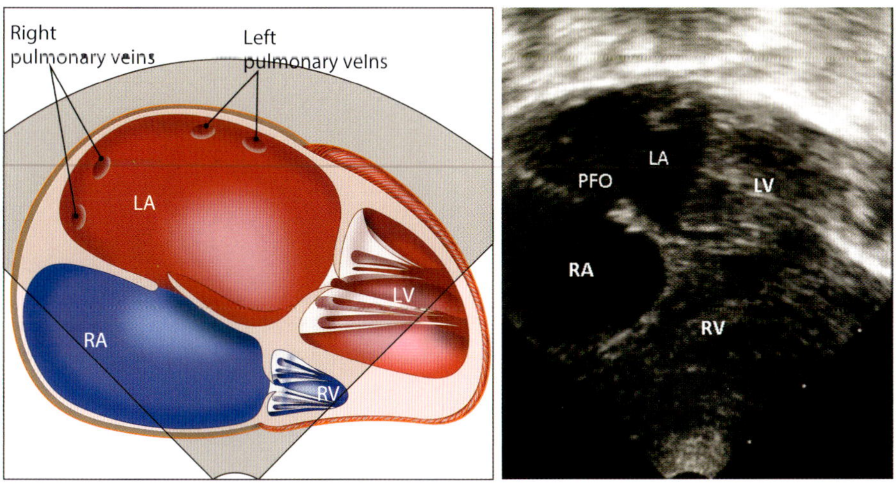

FIGURE and VIDEO 9-3. Diagram of subcostal coronal view of atrial septum and corresponding subcostal coronal posterior echocardiogram. Abbreviations: PFO, patent foramen ovale; RA, right atrium; LA, left atrium; LV, left ventricle; RV, right ventricle.

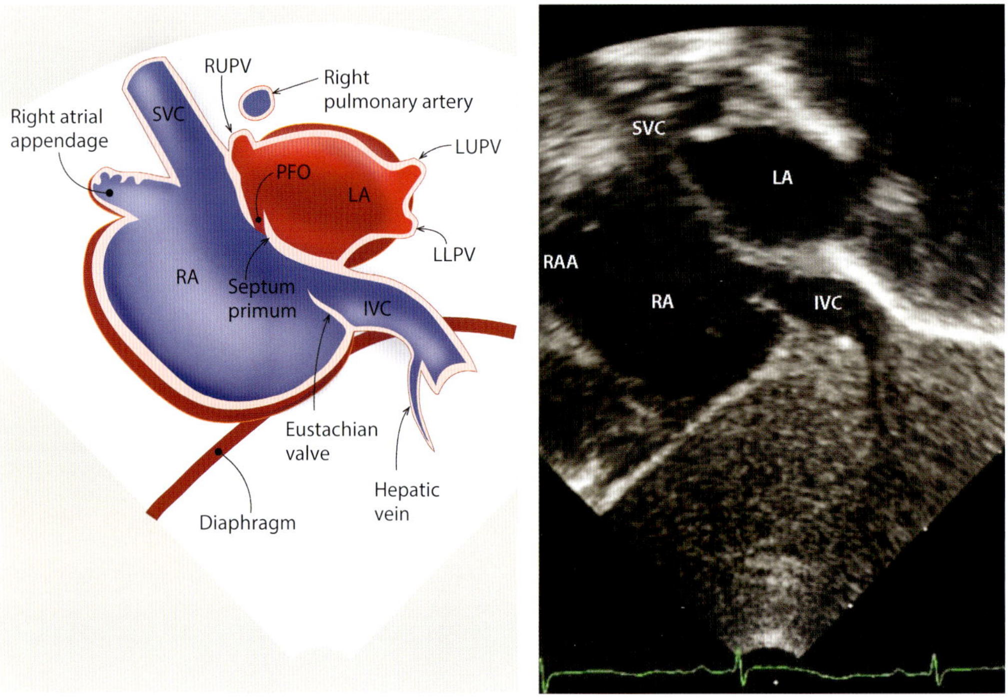

FIGURE and VIDEO 9-4. Diagram of subcostal sagittal bicaval and corresponding subcostal sagittal bicaval echocardiogram. Abbreviations: SVC , superior vena cava; RA, right atrium; IVC, inferior vena cava; LA, left atrium; PFO, patent foramen ovale; LLPV, left lower pulmonary vein; LUPV, left upper pulmonary vein; RUPV, right upper pulmonary vein.

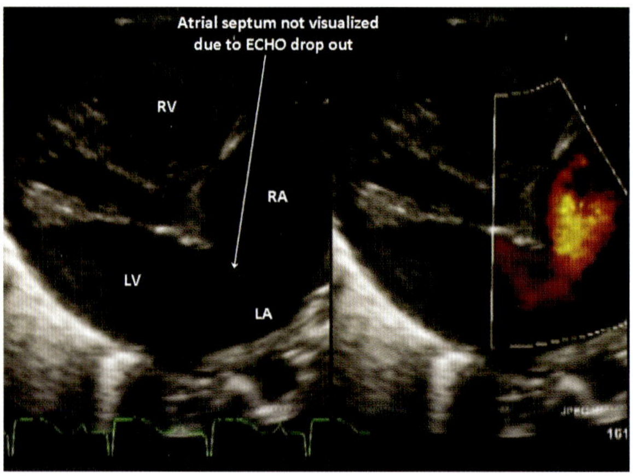

FIGURE and VIDEO 9-5. Parasternal long-axis four-chamber view showing left-to-right atrial shunting by color flow Doppler. Abbreviations: RV , right ventricle; RA, right atrium; LV, left ventricle; LA, left atrium.

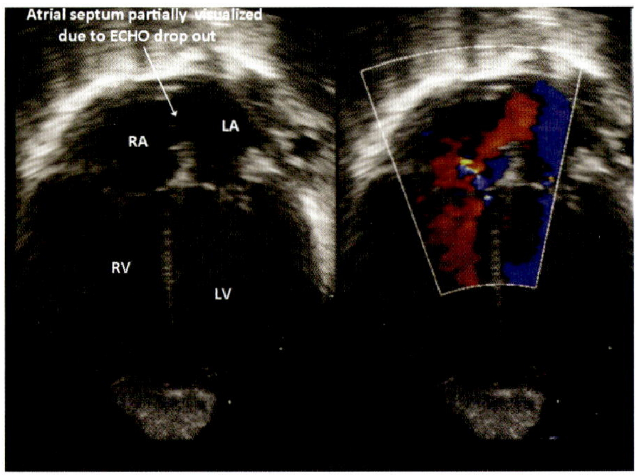

FIGURE and VIDEO 9-6. Apical four-chamber view. Atrial septum is partially visualized due to ECHO dropout. Color flow Doppler indicates left-to-right shunting through the PFO. Abbreviations: RV, right ventricle; RA, right atrium; LV, left ventricle; LA, left atrium.

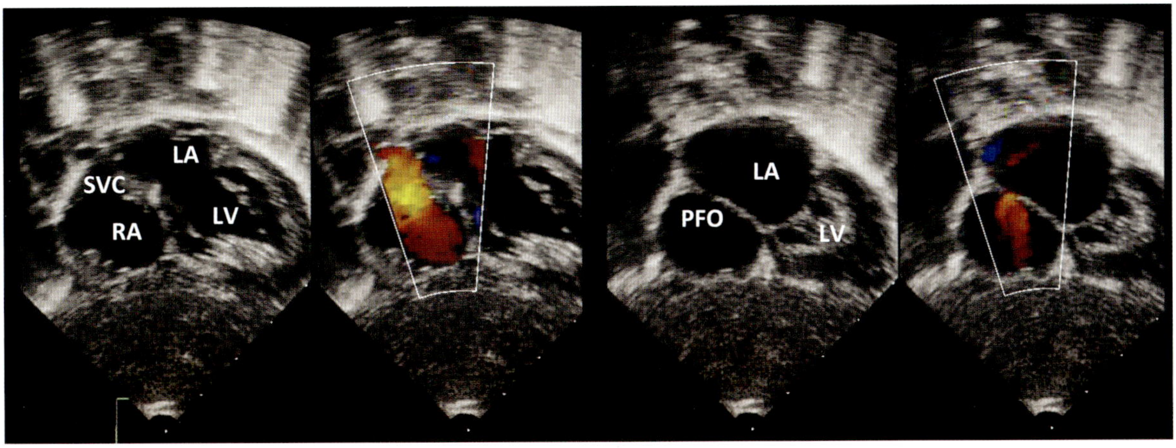

FIGURE and VIDEO 9-7. Subcostal coronal posterior view of atrial septum. A small PFO with left-to-right shunt is covered by a large superior vena cava (SVC) flow. However, on the right frames, a more posterior cut excludes SVC flow, revealing a small left-to-right atrial shunt. Abbreviations: PFO, patent foramen ovale; RA, right atrium; LV, left ventricle; LA, left atrium.

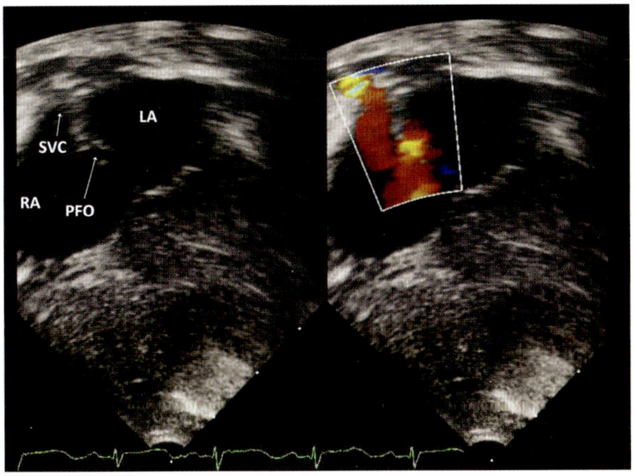

FIGURE 9-8. Subcostal coronal posterior view of atrial septum with large PFO shunt, which is well visualized in spite of a large of SVC flow. Abbreviations: SVC, superior vena cava; RA, right atrium; PFO, patent foramen ovale; LA, left atrium.

Large PFO flows are, however, often well visualized and easy to distinguish from SVC flow (Figure and Video 9-8). One important consideration when evaluating venous flows (including shunts through the atrial septum) is to set color flow gain to between 30 and 70 cm/sec and Doppler range gain to less than 100 cm/sec in order to detect low-velocity flows. Usually, pulsed Doppler with the region of interest gated to the area of the shunt is preferred for low-velocity flows.

ATRIAL SHUNTING DURING TRANSITIONAL CIRCULATION

Left-to-Right Shunting through PFO in Healthy Full-Term Neonates

Atrial septal shunting can be detected at birth with a significant right-to-left component. However, by 1 hour of life in almost all full-term neonates, color flow Doppler will detect shunting through a PFO that has a greater left-to-right component[7] (Figure 9-9). Although PFO shunting can be detected in all neonates up to 18 days of life,[8] it is usually so trivial that it is often difficult to detect beyond 5 days of age in more than 50% of neonates.[7] In most infants, PFO shunting disappears with time; however, in exceptional cases it can still be detected at 1 year of life.[9] As reported from autopsy studies, the incidence of patency of the foramen ovale is 80% at the end of first year of life.[3]

Left-to-Right Shunting through a PFO in Healthy Preterm Neonates

Shunting through a PFO in premature neonates without a patent ductus arteriosus (PDA) or significant lung disease is not much different from that in term neonates.

Left-to-Right Shunting through a PFO in Premature Neonates with a Patent Ductus Arteriosus or Chronic Lung Disease

The presence of a PDA with significant left-to-right shunting leads to increased blood flow into the left atrium,

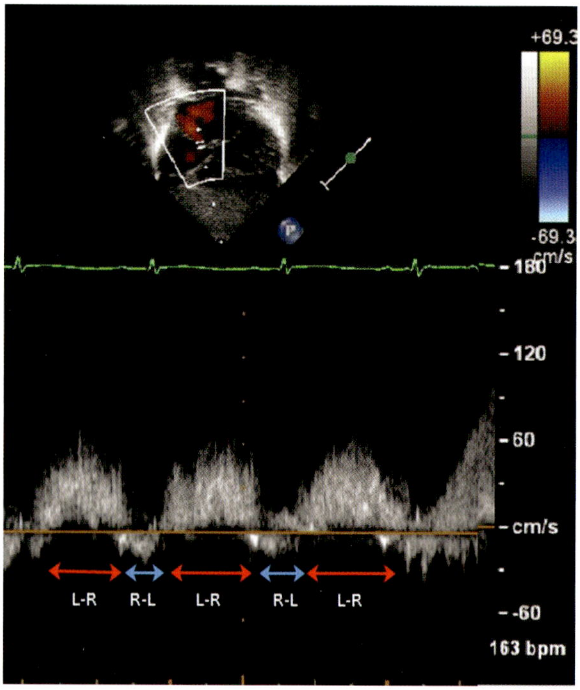

FIGURE 9-9. Directional color flow Doppler obtained as a guide, showing a mainly left-to-right (L-R) and a small right-to-left (R-L) atrial shunting.

leading to its distension and increased pressure, thereby facilitating a large left-to-right shunt through the PFO (Figure and Video 9-10). Some premature neonates, particularly extremely low-birth-weight infants who require prolonged assisted ventilation and supplemental oxygen administration, have a PFO with left-to-right shunting even beyond the neonatal period.[10] In most of these infants with significant L-R shunt through the PFO, systemic to pulmonary collateral vessels (Chapter 13) might be identified which again will lead to volume overload of the left atrium[11] (Figures and Videos 9-11 and 9-12). In the absence of a PDA or systemic to pulmonary collateral arteries in premature neonates, a trivial left-to-right shunt through the PFO might be detected.

ESTIMATION OF LEFT-TO-RIGHT SHUNT VOLUME

Pulmonary to Systemic Flow Ratios

Without any other cardiac shunts, left-to-right shunting through a PFO will increase right ventricular output, and since left ventricular output represents the systemic output, the difference between the two outputs will give a measure of the left-to-right shunt through the PFO. However, in most instances, the presence of shunting through a PDA

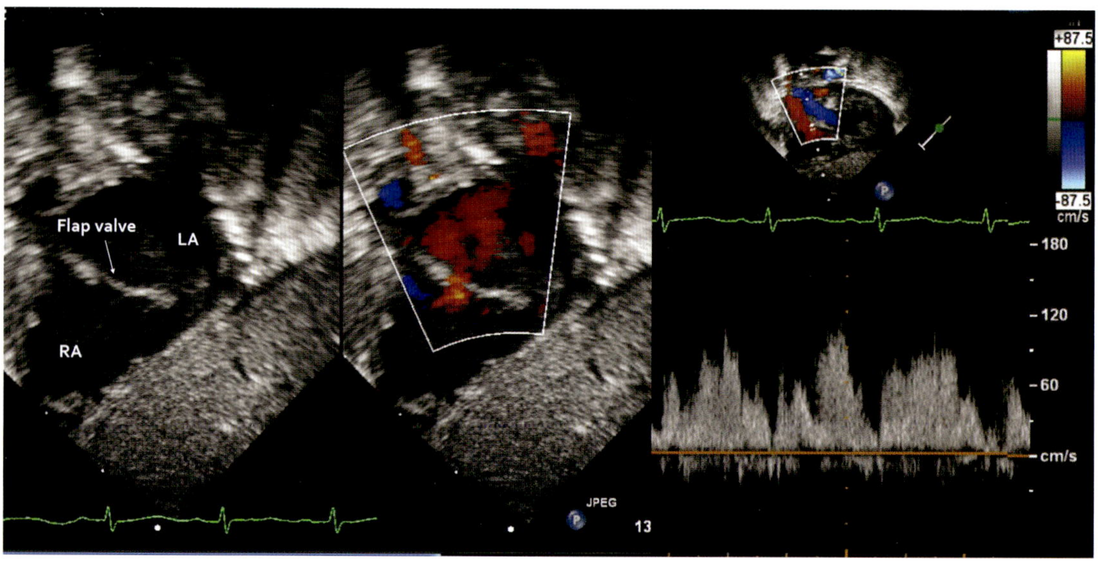

FIGURE and VIDEO 9-10. Subcostal sagittal bicaval view showing the PFO, patent foramen ovale, and its flap valve with high velocity left-to-right atrial shunting with a peak flow velocity exceeding 110 cm/sec. Abbreviations: RA, right atrium; LA, left atrium.

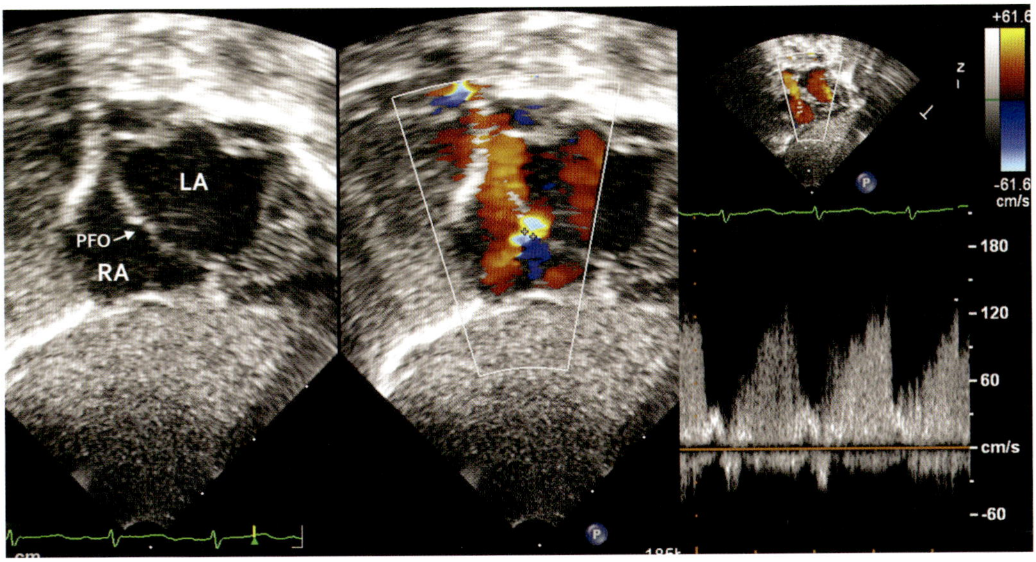

FIGURE and VIDEO 9-11. Subcostal sagittal bicaval view in a 3-month-old extremely low birth weight infant with systemic to pulmonary collateral arteries and a PFO (patent foramen ovale) with higher velocity left-to-right shunting shunt. Peak flow velocity exceeds 130 cm/sec. Abbreviations: LA, left atrium, RA, right atrium.

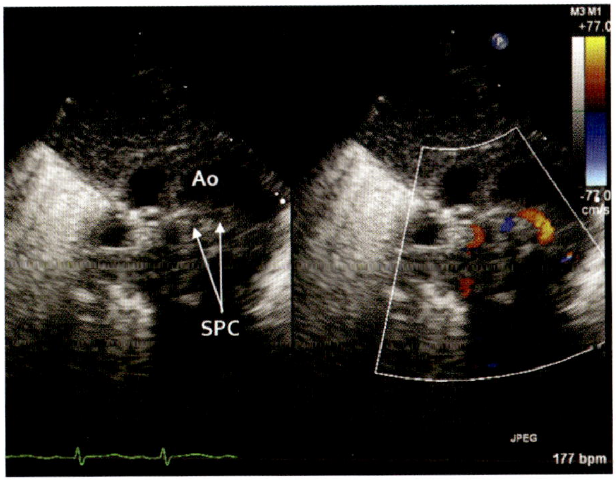

FIGURE and VIDEO 9-12. Suprasternal aortic arch echocardiogram in a 3-month-old extremely low birthweight infant revealing the presence of systemic to pulmonary artery shunts. Abbreviations: Ao, aorta; SPC systemic to pulmonary collateral artery/arteries.

or another site makes this measurement unreliable. In the presence of a left-to-right shunt through both a PDA and PFO, both right and left ventricular outputs are increased, thus making the calculation of the pulmonary to systemic flow ratio as a measure of left-to-right shunting impossible.

Diameter of Color Flow Doppler

The size and direction of interatrial shunt depends mainly on relative compliances of the right and left ventricles, the size of interatrial communication, and pressure gradients between the two atria. Except for neonates with persistent pulmonary hypertension, pulmonary artery and right ventricular pressures drop rapidly after birth, making left-to-right shunting the predominant flow through the PFO. The size of the color flow jet through atrial septal defects in adults has been shown to have a close correlation with pulmonary to systemic flow ratios.[12] However, several technical and practical factors should be considered: (1) Since the foramen ovale is oval in shape, the plane of sector cut can have significant effect on the size of the color flow jet. Usually the coronal subcostal sector will result in the largest color flow diameter (Figure and Video 9-13). For practical purposes, we consider the largest diameter obtained from any sector scan. (2) Peak flow velocity and Doppler gain should be optimized for low-velocity flows. (3) With significant bidirectional shunting, color flow size will overestimate left-to-right atrial shunting. (4) Unlike adults, there are no conclusive studies correlating the size of the color flow Doppler jet with the degree of left-to-right shunting during neonatal

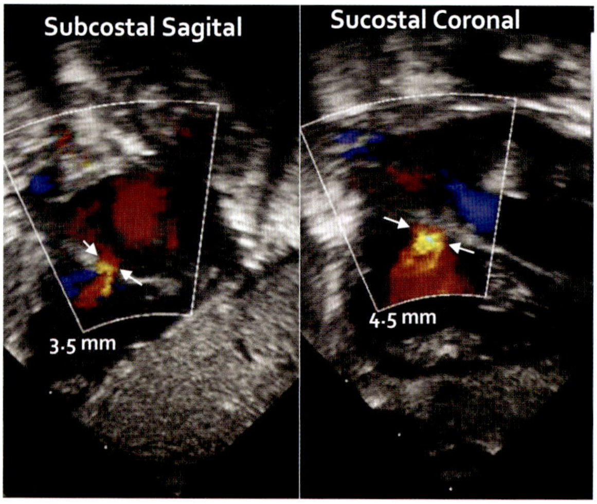

FIGURE and VIDEO 9-13. Subcostal sagittal and subcostal coronal images of atrial septum with left-to-right shunting through a PFO. Note that the subcostal coronal image provides a wider color flow Doppler jet width than the corresponding subcostal sagittal image.

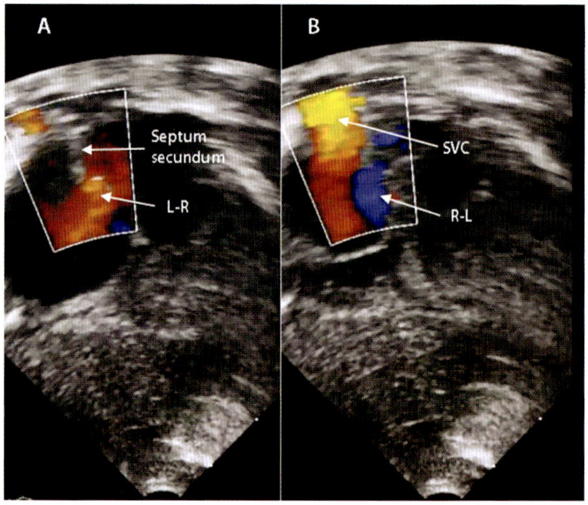

FIGURE and VIDEO 9-14. Subcostal coronal posterior echocardiogram of atrial septum with bidirectional shunt through a PFO. Abbreviations: SVC, superior vena cava; L-R, left to right; R-L, right to left.

and early infancy. In our experience, most premature infants with significant left-to-right shunting during the postnatal period also have systemic to pulmonary collateral arteries; this invalidates the use of pulmonary systemic flow ratios for documenting the size of a left-to-right shunt through the PFO. We use the following tentative guide for color flow width, estimating the size of a L-R shunt through the PFO: **<1mm, trivial; 1-1.9 mm, small; 2-4 mm, moderate; and >4 mm, large**. However, it should be noted that these values need to be validated with further studies.

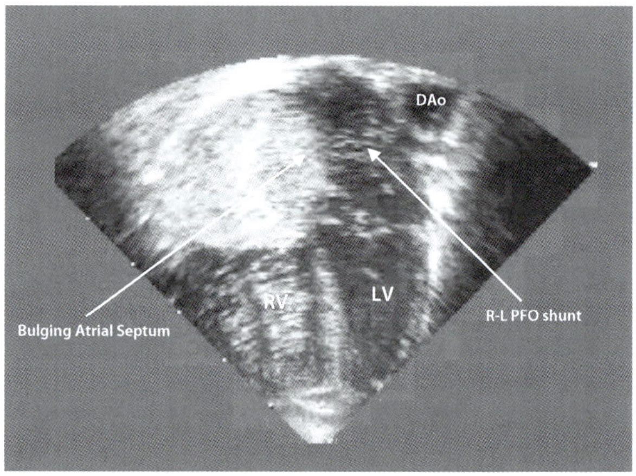

FIGURE and VIDEO 9-15. Apical four-chamber view during contrast echocardiography. Note bulging of atrial septum to left, and micro bubbles (contrast) entering the left atrium due to a right-to-left shunt through a PFO. There is a subsequent appearance of micro bubbles in the descending aorta. Abbreviations: RV, right ventricle; LV, left ventricle; Dao, descending aorta; R-L PFO, right-to-left patent foramen ovale.

RIGHT-TO-LEFT SHUNT THROUGH FORAMEN OVALE

Detection of R-L Right-to-Left Atrial Shunting

Color flow Doppler is often used to detect right-to-left atrial shunts. However, these types of atrial shunts are usually of very low velocity, and the color flow Doppler velocity range often needs to be decreased to less than 50 cm/sec to detect it (Figure and Video 9-14). It can also be detected by directional Doppler guided by color flow imaging (Figure 9-2). Contrast echocardiography is also a sensitive technique to detect small R-L atrial shunts: one ml of normal saline is injected rapidly into a peripheral vein while the 2D echocardiogram is recorded from an apical four-chamber view (Figure and Video 9-15).

Transient Right-to-Left Atrial Shunt Secondary to Crying, Valsalva Maneuver, and Deep Inspiration

During the inspiratory phase of respiration, systemic venous flow to the right atrium is accentuated due to increased negative intrathoracic pressure. Therefore, with

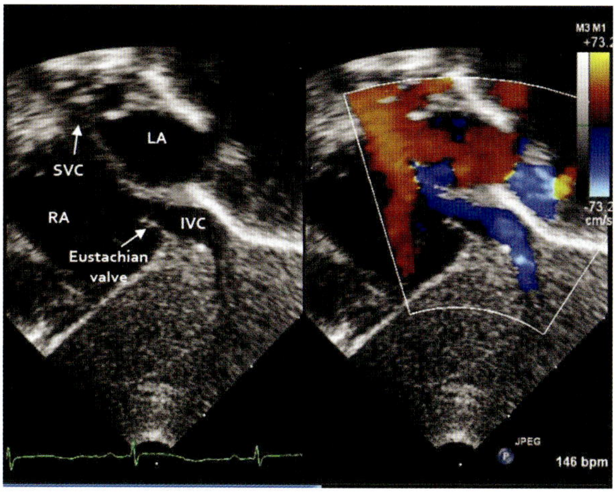

FIGURE and VIDEO 9-16. Subcostal sagittal bicaval echocardiogram revealing Eustachian valve with right-to-left shunt through the PFO (patent foramen ovale). Abbreviations: RA , right atrium; LA, left atrium; SVC, superior vena cava; IVC, inferior vena cava.

crying and a Valsalva maneuver, there can be an increase in right-to-left shunting through the PFO at the end of a deep inspiratory phase, especially if it coincides with the venous a-wave of atrial systole.

Cyanosis Secondary to Persistent Prominent Eustachian Valve

Infrequently, cyanosis encountered in a neonate can be secondary to a persistent, prominent Eustachian valve. In this instance, inferior vena cava flow is directed via the Eustachian valve through the PFO to the left atrium, leading to cyanosis (Figure and Video 9-16). A prominent Eustachian valve is often associated with persistent pulmonary hypertension or other congenital cardiac anomalies, and can accentuate the degree of cyanosis.[13,14]

Right-to-left Atrial Shunting Secondary to Persistent Pulmonary Hypertension, Right Ventricular Dysfunction, and Neonates with Severe Lung Disease

In healthy term neonates, a right-to-left atrial shunt occurring in up to 30% of the cardiac cycle is within the normal range.[7] In most neonates with persistent pulmonary hypertension (PPHN), although the PDA shunt is mainly right to left, the atrial shunt remains mainly left to right—as is seen in neonates without pulmonary hypertension (Figure and Video 9-17). In these instances, right ventricular function and its distensibility are preserved.

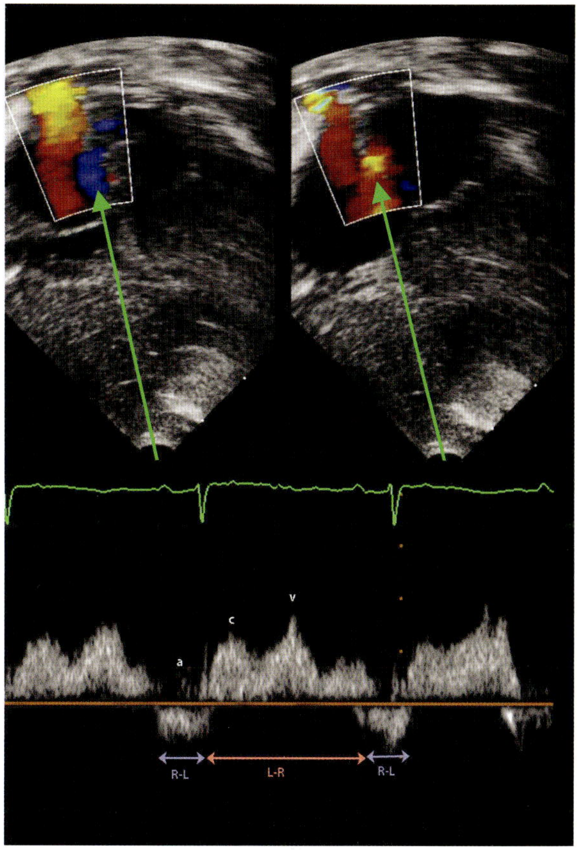

FIGURE and VIDEO 9-17. Subcostal coronal posterior with bidirectional shunt through the PFO indicated by two-dimensional still frames and directional spectral Doppler measurements. If the two-dimensional loop is frame advanced, it will reveal a very brief right-to-left shunt and a predominant left-to-right shunt, as indicated by directional spectral Doppler indicated by arrow.

However, if severe PPHN is associated with right ventricular myocardial dysfunction, or decreased right ventricular distensibility, an increased right-to-left atrial shunt is noted (Figure and Video 9-18), leading to increased severity of cyanosis. Right ventricular dysfunction is also associated with significant tricuspid regurgitation, which leads to increased right atrial pressure and a further increase in the right-to-left atrial shunt. Increased right atrial pressure and volume overload can also lead to a distended right atrium with the interatrial septum bulging into left atrium (Figure 9-19), and increased right-to-left atrial shunting.

Neonates with severe lung disease and PPHN on assisted ventilation may be at risk of adverse effects of high pressure settings. Although it has become axiomatic

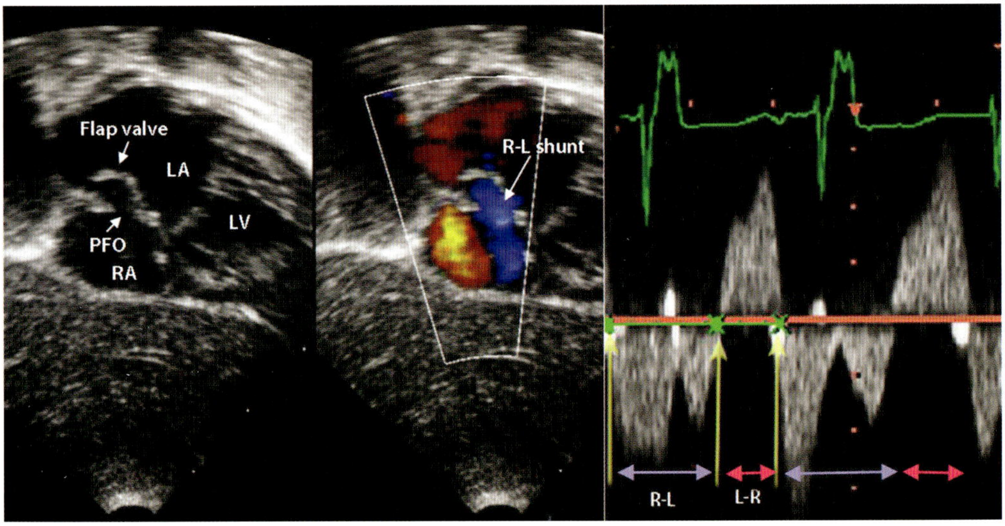

FIGURE and VIDEO 9-18. Subcostal coronal posterior echocardiogram of atrial septum with bidirectional shunt through PFO (patent foramen ovale) with a dominant right-to-left shunt as indicated by color flow and directional spectral Doppler images. Abbreviations: RV, right ventricle; RA, right atrium; LV, left ventricle; LA, left atrium.

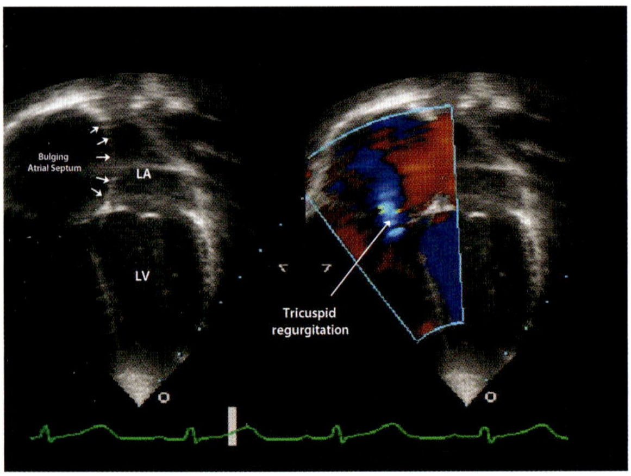

FIGURE 9-19. Apical four-chamber view indicating bulging of the atrial septum to the left and significant tricuspid insufficiency. Abbreviations: LV, left ventricle; LA, left atrium.

that increasing distending and mean airway pressure will improve oxygenation by reopening collapsed lungs, going beyond an optimal level of ventilator settings, which is often difficult to discern on clinical grounds, can actually lead to a worsening of oxygenation as follows: It will impede venous return to the right atrium, which in turn will decrease right ventricular output, probably will increase pulmonary vascular resistance, leading to a further increase in ductal right-to-left shunting, thereby severely decreasing pulmonary blood flow, resulting in decreased venous return to the left atrium. This in turn adversely affects the balance of left and right atrial pressures, resulting in an increased right-to-left atrial shunt (Figure and Video 9-20). Although in this situation further volume loading can improve venous return, decreasing the mean airway or distending pressure will also improve venous return, as well as improve pulmonary blood flow and decrease atrial and ductal right-to-left shunting.

INTERATRIAL SHUNTS IN NEONATES WITH CONGENITAL HEART DEFECTS

In most critical congenital cardiac defects, left-to-right or right-to-left atrial shunts are essential components of the overall physiology. These shunts are described in Chapter 15.

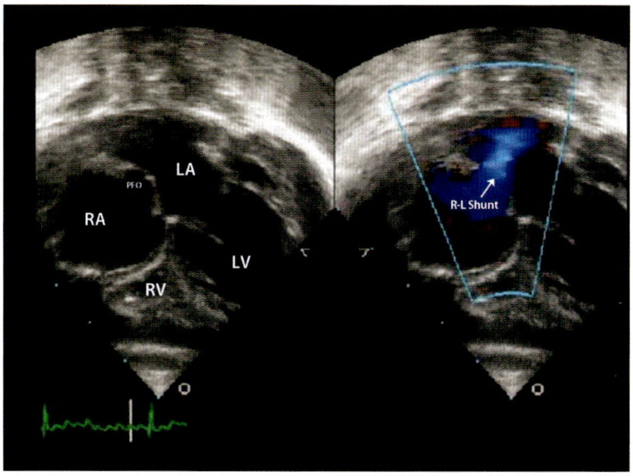

FIGURE and VIDEO 9-20. Subcostal coronal posterior echocardiogram of a neonate on high-frequency oscillatory ventilation with R-L (right-to-left) atrial shunt.

REFERENCES

1. Rojas CA, El-Sherief A, Medina HM, et al. Embryology and Developmental Defects of the Interatrial Septum. *AJR.* November 2010;195:1100–1104.
2. Patten BM. Closure of the foramen ovale. *Am J Anat.* 1931;48:19–44.
3. Hagen PT, Scholz DG, Edwards WD. Incidence and size of patent foramen ovale during the first 10 decades of life: an autopsy study of 965 normal hearts. *Mayo Clin Proc.* January 1984;59(1):17–20.
4. Lechat P, Mas JL, Lascault G, et al. Prevalence of patent foramen ovale in patients with stroke. *N Engl J Med* 1988;318:1148–52.
5. Sehra R, Ensing G, Hurwitz R. Persistent eustachian valves in infants: course and management in symptomatic patients. *Pediatr Cardiol.* 1998;19:221–224.
6. Raffa H, Al-Ibrahim K, Kayali M, Sorefan A, Rustom M. Central cyanosis due to prominence of the Eustachian and Thebesian valves. *Ann Thorac Surg.* 1992;54:159–160.
7. Hiraishi S, Agata Y, Saito K, et al. Interatrial shunt flow profiles in newborn infants: a color flow and pulsed Doppler echocardiographic study. *Br Heart J.* 1991;65:41–45.
8. Fugelseth D, Lindemann R, Liestøl K. Ultrasonographic study of ductus venosus in healthy neonates. *Arch Dis Child.* 1997;77:F131–F134.
9. Hannu H, Pentti K, Henrik E, et al. Patency of Foramen Ovale: does it influence hemodynamics in newborn infants? *Early Hum Dev.* 1989;20:281–287.
10. Evans N, Iyer P. Incompetence of the foramen ovale in preterm infants supported by mechanical ventilation. *J Pediatr.* November 1994;125(5 Pt 1):786–792.
11. Acherman RJ, Siassi B, Pratti-Madrid G, Luna C, Lewis AB, et al. Systemic to pulmonary collaterals in very low birth weight infants: color Doppler detection of systemic to pulmonary connections during neonatal and early infancy period. *Pediatrics.* 2000;105:528–532.
12. Pollick C, Sullivan H, Cujec B, et al. Doppler color flow imaging assessment of shunt size in Atrial Septal Defect. *Circulation.* 1988;78:522–528.
13. Sehra R, Ensing G, Hurwitz R. Persistent Eustacian valves in infants: course and management in symptomatic patients. *Pediatr Cardiol.* 1998;19:221–224.
14. Yasuda K, Iwashima S, Sugiura H, et al. Intermittent cyanosis due to prominent eustachian valve in a newborn Infant. *J Matern Fetal Neonatal Med.* 2009;22:812–815.

CHAPTER 10

Shock, Myocardial Dysfunction, and Heart Failure*

Shahab Noori and Tai Wei Wu

- INTRODUCTION
- BLOOD PRESSURE AND FLOW
- DETERMINANTS OF CARDIAC OUTPUT
  - Preload
  - Contractility
  - Afterload
- VASODILATORY SHOCK
  - Echocardiography Findings in Vasodilatory Shock
- CARDIOGENIC SHOCK
  - Myocardial Dysfunction and Postnatal Cardiovascular Maladaptation
  - Asphyxia
  - Sepsis
- HYPOVOLEMIC SHOCK
  - Hypovolemia
  - Pericardial Effusion and Cardiac Tamponade
- REFERENCES

INTRODUCTION

Shock is a pathophysiologic state characterized by poor tissue perfusion, resulting in a decrease in oxygen delivery that leads to tissue hypoxemia. If circulatory compromise is prolonged, it can lead to disrupted membrane pump function, energy failure, anaerobic metabolite accumulation, cell death, and eventually organ failure.

In the neonate, shock can be described by etiology (vasodilatory, cardiogenic, and hypovolemic shock), timing (immediate postnatal or out of transitional period), and progression of severity (compensated, uncompensated, and irreversible shock). This chapter focuses on the description of shock based upon pathogenesis, and the concomitant echocardiography findings. Understanding the developmental cardiovascular physiology along with the etiology of shock allows the clinician to arrive at a timely and appropriate therapy for this disease state.

It is important to point out that limited data are available on echocardiographic assessment of patients with shock in the neonatal period and early infancy. Nevertheless, systematic assessment of the cardiac function, preload, afterload, and systemic vascular resistance (SVR) can often direct the clinician to the underlying cause of cardiovascular compromise and help with formulating a treatment strategy based upon the pathophysiology. For patients in shock, it is prudent that echocardiographic evaluation be considered as an adjunct to clinical assessment rather than a replacement for it.

BLOOD PRESSURE AND FLOW

Understanding the interaction between blood pressure and flow is important in the assessment of the cause

*Videos can be accessed at http://PracticalNeonatalEcho.com.

of cardiovascular compromise. Poiseuille's law states that flow is directly related to the pressure gradient and the diameter of the tube, and inversely related to the viscosity of the fluid and the length of the tube. While Poiseuille's law is important in understanding the interaction between various factors that affect the flow, it cannot be used clinically. Instead, in clinical practice, Ohm's law is used to describe the interaction between flow and pressure. Accordingly:

$$\text{Blood pressure gradient (ie Mean systemic blood pressure} - \text{Mean right atrial pressure)} = \text{Flow} \times \text{SVR}$$

In this formula, SVR is a calculated factor. Therefore, by measuring the blood pressure and estimating cardiac output, one can calculate SVR. As atrial pressure is not routinely measured, the formula can be rewritten as:

$$\text{Blood pressure} \propto \text{Cardiac output} \times \text{SVR or Blood pressure} = \text{Cardiac output} \times \text{SVR index}$$

Given that blood pressure is routinely measured in the neonatal intensive care setting, the ability to assess cardiac output and, as a result, to estimate SVR would significantly enhance our understanding of the hemodynamic status. Unfortunately, estimation of cardiac output has its own limitation, especially during the transitional period when the fetal channels are open (see Chapter 7). Furthermore, the above measurements only describe central circulation and do not shed any light on the status of specific organ blood flow or microcirculation. As discussed in Chapter 7, Doppler assessment of large arteries supplying major organs can provide useful information about the status of specific organ blood flow. As for the assessment of microcirculation, other methodologies such as near-infrared or visible light spectroscopy, laser Doppler, or orthogonal polarization spectral imaging can be used.[1] Description of these techniques is beyond the scope of this book.

DETERMINANTS OF CARDIAC OUTPUT

Cardiac output is the product of stroke volume and heart rate. Stroke volume is in turn determined by the preload, contractility and afterload. Assessment of determinants of cardiac output can further assist the clinician in evaluation of the underlying cause of cardiovascular compromise (Figure 10-1). Below we will discuss echocardiographic assessment of the preload, contractility and afterload. It is important to point out that little is known about the effect of each of these factors on cardiac output in the neonatal period.

Preload

Preload is the amount of stretch of the myocardial sarcomere just prior to contraction. Therefore, preload can be described in terms of ventricular pressure or volume. For the purpose of assessment by echocardiography, preload can be defined as the volume of blood in the ventricle at the end of diastole. Using this definition, one can appreciate that preload is affected by a host of factors such as circulating blood volume and systolic and diastolic cardiac function, as well as extracardiac factors such as intrathoracic pressure. For assessment of systolic and diastolic function, refer to Chapter 8. Several indices have been used as a measure of preload. These include quantitative measures such as left atrium to aortic root ratio (see Chapter 11), left ventricular internal diameter at the end of diastolic (LVIDD), diameter of inferior vena cava (IVC), and IVC collapsibility index, as well as qualitative measures such as

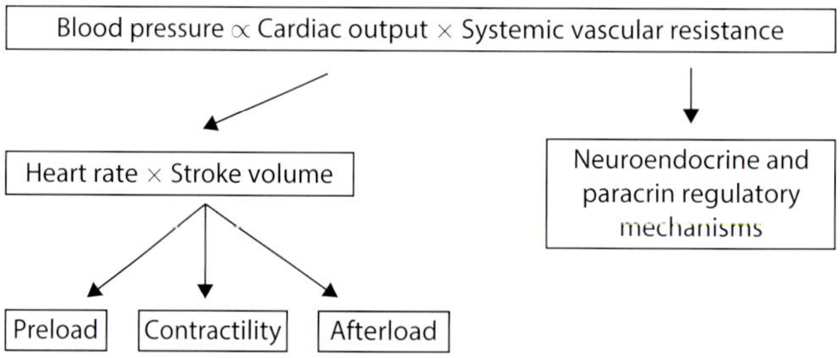

FIGURE 10-1. Blood pressure is the product of the interaction between cardiac output and systemic vascular resistance. Assessment of each component of this interaction is important and useful in identifying the underlying cause of cardiovascular compromise. Cardiac output is determined by the heart rate and stroke volume. Changes in preload, contractility, and afterload affect the stroke volume.

visual assessment of collapsibility of IVC during inspiration or appearance of an "underfilled" ventricle.

LVIDD. LVIDD is perhaps the most commonly used index of preload. LVIDD can be measured by M-mode or 2D echocardiography from the parasternal short- or long-axis view, as described for the measurement of the shortening fraction (Chapter 8). Normal LVIDD for a 3.5-kg infant is 18.8 ± 1.7 mm.[2] The reported LVIDD in preterm infants varies significantly.[3–5] The variation is most likely due to differences in the population studied and possibly due to the method used. In hemodynamically stable preterm infants ≤30 weeks' gestation, average LVIDD was 11.9 ± 1.3 mm (range 8.8–15.6) in the first 3 postnatal days and 11.3 ± 1.3 mm (range 9.3–15.6) from 4–14 days after birth.[5]

Given that LVIDD depends on the size of the patient, for comparison to other patients, adjustment for body weight is necessary. From this perspective, LVIDD adjusted for weight (aLVIDD) is a better index than unadjusted LVIDD. Dividing LVID by weight in kilogram yields aLVIDD. In hemodynamically stable preterm infants ≤30 weeks' gestation, aLVIDD was 15.2 ± 2.5 mm/kg in the first 3 postnatal days and 15.6 ± 2.3 mm/kg from 4–14 days after birth.[5] However, as discussed in Chapter 11, the size of heart structures and weight do not have a perfect positive linear relationship (ie, the size of heart structure does not increase by 2-fold if the weight is doubled). Therefore, adjusting for a fixed heart structure (eg, aortic root diameter) might be a better option. On the other hand, incorporating another measured diameter into the index will certainly introduce another potential error.

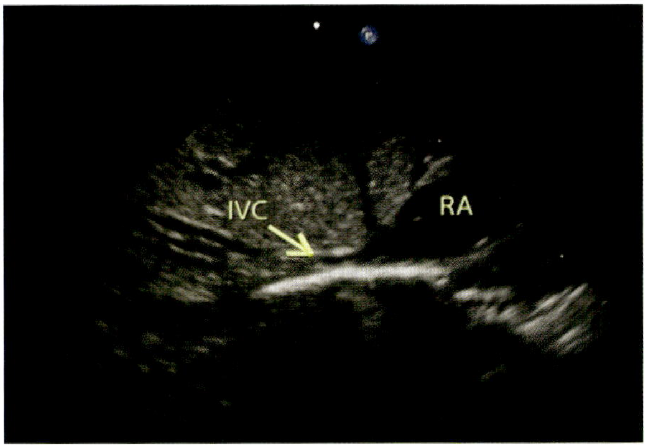

FIGURE and VIDEO 10-2. Collapsed inferior vena cava (IVC) in a preterm infant with lactic acidosis in the first postnatal day suggestive of low preload. Abbreviation: RA, right atrium.

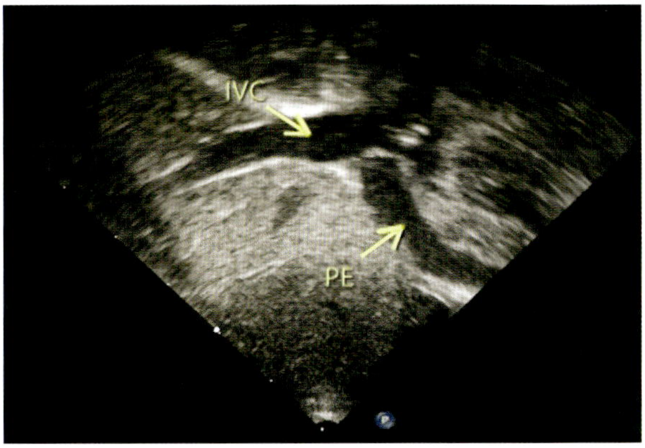

FIGURE and VIDEO 10-3. A dilated inferior vena cava (IVC) can be a sign of fluid overload, but in this case, the IVC is dilated because of an increase in pericardial pressure secondary to pericardial effusion. Abbreviation: PE, pericardial effusion.

IVC diameter and collapsibility index. The fluid status affects the IVC diameter (Figures and Videos 10-2 to 10-3). In hypovolemia, the IVC diameter is small and the IVC may collapse during inspiration in hypovolemic spontaneously breathing patients. IVC diameter is usually measured just below the diaphragm after the connection with the hepatic veins, using the subcostal longitudinal (sagittal) view. For the IVC diameter to be meaningful, it needs to be indexed to other cardiac structures. In older children and adults, IVC diameter is divided by aortic (Ao) diameter (measured in the same view as IVC). This IVC to Ao ratio has been found to be a useful tool in the assessment of fluid status in children with dehydration and in adults with septic shock.[6,7] Another measure of fluid status using IVC diameter is the collapsibility index: diameter in expiration–diameter in inspiration divided by diameter in expiration. This is based on the principle that the IVC is prone to collapse during inspiration and even more so when circulating blood volume is decreased. In adults, even a visual estimate of changes in IVC diameter with respiration has been found to be helpful in the assessment of fluid status.[8] However, none of these measurements or indices has been validated in the neonatal population, and therefore their utility is unknown.[9] Apart from changes in intravascular volume, many other factors can affect the IVC diameter and collapsibility index, including cardiac function, pericardial and pleural pressure, and positive pressure ventilation.

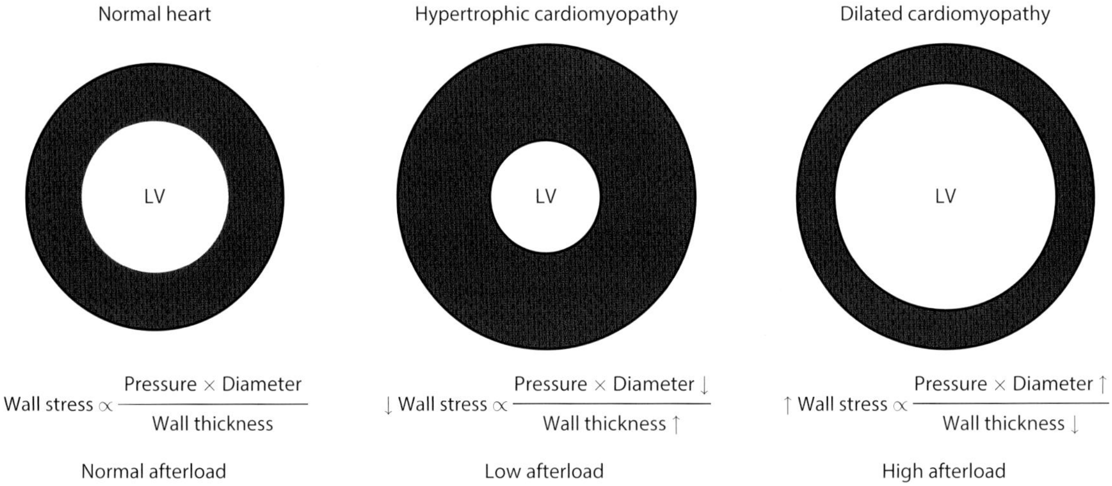

FIGURE 10-4. End-systolic wall stress is considered a good measure of the afterload. Left ventricular (LV) wall stress is directly related to LV diameter and LV pressure (which in turn is related to systemic blood pressure) and inversely proportional to LV wall thickness. In hypertrophic cardiomyopathy, the afterload is very low promoting a hyperdynamic state, while in the case of dilated cardiomyopathy, the afterload is very high, further compromising systolic function.

Contractility

One can describe contractility in terms of myocardial fiber shortening without any regards to the preload and afterload. Such load-dependent measures of contractility include shortening fraction and heart rate-corrected velocity of circumferential fiber shortening (VCF_C). Alternatively, and perhaps more appropriately, contractility can be defined as the ability of myocardium to contract when adjustment for variability in preload and afterload are made. This is considered true or load-independent contractility. Stress-velocity index, the relationship between VCF_C and wall stress, is thought to be relatively load-independent. Both load-dependent and -independent measures of contractility provide us with important clinically relevant information. Using a load-dependent index, the clinician gains insight on how the myocardium fares under current loading conditions; assessment by a load-independent index might help the clinician in ascertaining if an inherent contractility problem is the cause of cardiovascular compromise (irrespective of any abnormalities in preload or afterload). The pros and cons of each method, as well as measurement techniques, have been discussed in detail in Chapter 8.

Afterload

In Chapter 8 we discussed that left ventricular wall stress (WS) is a measure of afterload and that WS is directly related to left ventricular diameter and pressure and inversely related to ventricular wall thickness (by the law of Laplace). WS changes during the cardiac cycle, and end-systolic WS is considered the best indicator of afterload. Figure 10-4 illustrates the effect of left ventricular diameter and thickness on WS. In patients with a dilated ventricle secondary to heart failure or dilated cardiomyopathy, for the same blood pressure, the afterload is much greater than in a patient with a normally sized ventricle. On the other hand, a thick myocardium or a ventricle with a small cavity would have lower afterload for a given blood pressure. Finally, the higher the blood pressure, the higher the afterload for a given ventricular size and thickness. It is important to distinguish SVR from afterload; while related (primarily via SVR's effect on blood pressure), they are not the same and should not be used interchangeably (for further discussions see "Wall Stress" in Chapter 8).

■ VASODILATORY SHOCK

Normal vascular tone is maintained by a myriad of cellular signals, which can be hormonal, neuronal, or local. These mediators modulate vascular tone by inducing changes in the amount of intracellular calcium via second messengers or by direct activation of enzymes. Most of the mediators involved in regulation of vascular tone such as nitric oxide also play a role in pathogenesis of vasodilatory shock. Under physiologic conditions, there is a balance

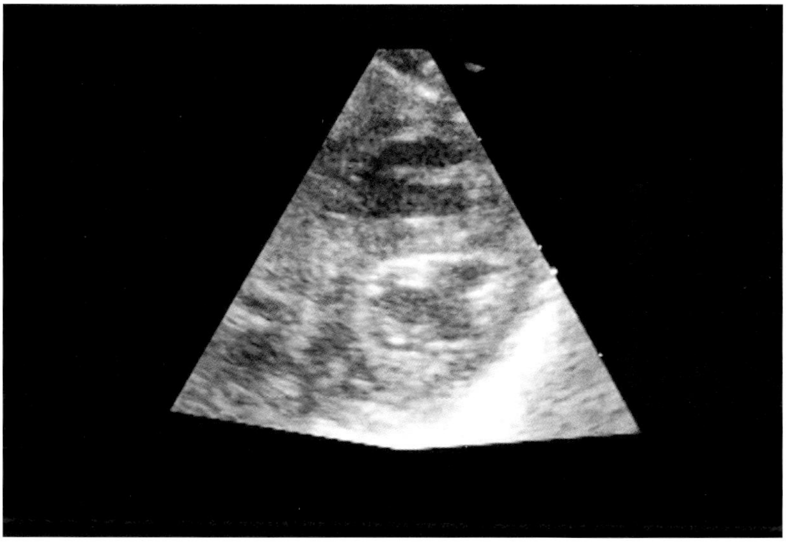

FIGURE and VIDEO 10-5. Parasternal short-axis view showing hyperdynamic myocardium in a hypotensive extremely preterm infant with necrotizing enterocolitis receiving high-dose dopamine. Despite cardiac output being in the high normal range (250 ml/kg/min), the patient was severely hypotensive. This suggests that despite some degree of compensatory increase in cardiac output, the pathological peripheral vasodilation was severe enough to result in hypotension.

between the vasodilator and vasoconstrictor forces. In a pathologic condition, the balance might favor excessive vasoconstriction over vasodilation.

The conditions that can lead to vasodilatory shock in the neonatal period include sepsis, respiratory distress syndrome, necrotizing enterocolitis, and absolute/relative adrenal hypoplasia. In addition, severe peripheral vasodilatation causing vasodilatory shock can ensue after prolonged and severe shock from other causes.

Clinically, vasodilatory shock is characterized by hypotension, warm and pink extremities, bounding pulses, and a relatively rapid capillary refill time.

Echocardiography Findings in Vasodilatory Shock

The echocardiographic findings of vasodilatory shock depend upon the adequacy of compensatory function. Without compensation, the findings are mainly secondary to a decreased return of venous blood to the heart and a relatively inadequate volume status due to maldistribution (ie, decreased preload). However, in the neonatal population one often encounters some degree of compensation with a hyperdynamic myocardium and high cardiac output. The calculated SVR is low and blood pressure is low despite the high cardiac output (incomplete compensation) (Figure and Video 10-5). Depending on the cause of vasodilatory shock and the stage of shock, myocardial contractility might also be affected. For example, in the late stage of septic shock, echocardiography can show an abnormally low shortening fraction and/or stress-velocity index.

Timely recognition of septic shock can reduced mortality.[10] There are limited data on cardiac function in neonates with shock.[11,12] In one study, preterm infants with sepsis were found to have high cardiac output and low vascular resistance.[12] While as a group, the survivors maintained their cardiac output and mildly raised their SVR, there was significant hemodynamic variability among individual patients. On the other hand, the nonsurvivors had a drop in cardiac output and abrupt rise in SVR. It is unclear if the drop in cardiac output was the result of excessive increase in SVR or the rise in SVR was a last-ditch effort by the body to maintain perfusion pressure in the setting of low cardiac output.

■ CARDIOGENIC SHOCK

In extremely preterm infants, myocardial dysfunction can be due to maladaptation during the transitional period, perinatal depression, or septic shock. All of these can lead to cardiogenic shock. The heart pump failure can be the only underlying cause of shock, or it can be associated with other pathophysiology such as vasodilation, as seen in septic shock. In this chapter, we will not discuss other causes of cardiogenic shock, such as congenital heart diseases, cardiomyopathies, and arrhythmias.

Myocardial Dysfunction and Postnatal Cardiovascular Maladaptation

Significant cellular, mechanistic, and functional differences in myocardial contraction during development explain contractility differences in the preterm, term, and adult heart. The immature myocytes during fetal life and at birth are smaller in size, more spherical in shape, and higher in water content, and they have fewer contractile elements and myofibril content per cross-sectional area. Disorganized myofibril orientation and internal cellular components also result in slower and less efficient contraction. In addition, immature myocytes depend mainly on extracellular calcium influx through the L-type calcium channels for myocardial contraction. Their higher cell surface-area-to-volume ratio perhaps compensate for the underdeveloped T-tubule system. In contrast, the L-type calcium channels of mature adult myocytes act only as a trigger to signal release of calcium from the more developed sarcoplasmic reticulum for contraction. These cumulative molecular and structural changes in cardiac development might account for the diminished ability of the immature heart to counter acute changes in preload or afterload. As shown in Figure 10-6, there are differences between the newborn heart and older children in contractility and afterload relationship.[13] There is a more significant drop in VCF_C (a measure of contraction) with increase in wall stress (an index of afterload) in neonates compared to older children. This higher sensitivity of the myocardium to increase in afterload has been implicated in the pathogenesis of shock in the immediate postnatal period in a subset of preterm infants who later develop brain hemorrhage. With the clamping of the cord and removal of low-resistance placental circulation, the SVR increases abruptly. This increase in SVR is thought to increase the left ventricular afterload and compromise left ventricular output. When superior vena cava (SVC) flow was used as a surrogate for systemic and brain blood flow, preterm infants with low SVC flow as a group had a steeper correlation coefficient line in the VCF_C and WS relationship.[14] This suggests that the higher sensitivity to afterload is associated with low systemic flow and may contribute to the development of low flow state immediately after birth

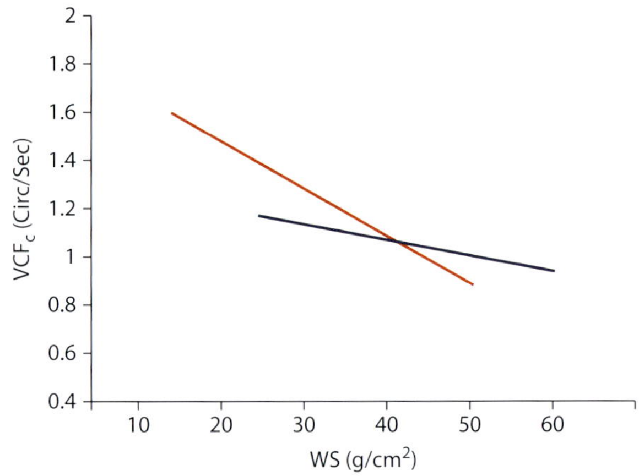

FIGURE 10-6. The blue line represents the normal inverse relationship that exists between the heart rate-corrected velocity of circumferential shortening (VCF_C, myocardial contractility) and the wall stress (WS, afterload) in children. In neonates the y-intercept of the regression line (red) is higher and the slope is steeper than in older children. In other words, the myocardium functions at a higher baseline contractile state, and with an increase in afterload, the contractility of immature myocardium decreases more than that of the mature heart of older children. (Adapted with permission from Rowland DG and Gutgesell HP. Noninvasive assessment of myocardial contractility, preload, and afterload in healthy newborn infants. *Am J Cardiol.* 1995 Apr;75(12):818–821.)

at least in a subset of extremely preterm infants. As low cardiac output and SVC flow have been implicated in the pathogenesis of peri/intraventricular hemorrhage,[15,16] and low SVC flow is predictive of poor neurodevelopmental outcome, [17] recognition of myocardial dysfunction in this setting becomes important.

Asphyxia

A neonate who has sustained a perinatal hypoxic-ischemic injury can present with cardiogenic shock. Recognition of this cause of myocardial dysfunction can be challenging for several reasons. First, the underlying etiology of asphyxia can mask and delay a clinical suspicion of myocardial dysfunction, as metabolic acidosis might be attributed to the initial insult. Second, the compensatory increase in SVR aiming at maintaining perfusion pressure can keep blood pressure in the normal range despite low cardiac output and poor organ blood flow (Figure and Video 10-7). Therefore, routine assessment of cardiac function by echocardiography can help in early detection of cardiogenic shock.[18] Furthermore, functional echocardiography can be helpful in guiding cardiovascular

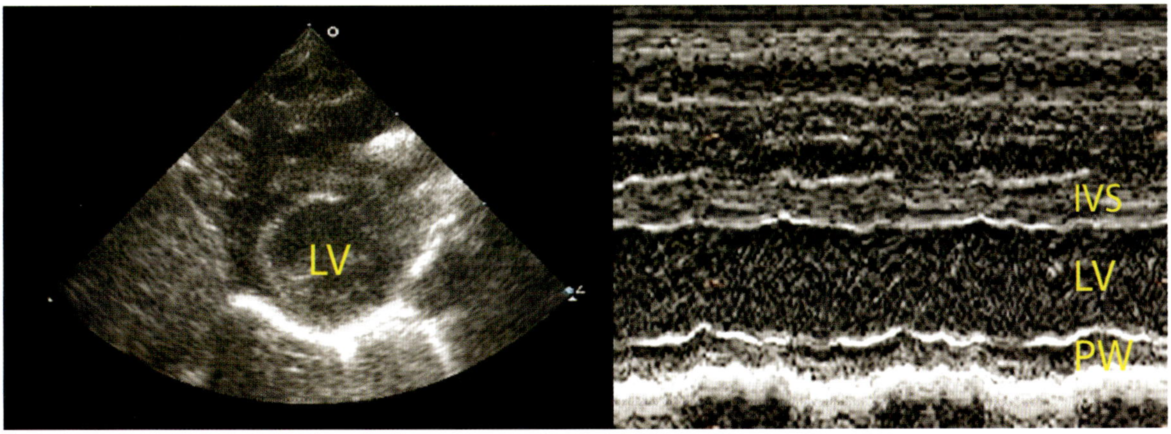

FIGURE and VIDEO 10-7. Parasternal short-axis view of the left ventricle in a preterm infant with very low Apgar scores. Note the poor approximation of the intraventricular septum (IVS) and the left ventricular (LV) posterior wall (PW) on the M-mode and the 2D mode (video). The patient had normal blood pressure despite having extremely low cardiac output (50 ml/kg/min). The compensatory increase in systemic vascular resistance had resulted in normal blood pressure, which could give a false reassurance of stable hemodynamic status in the situation where significant circulatory compromise is present.

support and choice of inotropes/vasopressors, and also in the management of pulmonary hypertension that is commonly associated with perinatal hypoxic-ischemic injury.

Myocardial dysfunction is fairly common in the asphyxiated neonate.[19] About a third of patients with asphyxia may have clinical or electrocardiographic evidence of cardiac involvement.[20,21] However, the incidence of myocardial dysfunction detectable by echocardiography varies significantly in the literature. In general, measures of myocardial systolic function such as shortening fraction (SF) and VCF_C are expected to be lower than normal. Similarly, left ventricular output (LVO) will be low in cardiogenic shock. Conversely, SVR can vary significantly depending on the stage and severity of the initial insult, the level of neurohormonal compensatory mechanisms, and the degree of ongoing acidosis and hypoxia. Therefore, SVR can be high, normal, or low. In addition, evidence of pulmonary hypertension (right-to-left flow through a patent ductus arteriosus and/or patent foramen ovale, tricuspid regurgitation with a high gradient, decreased right ventricular output, ventricular septal flattening or bowing toward the left ventricle) can often be seen in cases of asphyxia.

Several studies have shown a significant decrease in the shortening fraction in cases of asphyxia, while others have found the shortening fraction to be less valuable in defining myocardial involvement.[22-26] Similarly, low LVO is reported to be prevalent in some but not all studies.[23-25] Recent studies have suggested that tissue Doppler indices might be more sensitive than conventional echocardiographic measurements (eg, M-mode or 2D) in detecting myocardial dysfunction in asphyxiated neonates. For example, systolic velocity of the mitral annulus and myocardial peak systolic strain and strain rate have been found to be low in asphyxiated neonates, even when the shortening fraction and other conventional measures of systolic function were normal.[26,27] However, further studies on these new modalities are needed to define their clinical relevance. This is also true with regard to biomarkers such as troponin I and T; these markers may be more sensitive than echocardiography in detecting myocardial involvement,[23,24,27] but their relevance for guiding cardiovascular supportive care is unclear.

The effect of asphyxia on Doppler indices of anterior and middle cerebral arteries is variable. Most studies show an increase in indices of blood flow in the first postnatal day with a greater increase in severe cases.[28-30] Others have shown the opposite effect.[25] The differences in these studies are likely due (at least in part) to differences in the definition of asphyxia, as well as the severity and stage of disease and the timing of the study. In general, there is a reperfusion phase with an increase in flow after the initial ischemia. Whether cerebral blood flow increases or decreases likely depends on the severity of myocardial involvement, the amount of ongoing metabolic derangement, and the degree of impairment of cerebral autoregulation.

Sepsis

As mentioned earlier, in addition to pathologic vasodilation, myocardial function can also be affected in septic shock. Decreased systolic function and myocardial dysfunction are believed to be primarily due to cytokine-mediated myocardial depression, although myocardial ischemia also plays a role.[31,32] It is unknown whether cardiogenic shock due to sepsis-associated myocardial dysfunction is prevalent in the neonatal population. In older children, low cardiac output and elevated SVR (cardiogenic shock) were the dominant presentation of community-acquired septic shock as compared to high cardiac output and low SVR (vasodilatory) shock in hospital-acquired septic shock.[33]

In assessing infants with severe sepsis or septic shock, in addition to estimation of cardiac output and SVR, myocardial function should be evaluated. While conventional measures of systolic function (eg, SF) might not be affected, newer and more sensitive indices such as myocardial strain are found to be depressed in pediatric patients with septic shock.[34,35]

HYPOVOLEMIC SHOCK

Hypovolemia

In the pediatric population, treatment of shock commonly centers on correction of the circulatory imbalance, with empiric fluid resuscitation. Although hypovolemia might be the etiology underlying most children with shock, it is less common in neonates. In the setting of acute gastrointestinal fluid loss (vomiting, diarrhea), acute blood loss (uterine rupture, procedural blood loss, placental abruption), transepidermal water loss, or increased urine output (diabetes insipidus), hypovolemic shock can occur and should be treated accordingly with fluid resuscitation. Clinically, severe hypovolemia can result in decreased preload and hence decreased cardiac output (steep portion on the Frank-Starling curve). The decreased cardiac output is secondary to decreased stroke volume. With inadequate stretch of baroreceptors in the aortic arch and carotid sinus, sympathetic activity is increased with resultant compensatory peripheral vasoconstriction (to help increase preload) and tachycardia (to maintain adequate cardiac output). The infant presents with cool and pale extremities, high heart rate, and low blood pressure.

The echocardiographic findings include evidence of low preload, low cardiac output, and in more extreme cases, low SF due to poor myocardial stretch (Frank-Starling mechanisms).

Pericardial Effusion and Cardiac Tamponade

Pericardial effusion can be iatrogenic or caused by a host of pathologies such as infectious and autoimmune mechanisms. In neonates, common causes of pericardial effusion include hydrops fetalis, a complication of central venous catheters, and post-pericardiotomy syndrome. Whether a pericardial effusion leads to cardiac tamponade depends upon several factors including the amount of the effusion and how fast it develops. Clinically, significant pericardial effusion that evolves to cardiac tamponade is characterized by hypotension with a narrow pulse pressure (due to small stroke volume), muffled heart sounds, and pulsus paradoxus. It is quite easy to diagnose pericardial effusion with echocardiography (Figures and Videos 10-8 to 10-9). However, echocardiographic diagnosis of cardiac tamponade requires significant experience. Pericardial effusions can be assessed from parasternal, apical and subcostal view. There is no standard method of measurement of the amount of effusion. For the sake of consistency, it is recommended to measure the fluid from the subcostal view, from the epicardial surface to its maximal dimension in 2D imaging at end-diastole.[36] However,

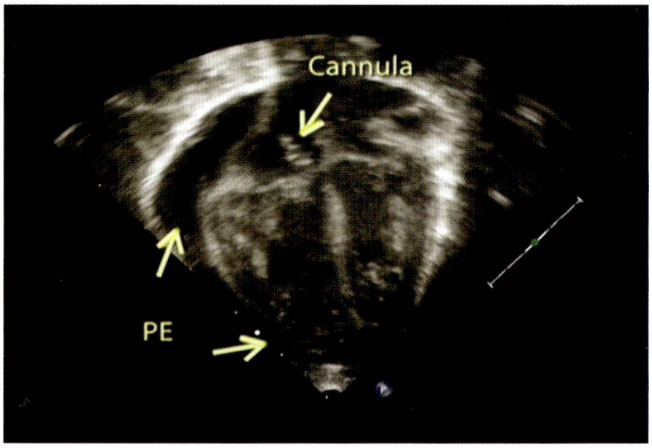

FIGURE and VIDEO 10-8. Apical view demonstrating a pericardial effusion in a full-term infant with meconium aspiration syndrome, several hours after placement of veno-venous extracorporeal membranous oxygenation. Note the misplaced cannula position deep in the right atrium. The cannula was likely pushing on the right atrial wall, causing the pericardial effusion. Abbreviation: PE, pericardial effusion.

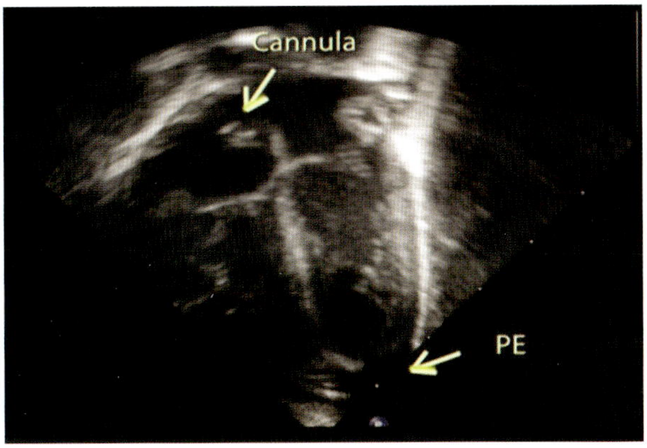

FIGURE and VIDEO 10-9. Same patient as in Figure and Video 10-8. 12 hours after adjustment of the cannula. Note that the pericardial effusion is almost completely resolved. Abbreviation: PE, pericardial effusion.

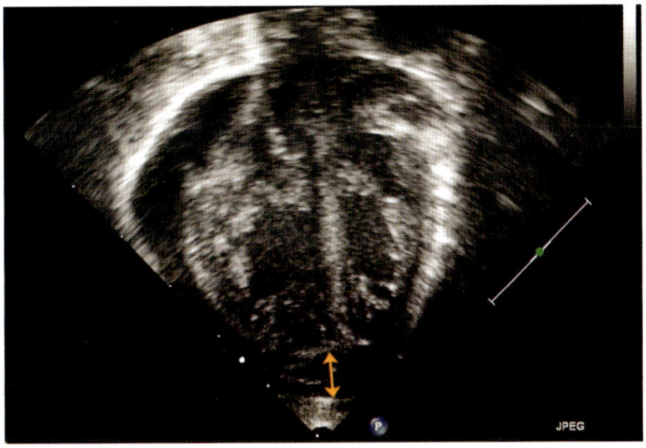

FIGURE 10-10. The arrow points to the pericardial effusion from the epicardial surface to its maximal dimension in the apical view. Any measurement of pericardial effusion in 2D should be used as a rough estimate, as the changes in the amount of pericardial effusion can vary significantly in different views (compare Videos 10-7 and 10.8).

other views are acceptable as long as repeated measurements are performed in the same area, and from the same view at end-diastole (Figure 10-9). In the presence of a significant pericardial effusion, the associated increase in pericardial pressure can result in dilatation of IVC (Figure and Video 10-3). However, a dilated IVC is a non-specific sign and can occur in other conditions as well. Evidence of cardiac tamponade includes right atrial collapse at the onset of systole, right ventricular collapse in diastole, and increased respiration-associated variation in mitral and tricuspid inflow Doppler velocities. In spontaneously breathing normal children, during inspiration, mitral and tricuspid peak E waves are decreased and increased by average of 8% and 26%, respectively.[37] However, mitral and tricuspid flow velocities can be difficult to interpret in mechanically ventilated infants.

REFERENCES

1. Noori S, Seri I. Evidence-based versus pathophysiology-based approach to diagnosis and treatment of neonatal cardiovascular compromise. *Semin Fetal Neonatal Med.* 2015;20:238–245.
2. Kampmann C, Wiethoff CM, Wenzel A, et al. Normal values of M mode echocardiographic measurements of more than 2000 healthy infants and children in central Europe. *Heart.* 2000;83:667–672.
3. Harada K, Takahashi Y, Tamura M, Orino T, Takada G. Serial echocardiographic and Doppler evaluation of left ventricular systolic performance and diastolic filling in premature infants. *Early Hum Dev.* 1999;54:169–180.
4. Zecca E, Romagnoli C, Vento G, De Carolis MP, De Rosa G, Tortorolo G. Left ventricle dimensions in preterm infants during the first month of life. *Eur J Pediatr.* 2001;160:227–230.
5. Noori S, Wu T-W, Seri I. pH effects on cardiac function and systemic vascular resistance in preterm infants. *J. Pediatr.* 2012. doi:10.1016/j.jpeds.2012.10.021.
6. Chen L, Kim Y, Santucci KA. Use of ultrasound measurement of the inferior vena cava diameter as an objective tool in the assessment of children with clinical dehydration. *Acad Emerg Med.* 2007;14:841–845.
7. Schefold JC, Storm C, Bercker S, et al. Inferior vena cava diameter correlates with invasive hemodynamic measures in mechanically ventilated intensive care unit patients with sepsis. *J Emerg Med.* 2010;38:632–637.
8. Weekes AJ, Tassone HM, Babcock A, et al. Comparison of serial qualitative and quantitative assessments of caval index and left ventricular systolic function during early fluid resuscitation of hypotensive emergency department patients. *Acad Emerg Med.* 2011;18:912–921.
9. Lopez L, Colan SD, Frommelt PC, et al. Recommendations for quantification methods during the performance of a pediatric echocardiogram: a report from the Pediatric Measurements Writing Group of the American Society of Echocardiography Pediatric and Congenital Heart Disease Council. *J Am Soc Echocardiogr.* 2010;23:465–495–577.
10. Davis AL, Carcillo JA, Aneja RK, et al. American College of Critical Care Medicine Clinical Practice Parameters for Hemodynamic Support of Pediatric and Neonatal Septic Shock. *Cri Care Med.* 2017;45:1061–1093.

11. Saini SS, Kumar P, Kumar RM. Hemodynamic changes in preterm neonates with septic shock: a prospective observational study*. *Pediatr Crit Care Med.* 2014;15: 443–450.

12. de Waal K, Evans N. Hemodynamics in preterm infants with late-onset sepsis. *J Pediatr.* 2010;156:918–922, 922.e1.

13. Rowland DG, Gutgesell HP. Noninvasive assessment of myocardial contractility, preload, and afterload in healthy newborn infants. *Am J Cardiol.* 1995;75:818–821.

14. Osborn DA, Evans N, Kluckow M. Left ventricular contractility in extremely premature infants in the first day and response to inotropes. *Pediatr Res.* 2007;61:335–340.

15. Kluckow M, Evans N. Low superior vena cava flow and intraventricular haemorrhage in preterm infants. *Arch Dis Child Fetal Neonatal Ed.* 2000;82:F188–F194.

16. Noori S, McCoy M, Anderson MP, Ramji F, Seri I. Changes in cardiac function and cerebral blood flow in relation to peri/intraventricular hemorrhage in extremely preterm infants. *J Pediatr.* 2014;164:264–270–273.

17. Hunt RW, Evans N, Rieger I, Kluckow M. Low superior vena cava flow and neurodevelopment at 3 years in very preterm infants. *J Pediatr.* 2004;145:588–592.

18. Kluckow M. Functional echocardiography in assessment of the cardiovascular system in asphyxiated neonates. *J Pediatr.* 2011;158:e13–e18.

19. Armstrong K, Franklin O, Sweetman D, Molloy EJ. Cardiovascular dysfunction in infants with neonatal encephalopathy. *Arch Dis Child.* 2012;97:372–375.

20. Martín-Ancel A, García-Alix A, Gayá F, Cabañas F, Burgueros M, Quero J. Multiple organ involvement in perinatal asphyxia. *J Pediatr.* 1995;127:786–793.

21. Kanik E, Ozer EA, Bakiler AR, et al. Assessment of myocardial dysfunction in neonates with hypoxic-ischemic encephalopathy: is it a significant predictor of mortality? *J Matern Fetal Neonatal Med.* 2009;22:239–242.

22. Barberi I, Calabrò MP, Cordaro S, et al. Myocardial ischaemia in neonates with perinatal asphyxia. Electrocardiographic, echocardiographic and enzymatic correlations. *Eur J Pediatr.* 1999;158:742–747.

23. Szymankiewicz M, Matuszczak-Wleklak M, Hodgman JE, Gadzinowski J. Usefulness of cardiac troponin T and echocardiography in the diagnosis of hypoxic myocardial injury of full-term neonates. *Biol Neonate.* 2005;88:19–23.

24. Costa S, Zecca E, De Rosa G, et al. Is serum troponin T a useful marker of myocardial damage in newborn infants with perinatal asphyxia? *Acta Paediatr.* 2007;96:181–184.

25. Liu J, Li J, Gu M. The correlation between myocardial function and cerebral hemodynamics in term infants with hypoxic-ischemic encephalopathy. *J Trop Pediatr.* 2007; 53:44–48.

26. Nestaas E, Støylen A., Brunvand L, Fugelseth D. Longitudinal strain and strain rate by tissue Doppler are more sensitive indices than fractional shortening for assessing the reduced myocardial function in asphyxiated neonates. *Cardiol Young.* 2011;21:1–7.

27. Wei Y, Xu J, Xu T, Fan J, Tao S. Left ventricular systolic function of newborns with asphyxia evaluated by tissue Doppler imaging. *Pediatr Cardiol.* 2009;30:741–746.

28. van Bel F, van de Bor M, Stijnen T, Baan J, Ruys JH. Cerebral blood flow velocity pattern in healthy and asphyxiated newborns: a controlled study. *Eur J Pediatr.* 1987;146:461–467.

29. Levene MI, Fenton AC, Evans DH, Archer LN, Shortland DB, Gibson NA. Severe birth asphyxia and abnormal cerebral blood-flow velocity. *Dev Med Child Neurol.* 1989;31:427–434.

30. Ilves P, Talvik R, Talvik T. Changes in Doppler ultrasonography in asphyxiated term infants with hypoxic-ischaemic encephalopathy. *Acta Paediatr.* 1998;87:680–684.

31. Court O, Kumar A, Parrillo JE, Kumar A. Clinical review: Myocardial depression in sepsis and septic shock. *Crit Care.* 2002;6:500–508.

32. Joulin O, Petillot P, Labalette M, Lancel S, Neviere R. Cytokine profile of human septic shock serum inducing cardiomyocyte contractile dysfunction. *Physiol Res.* 2007;56:291–297.

33. Brierley J, Peters MJ. Distinct hemodynamic patterns of septic shock at presentation to pediatric intensive care. *Pediatrics.* 2008;122:752–759.

34. Fenton KE, Sable CA, Bell MJ, Patel KM, Berger JT. Increases in serum levels of troponin I are associated with cardiac dysfunction and disease severity in pediatric patients with septic shock. *Pediatr Crit Care Med.* 2004;5:533–538.

35. Basu S, Frank LH, Fenton KE, Sable CA, Levy RJ, Berger JT. Two-dimensional speckle tracking imaging detects impaired myocardial performance in children with septic shock, not recognized by conventional echocardiography. *Pediatr Crit Care Med.* 2012;13:259–264.

36. Mertens L, Seri I, Marek J, et al. Targeted neonatal echocardiography in the neonatal intensive care nit: practice guidelines and recommendations for training. Writing Group of the American Society of Echocardiography (ASE) in collaboration with the European Association of Echocardiography (EAE) and the Association for European Pediatric Cardiologists (AEPC). *J Am Soc Echocardiogr.* 2011;24:1057–1078.

37. Riggs TW, Snider AR. Respiratory influence on right and left ventricular diastolic function in normal children. *Am J Cardiol.* 1989;63:858–861.

CHAPTER 11

Patent Ductus Arteriosus*

Shahab Noori

- INTRODUCTION
- HEMODYNAMIC EFFECTS OF A PDA
  - Cardiac Function
  - Pulmonary Blood Flow
  - Cerebral Blood Flow
  - Superior Mesenteric and Celiac Artery Blood Flow
  - Renal Blood Flow
- HEMODYNAMIC EFFECTS OF PDA LIGATION
  - Cardiac Effects
  - Effects on Cerebral Blood Flow
  - Effects on Blood Flow to Other Organs
- ECHOCARDIOGRAPHIC EVIDENCE OF A HEMODYNAMICALLY SIGNIFICANT PDA
  - Indicators of the Hemodynamic Significance of a PDA
  - PDA Diameter
  - PDA Flow Pattern
  - Left Atrium to Aortic Root Ratio
  - Flow Reversal in Descending Aorta
  - Left Pulmonary Artery Diastolic Flow
  - Left Ventricular Output
  - Absent or Reversal Diastolic Flow in MCA, SMA, and RA
  - Other Indices
- REFERENCES

INTRODUCTION

In this chapter, the impact of a patent ductus arteriosus (PDA) will be discussed in the clinical setting of a neonate with an otherwise structurally normal heart (± a patent foramen ovale). Specific emphasis will be placed on preterm infants with relatively low pulmonary vascular resistance and ductal shunting that is predominantly or completely left to right.

Until recently, because the harmful effects of a PDA were thought to be self-evident, the prevailing opinion was that PDA closure was indicated in all preterm infants. The predominant question was the best method to close a PDA in such patients, and this was the subject of numerous randomized clinical trials.[1,2] However, over the last decade, the rationale for the treatment of a PDA, in general, and ligation, in particular, has been increasingly challenged. The current trend is to recommend a less aggressive approach to the pharmacologic and surgical treatment of a PDA. This in turn has made the recognition of a hemodynamically significant patent ductus arteriosus (hsPDA) even more important. In this chapter, the hemodynamic effects of a PDA and its ligation will be reviewed, followed by a detailed description of the echocardiographic indices that can be helpful

*Videos can be accessed at http://PracticalNeonatalEcho.com.

in identifying an hsPDA. Finally, the use of PDA flow to estimate relative pulmonary vascular resistance in the setting of pulmonary hypertension will be briefly discussed.

HEMODYNAMIC EFFECTS OF A PDA

Cardiac Function

In the presence of a PDA with left-to-right shunting, pulmonary blood flow increases, leading to an increase in pulmonary venous return to the left atrium (LA). This increase in LA volume can augment the left ventricular (LV) preload, provided no significant shunt at the patent foramen ovale (PFO) is present (see below). The increase in LV preload will increase the stroke volume according to the Starling curve.[3–6] However, a PFO can significantly alter the effects of a PDA on LV stroke volume by decompressing the LA. Indeed, in the presence of a significant PFO (diameter >4 mm), right ventricular output (RVO) can even be greater than left ventricular output (LVO) despite the presence of a significant left-to-right PDA shunt.[7] Despite the inherent vulnerability of the immature myocardium and the potential for decreased myocardial perfusion due to low diastolic pressure, myocardial contractility appears not to be affected by an hsPDA. With short exposure (days) to an hsPDA, both load-dependent (LV shortening fraction, or SF) and load-independent (stress-velocity index) measures of systolic function are found to be normal.[8]

In the presence of a PDA, the heart rate does not change; therefore, the increase in LVO is solely the result of an increase in stroke volume. As systolic blood pressure is primarily affected by changes in stroke volume and diastolic blood pressure is mainly reflective of changes in systemic vascular resistance (SVR), the PDA-associated increase in stroke volume and decrease in SVR causes systolic blood pressure to be maintained or minimally decreased compared to a significant drop in diastolic blood pressure. This results in a wide pulse pressure, the hallmark of an hsPDA. However, in the first few days of postnatal life, both systolic and diastolic blood pressure can be affected to the same degree, thereby maintaining an unchanged pulse pressure.[9,10] This may be the result of inadequate compensatory increase in stroke volume and/or low amount of left-to-right PDA shunting during the early postnatal period. In animals, a left-to-right PDA shunt decreases diastolic and mean blood pressure, while only a moderate to large left-to-right PDA shunt reduces systolic blood pressure.[4]

The increase in LVO may compensate for the shunt, but as discussed below, this compensation may not be adequate and distal organ blood flow distribution is often significantly altered. Animal studies suggest that systemic blood flow is redistributed even in the presence of a small PDA.[4] The effect of blood flow diversion from the "steal phenomenon" of an hsPDA on organ blood flow varies. In general, blood flow to the brain is preserved better than any other organ. Skin, bone, and skeletal muscle are among the first organs to be adversely affected by an hsPDA. Next, the blood flow to the gastrointestinal system and kidneys is compromised. Importantly, organ blood flow can be compromised without any signs of left ventricular failure.[11,12]

Pulmonary Blood Flow

Pulmonary blood flow is derived from RVO and supplemented by the left-to-right PDA shunt (both during systole and diastole). In the presence of an hsPDA, the systemic flow (effective left cardiac output) can be compromised, leading to a decrease in venous return to the right side of heart and consequently a decrease in RVO. Despite this decrease in RVO, the net pulmonary blood flow increases in the presence of a left-to-right PDA shunt. Furthermore, with a significant PFO or atrial septal defect, the RVO is maintained despite a reduction in systemic venous return. In fact, with a significant PFO, the larger the PDA, the greater will be the RVO.

Cerebral Blood Flow

The PDA effect on cerebral blood flow (CBF) varies from one patient to another, depending upon the adequacy of a compensatory increase in left ventricular output and decrease in cerebral vascular resistance. In most patients, the compensatory increase in stroke volume results in an increase in CBF during systole,[12,13] and the steal phenomenon leads to a decrease, absent, or reversal of flow during diastole.[14,15] The net effect is an abnormal flow pattern but maintenance of a normal amount of CBF. Interestingly, in a subset of infants, there appears to be an effective compensatory vasodilation in the brain, as evidenced by a normal diastolic flow pattern in the large cerebral arteries.

The compensatory increase in stroke volume appears to be the key in maintaining CBF.[16] This compensatory mechanism may not be fully in place in the first few hours after birth. In term neonates, during the first 20 minutes after birth, there is an strong inverse relationship between middle cerebral artery (MCA) mean velocity (a surrogate for CBF) and the net left-to-right shunt through the PDA.[17] Similarly, in preterm infants, a significant PDA is an independent predictor of low superior vena cava flow, a surrogate for CBF, only during the first 12 hours after birth.[18]

In other words, the adverse effect of a PDA on CBF is most prominent during the early postnatal period before the compensatory increase in LVO is yet fully operational.

Superior Mesenteric and Celiac Artery Blood Flow

Blood flow to the abdominal organs is decreased in the presence of an hsPDA. Even a small ductal shunt has been shown to cause significant reductions in blood flow to the abdominal organs in preterm lambs.[4] Assessment of superior mesenteric and celiac arteries by Doppler shows a decrease in flow as well as an abnormal pattern: a decreased, absent, or reversed flow during diastole.[15,19,20] Importantly, this reduction in abdominal organ blood flow occurs despite a compensatory increase in LVO.[12] Therefore, while a compensatory increase in LVO might maintain adequate CBF (albeit with an abnormal pattern), it does not result in normal blood flow to the organs supplied by the abdominal aorta. Interestingly, in premature primates, not only is the baseline intestinal blood flow decreased, but also the normal postprandial increase in intestinal flow is blunted.[21]

Renal Blood Flow

Similar to SMA flow, renal blood flow is affected by an hsPDA. A reduced overall flow with absent or reversed diastolic flow mark the effect of an hsPDA on renal artery flow.

■ HEMODYNAMIC EFFECTS OF PDA LIGATION

Up to 45% of the preterm infants undergoing surgical ligation of their PDA develop a period of cardiopulmonary deterioration after the procedure.[22] This deterioration—marked by hypotension, increased vasopressor and/or inotrope treatment, and increased respiratory support—usually presents a few hours after the procedure, with the patient's condition improving by 24 to 48 hours.[22–28] While the exact cause of this deterioration is not clear, cardiac dysfunction and adrenal insufficiency play a role, as will be discussed below.[22,24,27,29]

Cardiac Effects

With ligation of a PDA, the LV preload decreases, resulting in a reduction in LVO. The heart rate does not change after ligation. Therefore, the decrease in LVO is solely due to a decrease in stroke volume. In the presence of a PDA, the vascular resistance against which the LV pumps includes both the systemic and pulmonary vascular beds. Following ligation of the PDA, the contribution of the low-resistance pulmonary vascular bed is eliminated; therefore, the calculated vascular resistance increases. However, despite the increase in vascular resistance, the LV afterload, as assessed by the wall stress, does not change.[24,30] The lack of increase in afterload is due to the fact that afterload depends on blood pressure, ventricular diameter, and ventricular wall thickness (see Chapter 8). Therefore, the increase in blood pressure due to elevated vascular resistance is counterbalanced by the reduction in LV diameter and increase in ventricular wall thickness as a result of decreased LV preload.[24] Regarding myocardial contractility, overall there are no significant changes in either load-dependent (SF, corrected velocity of circumferential fiber shortening) or load-independent (stress-velocity index) measures of contractility.[24,30] Among those presenting with hemodynamic instability after ligation, some have poor systolic function (low SF and cardiac output), while others have primarily vasodilation most probably secondary to relative adrenal insufficiency.[22,29] A very small subset of patients presents with a dramatic reduction of the interventricular septal wall motion after ligation (Figures and Videos 11-1 and 11-2).[1] More commonly, a subtle deterioration in global myocardial function is noted by measurement of the myocardial performance index (MPI) immediately after ligation, with partial recovery by 24 hours.[24] This deterioration in myocardial performance might be reflective of "resetting" the set point of the Starling curve of the myocardium after a prolonged period of stretch so that the decrease in end-diastolic fiber length following ligation will result in a decrease in contractile force. Therefore, the post-ligation decrease in LVO results not only from a decrease in preload but also as a consequence of transient myocardial dysfunction. In other words, after ligation, the LVO decreases in excess of what is expected by removal of the shunt alone. It is interesting that the pattern of changes in MPI mimics the changes in LVO (Figure 11-3). Furthermore, it was the MPI—rather than the preload, contractility, or afterload—that was most predictive of the LVO after ligation.[24] It is possible that MPI is more sensitive than conventional indices of cardiac function. Similarly, decreased LV performance, as defined by either a LVO of <170 mL/kg/min, fractional shortening of <25%, or systolic blood pressure less than the 3rd percentile, was found to be prevalent in patients with hemodynamic instability at 8 hours after PDA ligation.[27]

Given the complexity of the effect of ligation on cardiac function and the significant incidence of cardiovascular compromise, assessment of cardiovascular function by echocardiography can be helpful in guiding the treatment strategy in these patients.

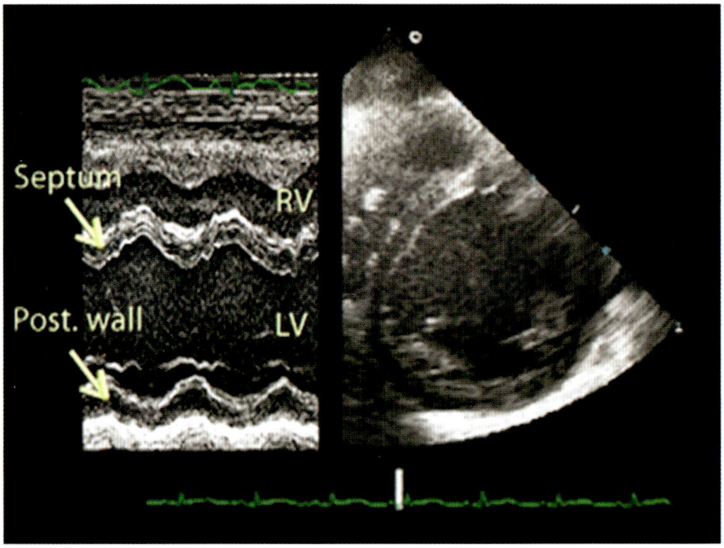

FIGURE and VIDEO 11-1. Parasternal short-axis view of the left ventricle at the level at the tips of mitral valve in an extremely preterm infant with a large PDA. The left ventricle is dilated as the result of the high preload secondary to the left-to-right PDA shunting. Note the normal motion of intraventricular septum during systole and diastole in M-mode. Abbreviations: RV, right ventricle; LV, left ventricle.

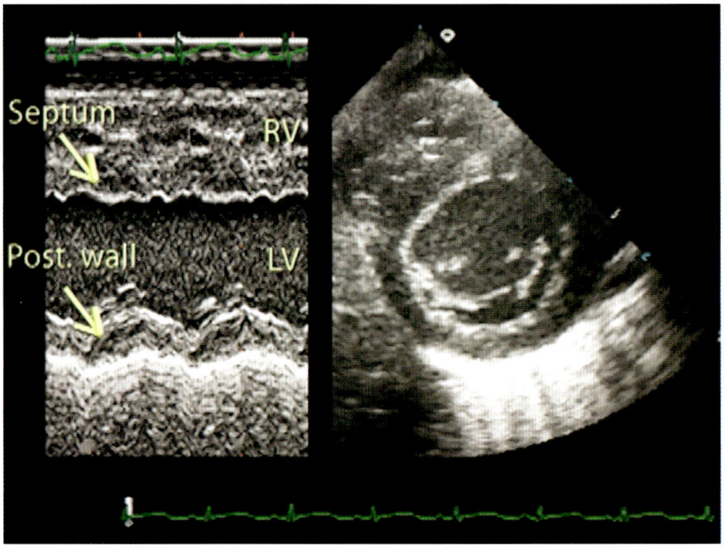

FIGURE and VIDEO 11-2. Parasternal short-axis view of the left ventricle at the level of the tips of mitral valve in the extremely preterm infant (same patient as in Figure and Video 11-1) after ligation of the large PDA. The left ventricular cavity is small and the M-mode tracing clearly demonstrates the minimal motion of the intraventricular septum during the cardiac cycle. Abbreviations: RV, right ventricle; LV, left ventricle.

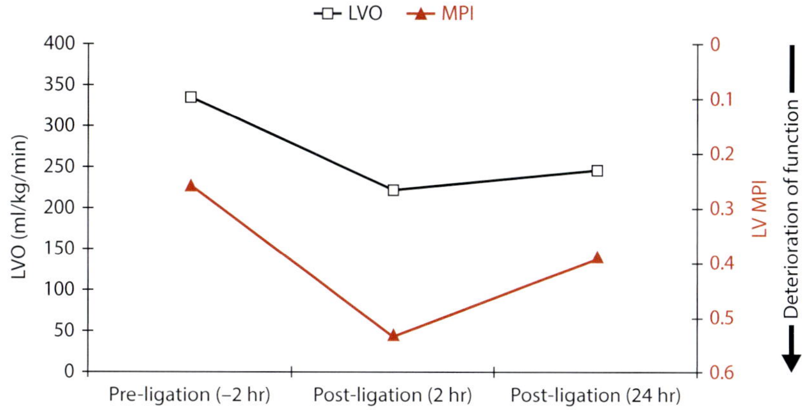

FIGURE 11-3. Changes in left ventricular output (LVO) and myocardial performance index (MPI) after PDA ligation are shown. Note that changes in MPI, a measure of global function, follow a similar pattern to the changes in LVO, supporting the notion that myocardial dysfunction may have played a role in the drop in cardiac output after ligation. (Data from Noori S, Friedlich P, Seri I, et al. Changes in myocardial function and hemodynamics after ligation of the ductus arteriosus in preterm infants. *J Pediatr*. 2007 Jun;150(6):597-602.)

Effects on Cerebral Blood Flow

The effects of ligation on CBF depend upon the pre-ligation CBF pattern and post-ligation cardiovascular function. As discussed earlier, the typical cerebral artery Doppler pattern in which the LV has compensated for the left-to-right PDA shunt shows high systolic flow and a reduced, absent, or reversal flow in diastole. With the decrease in stroke volume following ligation, and the accompanying increase in SVR, generally the systolic flow decreases while the diastolic flow increases. Depending on the relative changes in flow during the systole and diastole, mean or total blood flow can increase, decrease, or stay the same.

In most cases, prior to ligation, the compensatory increase in stroke volume has resulted in normal CBF; following ligation, the relative changes in systolic and diastolic flow cancel each other out, with the net result being little or no change in mean blood flow velocity. Conversely, in a small subset where pre-ligation compensatory increase in CBF during systole was not present prior to ligation, the improvement in diastolic flow would then result in an increase in CBF after ligation. Furthermore, in a subset of preterm infants, the CBF decreases post-ligation either due to an excess of pre-ligation systolic flow or because of post-ligation myocardial dysfunction and/or hypotension. Therefore, CBF status after ligation depends on the degree of pre-ligation compensatory increase in CBF and whether or not post-ligation cardiovascular compromise develops. This might explain some of the inconsistency in the literature on changes in CBF after ligation.[31–37]

Effects on Blood Flow to Other Organs

With the removal of a left-to-right PDA shunt, RVO increases but the total pulmonary blood flow decreases. The flow to all other organs, except for the brain, improves after ligation, provided no significant post-ligation cardiovascular compromise develops. The improvement in flow is primarily the result of an increase in diastolic blood flow.[33]

■ ECHOCARDIOGRAPHIC EVIDENCE OF A HEMODYNAMICALLY SIGNIFICANT PDA

The definition of hsPDA remains controversial. A hsPDA is a PDA that alters organ blood flow and could potentially contribute to pathogenesis of common disease of prematurity such as bronchopulmonary dysplasia and necrotizing enterocolitis. As discussed above, a PDA can have a variable effect on different organs. The symptomatology and adverse hemodynamic effect depends upon the size of the ductus arteriosus, the relative pulmonary to systemic resistance, and compensatory mechanisms within the heart and the other organ(s). While a PDA might be "significant" for the lung (ie, cause pulmonary edema), it might not be "significant" for the brain or kidney. On the other hand, a PDA might have minimal effects on the lung, yet have a profound effect on the gut or renal blood flow. Therefore, whenever one asks the question as to whether a PDA is hemodynamically significant, one should always clarify the target organ in question. Moreover, while the potential hemodynamic effect of a PDA on organ blood

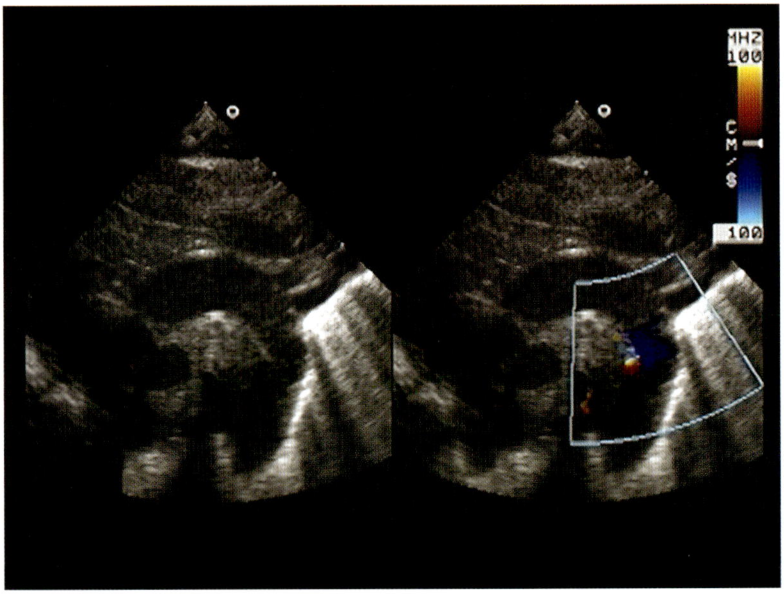

FIGURE and VIDEO 11-4. To visualize the PDA from the suprasternal view, first identify the aortic arch. Then with a slight counterclockwise rotation and anterior angulation, the operator will view the ductus arteriosus, as shown in this video clip. Further anterior angulation and minor adjustment of the transducer will yield the pulmonary artery and the ductus in its entirety (Figure and Video 11-5).

flow can be evaluated, it can be difficult to assess the adequacy of the organ's compensatory mechanisms.

Among the indicators of an hsPDA discussed below, ductal diameter has been consistently shown to be the most important parameter. However, measurement of ductal diameter is often inadequate as the sole indicator of hemodynamic significance of a PDA. Other indices of hsPDA, when used in conjunction with ductal diameter, can help predict the degree of shunt.[38] To determine the best management strategy for an hsPDA, one needs to use multiple echocardiographic indicators[39,40] and consider these in the context of the clinical setting, gestational and chronological age, vulnerability of the target organ(s), and the risks and benefits of a treatment regimen.

Technique

Position. The patient should be placed supine. If the patient's condition allows, the placement of a roll underneath the shoulders can facilitate neck extension and provide a better access to the suprasternal window. Otherwise, turning the head to the side can be helpful.

Transducer. For better resolution, a high-frequency (10–12 MHz) probe is preferable.

View. The ductus arteriosus can best be assessed from suprasternal or high parasternal short-axis views.

Procedure. In the suprasternal view, after visualization of the aortic arch, place the color box over the distal part of the arch and rotate the transducer slightly counterclockwise and tilt anteriorly. This maneuver should enable visualization of the ductus arteriosus, descending aorta and the main pulmonary artery (Figure and Video 11-4). With a slight adjustment in position and orientation of the transducer, the ductus arteriosus can be seen in its entirety (Figure and Video 11-5). Further minor adjustments will yield the "three fingers": the PDA (uppermost), and the left (middle) and right (bottom) pulmonary arteries (Figure and Video 11-6). Alternatively, the PDA can be visualized from the high left parasternal parasagittal view ("ductal view") or the high parasternal short-axis view. Depending on the direction

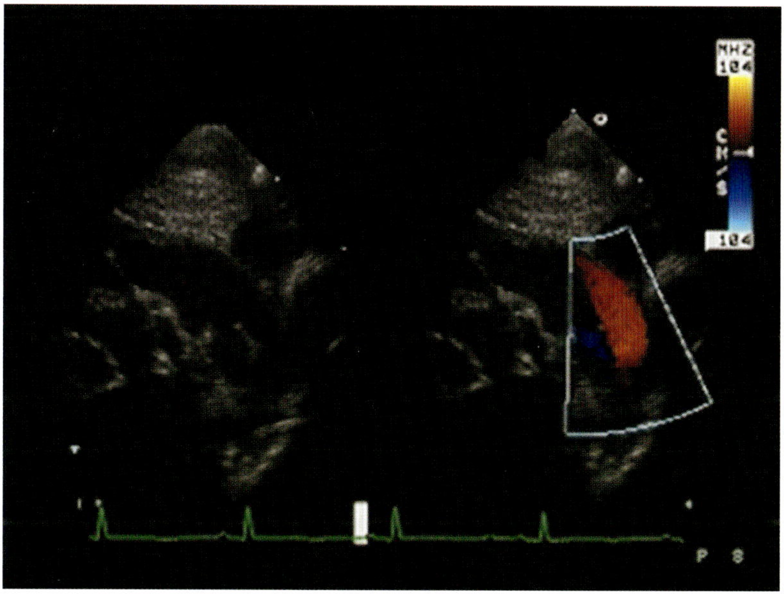

FIGURE and VIDEO 11-5. Ductal cut from suprasternal view. The PDA is seen in its entirety from the pulmonary to the aortic end.

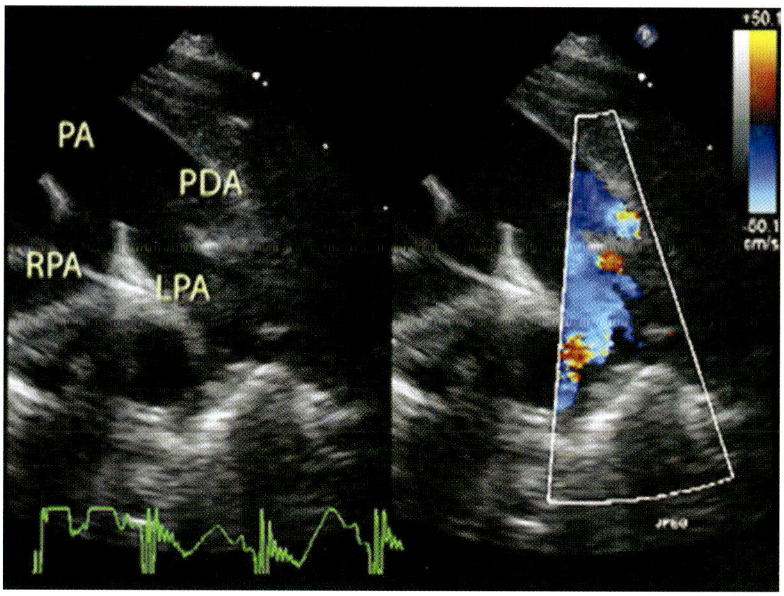

FIGURE and VIDEO 11-6. The "three fingers" cut from suprasternal view: PDA (upper most), and left (middle) and right (bottom) pulmonary arteries. Abbreviations: LPA, left pulmonary artery; PA, pulmonary artery; RPA, right pulmonary artery; PDA, patent ductus arteriosus.

of the shunt, the color flow can be blue (right-to-left; Figure and Video 11-7), red (left-to-right; Figure and Video 11-8), or blue and red (bidirectional; Figure and Video 11-9). Adjust (increase) the color scale to minimize oversaturation and reduce aliasing. However, when the flow velocity is low, too high of a scale will lead to poor visualization of ductal flow (Figure and Video 11-10).

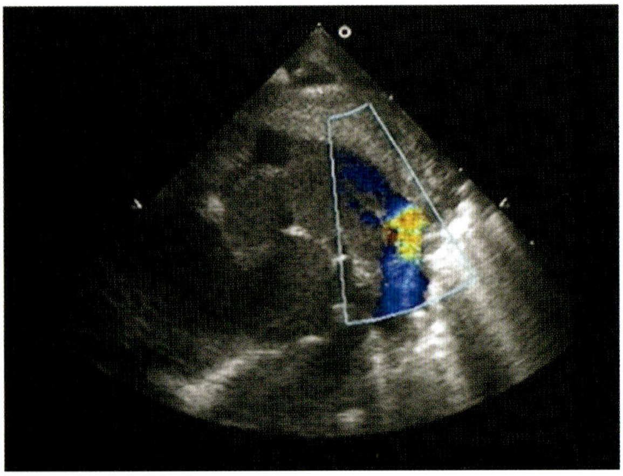

FIGURE and VIDEO 11-7. An extremely preterm infant with a constricted ductus arteriosus and right-to-left shunt (blue color).

Next, using pulsed wave (PW) Doppler, obtain a spectral Doppler flow envelope by placing the Doppler gate at the narrowest portion of the PDA. Since PW Doppler allows for estimation of flow velocity at a specific location (range resolution), it is the preferred mode of Doppler interrogation. However, when aliasing occurs because the flow velocity is too high (eg, with ductal constriction), continuous-wave (CW) Doppler should be used to quantify accurately the velocity across the PDA.

Measurement

It is customary to measure the PDA diameter at its narrowest point (usually the pulmonary end of the PDA) using color flow Doppler in suprasternal or high left parasternal view. Alternatively, if the ductal walls are clearly visible, PDA measurement can be performed with 2D imaging. Using 2D and color mode simultaneously (color compare mode) can help in identifying the course of the ductus, and therefore help in distinguishing between the ductal **flow** jet in the pulmonary artery and flow in the PDA. Alternatively, using "color suppress" with a still frame of a cine loop can be used to ensure that the diameter of the color flow jet being measured accurately represents the width of the vessel. For a discussion on the interpretation of PDA diameter and color flow Doppler patterns, see below.

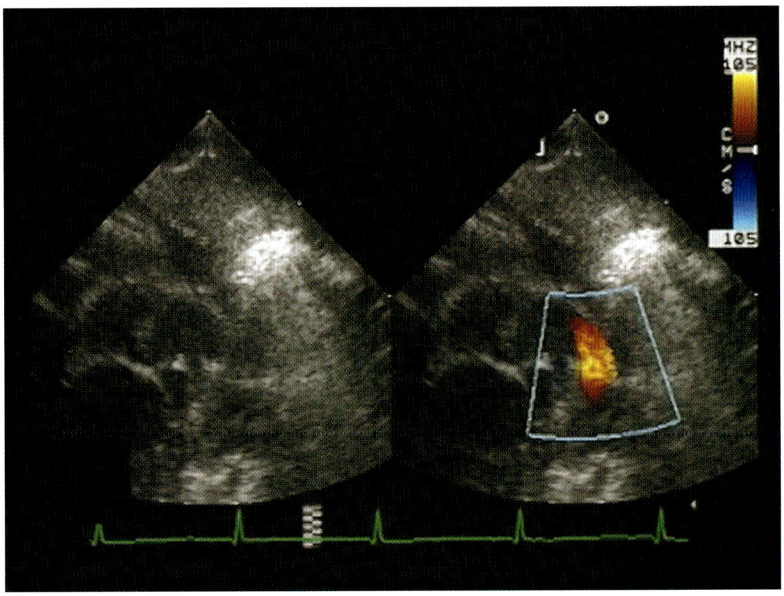

FIGURE and VIDEO 11-8. A large PDA with a left-to-right shunt (red color) in an extremely preterm infant at 16 hours after birth.

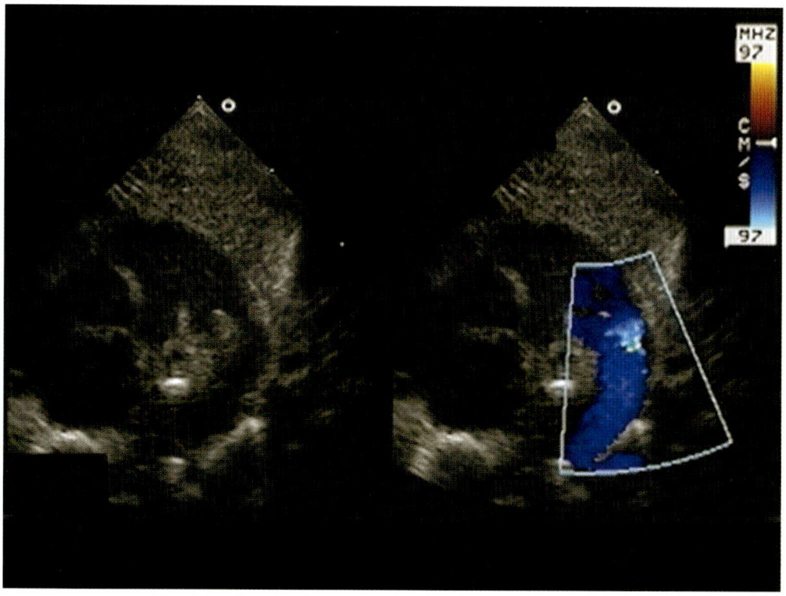

FIGURE and VIDEO 11-9. A large PDA with a bidirectional shunt (blue and red colors) in a 26 weeks' gestational age preterm infant at 5 hours after birth.

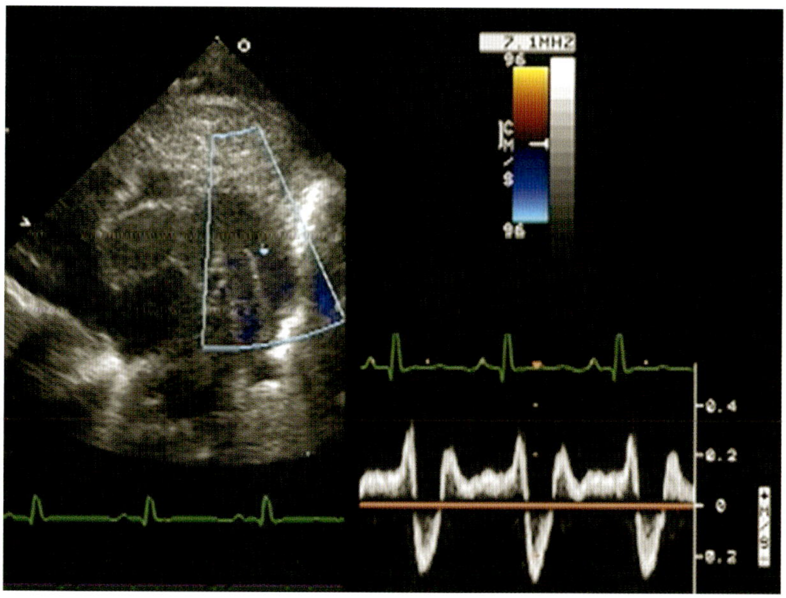

FIGURE and VIDEO 11-10. Adjustment of color scale is very important. Here, a large PDA with bidirectional shunt is shown with a suboptimal color scale. Too high of a scale has resulted in a very little color flow visualization in the large PDA. Spectral Doppler demonstrates the low blood flow velocity (about ± 0.25 m/s). Lowering the color scale from 96 to about 30 cm/s would have yielded a better visualization of ductal flow by color Doppler.

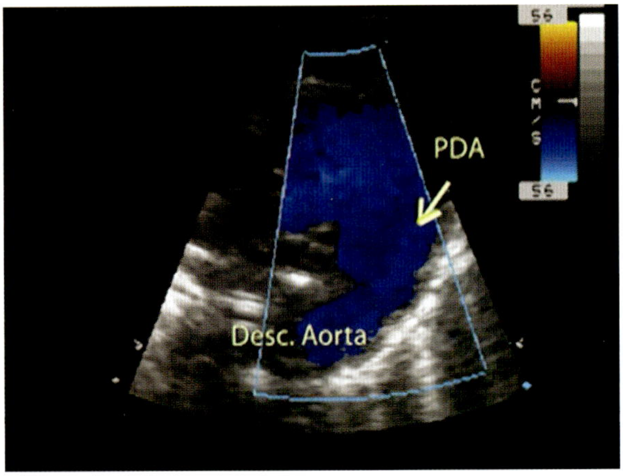

FIGURE and VIDEO 11-11. In the case of a complete right-to-left shunt, it can be more difficult to recognize the PDA flow. This large PDA with a right-to-left shunt in a term infant was missed by the sonographer and read as a closed ductus arteriosus.

Limitations

While it is often quite easy to visualize a PDA if the shunt is left-to-right or bidirectional, a completely right-to-left shunt can readily be missed (Figure and Video 11-11). In this case, because the direction of right-to-left ductal flow is similar to that of the distal aortic arch and left pulmonary artery, the blue ductal flow can be mistaken for one of these structures. Therefore, whenever the ductus arteriosus appears to be closed in a clinical setting in which it might otherwise be expected to be open (eg, early postnatal period), or in which one might expect a right-to-left shunt (eg, pulmonary hypertension or ductal-dependent congenital heart disease such as hypoplastic left heart syndrome), extra attention should be paid to identify the aortic arch, and left and right pulmonary arteries, before concluding that the ductus arteriosus is closed. The large PDA with right-to-left shunting in the above settings is often referred to as "ductal arch" to emphasize it arch-like appearance.

Indicators of the Hemodynamic Significance of a PDA

PDA Diameter

As mentioned earlier, ductal diameter is the most important predictor of hemodynamic significance of the PDA.[41,42] In the very preterm infants, a ductal size of <1.5 mm is generally considered not significant. However, given the relative size, the effects of a 1.5 mm PDA in a 0.5 kg and 1.4 kg neonates are different. As a result, attempts have been made at correcting the diameter for weight or another structure in the heart. Dividing the ductal diameter by weight is not appropriate as the heart structures including the ductus do not grow by the same proportion as the weight. For example, the diameter of aortic annulus in a 0.5 kg baby is about 3.5 mm as compared to 8 mm (not 21 mm) in a 3-kg infant. Some have used ductal diameter to left pulmonary artery ratio as an indicator of significance. This index is more appropriate; however, given the fact that available echocardiographic data on PDA are primarily based on ductal diameter; interpretation of the PDA/LPA index can be problematic.

PDA Flow Pattern

Five flow patterns have been described (Figure 11-12).[43] In the *pulmonary hypertension patterns* the PDA flow is either completely (Figure 11-12A) or predominately (Figure 11-12B) right-to-left. If the flow is bidirectional (Figure 11-12B), the right-to-left component occurs during systole and the left-to-right component happens in diastole. The pulmonary hypertension pattern is indicative of elevated pulmonary vascular resistance; the pure right-to-left shunting (Figure 11-12A) signifies a higher pulmonary vascular resistance than the bidirectional pattern (Figure 11-12B). The *growing pattern* (Figure 11-12C) signals a fall of pulmonary vascular resistance and is characterized by a bidirectional shunt with predominately left-to-right and a minimal right-to-left component. The *pulsatile pattern* (Figure 11-12D) is defined as purely left-to-right shunt with higher velocity during systole and lower velocity during diastole (hence the term pulsatile). Both growing and pulsatile patterns are associated with hsPDA. Finally, the *closing pattern* (Figure 11-12E) is characterized by continuous high-velocity left-to-right shunting (in the case of Figure 11-12E, above 2 m/s) during systole and diastole with a lack of pulsatility. The closing pattern is suggestive of a constricted PDA, as the flow through a narrow ductus would give a high velocity according to Bernoulli's equation (Chapter 6). It is important to note that the pulmonary hypertension pattern also has significant hemodynamic effects; however, the term hsPDA is in general reserved for when there is a significant left-to-right shunt.

Assessing the PDA flow pattern is important. The most important information concerns the relative pulmonary vascular resistance (ie, the difference between systemic

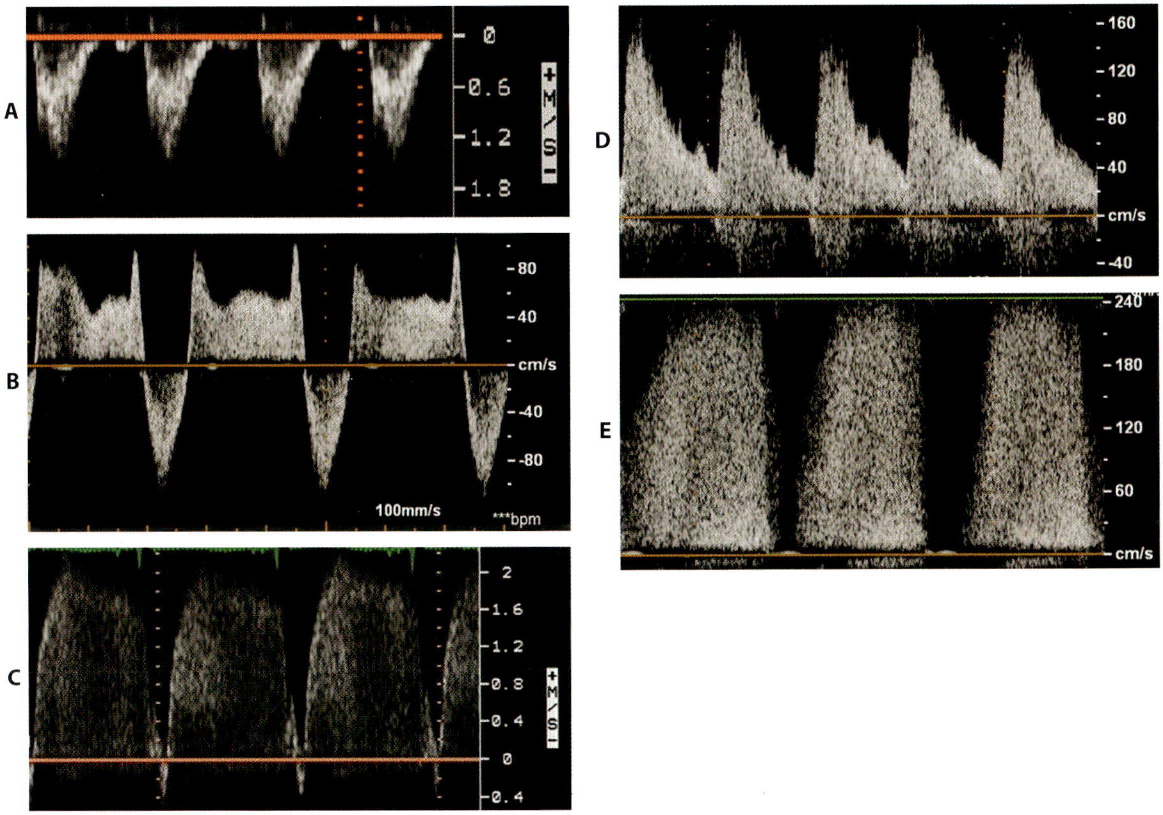

FIGURE 11-12. Examples of PDA flow pattern are shown. **A.** Pulmonary hypertension pattern with a pure right-to-left shunt, indicative of suprasystemic pulmonary arterial pressure; **B.** Bidirectional shunt suggestive of elevated systolic pulmonary arterial pressure, with right-to-left shunting during systole and left-to-right shunting in diastole ; **C.** Growing pattern: almost complete left-to-right shunt with minimal right-to-left, indicative of decreasing pulmonary arterial pressure; **D.** Pulsatile pattern, completely left-to-right shunt with a significant difference in systolic and diastolic velocities; **E.** Closing pattern: completely left-to-right shunt with high velocity and minimal or no difference between systolic and diastolic velocities. The flow in the closing pattern is continuous, but due to the small PDA size, there can be gaps (as in this example) with the cursor moving in and out of the ductus with heart motion or respiration.

and pulmonary vascular resistances). For example, it is important to identify the pulmonary hypertension pattern because PDAs exhibiting this pattern should not be closed. In such cases, the pulmonary vascular resistance is likely equal to or higher than the systemic vascular resistance, and closing the PDA could result in development of suprasystemic pulmonary arterial pressure and right heart failure. Identifying other patterns can be useful as an adjunct to ductal diameter in determining the hemodynamic significance of PDA. While there is generally good correlation between the ductal diameter and flow pattern,[44] it is important to note that assigning one of the five flow patterns to a given patient is not always possible. In one study, about 14% of cases had an ambiguous flow pattern.[44]

LA/Ao Ratio

The LA to aortic root (Ao) ratio is one of the oldest echocardiographic indices for diagnosis of hsPDA. At the early stages of development of cardiac sonography when 2D echocardiography and color flow Doppler were not available, the clinicians relied on the indirect sign of hsPDA (ie, increase in left-sided preload) using M-mode echocardiography. This ratio was the main method of diagnosis in the 1970s when direct visualization of the PDA was not possible.[45] In the calculation of this ratio, the larger the LA diameter relative to the constant Ao, the greater the index, and the more likely a significant PDA is present. The main limitation is that this ratio is nonspecific; the LA can increase in size due to other conditions, for example volume overload or mitral/LV dysfunction. Conversely, in the presence of a large PFO, the ratio might be small due to a large left-to-right PFO shunt, even in the presence of a significant hsPDA. Nevertheless, LA/Ao does provide additional information on hemodynamic significance of the ductus and can be used as an adjunct to PDA diameter. In general, an LA/Ao of >1.3–1.5 is considered significant.[46]

Measurement of LA/Ao ratio is described in Chapter 5. Briefly, LA diameter is measured in a standard short (or long) parasternal view with the M-mode line cutting through the aortic valve and left atrium. The LA diameter is measured in systole (largest distance) and Ao in diastole (when the valve is closed). The measurement of Ao for this ratio is different than measuring the diameter for calculation of the LVO. For the purpose of the LA/Ao ratio, the diameter is measured from the internal side (leading edge) of the anterior wall to the external side (leading edge) of posterior wall of the annulus (Figure 11-13). In contrast, in the calculation of the LVO, the hinge points of the aortic valve diameter (inner edge to inner edge) are measured during mid-systole (Chapter 5).

Flow Reversal in the Descending Aorta

With the ductus arteriosus closed, flow in descending aorta is anterograde during the whole cardiac cycle. The flow is predominantly during systole with an absent or low-velocity flow during diastole. In case of hsPDA, the stolic flow velocity may decrease while retrograde diastolic flow can occur. The degree and duration of retrograde diastolic flow has been used as an index of hemodynamic significance. Diastolic flow reversal in the descending aorta has been reported as early as 4 hours after birth in the very preterm infants, suggesting that a PDA can become hemodynamically significant shortly after birth.[47]

Doppler interrogation of the descending aorta can be performed from the suprasternal or subcostal views. The PW Doppler gate should be placed distal to the PDA. This can be challenging from the suprasternal view, and careful image optimization should be performed to visualize the distal descending thoracic aorta beyond the PDA. Alternatively, the subcostal approach provides a view of the descending thoracic aorta below the PDA, but Doppler interrogation at an angle <10° can be difficult from this perspective.

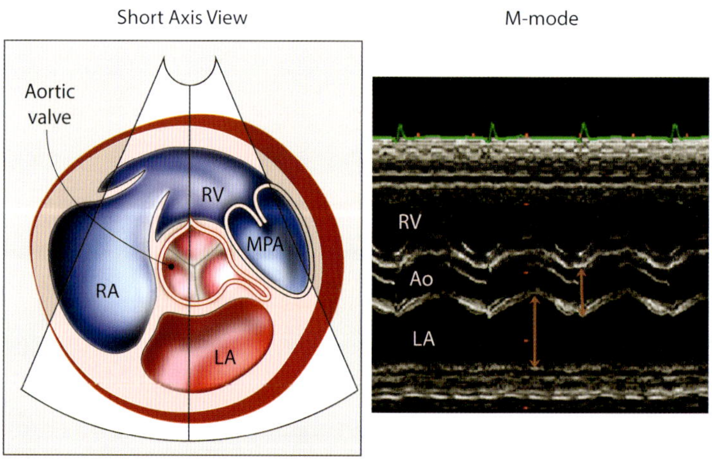

FIGURE 11-13. Measurement of the left atrium (LA) to the aortic root (Ao) ratio is shown. A schematic drawing of the short-axis view of the heart at the level of aortic root is depicted on the right. The dotted line on the drawing illustrates where the M-mode line is placed. The motion of various structures along this dotted line is displayed in the M-mode tracing (on the left). As shown, the aortic root is measured from the leading edge to leading edge.

Left Pulmonary Artery Diastolic Flow Velocity

Recently, left pulmonary artery (LPA) diastolic velocity has been used as an indicator of hsPDA. In the absence of a PDA, flow through the LPA is usually monophasic—that is, only occurring during systole—and if it is biphasic, the diastolic component is generally minimal. In the presence of continuous left-to-right PDA shunting, not only does flow velocity in the LPA increase during systole, but the flow also becomes biphasic—it is seen during both systole and diastole (Figure 11-14). The greater the left-to-right ductal shunting, the higher will be the diastolic flow velocity. In the literature, an arbitrary cutoff of 0.2 m/s end-diastolic velocity has been used to define an hsPDA. The main limitation of this index is that it does not provide any information on systemic flow. Therefore, when used for assessment of hemodynamic significance, it must be combined with the other indices.

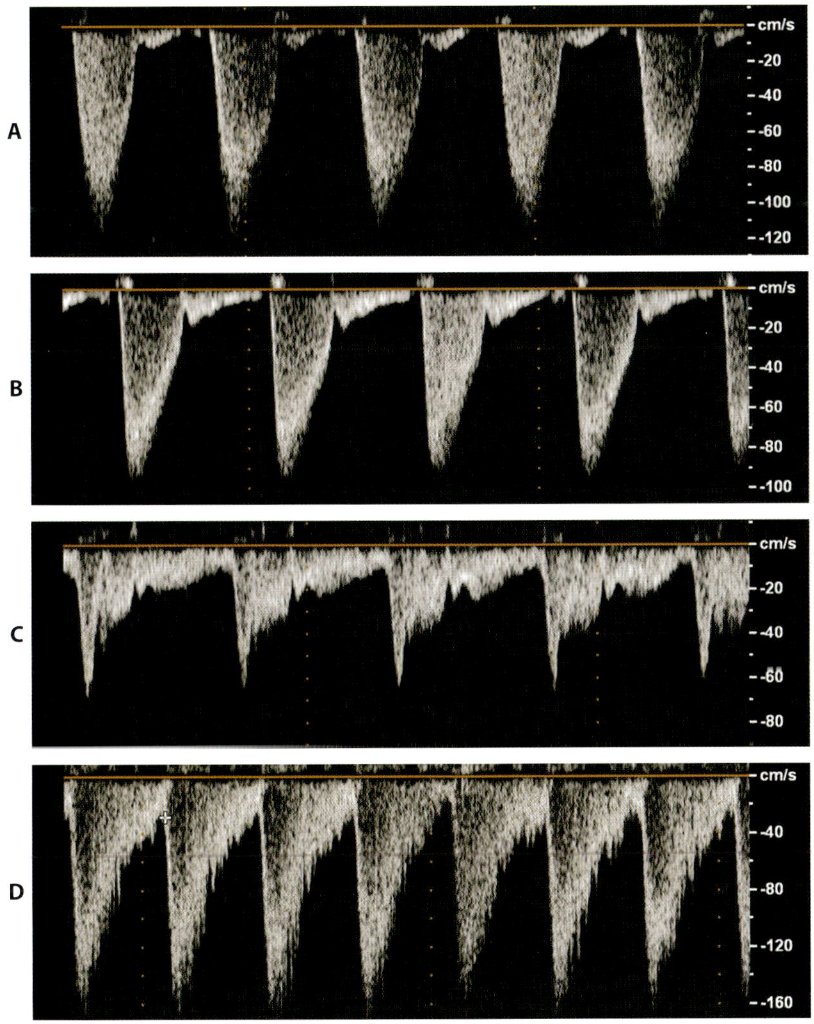

FIGURE 11-14. Examples of Doppler flow pattern in left pulmonary artery (LPA) are shown. **A.** A 4-day-old preterm infant born at 34 weeks' gestation with a closed ductus arteriosus; **B.** An 18-hour-old preterm infant born at 33 weeks' gestation with a small PDA with a left-to-right shunt. Note the small amount of diastolic flow that is present; **C.** A 2-hour-old preterm infant born at 33 weeks' gestation with a bidirectional shunt across a large PDA (right to left in systole, left to right in diastole). Note the significant diastolic flow in the LPA; **D.** A 21-day-old preterm infant born at 24 weeks' gestation with a large PDA with a left-to-right shunt.

As for the method of acquiring the LPA Doppler flow pattern, the standard parasternal short-axis or modified suprasternal view (ductal cut) can be used to visualize and interrogate the LPA with PW Doppler.

Left Ventricular Output

With increasing left-to-right PDA shunting, LVO increases. With a large-sized PDA, it is not uncommon to have an LVO in the range of 400–600 ml/kg/min (normal range 100–300 ml/kg/min). Therefore, the greater the LVO is above normal, the larger the PDA shunt. The use of LVO as an indicator of hsPDA has several limitations. In the presence of a large PFO or atrial septal defect, the LVO can be in normal range yet there can still be a significant PDA shunt, and some of the increased pulmonary venous return from the PDA is diverted through the atrial communication into the right atrium/right ventricle. Indeed, in the presence of a large PDA with a left-to-right shunt, systemic blood flow is more compromised when LVO is low or in the normal range. As such, a normal or low LVO signifies a lack of adequate compensation (see "Hemodynamic Effects of a PDA" at the beginning of this chapter. For measurement of LVO, refer to Chapter 7.

Absence or Reversal of Diastolic Flow in the MCA, SMA, and RA

As discussed earlier, in the presence of an hsPDA, both systolic and diastolic flow are affected in major arteries such as the middle cerebral artery (MCA), superior mesenteric artery (SMA), and renal artery (RA). In the case of the MCA, the systolic flow velocity usually increases but may remain the same or decrease depending upon whether a significant compensatory increase in stoke volume has occurred or not. The diastolic flow velocity can be decreased, absent, or reversed. With the above changes, the mean velocity in the MCA can be maintained. On the other hand, with arteries arising from the descending aorta such as SMA and RA, the systolic flow velocity is usually decreased, and diastolic velocity is either absent or reversed. The change in systolic and diastolic flow velocity patterns in these arteries results in a lower mean flow velocity and potential hypoperfusion to the organs supplied by these arteries. Of course, the above described changes in flow pattern are not unique to hsPDA and can occur in other conditions. Nevertheless, assessment of MCA, SMA, and RA flow patterns can be helpful in defining which organs are at risk.

For a description of the technique and details of flow assessment of the MCA, SMA, and RA, refer to Chapter 7.

Other Indices

Several other indices have been used to describe the hemodynamic significance of a PDA. Transductal flow velocity ratio is defined as the ratio of peak velocity at the pulmonary end of the PDA divided by peak velocity at the aortic origin of the PDA. This ratio has been shown to be greater in preterm infants with a significant PDA (as defined by larger PDA diameter, elevated LA/Ao, and absent or reversed diastolic flow in the descending aorta).[48] The utility of this ratio is based on the premise that ductal constriction first occurs at the pulmonary end. While transductal velocity ratio provides us with valuable information on ductal constriction, technical challenges can limit its utility. This index can be measured from a modified suprasternal view (the ductal cut) where the ductus can be visualized in its entirety. In order to measure the peak velocity, the PW Doppler gate is placed in both the pulmonary and aortic margins of the ductus arteriosus.

LV diameter at the end of diastole (LVIDD) is another index for hsPDA.[49,50] This index reflects LV overload as a result of left-to-right ductal shunting. The main limitation of LVIDD is its lack of specificity. The method of measurement of LVIDD is described in "Fractional Shortening" in Chapter 5.

Finally, there are other indices beside the ductal diameter (>1.5 mm) during the first few hours after birth that are found to be predictive of development of hsPDA later on. In a recent study in the very preterm infants, ductal length from aorta to pulmonary end (<5.2 mm) and from constriction to pulmonary insertion (<1.7 mm) at mean age of 9 hours were predictive of hsPDA at 72 hours after birth.[42]

REFERENCES

1. Noori S. Patent ductus arteriosus in the preterm infant: to treat or not to treat? *J Perinatol.* 2010;30(Suppl):S31–S37.
2. Benitz WE. Committee on Fetus and Newborn, American Academy of Pediatrics. Patent ductus arteriosus in preterm infants. *Pediatrics.* 2016:137.
3. Alverson DC, Eldridge MW, Johnson JD, et al. Effect of patent ductus arteriosus on left ventricular output in premature infants. *J Pediatr*. 1983;102:754–757.
4. Clyman RI, Mauray F, Heymann MA, Roman C. Cardiovascular effects of patent ductus arteriosus in preterm lambs with respiratory distress. *J Pediatr*. 1987;111:579–587.

5. Walther FJ, Kim DH, Ebrahimi M, Siassi B. Pulsed Doppler measurement of left ventricular output as early predictor of symptomatic patent ductus arteriosus in very preterm infants. *Biol Neonate*. 1989;56:121–128.
6. Lindner W, Seidel M, Versmold HT, Döhlemann C, Riegel KP. Stroke volume and left ventricular output in preterm infants with patent ductus arteriosus. *Pediatr Res*. 1990;27:278–281.
7. Evans N, Iyer P. Assessment of ductus arteriosus shunt in preterm infants supported by mechanical ventilation: effect of interatrial shunting. *J Pediatr*. 1994;125:778–785.
8. Barlow AJ, Ward C, Webber SA, Sinclair BG, Potts JE, Sandor GG. Myocardial contractility in premature neonates with and without patent ductus arteriosus. *Pediatr Cardiol*. 2004;25:102–107.
9. Ratner I, Perelmuter B, Toews W, Whitfield J. Association of low systolic and diastolic blood pressure with significant patent ductus arteriosus in the very low birth weight infant. *Crit Care Med*. 1985;13:497–500.
10. Evans N, Moorcraft J. Effect of patency of the ductus arteriosus on blood pressure in very preterm infants. *Arch Dis Child*. 1992;67:1169–1173.
11. Meyers RL, Alpan G, Lin E, Clyman RI. Patent ductus arteriosus, indomethacin, and intestinal distension: effects on intestinal blood flow and oxygen consumption. *Pediatr Res*. 1991;29:569–574.
12. Shimada S, Kasai T, Konishi M, Fujiwara T. Effects of patent ductus arteriosus on left ventricular output and organ blood flows in preterm infants with respiratory distress syndrome treated with surfactant. *J Pediatr*. 1994;125:270–277.
13. Baylen BG, Ogata H, Oguchi K, et al. The contractility and performance of the preterm left ventricle before and after early patent ductus arteriosus occlusion in surfactant-treated lambs. *Pediatr Res*. 1985;19:1053–1058.
14. Perlman JM, Hill A, Volpe JJ. The effect of patent ductus arteriosus on flow velocity in the anterior cerebral arteries: ductal steal in the premature newborn infant. *J Pediatr*. 1981;99:767–771.
15. Martin CG, Snider AR, Katz SM, Peabody JL, Brady JP. Abnormal cerebral blood flow patterns in preterm infants with a large patent ductus arteriosus. *J Pediatr*. 1982;101:587–593.
16. Baylen BG, Ogata H, Ikegami M, Jacob H, Jobe A, Emmanouilides GC. Left ventricular performance and regional blood flows before and after ductus arteriosus occlusion in premature lambs treated with surfactant. *Circulation*. 1983;67:837–843.
17. Noori S, Wlodaver A, Gottipati V, McCoy M, Schultz D, Escobedo M. Transitional changes in cardiac and cerebral hemodynamics in term neonates at birth. *J Pediatr*. 2012;160:943–948.
18. Kluckow M, Evans N. Low superior vena cava flow and intraventricular haemorrhage in preterm infants. *Arch Dis Child Fetal Neonatal Ed*. 2000;82:F188–F194.
19. Deeg KH, Gerstner R, Brandl U, et al. [Doppler sonographic flow parameter of the anterior cerebral artery in patent ductus arteriosus of the newborn infant compared to a healthy control sample]. *Klin Padiatr*. 1986;198:463–470.
20. Coombs RC, Morgan ME, Durbin GM, Booth IW, McNeish AS. Gut blood flow velocities in the newborn: effects of patent ductus arteriosus and parenteral indomethacin. *Arch Dis Child*. 1990;65:1067–1071.
21. McCurnin D, Clyman RI. Effects of a patent ductus arteriosus on postprandial mesenteric perfusion in premature baboons. *Pediatrics*. 2008;122:e1262–e1267.
22. Clyman RI, Wickremasinghe A, Merritt TA, et al. Hypotension following patent ductus arteriosus ligation: the role of adrenal hormones. *J Pediatr*. 2014;164:1449–1455.e1.
23. Moin F, Kennedy KA, Moya FR. Risk factors predicting vasopressor use after patent ductus arteriosus ligation. *Am J Perinatol*. 2003;20:313–320.
24. Noori S, Friedlich P, Seri I, Wong P. Changes in myocardial function and hemodynamics after ligation of the ductus arteriosus in preterm infants. *J Pediatr*. 2007;150:597–602.
25. Harting MT, Blakely ML, Cox CS Jr, Lantin-Hermoso R, Andrassy RJ, Lally KP. Acute hemodynamic decompensation following patent ductus arteriosus ligation in premature infants. *J Invest Surg*. 2008;21:133–138.
26. Teixeira LS, Shivananda SP, Stephens D, Van Arsdell G, McNamara PJ. Postoperative cardiorespiratory instability following ligation of the preterm ductus arteriosus is related to early need for intervention. *J Perinatol*. 2008;28:803–810.
27. McNamara PJ, Stewart L, Shivananda SP, Stephens D, Sehgal A. Patent ductus arteriosus ligation is associated with impaired left ventricular systolic performance in premature infants weighing less than 1000 g. *J Thorac Cardiovasc Surg*. 2010;140:150–157.
28. Noori S. Pros and cons of patent ductus arteriosus ligation: hemodynamic changes and other morbidities after patent ductus arteriosus ligation. *Semin Perinatol*. 2012;36:139–145.
29. Noori S, McNamara P, Jain A, et al. Catecholamine-resistant hypotension and myocardial performance following patent ductus arteriosus ligation. *J Perinatol*. 2015;35:123–127.
30. Kimball TR, Ralston MA, Khoury P, Crump RG, Cho FS, Reuter JH. Effect of ligation of patent ductus arteriosus on left ventricular performance and its determinants in premature neonates. *J Am Coll Cardiol*. 1996;27:193–197.

31. Sonesson SE, Lundell BP, Herin P. Changes in intracranial arterial blood flow velocities during surgical ligation of the patent ductus arteriosus. *Acta Paediatr Scand.* 1986;75:36–42.

32. Saliba EM, Chantepie A, Gold F, Marchand M, Pourcelot L, Laugier J. Intraoperative measurements of cerebral haemodynamics during ductus arteriosus ligation in preterm infants. *Eur J Pediatr.* 1991;150:362–365.

33. Hoodbhoy SA, Cutting HA, Seddon JA, Campbell ME. Cerebral and splanchnic hemodynamics after duct ligation in very low birth weight infants. *J Pediatr.* 2009;154:196–200.

34. Zaramella P, Freato F, Quaresima V, et al. Surgical closure of patent ductus arteriosus reduces the cerebral tissue oxygenation index in preterm infants: a near-infrared spectroscopy and Doppler study. *Pediatr Int.* 2006;48:305–312.

35. Hüning BM, Asfour B, König S, Hess N, Roll C. Cerebral blood volume changes during closure by surgery of patent ductus arteriosus. *Arch Dis Child Fetal Neonatal Ed.* 2008;93:F261–F264.

36. Vanderhaegen J, De Smet D, Meyns B, Van De Velde M, Van Huffel S, Naulaers G. Surgical closure of the patent ductus arteriosus and its effect on the cerebral tissue oxygenation. *Acta Paediatr.* 2008;97:1640–1644.

37. Lemmers PMA, Molenschot MC, Evens J, Toet MC, van Bel F. Is cerebral oxygen supply compromised in preterm infants undergoing surgical closure for patent ductus arteriosus? *Arch Dis Child Fetal Neonatal Ed.* 2010;95:F429–F434.

38. El Hajjar M, Vaksmann G, Rakza T, Kongolo G, Storme L. Severity of the ductal shunt: a comparison of different markers. *Arch Dis Child Fetal Neonatal Ed.* 2005;90:F419–F422.

39. Sehgal A, Paul E, Menahem S. Functional echocardiography in staging for ductal disease severity:role in predicting outcomes. *Eur J Pediatr.* 2013;172:179–184.

40. El-Khuffash A, James AT, Corcoran JD, et al. A patent ductus arteriosus severity score predicts chronic lung disease or death before discharge. *J Pediatr.* 2015;167:1354–1361.e2.

41. Kluckow M, Evans N. Early echocardiographic prediction of symptomatic patent ductus arteriosus in preterm infants undergoing mechanical ventilation. *J Pediatr.* 1995;127:774–779.

42. Polat TB, Celik IH, Erdeve O. Early predictive echocardiographic features of hemodynamically significant patent ductus arteriosus in preterm VLBW infants. *Pediatr Int.* 2016;58:589–594.

43. Su BH, Watanabe T, Shimizu M, Yanagisawa M. Echocardiographic assessment of patent ductus arteriosus shunt flow pattern in premature infants. *Arch Dis Child Fetal Neonatal Ed.* 1997;77:F36–F40.

44. Condò M, Evans N, Bellù R, Kluckow M. Echocardiographic assessment of ductal significance: retrospective comparison of two methods. *Arch Dis Child Fetal Neonatal Ed.* 2012;97:F35–F38.

45. Silverman NH, Lewis AB, Heymann MA, Rudolph AM. Echocardiographic assessment of ductus arteriosus shunt in premature infants. *Circulation.* 1974;50:821–825.

46. Iyer P, Evans N. Re-evaluation of the left atrial to aortic root ratio as a marker of patent ductus arteriosus. *Arch Dis Child Fetal Neonatal Ed.* 1994;70:F112–F117.

47. Groves AM, Kuschel CA, Knight DB, Skinner JR. Does retrograde diastolic flow in the descending aorta signify impaired systemic perfusion in preterm infants? *Pediatr Res.* 2008;63:89–94.

48. Davies MW, Betheras FR, Swaminathan M. A preliminary study of the application of the transductal velocity ratio for assessing persistent ductus arteriosus. *Arch Dis Child Fetal Neonatal Ed.* 2000;82:F195–F199.

49. Baylen B, Meyer RA, Korfhagen J, Benzing G 3rd, Bubb ME, Kaplan S. Left ventricular performance in the critically ill premature infant with patent ductus arteriosus and pulmonary disease. *Circulation.* 1977;55:182–188.

50. Hirschklau MJ, DiSessa TG, Higgins CB, Friedman WF. Echocardiographic diagnosis: pitfalls in the premature infant with a large patent ductus arteriosus. *J Pediatr.* 1978;92:474–477.

CHAPTER 12

Persistent Pulmonary Hypertension in Newborn Infants: Assessment of Pulmonary Artery Pressure*

Tina A. Leone

- INTRODUCTION
- TRANSITIONAL CIRCULATION AND PPHN
- ESTIMATING PULMONARY ARTERY PRESSURE
  - Tricuspid Regurgitation Jet
  - Patent Ductus Arteriosus
- OTHER ECHOCARDIOGRAPHIC INDICES OF ELEVATED PULMONARY PRESSURE
  - Flow Pattern at Patent Foramen Ovale
  - Systolic Time Intervals
  - Position of Interventricular Septum
  - Ventricular Function
  - Myocardial Performance Index
  - TAPSE
- REFERENCES

INTRODUCTION

Pulmonary hypertension exists as a pathologic finding in newborn infants in several clinical settings. In the early newborn period, the syndrome of persistent pulmonary hypertension of the newborn (PPHN) can occur, consisting of failure of the fetal circulation to adapt to postnatal newborn physiology, mainly because of a persistent elevation in pulmonary vascular resistance. PPHN can occur as a primary pathology or secondary to pulmonary diseases such as meconium aspiration syndrome, pneumonia, pulmonary hypoplasia, or pulmonary/intrathoracic anomalies. Pulmonary hypertension can also occur after the early newborn period as a consequence of chronic pulmonary diseases such as bronchopulmonary dysplasia, or in association with congenital heart disease. At a physiologic level, pulmonary hypertension can be caused by increased pulmonary vascular resistance, by increased pulmonary blood flow, or by obstruction to pulmonary venous drainage. While the measurements of pulmonary artery pressure are similar no matter what the cause, some of the associated echocardiographic findings and the clinical scenarios will differ. The primary problem might not be easily discernible by echocardiography alone. However,

*Videos can be accessed at http://PracticalNeonatalEcho.com.

assessment of the hemodynamics can often assist the clinician in choosing appropriate therapies.

Understanding the physiology of normal transition and of pulmonary hypertension is essential for interpreting the echocardiographic findings. Fetal circulation is characterized by high pulmonary vascular resistance and low pulmonary blood flow. Pulmonary pressures in the fetus are higher than those of the post-transitional newborn circulation. The normal transitional circulation involves a decreasing pulmonary vascular resistance and pulmonary artery pressure over the first 3 days of life. In a study of normal-term infants catheterized in the first 3 days of life, peak systolic pulmonary pressures were approximately equal to systemic pressures in the first 10 hours of life. Pulmonary pressures were lower in infants with increasing age over the first 3 days of life.[1] PPHN was previously referred to as persistent fetal circulation (PFC) because the circulatory pattern does not transition from the fetal to newborn pattern along the normal timeline, and the baby becomes hypoxemic.

It is important to understand the expected findings in normal transition in order to interpret the echocardiogram in the clinical setting of PPHN. The physiology of PPHN includes elevated pulmonary pressures and decreased pulmonary blood flow due to high pulmonary vascular resistance. A higher force from the right ventricle is required to overcome the resistance of the pulmonary vessels. With decreased pulmonary blood flow, there will be decreased pulmonary venous return to the left atrium and therefore decreased left ventricular preload. Because of the increased pressure in the right ventricle, the interventricular septum can be pushed toward the left, potentially impairing function of the left ventricle. The systemic blood flow can be decreased as a result of the combination of these factors. The echocardiogram can be used to estimate the pulmonary artery pressure, provide information about the relative pulmonary to systemic pressure gradients, and evaluate the overall hemodynamic consequences. The echocardiogram is also critical in differentiating the diagnosis of pulmonary hypertension from other causes of cyanosis.

In this chapter, the specific echocardiographic findings in pulmonary hypertension compared to the normal newborn is reviewed. Though each measure is discussed individually, the clinician must look at all of the information from the echocardiogram (including anatomy and function) and interpret the imaging data in conjunction with the clinical information, in order to make the best management decisions.

ESTIMATING PULMONARY ARTERY PRESSURE

Tricuspid Regurgitation Jet

Pulmonary artery pressure can be estimated by echocardiography in several ways. The most direct and accurate measure of systolic pulmonary artery pressure uses the tricuspid regurgitation (TR) jet. Tricuspid regurgitation occurs because the tricuspid valve is not able to contain all of the blood in the right ventricle when under pressure during systole. The speed with which blood escapes the right ventricle through the tricuspid valve can be measured by Doppler echocardiography. The modified Bernoulli equation is used to estimate the pressure difference between two chambers from the velocity of blood flow between the two chambers:

$$\Delta P = 4v^2$$

where P = pressure, v = velocity (measured by Doppler).

Since the modified Bernoulli equation estimates the pressure difference between the right ventricle (RV) and right atrium (RA), an estimate of right atrial pressure must be added to this value in order to determine an estimate of the pulmonary artery pressure.[2,3] Since RA pressure is not actually measured, a factor of 5-10 mmHg is often used as an estimate. It is important to understand that the estimation of pulmonary artery pressure from the tricuspid regurgitation jet assumes that the pressures in the pulmonary artery (PA) and right ventricle are equal. This is only true when there is no obstruction between the RV and PA. Therefore, to interpret the significance of the TR jet, one must know that the anatomy at the pulmonary valve and right ventricular outflow tract is normal. The tricuspid regurgitation jet is not always present or measurable when the pulmonary pressure is elevated. In one reported series of infants with PPHN, the TR jet was measurable in 70 to 80% of infants studied.[4,5] When present, it provides one of the most accurate and repeatable noninvasive measures of pulmonary artery pressure.[6,7]

Imaging

Tricuspid regurgitation can be imaged from several views. It is often easily identified and best measured from either the parasternal long-axis right ventricular inflow view (Figure and Video 12-1) or the apical four-chamber view (Figure and Video 12-2). The tricuspid regurgitation jet

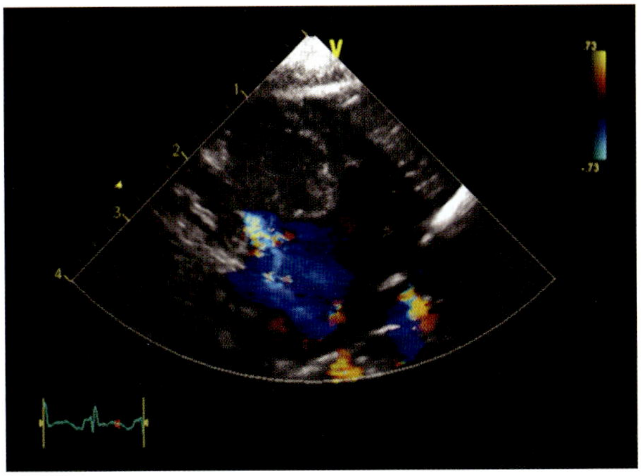

FIGURE and VIDEO 12-1. Tricuspid regurgitation seen in the parasternal long-axis right ventricular inflow view.

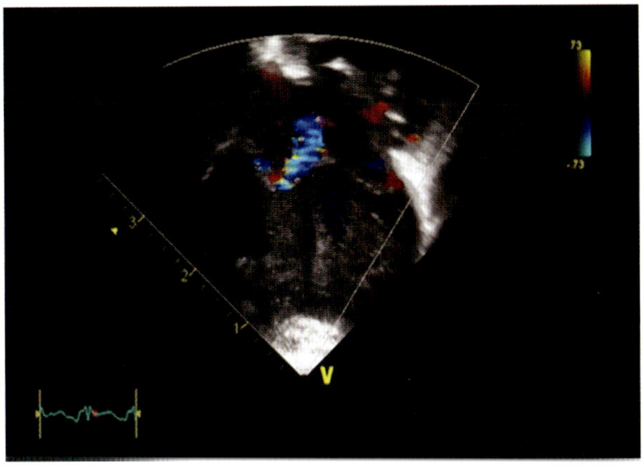

FIGURE and VIDEO 12-2. Tricuspid regurgitation seen in the apical four-chamber view.

is identified with color flow Doppler, and the velocity is then measured by positioning the continuous-wave Doppler sample in line with the jet. Continuous-wave Doppler is usually necessary because the TR jet velocity will be too high to be measured with pulsed wave Doppler. Since the TR jet can be multidirectional, the Doppler sampling beam might need to be maneuvered into an optimal location. For an accurate measurement of velocity, the spectral Doppler signal should be complete throughout the systolic phase of the cardiac cycle and should reach a clear peak. An example of a complete Doppler signal is shown in the last cycle of the tracing in Figure 12-3. In contrast, when the complete Doppler signal is not obtained, the velocity will be falsely low. An example of an incomplete Doppler signal is shown in Figure 12-4.

Tricuspid regurgitation has been evaluated in healthy term and preterm infants in the first days of life.[8] In a group of healthy transitioning infants, all preterm infants had some identifiable TR in the first three days of life, half of which were measurable. The TR was no longer seen in these healthy infants after 72 hours of life. About 70% of term infants had some identifiable TR during this period, but only 20 to 30% were measurable. In a comparison between healthy infants and infants with respiratory distress syndrome (RDS), those with RDS were more likely to have TR present at 72 hours of life and had higher estimates of pulmonary artery pressure between 12 and 48 hours of life.[9]

Patent Ductus Arteriosus

The pulmonary artery pressure can also be estimated from the Doppler examination of the patent ductus arteriosus (PDA). If the PDA flow is bidirectional, the relative difference between the systemic and pulmonary pressures can be estimated by the percentage of time that blood is flowing right to left compared with the entire cardiac cycle length. If the right-to-left component of a bidirectional shunt is greater than 60% of systole or greater than 30% of the total cycle, the peak pulmonary artery pressure is likely to be suprasystemic.[10] Figure 12-5 shows a pulsed wave Doppler tracing of a bidirectional PDA with the right-to-left component that is approximately 30% of the cycle. Figure and Video 12-6 shows the color Doppler image of this PDA. Note that it is difficult to see the blue (right-to-left) component when the video is playing at full speed. Slowing the video down and reviewing it frame by frame allows for identification of blue followed by red flow patterns. The small left-to-right component of the shunt can also be visualized by spectral Doppler.

An estimate of the pulmonary artery pressure can also be determined by measuring the peak velocity of the PDA flow. Once the peak velocity of the PDA flow is measured, the pressure difference between the aorta and pulmonary artery can then be calculated from the modified Bernoulli equation. With pure left-to-right PDA flow, the systemic systolic pressure minus the pressure difference between the aorta and the pulmonary artery (as calculated by Doppler velocity) will be an estimate of the systolic

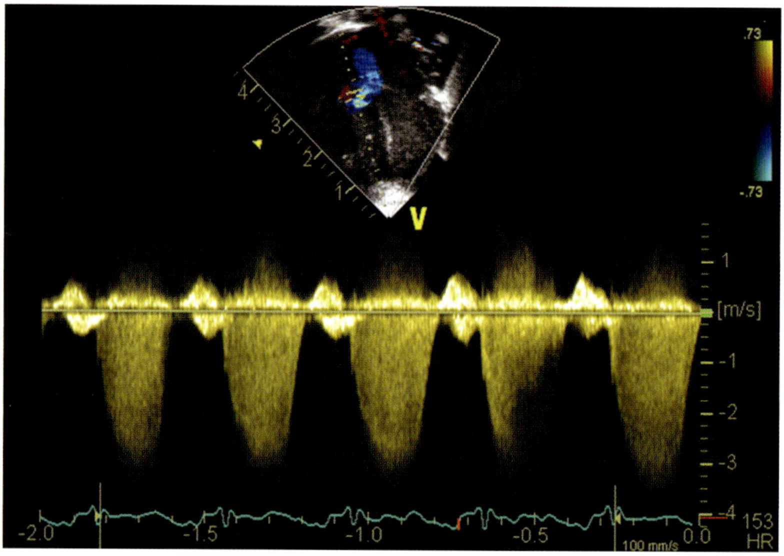

FIGURE 12-3. An example of a complete Doppler signal is shown in the last cycle of the tracing.

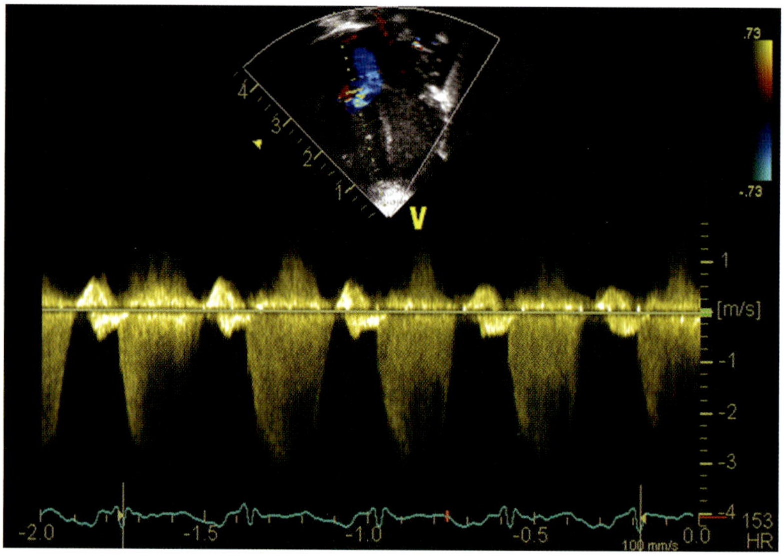

FIGURE 12-4. An example of an incomplete Doppler signal is shown.

pulmonary artery pressure. Figure 12-7 shows a pulsed wave Doppler image of a pure left-to-right PDA. The peak velocity of the left-to-right component is measured at 2.11 m/s, and the pressure difference between the aorta and the pulmonary artery is calculated as 17.75 mmHg (calculated by machine software using the modified Bernoulli equation). The infant's systemic systolic blood pressure was 68 mmHg. Therefore, the peak pulmonary pressure can be estimated to be 50.25 mmHg. Conversely, with pure right-to-left flow, the systolic systemic blood pressure plus the pressure difference between the aorta and the pulmonary artery will be an estimate of the systolic pulmonary artery pressure. In clinical practice, knowledge about the relative pressure differences between the systemic and pulmonary

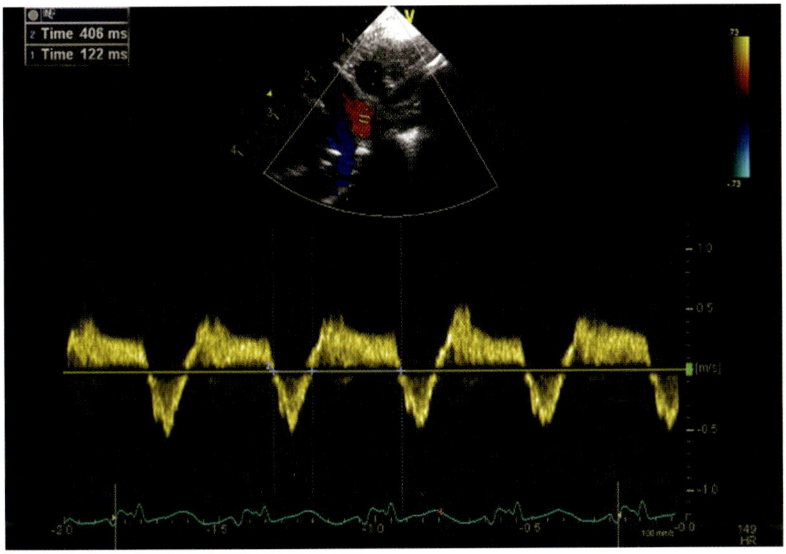

FIGURE 12-5. A pulsed wave Doppler tracing of a bidirectional PDA with the right-to-left component that is approximately 30% of the cycle.

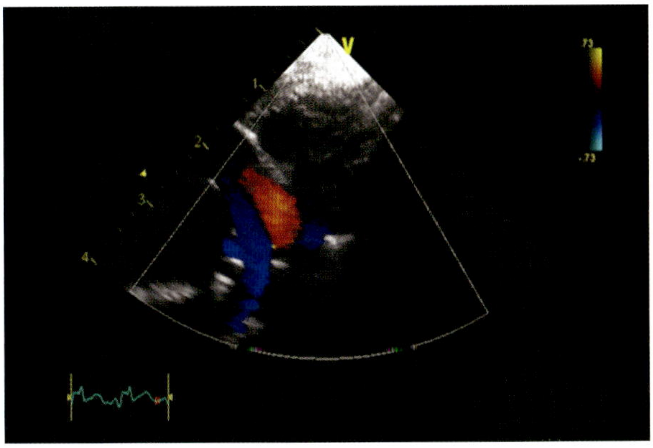

FIGURE and VIDEO 12-6. The color Doppler of a bidirectional PDA. In this figure, the left-to-right component is shown.

circulations adds to the overall assessment that a clinician makes when evaluating an infant.

Imaging

The PDA is best imaged from the suprasternal ductal cut (Chapter 3). Once a good 2D image is obtained (Figure and Video 12-8), color Doppler is applied and a visual assessment of the direction of flow through the PDA can be made. It is generally best to take a clip of the color Doppler imaging and review the clip in a frame-by-frame approach to identify the color at each point in the cardiac cycle. A color signal cycling between blue and red suggests bidirectional shunting, whereas a color signal that incorporates multiple colors in the same stream suggests high-velocity, turbulent flow with color aliasing. Figure and Video 12-9 shows a PDA that is mostly right to left, indicated by the mostly blue color. Intermittently there is a small amount of red seen, indicating the left-to-right portion of the flow. Compare this with Figure 12-6, which shows a bidirectional PDA with more left-to-right flow and Figure and Video 12-10, which shows a completely left-to-right PDA that has many different colors due to constriction resulting in high velocity with color aliasing. With live imaging, once a good color image visualizing the entire length of the PDA has been obtained, pulsed and continuous-wave Doppler evaluation can be performed in line with the PDA to obtain the velocity and pattern of the flow.

In term infants, immediately after birth the direction of PDA shunting is often bidirectional. As discussed previously, values of greater than 30% right-to-left flow throughout the cardiac cycle correlate with significantly elevated pulmonary artery pressure. By 12 hours of life the PDA is completely left-to-right in most healthy-term newborn infants.[11] Assessment of the PDA shunt direction and character is helpful to the clinician caring for infants with PPHN, but once the PDA is closed, pulmonary artery pressure can no longer be estimated using these methods.

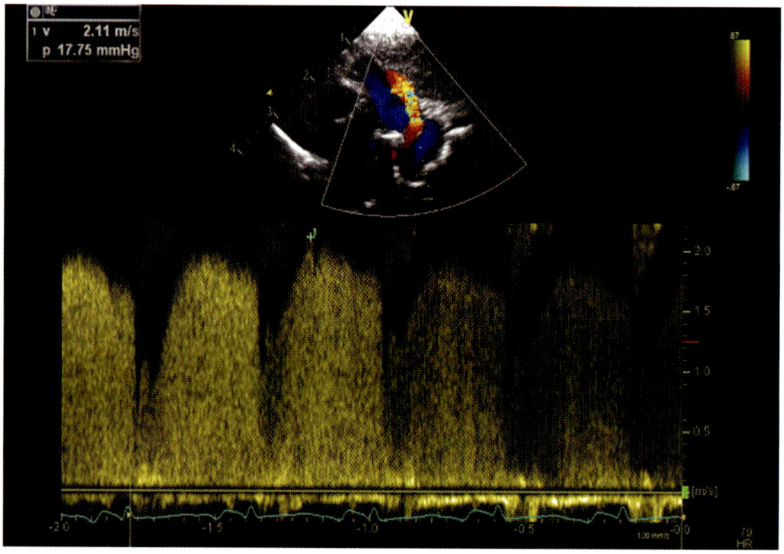

FIGURE 12-7. A pulsed wave spectral Doppler image of a pure left-to-right PDA. The peak velocity is measured at 2.11 m/s.

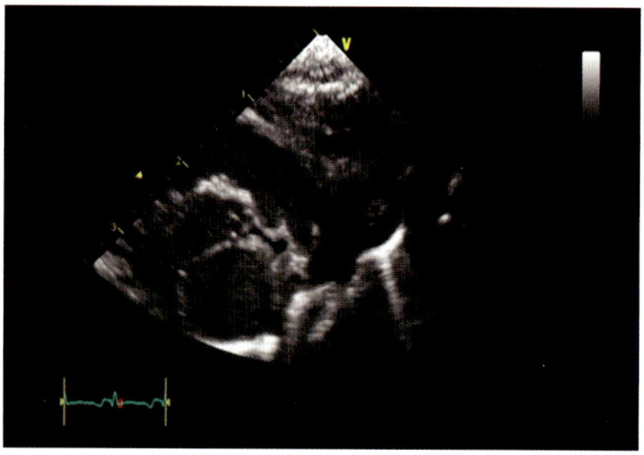

FIGURE and VIDEO 12-8. A 2D image of PDA in suprasternal view.

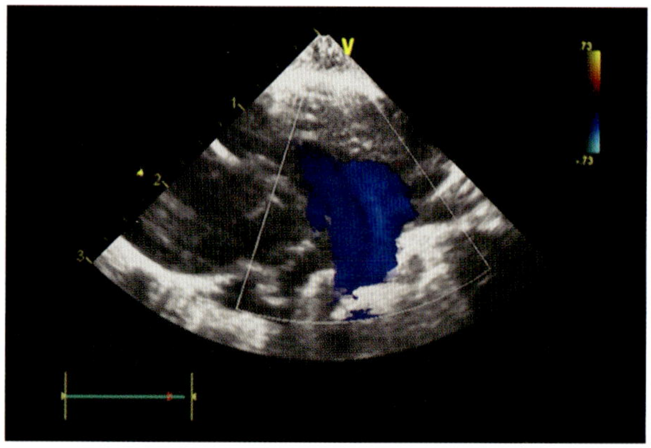

FIGURE and VIDEO 12-9. A color Doppler image of a PDA with mostly right-to-left shunt. In the figure, only right-to-left component is seen.

OTHER ECHOCARDIOGRAPHIC INDICES OF ELEVATED PULMONARY PRESSURE

Flow Pattern at the Patent Foramen Ovale

The clinician should also evaluate the patent foramen ovale (PFO) flow in the assessment of pulmonary hypertension. The best images of the atrial septum can be obtained from the subcostal coronal posterior view with the probe angled slightly posteriorly and superiorly (Chapter 3). Figure and Video 12-11 shows an example of the atrial septum imaged from this window. In this example, the septum is bulging toward the right. Once a good 2D image is obtained, color Doppler should be used to identify flow across the septum. Figure and Video 12-12 shows the color Doppler imaging of this atrial septum. Note that the flow is left-to-right and higher velocity. However, when imaging the atrial septum, the clinician should keep the Doppler scale low enough to identify low-velocity flow. An atrial shunt from the same baby with the scale set lower is shown in

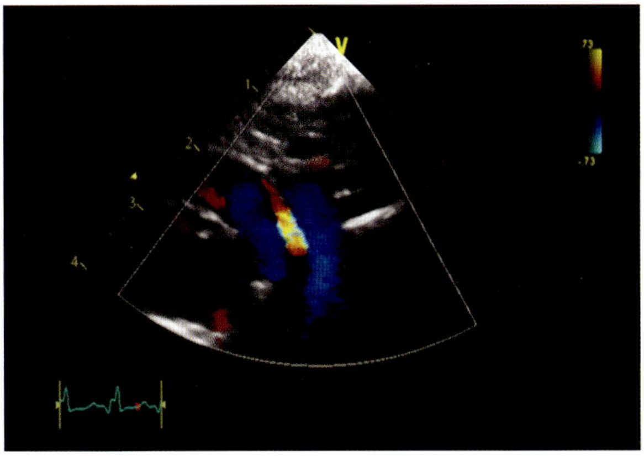

FIGURE and VIDEO 12-10. A color Doppler image of a PDA with a complete left-to-right shunt. The many different colors are due to PDA constriction, resulting in high velocity with color aliasing.

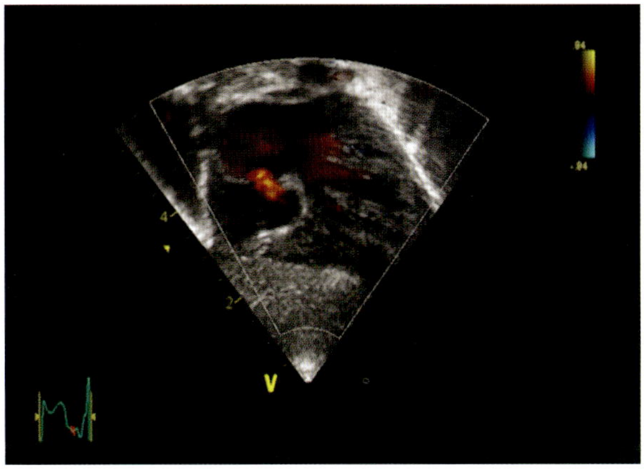

FIGURE and VIDEO 12-12. A color Doppler imaging of atrial septum from the subcostal coronal posterior view. Note that the flow is left-to-right and higher velocity.

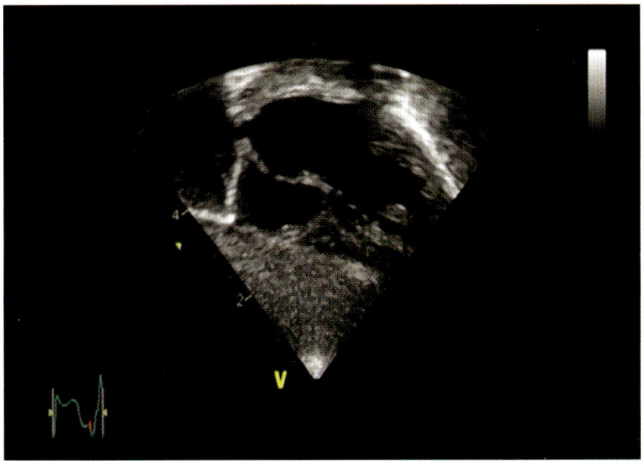

FIGURE and VIDEO 12-11. An example of the atrial septum imaged from the subcostal coronal posterior view with the probe angled slightly posteriorly and superiorly.

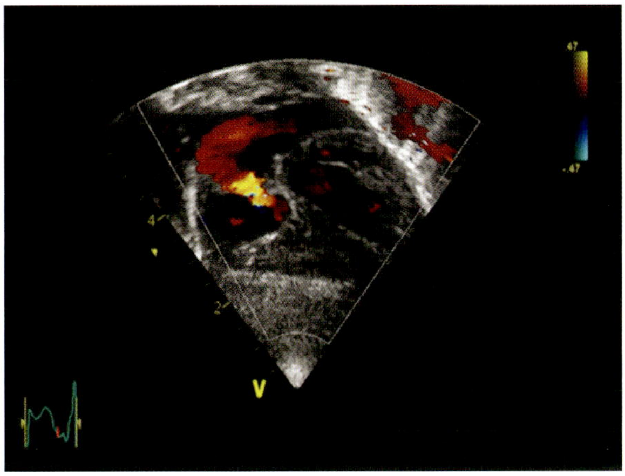

FIGURE and VIDEO 12-13. The same view as in Figure and Video 12-12, but the Doppler scale was decreased to better identify low-velocity flow.

Figure and Video 12-13. A pulsed wave Doppler signal at the foramen should also be obtained to best identify the direction of flow. An example of the pulsed wave Doppler signal from the same study is shown in Figure 12-14. The flow through the PFO is frequently bidirectional though predominantly left-to-right in the first 24 hours of life in most term and preterm newborn infants.[12,13] However, term infants with pulmonary hypertension have a longer right-to-left component of the shunt throughout the cardiac cycle. Additionally, the bidirectional shunting at the PFO can last for several days in infants with PPHN, even after the PDA closes.[12] Changes in direction of flow of both the PDA and PFO can be a useful guide in monitoring a baby's progress throughout the course of PPHN.

Systolic Time Intervals

Another method of evaluating pulmonary hypertension involves using ventricular systolic time intervals. Systolic time intervals were initially described to measure ventricular function but have been extensively evaluated in pulmonary hypertension. A ventricle working against a high afterload will take a longer time to build up enough

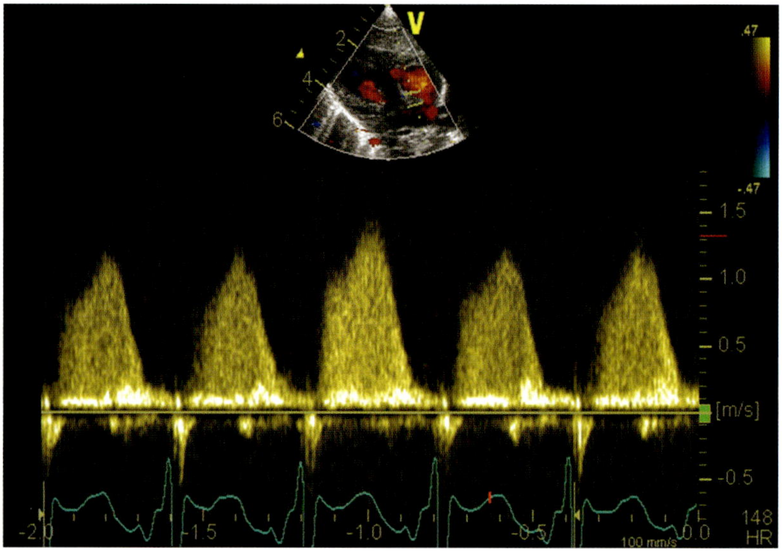

FIGURE 12-14. The pulsed wave spectral Doppler of the atrial shunt of the same patient as in the Figure and Video 12-13.

force to open the outflow valve once the electrical impulse has been generated and will then eject blood more quickly. The influence of afterload on these measures is what makes them useful in the evaluation of pulmonary hypertension. Systolic time intervals can be measured for each ventricle and can be determined from M-mode or Doppler tracings at the pulmonary and aortic valves. Though these methods are not used extensively in clinical practice, it is helpful to understand them and to have them available as some of the many tools that can be used in the evaluation of pulmonary hypertension. The main advantage of systolic time intervals is that they can be obtained in any baby. They do not correlate as well with pulmonary artery pressures as the other methods described, and they do not give a quantitative estimate of pulmonary artery pressure.

RPEP:RVET

The right ventricular pre-ejection period to right ventricular ejection time ratio (RPEP:RVET) is determined by using the electrocardiogram (ECG) tracing in conjunction with the Doppler tracing (or M-mode tracing) obtained at the pulmonary valve. The pre-ejection period is the time from the start of the Q wave to the time when the pulmonary valve opens. It is a measure of the ventricular isovolemic contraction time. If the ventricle is pushing against a higher afterload, it will take more time for the ventricle to generate the pressure needed to open the valve and the RPEP will be longer. The right ventricular ejection time is the time that the pulmonary valve is open and flow is measurable in the main pulmonary artery. The measurement of RPEP:RVET is demonstrated in Figure 12-15. In the setting of pulmonary hypertension, the RPEP:RVET ratio will be high because of the longer isovolemic contraction time needed prior to the opening of the pulmonary valve. In a group of healthy-term infants, the RPEP:RVET ratio decreased from an average of 0.39 ± 0.05 at 0-12 hours of life to 0.28 ± 0.03 at more than 48 hours of life.[14] In contrast, infants with PPHN at an average of 24 hours of life had a mean RPEP:RVET of 0.6 with both a longer RPEP and shorter RVET.[15] Infants who survived had decreasing RPEP:RVET consistent with clinical improvement.

TPV:RVET

Another measure of systolic time intervals that can be derived from the PA Doppler waveform alone is a ratio of the time to peak velocity to right ventricular ejection time (TPV:RVET). This is also sometimes called the pulmonary artery acceleration time to right ventricular ejection time (PAAT:RVET). The time to peak velocity is the time from the start of blood flow into the artery until the time when blood flow reaches its peak velocity. An example of this measurement is shown in Figure 12-16. In the setting of pulmonary hypertension, after the ventricle has built up a significant amount of force trying to push against

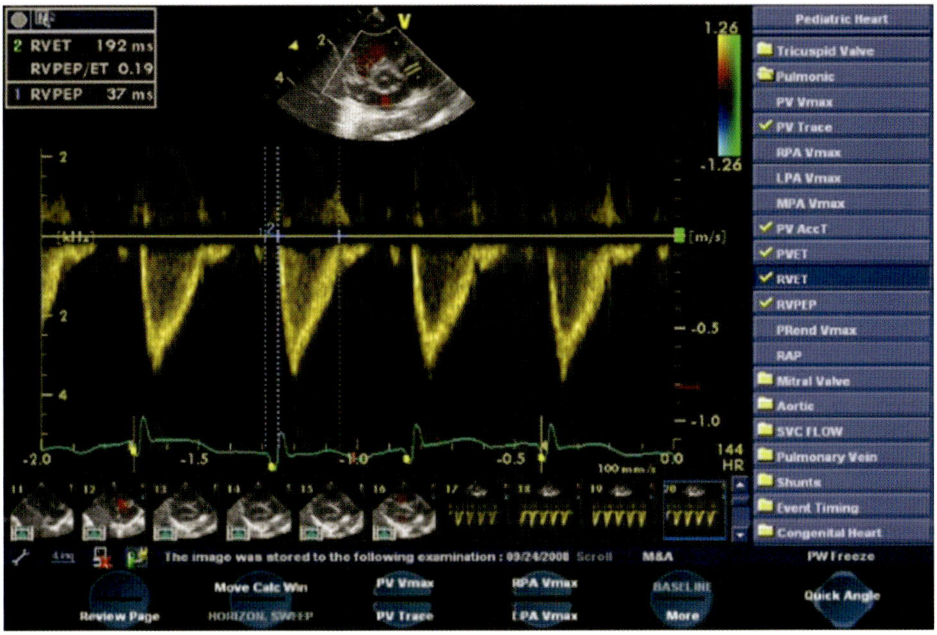

FIGURE 12-15. Measurement of the right ventricular pre-ejection period to right ventricular ejection time (RPEP:RVET) ratio.

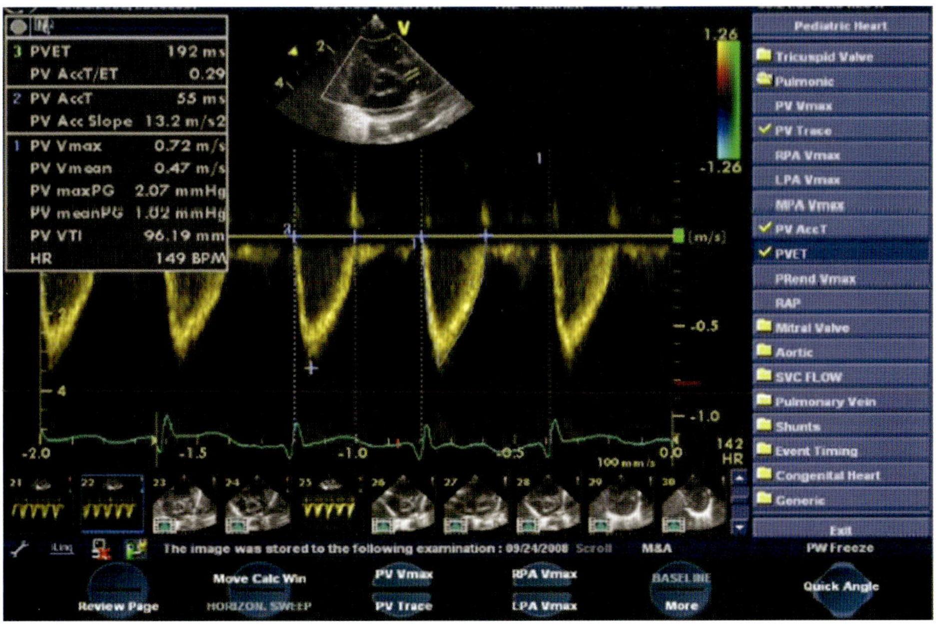

FIGURE 12-16. Measurement of the time to peak velocity to right ventricular ejection time (TPV:RVET) ratio.

a high afterload, blood flows out very quickly once the valve opens. It then slows down, coming back to baseline as the valve closes. The TPV:RVET ratio is, therefore, lower when the pulmonary pressure is higher. In normal transitioning newborns, the TPV:RVET increased from an average of 0.37 to 0.56 between 1 and 4 days of life. In the same infants the RPEP:RVET decreased from an average of 0.51 to 0.34 between 1 and 4 days of life.[16] In the first 6 hours of life, healthy-term and preterm infants had similar TPV:RVET with means (SD) of 0.23 (0.035) and 0.195 (0.042). The ratio increased over the first 30 hours of life; however, preterm infants took longer to reach a stable postnatal ratio.[17] Preterm infants with hyaline membrane disease had a TPV:RVET that remained low throughout the first 5 days of life, and was significantly less than healthy preterm babies at all time points except the first 5 hours of life.[18] Different studies have shown varying levels of accuracy of the systolic time intervals when correlated with catheter-derived pulmonary artery pressures. In a comparison of the repeatability of four different measures of pulmonary artery pressure (TR peak velocity, PDA peak velocity, TPV:RVET, and RPEP:RVET), the systolic time intervals had the worst inter- and intra-observer repeatability.[7] A recent study measuring PAAT in children of various ages found that the PAAT increased from an average of 81 ms in newborns to an average of 151 ms at 18 years of age.[19]

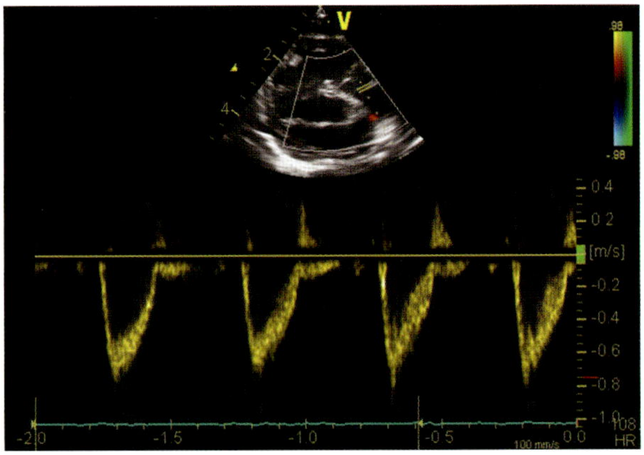

FIGURE 12-17. A normal pulsed wave Doppler tracing from the pulmonary artery.

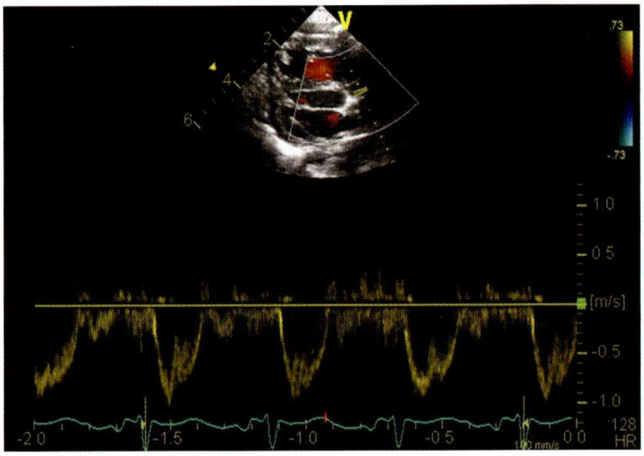

FIGURE 12-18. An abnormal pulsed wave Doppler tracing from the pulmonary artery. Note the notching pattern.

Pulmonary Artery Flow Pattern

The character of the Doppler tracing at the pulmonary valve can also be a qualitative indication of the presence of pulmonary hypertension. The pattern is normally a smooth upward and downward tracing indicating a steady increase followed by somewhat slower but also steady decrease in velocity throughout systole. Figure 12-17 shows a normal pulsed wave Doppler tracing from the pulmonary artery. In the case of pulmonary hypertension, the pattern is that of a rapid increase in velocity followed by a slow decrease in velocity, often with a stutter during deceleration. The stutter is displayed as a notch in the descending limb of the Doppler pattern. Figure 12-18 shows a Doppler trace with a notching pattern. Notching of the pulmonary valve was initially described using M-mode evaluation of the valve.[20] Studies have evaluated the waveform of the pulmonary valve as an indicator of pulmonary hypertension with varying degrees of success.[21] More recently, in a Doppler study of adult patients with pulmonary hypertension, the presence of mid-systolic notching was associated with a higher pulmonary vascular resistance. These findings suggest that this visual evaluation of the pulmonary artery Doppler pattern might help differentiate pulmonary hypertension caused by increased vascular resistance from that caused by increased pulmonary blood flow or other causes.[22]

Position of Interventricular Septum

The shape and size of the ventricles gives some indication of how the ventricle is functioning, including whether preload and afterload are affecting the ventricle. During the fetal life, the right ventricle performs a large portion of the total heart function and appears larger than it does after birth.[23] After birth and a normal circulatory transition, the left ventricle becomes dominant and appears larger

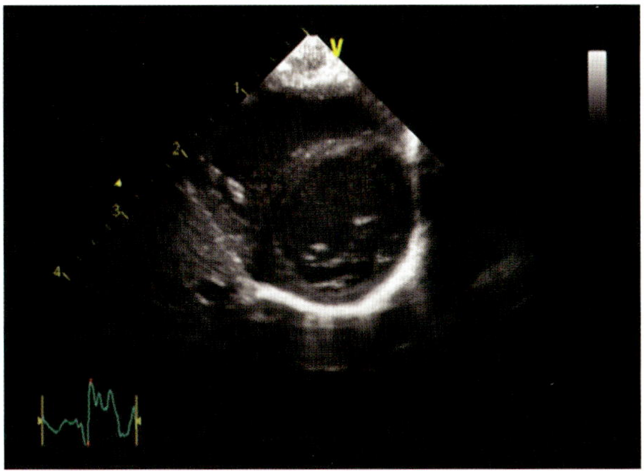

FIGURE and VIDEO 12-19. The normal circular shape of the LV after the transitional period.

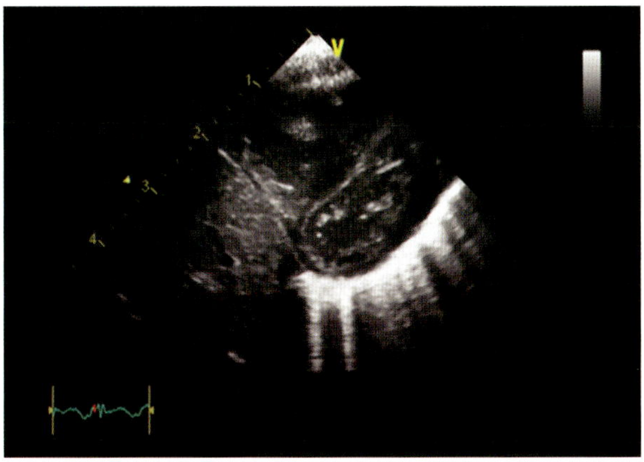

FIGURE and VIDEO 12-20. An example of a short-axis view of the heart from a baby with persistent pulmonary hypertension of newborn. Note the bulging of the right ventricle into the left ventricle.

than the right ventricle, with a more circular appearance in cross section. Figure and Video 12-19 shows the normal circular shape of the LV after the transitional period. In the normal term infant the left ventricle begins to look circular around 24 hours of life, whereas in the preterm infant the transition to the normal shape of the left ventricle can be delayed by several days to weeks.[24] The cross sectional appearance of the ventricles during pulmonary hypertension often shows a flattened septum distorting the circular appearance of the left ventricle.[25] An example of a short-axis view of the heart from a baby with PPHN is shown in Figures and Videos 12-20 and 12-21. The right ventricle can be seen bulging into the left ventricle in these images.

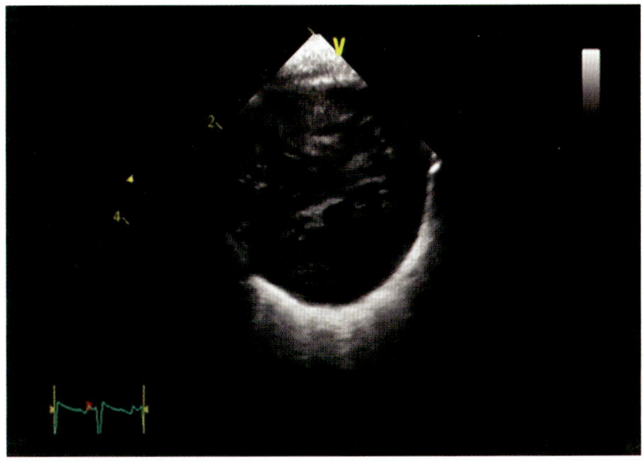

FIGURE and VIDEO 12-21. An example of a short-axis view of the heart from a baby with persistent pulmonary hypertension of newborn. Note the flattening of the interventricular septum.

Right Ventricular Function

Pulmonary hypertension can ultimately lead to RV dysfunction, which when present is associated with a worse prognosis. The function of the right ventricle is difficult to evaluate because of the shape of the ventricle and difficulty imaging the complete ventricle in a single view. A variety of measurements have been described to assess RV function, but all may be affected by multiple factors and should not be used to make clinical decisions in isolation. When determining the best course of action, the clinician should consider the entire clinical condition in conjunction with the echocardiography findings. We will discuss the measures of myocardial performance index and TAPSE for evaluating right ventricular function. TAPSE may be the most useful bedside measure for evaluating RV function in the newborn, as it is easy to perform has a high intra- and inter-observer reliability and correlates with important outcomes.[26,27]

Myocardial Performance Index

A measure of global myocardial function has been described and correlated with findings in pulmonary hypertension. This myocardial performance index (MPI) or Tei index can be calculated from the pulsed wave Doppler waveforms of either ventricle or from tissue Doppler imaging and is called a measure of global myocardial function because it includes measures of systole and diastole. The index is a measure of isovolumic contraction and isovolumic relaxation times divided by the ventricular ejection time. For the right ventricle, it is calculated by measuring the time from tricuspid valve closure

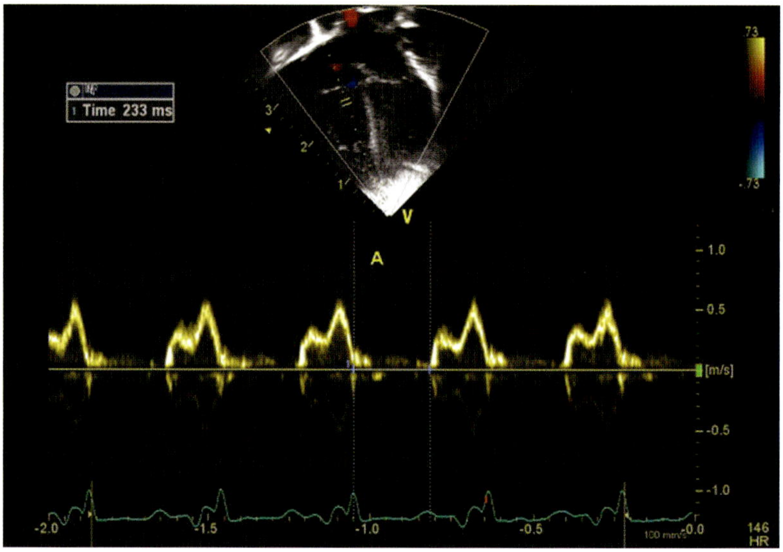

FIGURE 12-22. An example of spectral Doppler of the right ventricular inflow. The time from tricuspid valve closure to opening is shown here as A.

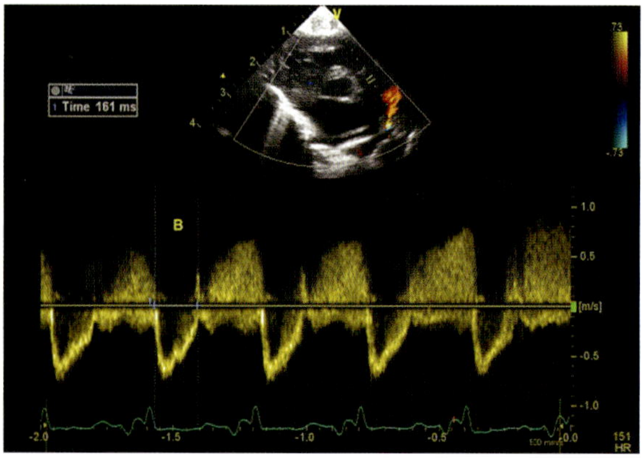

FIGURE 12-23. An example of spectral Doppler of the pulmonary artery flow. The right ventricular ejection time is shown here as B.

to opening. This is shown as time A in Figure 12-22. The RV ejection time (shown as time B in Figure 12-23) is subtracted from this value, and the result is divided by the ejection time. In the example shown the MPI is 0.45 (=233ms-161ms/161ms). The RV MPI is prolonged in cases of pulmonary hypertension.[28] In an evaluation of the MPI of both ventricles in fetal and early post-natal life, the index decreased over time during gestation, more in the left than the right ventricle, indicating that the right ventricle works against a higher afterload than the left ventricle in late fetal life. After birth there was an increase in the index followed by a rapid decline after 24 hours of life.[29] In infants with pulmonary hypertension, the RV MPI was higher (mean 0.55 ± 0.17) than in healthy term infants (mean 0.24 ± 0.09).[30]

TAPSE

Tricuspid annular plane systolic excursion (TAPSE) is a measurement of systolic function of the right ventricle. The ventricles are composed of both circumferential and longitudinal fibers, and longitudinal fibers comprise a significant portion of the right ventricular muscle fibers. As longitudinal fibers contract, the AV valves move toward the apex of the heart. TAPSE is a measurement of longitudinal contraction of the right ventricle. TAPSE is measured from a four-chamber apical view by the clinician placing an M-mode sample at the tricuspid annulus insertion points on the lateral ventricular wall. The distance that the ventricular wall moves in systole is the TAPSE (Figure). Normal measurements for TAPSE in the newborn period were evaluated in 50 healthy term newborns in the first 2 days of life, and the mean (SD) were found to be 0.92 cm (14) at an average of 15 hours of life and 0.91 (13) at an average of 35 hours of life.[31] In a single center retrospective review of newborns with PPHN, lower TAPSE values were associated with death or ECMO. A TAPSE < 4 mm combined with a predominantly right-to-left PDA, poor LV function, or an oxygenation index >20 was a highly specific measure for death or need for ECMO.[27]

SUMMARY

Assessment of pulmonary hypertension is important in the newborn period and includes a global evaluation of heart function in addition to specific measures of pulmonary artery pressure. It remains critical to use all aspects of the echocardiographic findings, in combination with the clinical findings, to make informed clinical decisions. It also remains important to reevaluate an individual infant on a regular, ongoing basis, since the findings of pulmonary hypertension are dynamic in the newborn period. Differentiating pulmonary hypertension caused by elevated pulmonary vascular resistance from pulmonary hypertension caused by elevated pulmonary blood flow can be difficult and truly requires integration of all of the associated findings, as well as the potential causes of the pulmonary hypertension. Clinicians who practice echocardiography will often develop intuitive skills in understanding these differences that are not as easily defined by specific measures.

REFERENCES

1. Emmanouilides GC, Moss AJ, Duffie ER, Adams FH. Pulmonary artery pressure changes in human newborn infants from birth to 3 days of age. *J Pediatr.* 1964;65:327–333.
2. Yock PG, Popp RL. Noninvasive estimation of right ventricular systolic pressure by Doppler ultrasound in patients with tricuspid regurgitation. *Circulation.* 1984;70:657–662.
3. Skinner JR, Stuart AGS, O'Sullivan J, Heads A, Boys RJ, Hunter S. Right heart pressure determination by Doppler in infants with tricuspid regurgitation. *Arch Dis Child.* 1993;69:216–220.
4. Skinner JR, Hunter SM, Hey EN. Haemodynamic features at presentation in persistent pulmonary hypertension of the newborn and outcome. *Arch Dis Child.* 1996;74:F26–F32.
5. Sehgal A, Athikarisamy SE, Adamopoulos M. Global myocardial function is compromised in infants with pulmonary hypertension. *Acta Paediatrica.* 2012;101:410–413.
6. Stevenson JG. Comparison of several non-invasive methods for estimation of pulmonary artery pressure. *J Am Soc Echocardiogr.* 1989;2:157–171.
7. Skinner JR, Boys RJ, Heads A, Hey EN, Hunter S. Estimation of pulmonary artery pressure in the newborn: study of the repeatability of four Doppler echocardiographic techniques. *Pediatr Cardiol.* 1996;17:360–369.
8. Skinner JR, Boys RJ, Hunter S, Hey EN. Non-invasive assessment of pulmonary arterial pressure in healthy neonates. *Arch Dis Child.* 1991;66:386–390.
9. Seppanen MP, Kaapa PO, Kero PO, Seraste M. Doppler-derived systolic pulmonary artery pressure in acute neonatal respiratory distress syndrome. *Pediatrics.* 1994;93:769.
10. Musewe NN, Poppe D, Smallhorn JF, et al. Doppler echocardiographic measurement of pulmonary artery pressure from ductal Doppler velocities in the newborn. *J Am Coll Cardiol.* 1990;15:446–456.
11. Walther FJ, Benders MJ, Leighton JO. Early changes in the neonatal circulatory transition. *J Pediatr.* 1993;123:625–632.
12. Hiraishi S, Agata Y, Saito K, et al. Interatrial shunt flow profiles in newborn infants: a colour flow and pulsed Doppler echocardiographic study. *Br Heart J.* 1991;65:41–45.
13. Evans N, Iyer P. Incompetence of the foramen ovale in preterm infants supported by mechanical ventilation. *J Pediatr.* 1994;125:786–792.
14. Riggs T, Hirschfeld S, Bormuth C, et al. Neonatal circulatory changes: an echocardiographic study. *Pediatrics.* 1977;59:338–344.
15. Riggs T, Hirschfeld S, Fanaroff A, et al. Persistence of fetal circulation syndrome: An echocardiographic study. *J Pediatr.* 1977;91:626–631.
16. Siraishi H, Yanagisawa M. Pulse Doppler echocardiographic evaluation of neonatal circulatory changes. *Br Heart J.* 1987;57:161–167.
17. Evans NJ, Archer LN. Postnatal circulatory adaptation in healthy term and preterm neonates. *Arch Dis Child.* 1990;65:24–26.
18. Evans NJ, Archer LN. Doppler assessment of pulmonary artery pressure and extrapulmonary shunting in the acute phase of hyaline membrane disease. *Arch Dis Child.* 1991;66:6–11.
19. Koestenberger M, Grangl G, Avian A, et al. Normal reference values and z scores of the pulmonary artery acceleration time in children and its importance for the assessment of pulmonary hypertension. *Circ Cardiovasc Imaging.* 2017;10(1):e005336.
20. Weyman AE, Dillon JC, Feigenbaum H, Chang S. Echocardiographic patterns of pulmonic valve motion with pulmonary hypertension. *Circulation.* 1974;50:905–910.
21. Oberhänsli I, Branden G, Girod M, Friedli B. Estimation of pulmonary artery pressure by ultrasound. A study comparing simultaneously recorded pulmonary valve echogram and pulmonary artery pressures. *Pediatr Cardiol.* 1982;2:123–130.
22. Arkles JS, Opotowsky AR, Ojeda J, et al. Shape of the right ventricular Doppler envelope predicts hemodynamics and right heart function in pulmonary hypertension. *Am J Respir Crit Care Med.* 2011;183:268–276.

23. Azancot A, Caudell TP, Allen HD, et al. Analysis of ventricular shape by echocardiography in normal fetuses, newborns, and infants. *Circulation*. 1983;68:1201–1211.

24. Lee LA, Kimball TR, Daniels SR, et al. Left ventricular mechanics in the preterm infant and their effect on the measurement of cardiac performance. *J Pediatr*. 1992;120:114–119.

25. King ME, Braun H, Goldblatt A, Liberthson R, Weyman AE. Interventricular septal configuration as a predictor of right ventricular systolic hypertension in children: a cross-sectional echocardiographic study. *Circulation*. 1983;68:68–75.

26. Richardson C, Amirtharaj C, Gruber D, Hayes DA. Assessing myocardial function in infants with pulmonary hypertension: the role of tissue Doppler imaging and tricuspid annular plane systolic excursion. *Pediatr Cardiol*. 2017;38:558–565.

27. Malowitz JR, Forscha DE, Smith PB, et al. Right ventricular echocardiographic indices predict poor outcomes in infants with persistent pulmonary hypertension of the newborn. *Eur Heart J Cardiovasc Imaging*. 2015;16:1224–1231.

28. Yeo TC, Dujardin KS, Tei C, et al. Value of a Doppler-derived index combining systolic and diastolic time intervals in predicting outcome in primary pulmonary hypertension. *Am J Cardiol*. 1998;81:1157–1161.

29. Tsutsumi T, Ishii M, Eto G, et al. Serial evaluation for myocardial performance in fetuses and neonates using a new Doppler index. *Pediatr Int*. 1999;41:722–727.

30. Patel N, Mills JF, Cheung MMH. Use of the myocardial performance index to assess right ventricular function in infants with pulmonary hypertension. *Pediatr Cardiol*. 2009;30:133–137.

31. Jain A, Mohamed A, El-Kaffash A, et al. A comprehensive echocardiographic protocol for assessing neonatal right ventricular dimensions and function in the transitional period: Normative data and z-scores. *J Am Soc Echocardiogr*. 2014;27:1293–1304.

CHAPTER 13

Desaturation and Cyanosis in the Newborn Infant without Congenital Heart Disease*

Tina A. Leone

- INTRODUCTION
- DIFFERENTIATING THE PRIMARY CAUSE OF HYPOXEMIA
- ECHOCARDIOGRAPHIC FINDINGS IN SPECIFIC CAUSES OF HYPOXEMIA
  - Respiratory Distress Syndrome
  - Infants of Diabetic Mothers
  - Fetal Ductus Arteriosus Closure
  - Meconium Aspiration Syndrome
- ECHOCARDIOGRAPHIC EVALUATION OF THERAPEUTIC RESPONSES
  - Oxygen
  - Ventilation
  - Surfactant
- A SYSTEMATIC APPROACH TO PERFORMING THE ECHOCARDIOGRAM
  - Parasternal Window
  - Parasternal Short-Axis Views
  - Apical Window
  - Suprasternal Window
  - Subcostal Window
  - Global Assessment
- SUMMARY
- REFERENCES

INTRODUCTION

The physical signs of cyanosis and decreased oxygen saturation are usually the result of hypoxemia, and can be found in newborn infants with a variety of pathologies. Hypoxemia can be the result of shunting of deoxygenated blood from the venous to the arterial circulation. This can occur at many levels including intracardiac, extracardiac, and intrapulmonary locations. The primary causes of hypoxemia in infants without congenital heart disease vary and include pulmonary problems such as pneumonia, respiratory distress syndrome (RDS), congenital anomalies, pneumothorax, and meconium aspiration syndrome (MAS). Additionally, the primary cause of hypoxemia could be persistent pulmonary hypertension of the newborn (PPHN), a failure or delay in making the circulatory transition from fetal to newborn life leading to persistently elevated pulmonary vascular resistance, and continued shunting through the fetal channels. In most cases, PPHN is secondary to another respiratory disease, and therefore these findings do not usually occur in isolation. Certain conditions predispose infants to having a more prolonged

*Videos can be accessed at http://PracticalNeonatalEcho.com.

circulatory transition. Infants at higher risk include infants of diabetic mothers, infants with trisomy 21, and fetal exposure to nonsteroidal anti-inflammatory agents or selective serotonin reuptake inhibitors. Preterm infants may have a variety of transitional problems after birth leading to hypoxemia. Both RDS and prolonged premature rupture of membranes (PPROM) are associated with PPHN. Additionally, a significant patent ductus arteriosus (PDA) is often associated with increasing oxygen and ventilator requirements. Echocardiography can be helpful in the diagnosis and management of many of these problems.

To differentiate the causes of hypoxemia, the neonatologist should perform and interpret a complete, comprehensive echocardiographic study to exclude congenital heart disease. When interpreting the echocardiogram, one must consider the clinical circumstances associated with the presentation. The neonatologist is in a unique position to be thoroughly involved with the clinical care of the infant and can determine whether the clinical course and the echocardiography findings are congruent. When the clinical course and the echocardiography findings are inconsistent, it is important for the neonatogolist to further evaluate all of the findings. The neonatologist performing echocardiography should readily refer to a pediatric cardiologist whenever congenital heart disease is suspected. In recent years, routine oxygen saturation screening of the newborn prior to discharge from the hospital has been recommended to detect otherwise silent critical congenital heart disease that could cause serious complications if left undetected.[1,2] These screens have frequently identified infants with hypoxemia not caused by critical congenital heart disease. Approximately one-third of the infants with a positive screen result that is not associated with critical congenital heart disease will have another illness requiring treatment.[3,4]

In addition to assessment of the immediate transitional problems that cause hypoxemia, echocardiography can be helpful in evaluating infants at any time during the neonatal intensive care unit course when clinical deterioration occurs. Infants on the ventilator may have impaired cardiac function because of excessive intrathoracic pressure. Pleural and pericardial effusions can develop as complications from invasive central lines and are easily identified on the ultrasound examination. Infants with bronchopulmonary dysplasia or sepsis can have hemodynamic compromise that can be evaluated by echocardiography. Thus, echocardiography should be considered an important tool to assist in the intensive care management of any newborn infant. Many treatment strategies for neonatal diseases vary by institution and geographic location. Particularly in the case of PPHN treatment, strategies have been documented to be quite variable.[5] Using echocardiography to guide therapy is a useful approach to individualizing treatment. However, many challenges in consistently accomplishing such an approach continue to exist, including the lack of evidence for specific treatments in relation to echocardiographic findings.

In this chapter, the constellation of echocardiographic findings in a variety of disease states will be reviewed. Whenever available, currently existing evidence for echocardiography-guided treatment will be discussed. The echocardiographic findings for each standard view that might be seen in infants with hypoxemia will be reviewed. The specific findings of congenital heart disease will not be discussed except for a few key features that should trigger a more thorough anatomic evaluation. Echocardiographic findings that can be used to influence management will also be presented.

DIFFERENTIATING THE PRIMARY CAUSE OF HYPOXEMIA

Since the establishment of echocardiography as a superior, noninvasive, and readily available diagnostic modality, investigators have evaluated a variety of methods that can utilize this technique to help differentiate the causes of hypoxemia and predict the outcome and response to therapy. Decades ago, Johnson et al[6] evaluated 16 infants with primary pulmonary disease (pneumonia, MAS, and RDS) requiring 100% oxygen. Systolic time intervals, right ventricular pre-ejection period/right ventricular ejection time ratio (RPEP/RVET), and left ventricular pre-ejection period/left ventricular ejection time ratio (LPEP/LVET) were compared among infants who responded to tolazoline and those who did not. Half of the infants responded to tolazoline; this cohort had prolonged RPEP/RVET and LPEP/LVET ratios compared with those who did not. This suggests that infants with a responsive pulmonary vasculature such as in PPHN are more likely to have prolonged ventricular systolic time intervals. Walther et al[7] compared 33 infants treated with high oxygen concentrations and mechanical ventilation in the first day of life with 32 control infants. Half of the infants with high oxygen requirements met criteria for extracorporeal membrane oxygenation (ECMO). Compared with controls, those with high oxygen requirements had lower aortopulmonary pressure differences, larger diameter and more prolonged patency of the ductus arteriosus, and more right-to-left ductal shunting. Infants meeting ECMO criteria had very low aortopulmonary pressure differences. Similarly, Evans et al[8] used serial echocardiography to evaluate 32 term infants requiring more than 70% oxygen. Echocardiograms were performed at presentation, and then daily until the oxygen requirement was less than 30%. Infants were divided into a primary respiratory pathology group and a primary PPHN group. Those with primary PPHN had a higher incidence of PDA and larger PDAs. Similar numbers of infants in each group had bidirectional or pure right-to-left shunting at the PDA. Both groups had a frequent occurrence of low ventricular output (both right and left ventricles), which increased with the clinical improvement of the infants. Overall, in both groups only approximately 50% of the infants had suprasystemic pulmonary artery pressures, and pulmonary artery pressure decreased before the hypoxemia improved. The authors concluded that most of the hypoxemia in these infants was caused by intrapulmonary right-to-left shunting rather than shunting through the PDA and patent foramen ovale (PFO).

These studies show that the constellation of echocardiographic findings in infants with high oxygen requirements frequently includes abnormal systolic time intervals (a sign of increased afterload), prolonged patency of the ductus arteriosus, smaller aortopulmonary pressure differences with more right-to-left shunting through the PDA (a sign of higher pulmonary artery pressures), and decreased ventricular outputs.

ECHOCARDIOGRAPHIC FINDINGS IN SPECIFIC CAUSES OF HYPOXEMIA

Respiratory Distress Syndrome

Many studies have shown that infants with RDS have delayed transitional circulation with evidence of higher pulmonary artery pressure and lower aortopulmonary pressure differences in the first several days after birth. In 1977, Halliday et al[9] published an echocardiographic evaluation of infants with RDS over the first 5 days of life finding prolonged RPEP:RVET in infants with more severe clinical disease. Randala et al[10] found that preterm infants with RDS treated with surfactant had a lower systemic to pulmonary artery pressure difference than preterm infants without RDS and term infants at 48 and 72 hours of age, yet all groups were similar at 24 hours of age. Evans and Archer[11] found that preterm infants with RDS had signs of increased pulmonary artery pressure estimated by right ventricular systolic time intervals compared with infants without respiratory distress. The systolic time intervals did not correlate well with clinical disease but did correlate with the level of bidirectional shunting at the PDA and PFO. These authors also showed that the ductus arteriosus closed more slowly in infants with RDS. Bidirectional PDA flow occurred in 40% of infants with RDS at 19 hours of life, but most had become completely left to right by 60-79 hours of life. In preterm infants, Seppanen et al[12] showed that those with RDS more frequently had tricuspid regurgitation (TR) than healthy preterm infants, and pulmonary artery pressure decreased more slowly in infants with RDS. Evans and Kluckow[13] documented a higher incidence of low right ventricular output (<150 ml/kg/min) in preterm infants with more severe RDS. Taken together, these studies show evidence of relatively elevated pulmonary arterial pressure and prolonged ductal patency in infants with RDS.

Infants of Diabetic Mothers

It is well known that poor glycemic control during pregnancy is associated with hypertrophic cardiomyopathy.[14,15] The echocardiogram will show an increased interventricular septum thickness. The ventricular free wall thickness may also be increased but often not as much as the septal wall (asymmetric septal hypertrophy). Functional ventricular outflow obstruction can be seen with decreased left ventricular output.[16] Infants of diabetic mothers are also at risk for delayed circulatory transition with increased pulmonary artery pressure and prolonged persistence of the ductus arteriosus.[17,18] Even when glucose levels are tightly managed during pregnancy, infants show signs of delayed circulatory transition with lower right ventricular output than control infants.[19]

Fetal Ductus Arteriosus Closure

Another condition that can be associated with hypertrophic cardiomyopathy is fetal closure of the ductus arteriosus. Gewilling et al[20] reviewed the echocardiographic findings in 12 cases of fetal ductus arteriosus closure. Important abnormalities included right ventricular hypertrophy, tricuspid and pulmonary regurgitation, and right atrial dilation. Such findings demonstrate the consequences of prolonged exposure to excessive afterload during fetal life on the right ventricle. These patients are at increased risk of hypoxemia due to right-to-left shunting at the fetal channels secondary to pulmonary hypertension.

Meconium Aspiration Syndrome

Fewer echocardiographic studies have focused on the findings associated with MAS, even though this is one of the more common diseases leading to PPHN. However, in one study, Korhonen et al[21] compared serial echocardiography findings in 17 infants with mild to moderate MAS with those in 16 healthy matched control infants over the first 3 days of life. They found more frequent bidirectional shunting at the ductus arteriosus at 12 hours of life in infants with MAS. Additionally, infants with MAS had a lower aortopulmonary pressure gradient over the first 12 hours of life. In this population of infants, none had pure right-to-left ductal shunting and the left ventricular output was not compromised. On the other hand, infants with MAS had a lower-velocity time integral in the left pulmonary artery. Therefore, hypoxemia in the setting of MAS is multifactorial, which includes low pulmonary flow, right-to-left shunting at the fetal channels, and intrapulmonary V:Q mismatch.

ECHOCARDIOGRAPHIC EVALUATION OF THERAPEUTIC RESPONSES

Oxygen

Oxygen is often recognized as a pulmonary vasodilator, although in excess can blunt vasodilation response to nitric oxide. To determine the hemodynamic response to different levels of oxygenation, Skinner et al[22] performed echocardiograms on 18 preterm infants with respiratory failure at three levels of arterial oxygen saturation (SpO_2): 86%, 96%, and 100%. The level of oxygenation was adjusted in each infant by changing FiO_2 and maintaining the SpO_2 at the desired level for 15 minutes. Infants with lower SpO_2 had more signs of elevated pulmonary artery pressure as evidence by lower aortopulmonary pressure differences from Doppler assessment of the PDA flow. Higher oxygen saturation levels were also associated with greater constriction of the ductus arteriosus. In contrast, in a group of 13 preterm infants, Bard et al[23] found no differences in pulmonary artery pressure measured by velocity of the TR jet between SpO_2 levels of 95% versus 90%. The differences in findings between these studies may be related to the sensitivity of the marker evaluated in each study or to the differences in oxygen saturation levels.

Ventilation

Assisted ventilation has the potential to alter neonatal hemodynamics in several ways. Increasing intrathoracic pressure may increase pulmonary vascular resistance, decrease pulmonary blood flow, and decrease systemic venous return. Alternatively, optimizing lung volume could decrease pulmonary vascular resistance and increase pulmonary blood flow. The actual effects of changes in intrathoracic pressure from assisted ventilation can most depend upon the level of illness of the lungs. De Waal et al[24] evaluated the hemodynamic effects of altering the positive end expiratory pressure (PEEP) level between 5 and 8 cm H_2O in 50 ventilated infants. Increasing PEEP to 8 cm H_2O was associated with a significant change in superior vena cava (SVC) flow in 36% of infants, but the direction of change increased in half of those and decreased in the other half. Improving pulmonary compliance tended to improve systemic blood flow measures. The right ventricular output was decreased on average with increasing PEEP. One of the risk factors for low SVC flow in preterm infants is higher mean airway pressure.[25] Osborn and Evans[26] performed a randomized controlled trial comparing the hemodynamic effects of high-frequency oscillatory ventilation (HFOV) with conventional ventilation. There were no statistically significant differences found in the SVC flow or right ventricular output. However, a nonsignificant trend in terms of increased incidence of low SVC flow was found with HFOV, and more infants in the HFOV group were treated with dobutamine.

Surfactant

The hemodynamic response to surfactant dosing remains incompletely understood. Hamdan and Shaw[27] evaluated the ratio of pulmonary artery acceleration time (PAAT) to RVET (PAAT:RVET) in infants immediately before each of 2 doses of exosurf were given to a group of preterm infants. They then repeated measures 1 and 6 hours after each dose and 12, 36, and 60 hours after the second dose. They found that pulmonary artery acceleration time to right ventricular ejection time (PAAT:RVET) steadily increased over this time period but the rate of increase was higher at 1 hour after each surfactant dose. Kaapa et al[28] found a decrease in pulmonary artery pressure and an increase in left-to-right PDA flow after surfactant dosing as compared to infants undergoing endotracheal suctioning who did not have these changes. By contrast, Bloom et al[29] evaluated 12 preterm infants with severe RDS treated with natural surfactant and 25 preterm infants with mild RDS. They found significantly lower aortopulmonary pressure difference in infants with severe RDS compared with those with mild RDS. These aortopulmonary pressure differences did not increase immediately after surfactant administration but became similar to infants with mild RDS by 48 hours of age. They also found lower levels of left pulmonary artery blood flow in infants with more severe RDS. More recently, in a study of delivery room surfactant administration to preterm infants less than 30 weeks' gestation, Sehgal et al[30] found that PDA shunting became all left to right after surfactant dosing given within 30 minutes of birth. In summary, these studies show that infants with RDS have signs of increased pulmonary artery pressure compared with infants who do not have RDS. Surfactant therapy is associated with a reduction in pulmonary artery pressure at varying time frames after dosing.

A SYSTEMATIC APPROACH TO PERFORMING THE ECHOCARDIOGRAM

Each clinician must have an organized and standardized approach to performing an echocardiogram. This same approach should be followed with each examination, so that no images/views are missed. Similarly, clinicians should follow a standardized approach when reviewing the images to ensure that all aspects were assessed. The following is one approach that can be used. Individual clinicians may choose a different order of imaging as long as all areas are addressed. The discussion of each of the following images focuses on the findings associated with diseases causing hypoxemia. A set of images taken from newborn infants with a variety of clinical conditions will follow each description. In interpreting the echocardiographic images, it is critical for the clinician to remember that the findings are very dynamic over the first several days of life. Therefore, when evaluating the sick infant, one must consider the normal changes that can occur during that same time frame. In the first 3 days of life, knowledge of the age of the patient is very important for the interpretation of the echocardiogram.

Parasternal Window

Parasternal Long-Axis View

In the parasternal long-axis view, it is important to evaluate the relative size of the chambers and the function of the ventricles. In PPHN, pulmonary blood flow is low and therefore pulmonary venous return is decreased and the left atrium and left ventricle can appear underfilled. An interventricular septum that is flattened or bulging into the left side can often be seen in the long-axis view. Myocardial hypertrophy can also be evaluated from this view. Measures of systolic function such as shortening fraction can be obtained using an M-mode tracing through the interventricular septum at the level of the mitral valve (see Chapters 5 and 8). It should be remembered that these measures are not reliable when the ventricular motion is not uniform or the shape is distorted. Decreased left ventricular systolic function is not a frequent finding in PPHN. The relative size of the left atrium and aortic root can also be measured in this view. The aortic valve diameter should be measured in this view for calculation of the left ventricular output. In infants with impairment of myocardial systolic function, mitral insufficiency can often be identified in this view using color flow Doppler.

Figure and Video 13-1 is an example of a long-axis view from a 30-week preterm infant with mild RDS at 4 hours of life. This image shows normal cardiac anatomy (from this perspective) and function. Figure and Video 13-2 is an example of this view in a 25-week preterm infant with a large mostly left-to-right PDA at

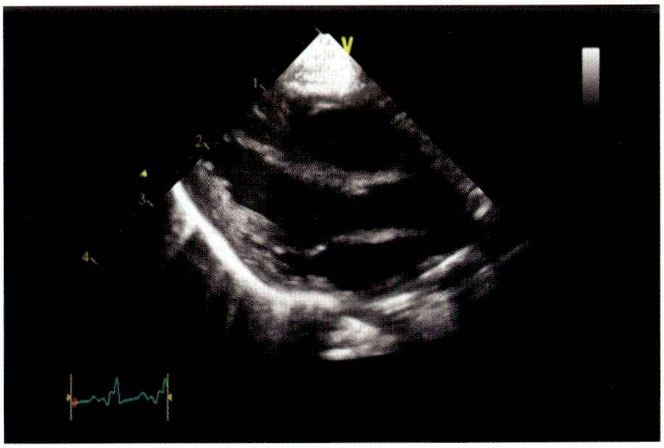

FIGURE and VIDEO 13-1. An example of a long-axis view from a 30-week preterm infant with mild respiratory distress syndrome at 4 hours of life. This image shows normal cardiac anatomy (from this perspective) and function.

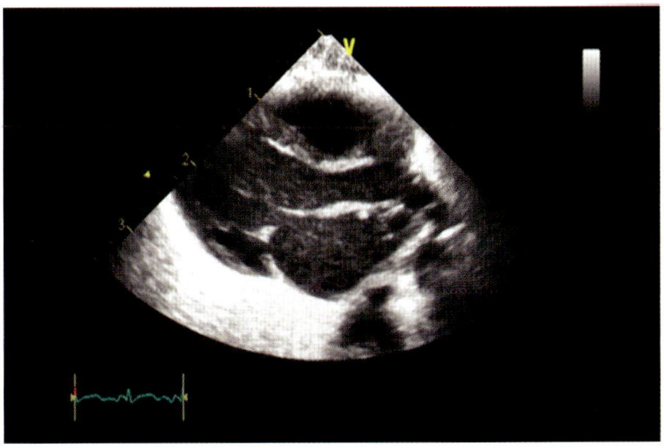

FIGURE and VIDEO 13-2. An example of a long-axis view in a 25-week preterm infant with a large mostly left-to-right patent ductus arteriosus at approximately 4 hours of life.

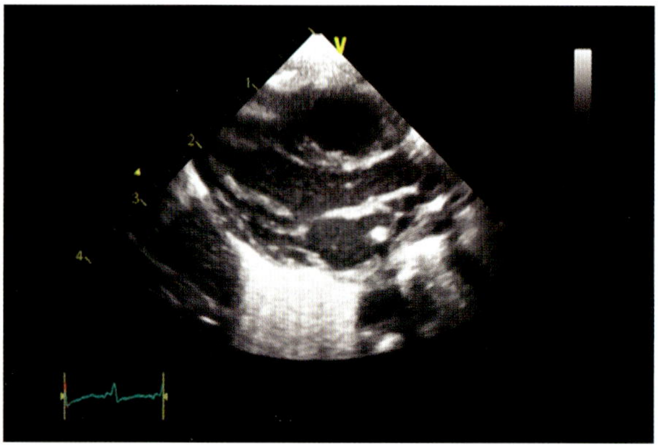

FIGURE and VIDEO 13-3. The same infant as in Figure and Video 13-2 at 20 hours of life with a closed ductus arteriosus after 1 dose of indomethacin. Notice the difference between the two videos in the size of left atrium.

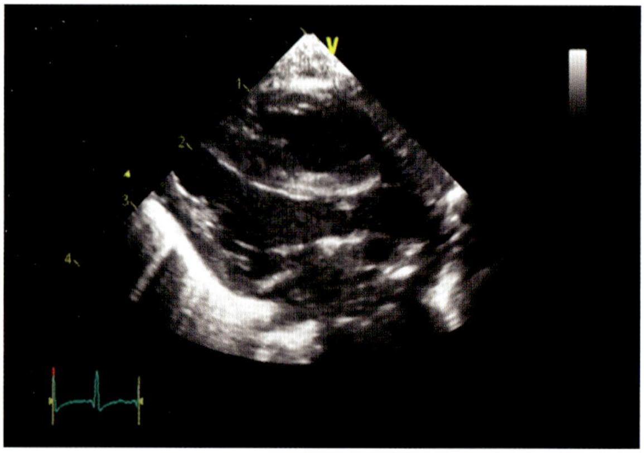

FIGURE and VIDEO 13-4. An example of a long-axis view in an infant with prolonged premature rupture of membrane at 2 hours of life. Note the somewhat thickened interventricular septum and the small left atrium.

approximately 4 hours of life. Figure and Video 13-3 shows the same infant at 20 hours of life with a closed PDA after 1 dose of indomethacin. Notice the difference between the two clips in the size of left atrium. Figure and Video 13-4 shows this view from an infant with prolonged rupture of membranes at 2 hours of life. Note the somewhat thickened interventricular septum and the small left atrium. Figure and Video 13-5 shows the long-axis view from a term infant who failed the oxygen saturation screen and was thought to have fetal closure of the ductus arteriosus. Note the hypertrophied right ventricle. Figure and Video 13-6 shows the long-axis view from an infant with severe oligohydramnios associated with renal anomalies at 3 hours of life. Figure and Video 13-7

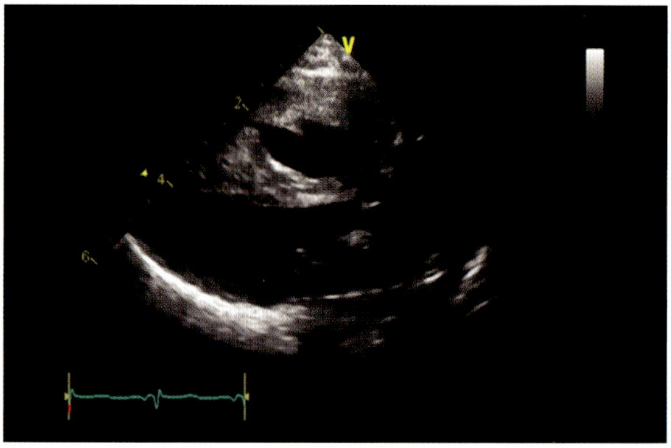

FIGURE and VIDEO 13-5. A long-axis view from a term infant who failed the oxygen saturation screen and was thought to have fetal closure of the ductus arteriosus. Note the hypertrophied right ventricle.

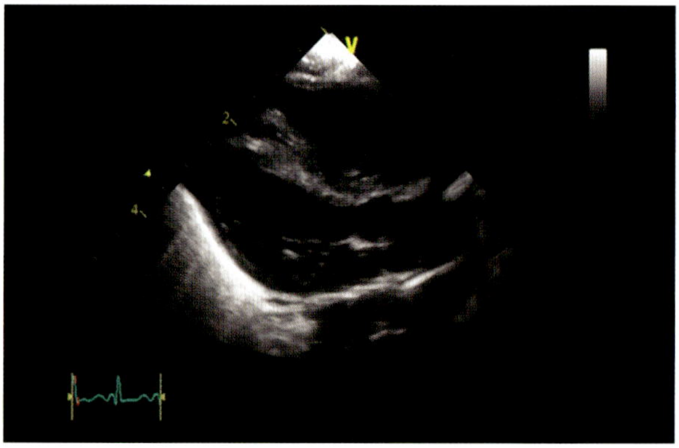

FIGURE and VIDEO 13-6. A long-axis view from an infant with severe oligohydramnios associated with renal anomalies at 3 hours of life.

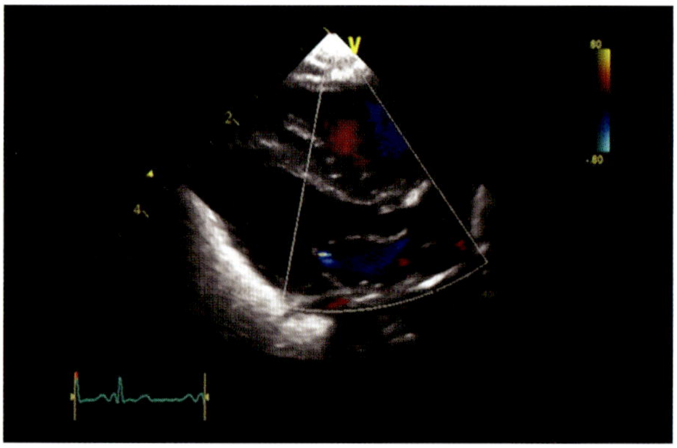

FIGURE and VIDEO 13-7. A color Doppler imaging of the long-axis view of same patient as in Figure and Video 13-6. Note the mitral regurgitation that is present at this time.

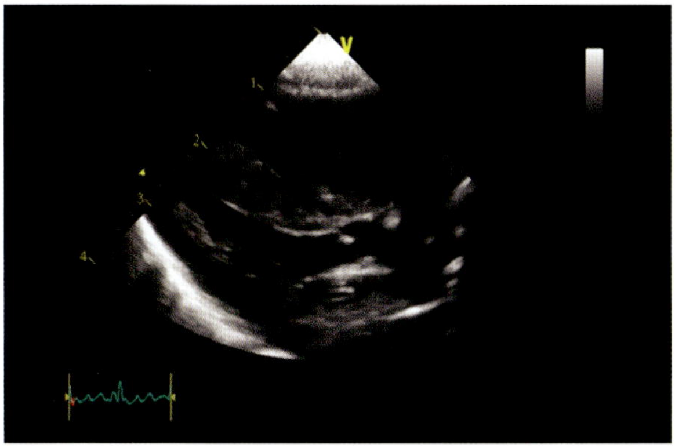

FIGURE and VIDEO 13-8. A long-axis view from the same patient as in Figures and Videos 13-6 and 13-7 at 13 hours of life at a time when the infant developed higher oxygen requirements and increasing acidosis. Note the visibly poor function in this clip with the infant on high-frequency ventilation.

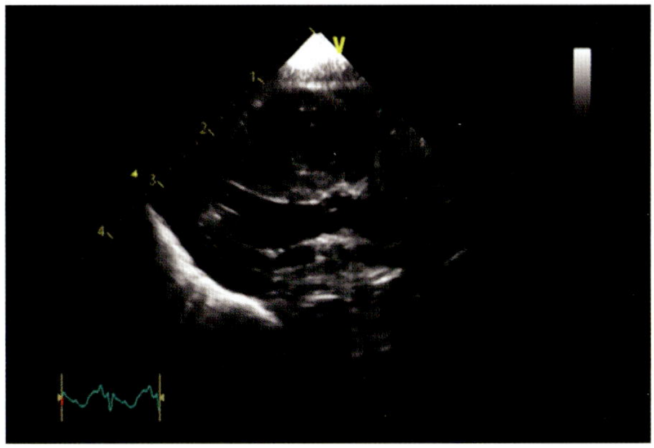

FIGURE and VIDEO 13-10. A long-axis view from the same patient as in Figures and Videos 13-6 to 13-9 after 7 hours and on an epinephrine drip.

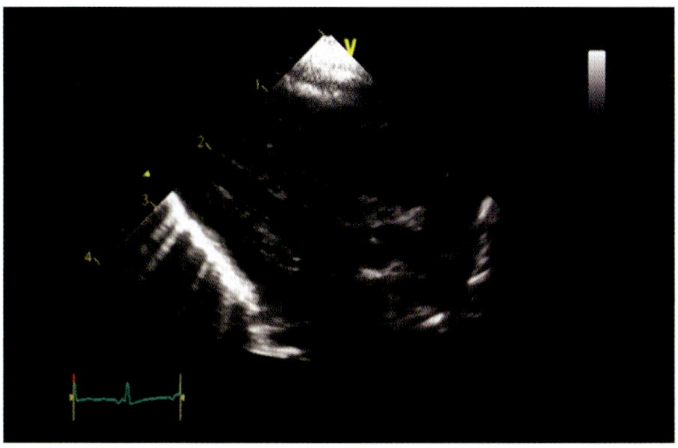

FIGURE and VIDEO 13-9. A long-axis view from the same patient as in Figures 12-6 to 12-8, now on a brief trial of conventional mechanical ventilation.

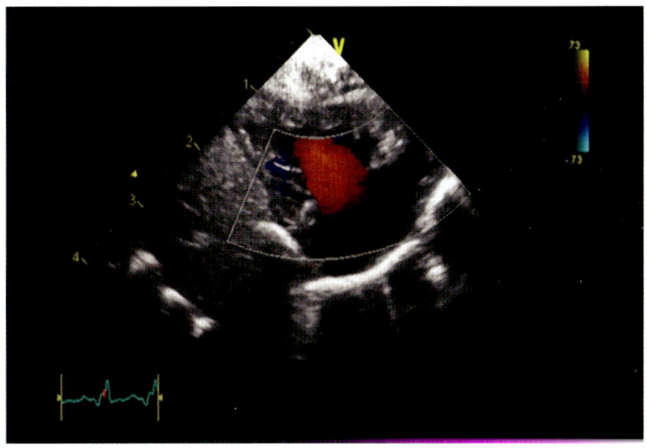

FIGURE and VIDEO 13-11. A right ventricular inflow view using color Doppler of a 30-week preterm infant with mild respiratory distress syndrome at 4 hours of age.

shows the color Doppler imaging from this view in the same infant. Note the mitral regurgitation that is present at this time. In Figure and Video 13-8 we see the long-axis view from this infant at 13 hours of life at a time when the infant developed higher oxygen requirements and increasing acidosis. Note the visibly poor function in this clip with the infant on HFOV. Figure and Video 13-9 shows this infant on a brief trial of conventional mechanical ventilation. Finally, in Figure and Video 13-10 we see imaging from the same infant after 7 hours on a continuous epinephrine infusion. This series of clips demonstrates a range of findings that can be observed in this single view even in an individual infant followed over time as the disease progresses.

Right Ventricular Inflow View

With color Doppler, TR can be identified and with CW Doppler the velocity of the TR jet can be measured. With the modified Bernoulli equation, the pressure difference between the right ventricle and right atrium can be calculated and the pulmonary artery pressure can be estimated (see Chapter 12). Figure and Video 13-11 shows the right ventricular inflow view using color Doppler of a 30-week preterm

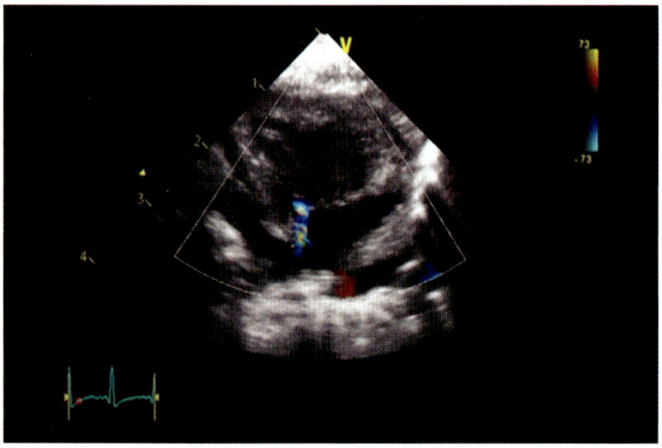

FIGURE and VIDEO 13-12. A right ventricular inflow view from an infant with prolonged premature rupture of membrane at 2 hours of life. Note the tricuspid regurgitation.

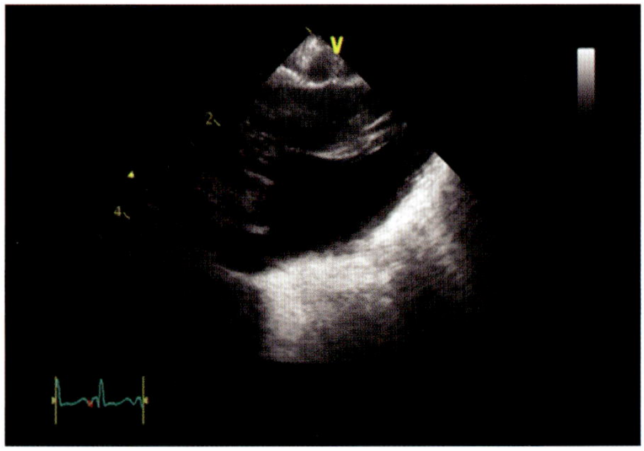

FIGURE and VIDEO 13-14. A 2D imaging of the right ventricular inflow view in an infant with severe oligohydramnios.

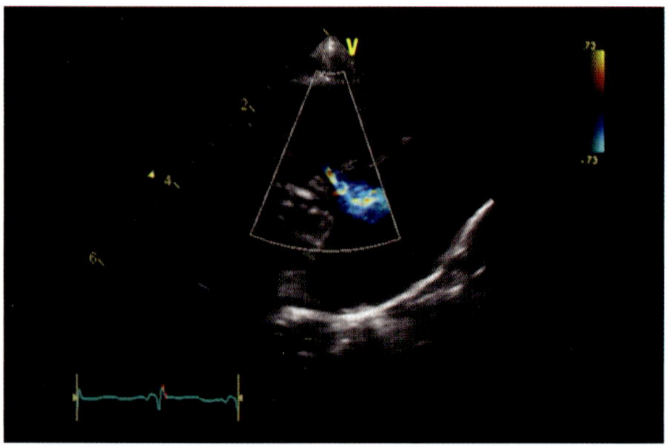

FIGURE and VIDEO 13-13. A right ventricular inflow view from an infant with fetal closure of the ductus arteriosus. Note the tricuspid regurgitation.

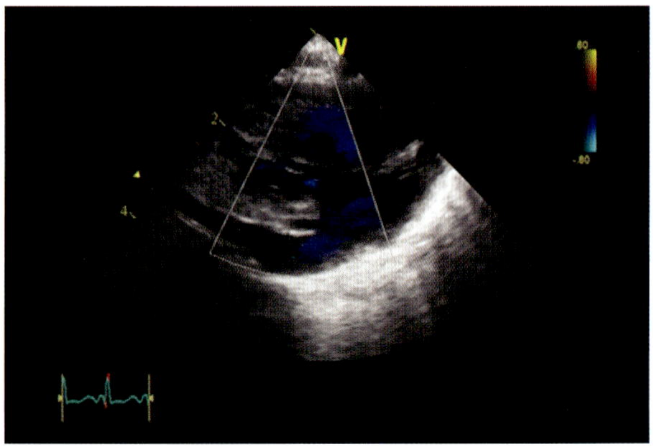

FIGURE and VIDEO 13-15. A color Doppler imaging of the right ventricular inflow view in an infant with severe oligohydramnios.

infant with mild RDS at 4 hours of age. Figure and Video 13-12 shows the right ventricular inflow view from an infant with PPROM at 2 hours of life. Figure and Video 13-13 shows this view from an infant with fetal closure of the ductus arteriosus. Note the tricuspid regurgitation (TR) in Figures and Videos 13-12 and 13-13. Figures and Videos 13-14 and 13-15 show the two-dimensional (2D) and color Doppler imaging of the right ventricular inflow view in an infant with severe oligohydramnios. Figure 13-16 shows the CW Doppler trace from an infant with significant TR.

Right Ventricular Outflow View

When the pulmonary valve is visualized, the leaflets should be seen opening and closing. With color Doppler the blood flow out of the right ventricle can be evaluated. Normal flow should be laminar, and this is seen as a uniform color hue. Turbulent flow suggests a physical obstruction to flow. A hypertrophic ventricle can lead to ventricular outflow tract obstruction leading to turbulent flow with increased velocity seen distal to the obstruction. A pulsed wave (PW) Doppler tracing is obtained with the range gate placed just distal to the pulmonary

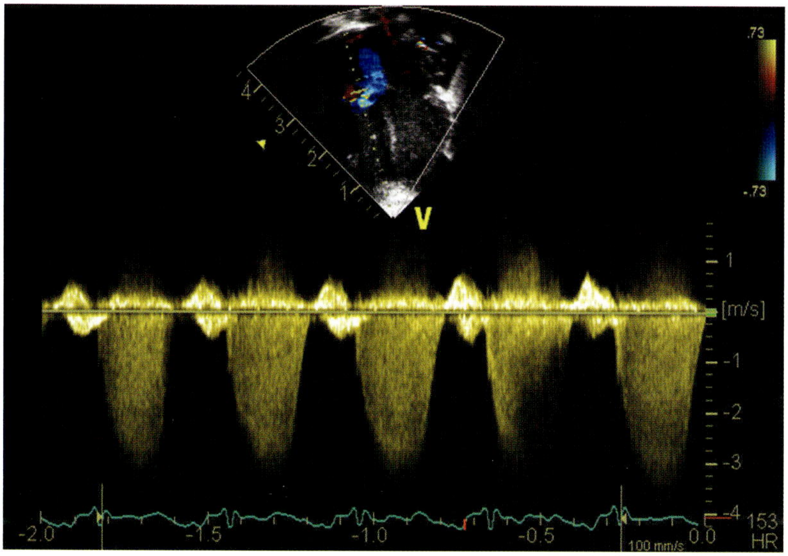

FIGURE 13-16. A CW Doppler tracing from an infant with significant tricuspid regurgitation.

valve. The shape of the waveform can give an indication of the presence of pulmonary hypertension with a rapid acceleration limb and notching on the deceleration limb. The RPEP:RVET and time to peak velocity (TPV) to RVET ratio (TPV:RVET) can be measured as previously described (Chapter 12), and if abnormal, these measures give an indication of the presence of increased afterload. If a PDA with left-to-right shunting is present, the color Doppler signal from the PDA can be seen coming into the main pulmonary artery and can cause a signal of continuous systolic/diastolic flow into the main and branch pulmonary arteries by PW and continuous-wave (CW) Doppler.[31] The right ventricular output will be measured in this view using the diameter of the pulmonary valve and the velocity time integral and heart rate from the PW Doppler tracing.

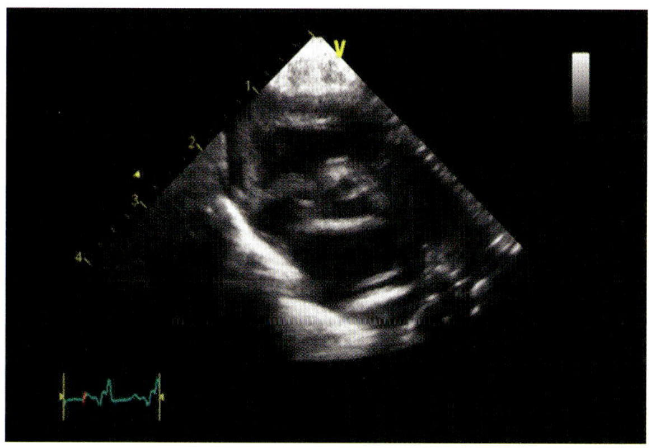

FIGURE and VIDEO 13-17. A right ventricular outflow view from a 30-week preterm infant with mild respiratory distress syndrome at 4 hours of life.

Figure and Video 13-17 shows the right ventricular outflow view from a 30-week preterm infant with mild RDS at 4 hours of life. Figure 13-18 show the PW Doppler trace in the main pulmonary artery in this infant. The diastolic flow reflects PDA left-to-right shunting into the pulmonary artery. Figure and Video 13-19 shows the right ventricular outflow view from the recipient infant of TTTS. Note the more hypertrophied appearance of the RV. Figure and Video 13-20 shows the pulmonary artery from an infant with PPROM. Figures and Videos 13-21 and 13-22 show the 2D and color flow Doppler imaging of the right ventricular outflow from an infant with fetal closure of the ductus arteriosus. Figure 13-23 shows the PW Doppler in the main pulmonary artery of this infant demonstrating a notching pattern with a rapid acceleration limb of the tracing, signifying elevated pulmonary

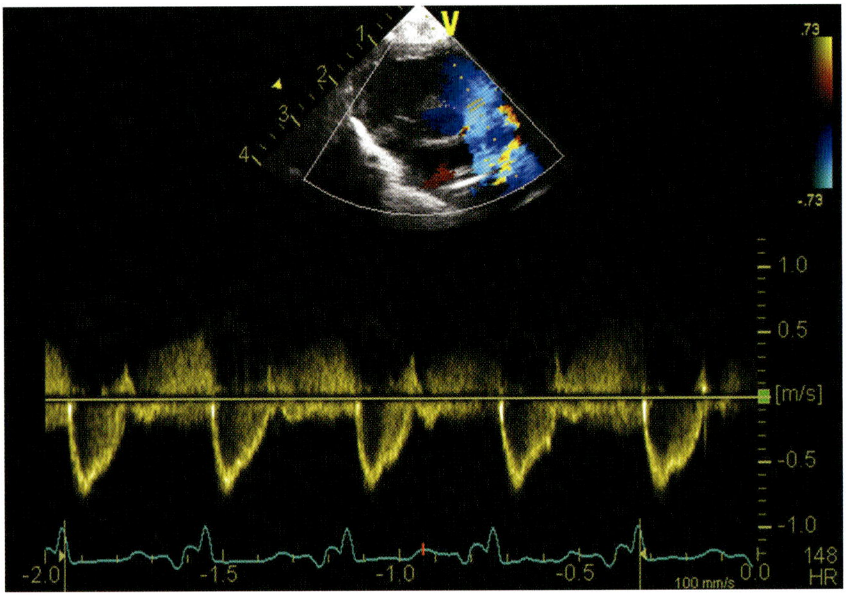

FIGURE 13-18. A PW Doppler tracing in the main pulmonary artery in the same patient as in Figure and Video 13-17. The diastolic flow reflects PDA left-to-right shunting into the pulmonary artery.

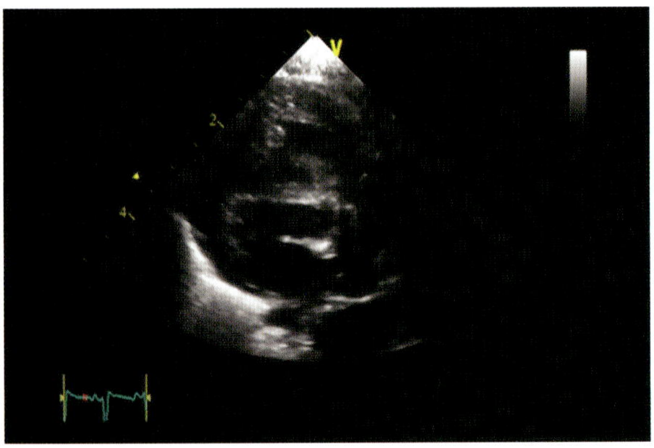

FIGURE and VIDEO 13-19. A right ventricular outflow view from the recipient infant of twin-to-twin transfusion. Note the more hypertrophied appearance of the right ventricle.

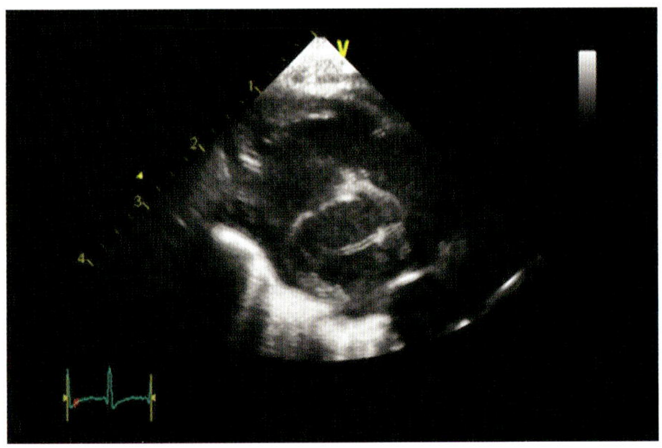

FIGURE and VIDEO 13-20. A right ventricular outflow view from an infant with prolonged premature rupture of membrane showing pulmonary artery.

artery pressure (pulmonary hypertension). Figures and Videos 13-24 and 13-25 show the 2D and color flow Doppler imaging from an infant with severe oligohydramnios at 3 hours of life. Compare these with Figure and Video 13-26 taken from this infant at 13 hours of life and Figure and Video 13-27 once the infant had been treated with a continuous epinephrine infusion. Figures 13-28 and 13-29 show the PW Doppler tracing from this infant at 13 hours of life when the function was at its worst, and at 20 hours after treatment with epinephrine.

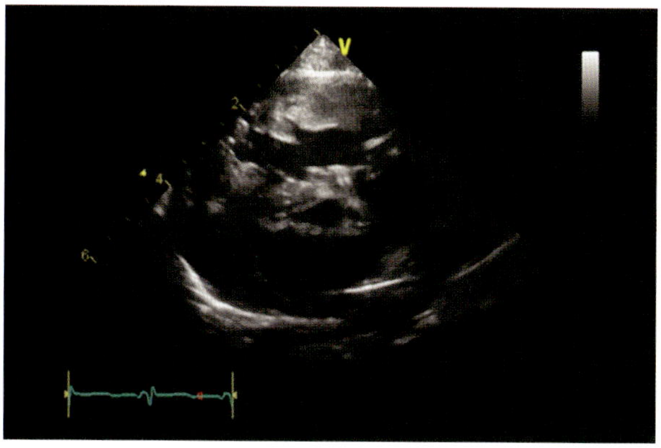

FIGURE and VIDEO 13-21. A 2D imaging of the right ventricular outflow from an infant with fetal closure of the ductus arteriosus.

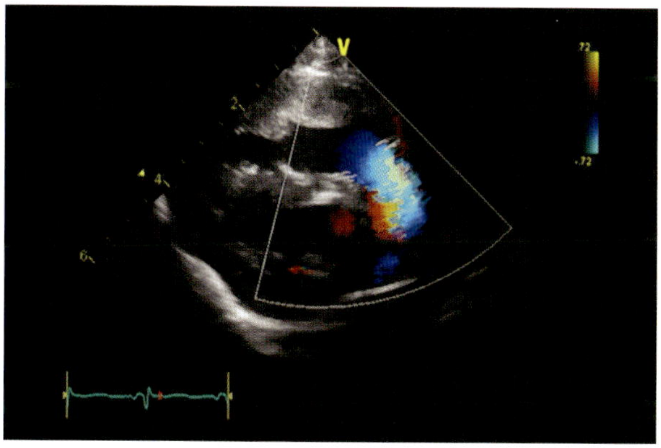

FIGURE and VIDEO 13-22. A color Doppler imaging of the right ventricular outflow from an infant with fetal closure of the ductus arteriosus.

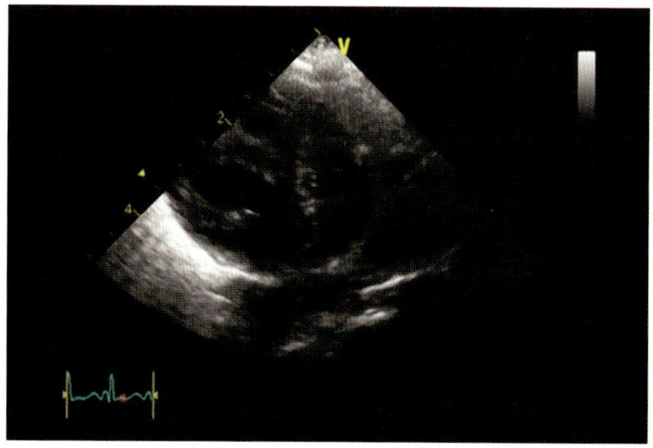

FIGURE and VIDEO 13-24. A 2D imaging of right ventricular outflow from an infant with severe oligohydramnios at 3 hours of life.

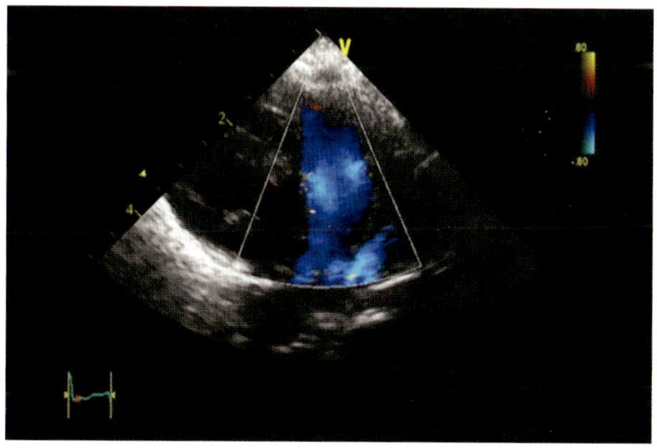

FIGURE and VIDEO 13-25. A color Doppler imaging of right ventricular outflow from an infant with severe oligohydramnios at 3 hours of life.

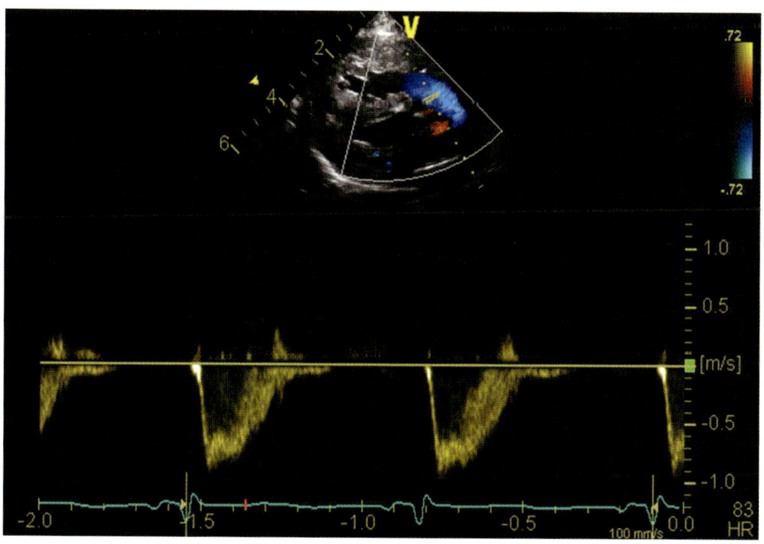

FIGURE 13-23. A PW Doppler tracing of the main pulmonary artery of the patient in Figure and Video 13-22 demonstrating a notching pattern with a rapid acceleration limb of the tracing, signifying elevated pulmonary artery pressure (pulmonary hypertension).

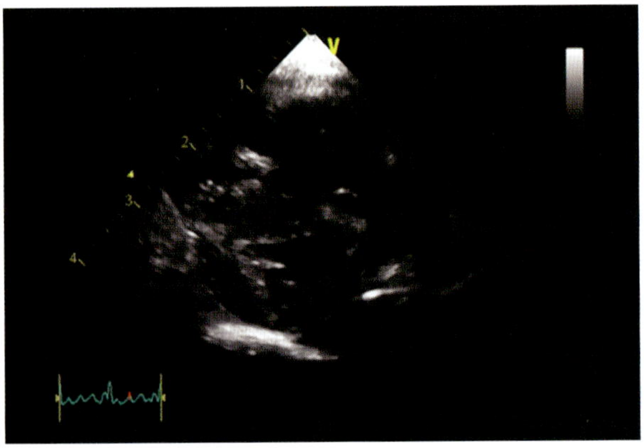

FIGURE and VIDEO 13-26. A 2D imaging of right ventricular outflow of the same patient as in Figures and Videos 13-24 and 13-25 taken at 13 hours of life.

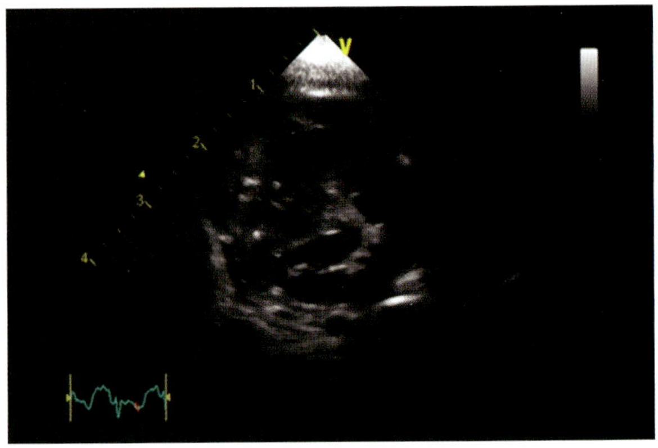

FIGURE and VIDEO 13-27. A color Doppler imaging of right ventricular outflow of the same patient as in Figures and Videos 13-24 to 13-26 once the infant had been treated with continuous epinephrine infusion.

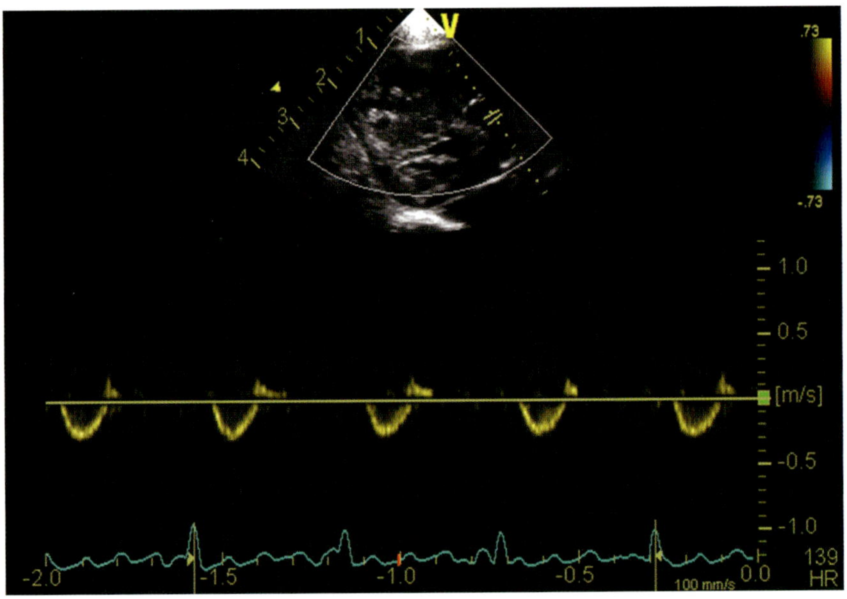

FIGURE 13-28. A PW Doppler tracing of pulmonary artery of same patient as in Figures and Videos 13-24 to 13-27 at 13 hours of life when the cardiac function was at its worst.

Parasternal Short-Axis Views

Base of Heart View

In this view the aortic valve is visualized in cross section with the three leaflets seen clearly. The relative size of the left atrium and aortic valve can also be evaluated from this view. In this view, TR can also be seen.

Figure and Video 13-30 shows the short-axis base of heart view from a 30-week preterm infant with mild RDS making a healthy transition. Figure and Video 13-31 shows this view from an infant with PPROM. It is possible to see the umbilical venous catheter in the left atrium in this image, a finding that would prompt repositioning of the catheter. Figures and Videos 13-32

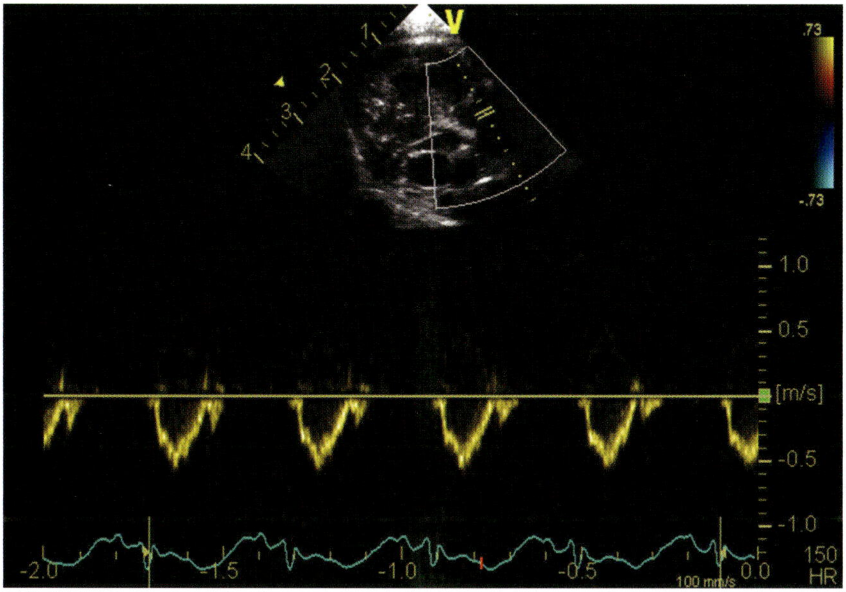

FIGURE 13-29. A PW Doppler tracing of pulmonary artery of same patient as in Figures and Videos 13-24 to 13-28 at 20 hours of life after treatment with epinephrine.

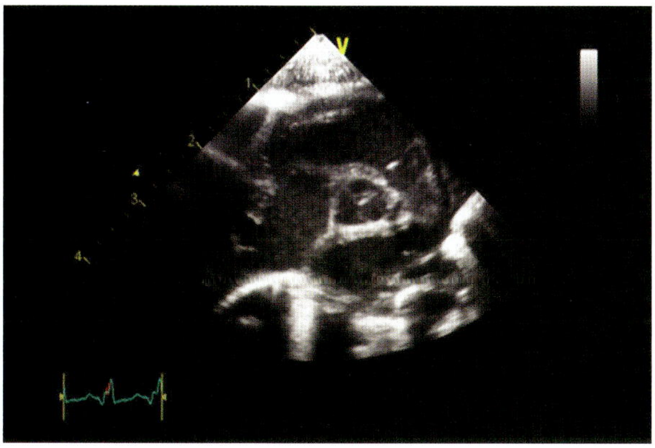

FIGURE and VIDEO 13-30. A short-axis base of heart view from a 30-week preterm infant with mild respiratory distress syndrome making a healthy transition.

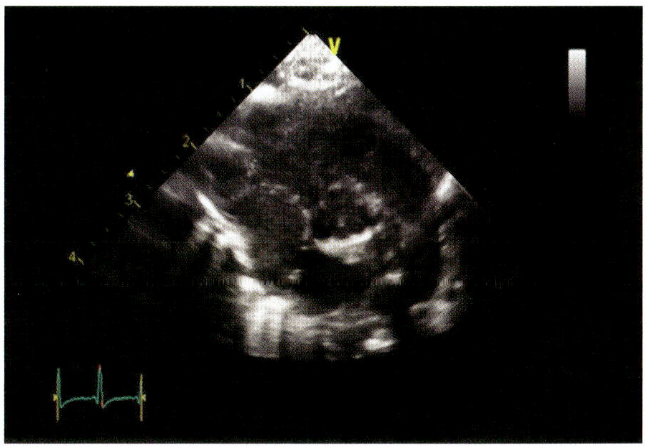

FIGURE and VIDEO 13-31. A short-axis base of heart view from an infant with prolonged premature rupture of membrane. It is possible to see the umbilical venous catheter in the left atrium in this image.

and 13-33 show this view from an infant with severe oligohydramnios at 3 and 13 hours of life. With increasing severity of PPHN, the left atrium often appears smaller in these images, reflecting the decreased pulmonary blood flow.

Mitral Level View

In this view the mitral valve is evaluated in cross section, creating the "fish mouth" appearance. This view is important for evaluating the ventricular shape. In the normal post-transitional heart, the left ventricle in cross section

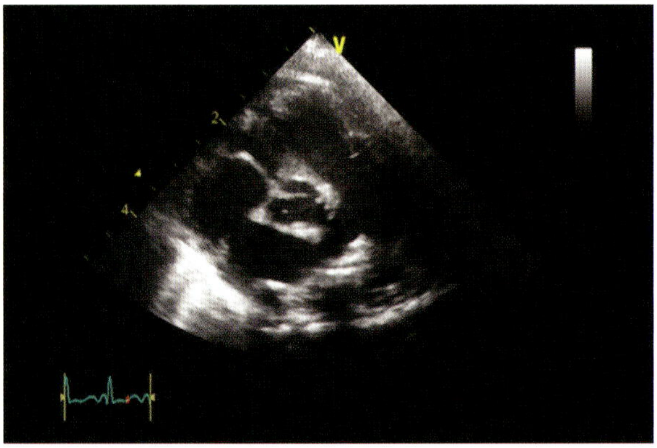

FIGURE and VIDEO 13-32. A short-axis base of heart view from an infant with severe oligohydramnios at 3 hours of life.

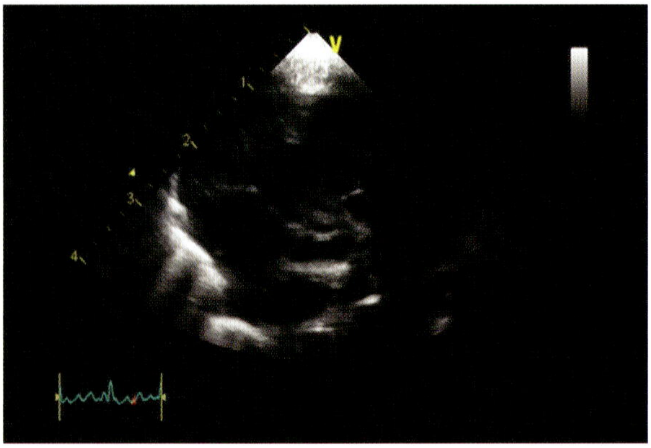

FIGURE and VIDEO 13-33. A short-axis base of heart view from the same patient as in Figure and Video 13-32 at 13 hours of life. With increasing severity of PPHN the left atrium often appears smaller in these images reflecting the decreased pulmonary blood flow.

should have the shape of a circle. However, immediately after birth or with PPHN, the right ventricle will have elevated pressure, causing the interventricular septum to appear flattened (see below). In more severe PPHN, the right ventricle will bulge into the left ventricle. If the myocardium is not functioning well, it might be possible to visualize asymmetric ventricular wall motion.

Figure and Video 13-34 shows the normal short-axis mitral level view demonstrating the LV appearing as a circle. The next few clips all show a degree of right ventricular prominence distorting the shape of the left ventricle. Figure and Video 13-35 shows the short-axis mitral valve view from the recipient infant of TTTS. Figure and Video 13-36 shows this view from an infant with PPROM.

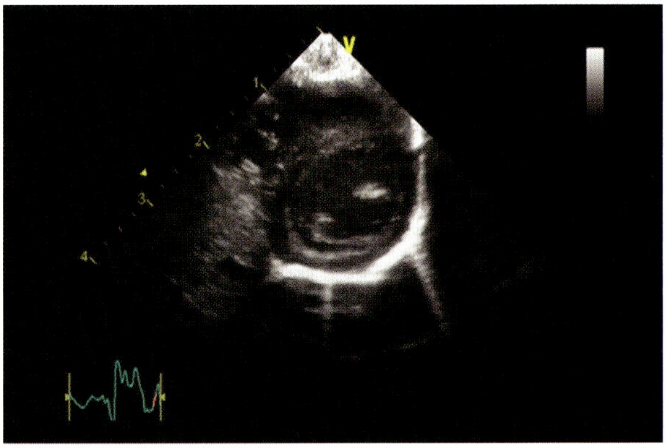

FIGURE and VIDEO 13-34. A normal short-axis mitral-level view demonstrating the left ventricle appearing as a circle.

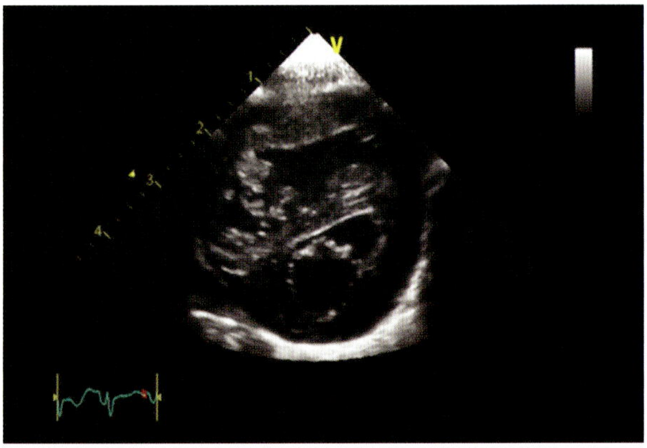

FIGURE and VIDEO 13-35. A short-axis mitral valve view from the recipient infant of twin-to-twin-transfusion. Note the right ventricular prominence distorting the shape of the left ventricle.

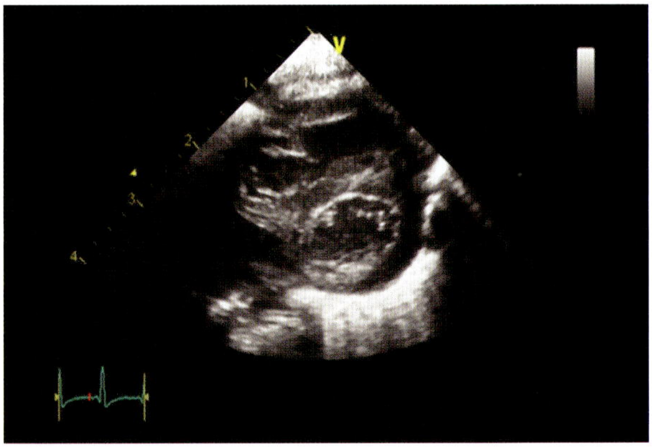

FIGURE and VIDEO 13-36. A short-axis mitral valve view from an infant with prolonged premature rupture of membrane. Note the right ventricular prominence distorting the shape of the left ventricle.

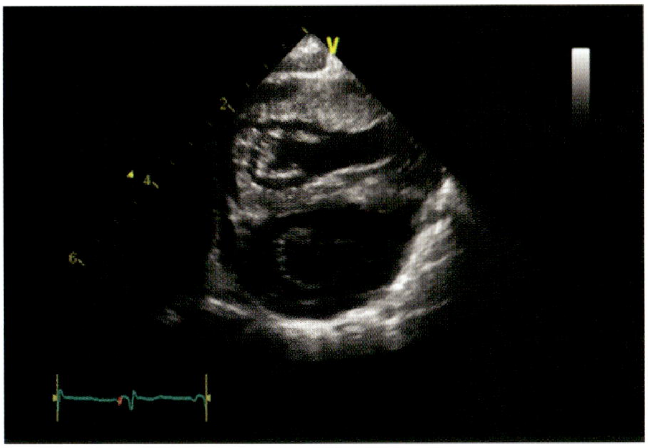

FIGURE and VIDEO 13-37. A short-axis mitral valve view from an infant with fetal closure of the ductus arteriosus. Note the right ventricular prominence distorting the shape of the left ventricle.

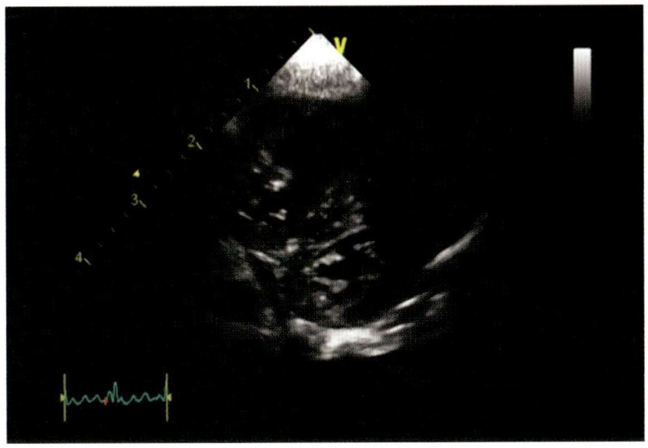

FIGURE and VIDEO 13-39. A short-axis mitral valve view from the same patient as in Figure and Video 13-37 at 13 hours of life. Note the dramatic difference in the appearance of contractile function at these 2 time points.

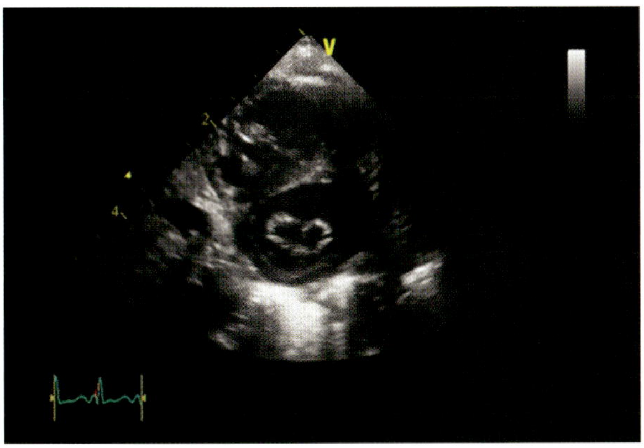

FIGURE and VIDEO 13-38. A short-axis mitral valve view from an infant with severe oligohydramnios at 3 hours of life. Note the right ventricular prominence distorting the shape of the left ventricle.

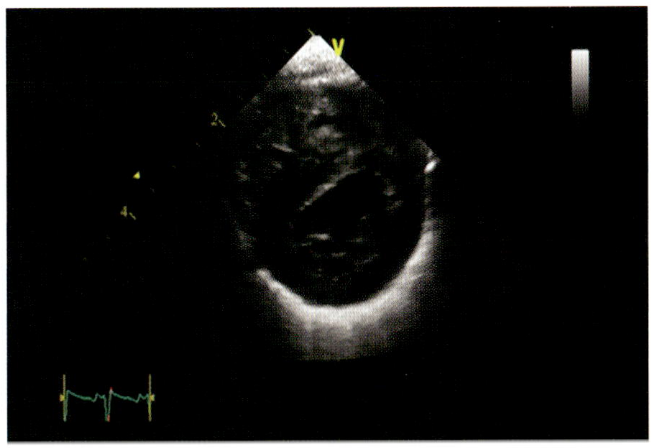

FIGURE and VIDEO 13-40. A papillary muscle view in the recipient infant of twin-to-twin-transfusion.

Figure and Video 13-37 is taken from an infant with fetal closure of the ductus arteriosus. Figures and Videos 13-38 and 13-39 show this view from an infant with severe oligohydramnios at 3 and 13 hours of life. Note the dramatic difference in the appearance of contractile function at these two time points.

Papillary Muscle View

These allow the clinician to continue evaluating the shape of the ventricle and movement of the ventricles. All of the short-axis views are important in the screening for congenital heart disease because ventricular septal defects can be identified by a sweep of the ventricular septum.

Figure and Video 13-40 shows the papillary muscle view in the recipient infant of TTTS. Figure and Video 13-41 shows the papillary muscle view in an infant with PPROM. Figure and Video 13-42 shows the papillary muscle view from an infant with severe oligohydramnios at 3 hours of life.

Apical Window

Four-Chamber View

From this view, the relative sizes of each chamber of the heart can be evaluated to determine whether there is symmetry, or if one side of the heart is more prominent. The atrioventricular valves can be evaluated using color flow

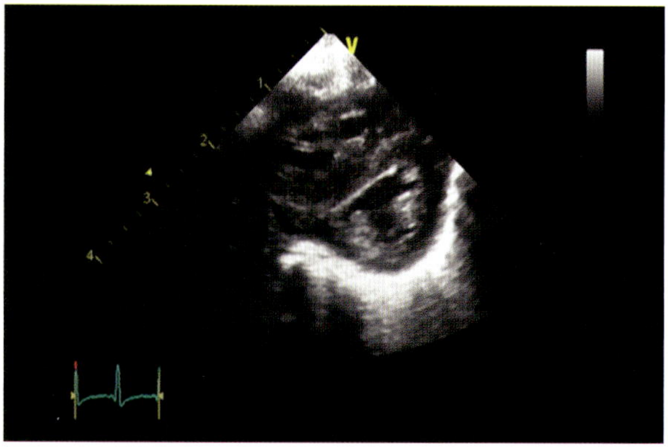

FIGURE and VIDEO 13-41. A papillary muscle view in an infant with prolonged premature rupture of membrane.

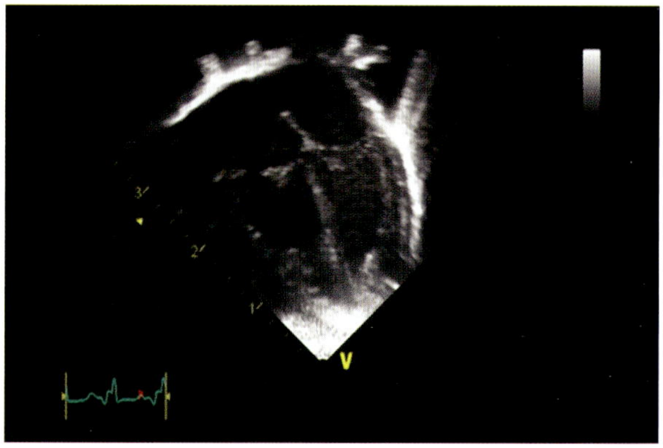

FIGURE and VIDEO 13-43. An apical four-chamber view from a 30-week preterm infant with mild respiratory distress syndrome.

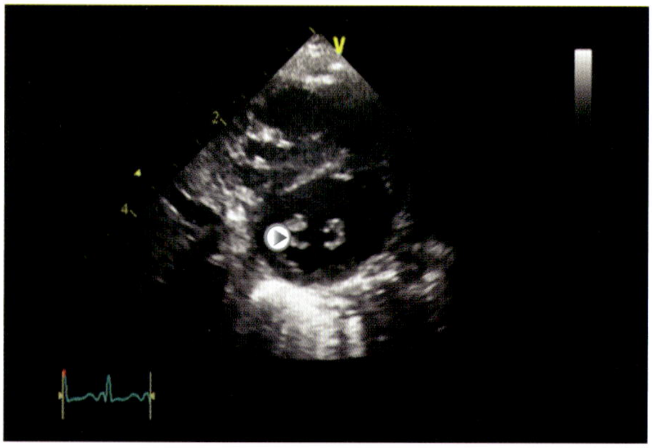

FIGURE and VIDEO 13-42. A papillary muscle view from an infant with severe oligohydramnios at 3 hours of life.

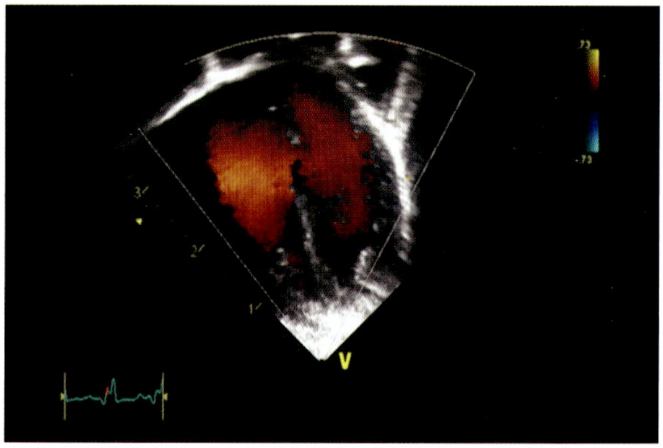

FIGURE and VIDEO 13-44. A color Doppler imaging of apical four-chamber view from a 30-week preterm infant with mild respiratory distress syndrome.

and spectral (CW/PW) Doppler. With color flow Doppler any valve insufficiency can be identified. The CW Doppler of the TR jet is often best measured in this view, as the angle of insonation is generally optimal from this view, though this can be variable depending upon the direction of the jet. Mitral insufficiency can also be identified in this view. When both valves are insufficient, the clinician must consider myocardial dysfunction. It should also be remembered that valvar insufficiency can result from a distal obstruction to flow, reinforcing the importance of a careful evaluation of anatomy. PW Doppler evaluation of each of the atrioventricular valves at the inflow into the ventricles gives an indication of the diastolic function of the respective ventricles (see Chapter 8).

Figure and Video 13-43 shows the apical four-chamber view from a 30-week preterm infant with mild RDS. Figure and Video 13-44 shows imaging from the same infant using color Doppler. Figure and Video 13-45 shows the apical four-chamber view from an infant with fetal ductus arteriosus closure. Figure and Video 13-46 shows this view from an infant with severe oligohydramnios at 3 hours of life. Figures 13-47 and 13-48 show the PW Doppler tracings of the tricuspid valve from 30-week preterm infant with mild RDS and from an infant with fetal closure of the ductus arteriosus, respectively. Figure 13-49 shows the PW Doppler trace of the mitral valve from the 30-week preterm infant with mild RDS.

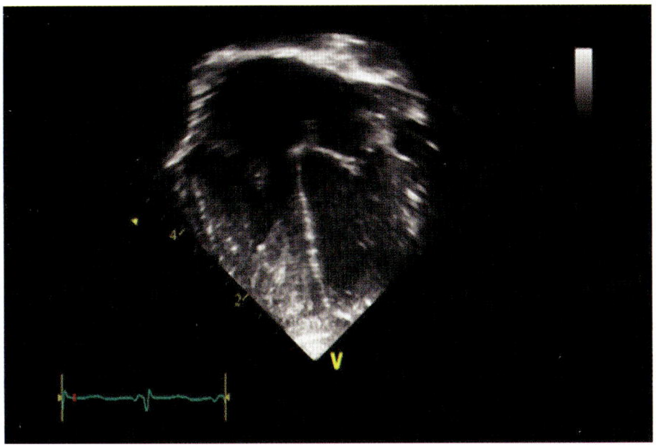

FIGURE and VIDEO 13-45. An apical four-chamber view from an infant with fetal ductus arteriosus closure.

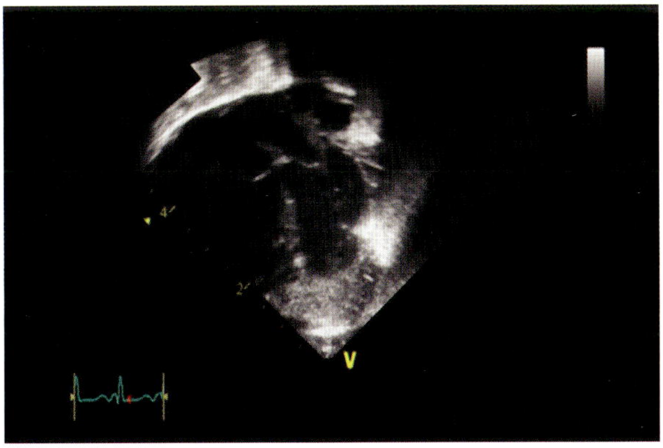

FIGURE and VIDEO 13-46. An apical four-chamber view from an infant with severe oligohydramnios at 3 hours of life.

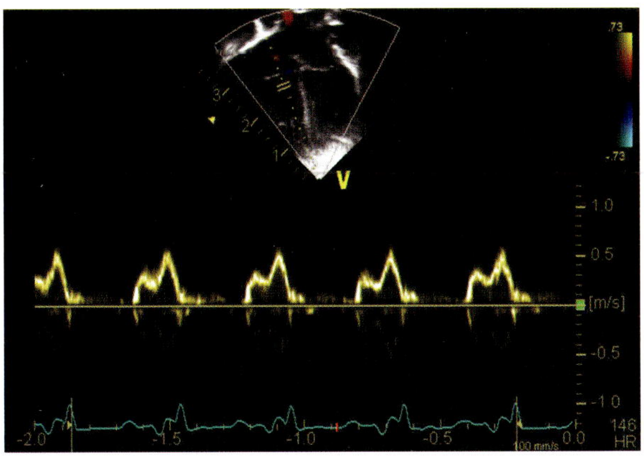

FIGURE 13-47. A PW Doppler tracing of the tricuspid valve from a 30-week preterm infant with mild respiratory distress syndrome.

Five-Chamber View

In this view, the left ventricular outflow tract and aortic valve can be evaluated with color and pulsed wave Doppler. Color flow Doppler will give an indication as to whether there is laminar versus turbulent flow. Turbulent flow would be a sign of outflow tract obstruction, which might be seen in hypertrophic cardiomyopathy with dynamic subaortic narrowing. PW Doppler just past the aortic valve allows for calculation of the left ventricular output.

The five-chamber view is shown in Figure and Video 13-50 with the PW Doppler (Figure 13-51) just distal to the aortic valve. These images are taken from a 1-hour-old term infant who presented with increased work of breathing and desaturation shortly after birth. The patient had no congenital heart defect and the PW Doppler appears normal.

Suprasternal Window

Aortic Arch View

It is important to visualize the entire arch including the initial branching of the head and neck vessels. With color flow Doppler the arch should be evaluated for laminar forward flow. Pulsed wave Doppler of the descending aorta distal to the ductus arteriosus should be performed to evaluate the flow in the distal aorta. Reversal of flow in the descending aorta during diastole suggests that a left-to-right PDA might be hemodynamically significant, potentially causing impaired distal systemic blood flow (see Chapter 11). Increased peak velocity distal to the aortic isthmus suggests a possible coarctation. If this finding is encountered a complete pediatric echocardiogram (interpreted by a pediatric cardiologist) should be obtained. Figure and Video 13-52 shows 2D imaging of the aortic arch.

Ductal Cut View

The PDA can be seen in this view throughout its course from the pulmonary artery to the aorta (see Chapters 3 and 11). The PDA should be evaluated using 2D imaging and color flow Doppler. The direction of flow can be evaluated with both color flow and spectral (PW/CW) Doppler. The direction of flow gives an indication of the relative pressure differences between the pulmonary and systemic circulations. The color flow Doppler images should be evaluated carefully because pure right-to-left flow can be confused with aortic blood flow if one does not carefully identify each vessel. Similarly, bidirectional flow can be mistaken as pure left-to-right flow because

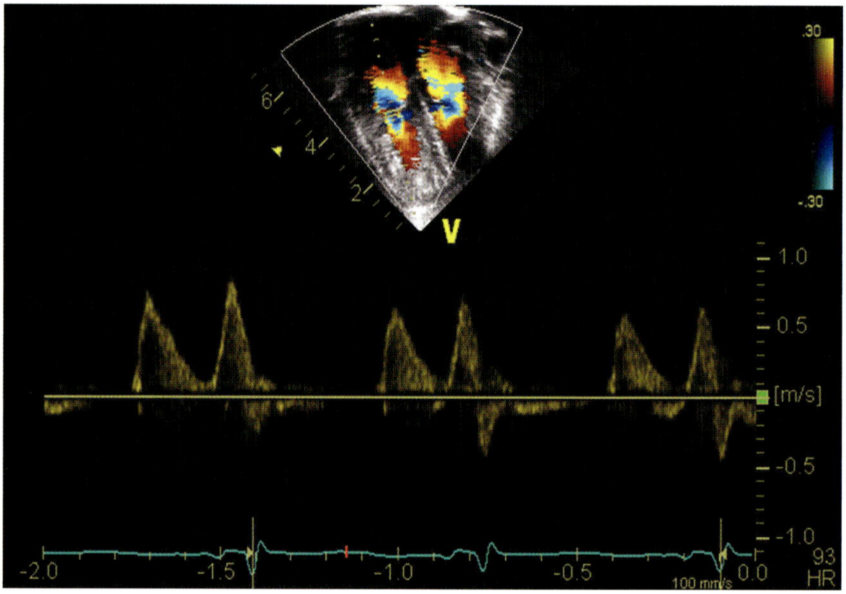

FIGURE 13-48. A PW Doppler tracing of the tricuspid valve from an infant with fetal closure of the ductus arteriosus.

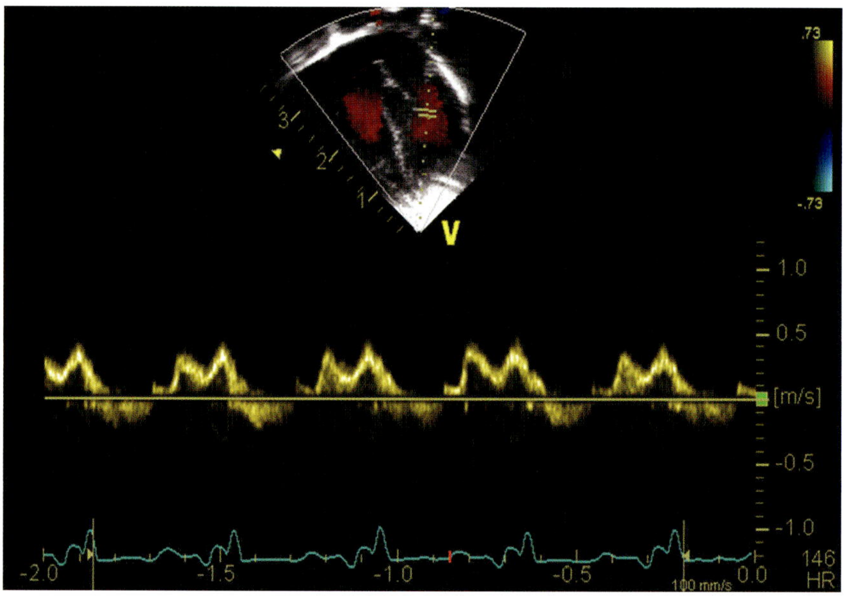

FIGURE 13-49. A PW Doppler tracing of the mitral valve from a 30-week preterm infant with mild respiratory distress syndrome.

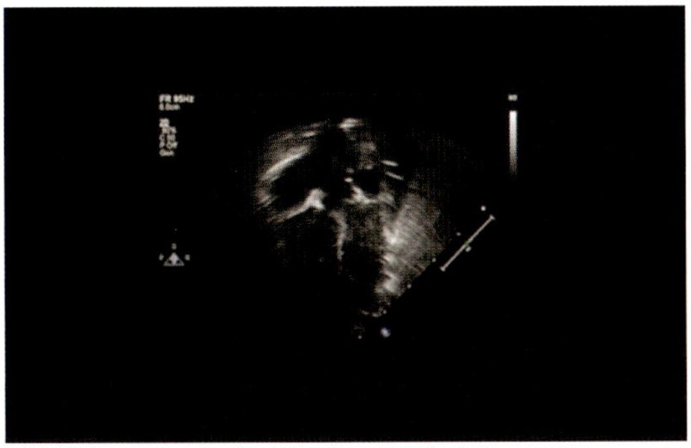

FIGURE and VIDEO 13-50. A five-chamber view from a 1-hour old term infant who presented with increased work of breathing and desaturation shortly after birth. The patient had no congenital heart defect.

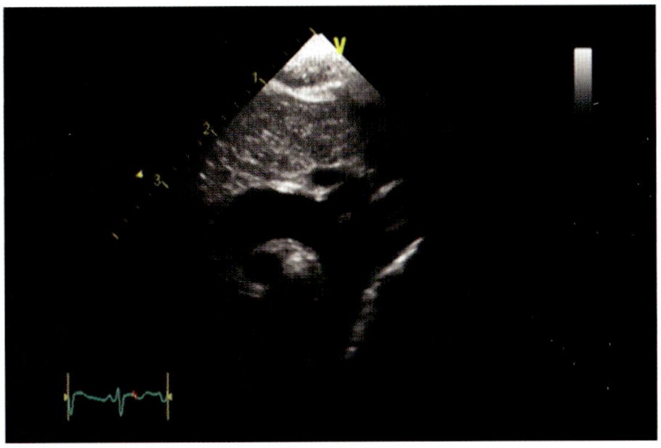

FIGURE and VIDEO 13-52. A 2D imaging of the aortic arch.

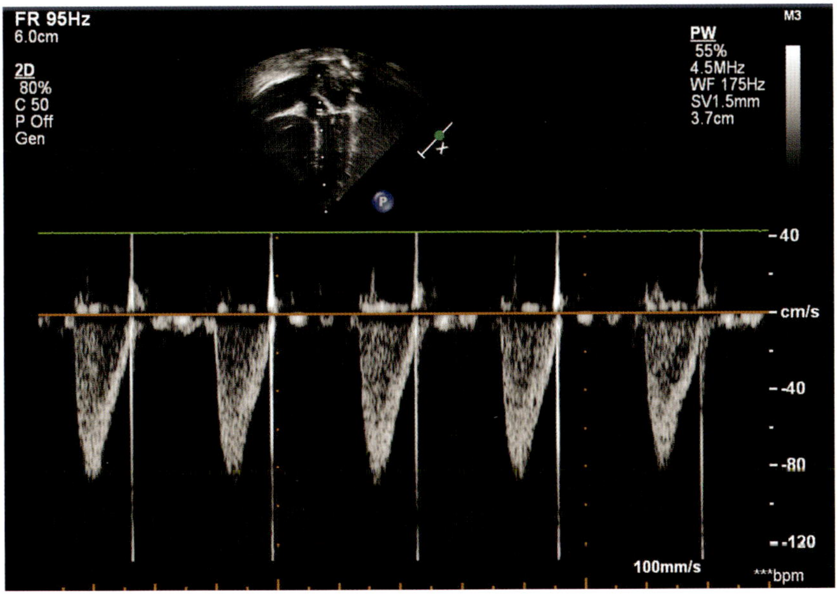

FIGURE 13-51. A PW Doppler tracing at aortic valve obtained from a five-chamber view of a 1-hour-old term infant who presented with increased work of breathing and desaturation shortly after birth. The patient had no congenital heart defect and the PW Doppler appears normal.

the blue (right-to-left) component moves so quickly through the cycle. Within the first 12 hours of life, the proportion of right-to-left flow that is greater than 30% of the entire cycle suggests elevated pulmonary pressure. The presence of bidirectional or pure right-to-left flow through the PDA should alert the clinician to the possibility of ductal-dependent systemic circulation from some type of left-sided obstructive congenital cardiac defect. A careful examination for a critical coarctation or some other form of left-sided obstructive congenital cardiac defect is essential before pharmacologic closure of the PDA is considered. A complete pediatric echocardiogram should be performed and interpreted by a pediatric cardiologist.

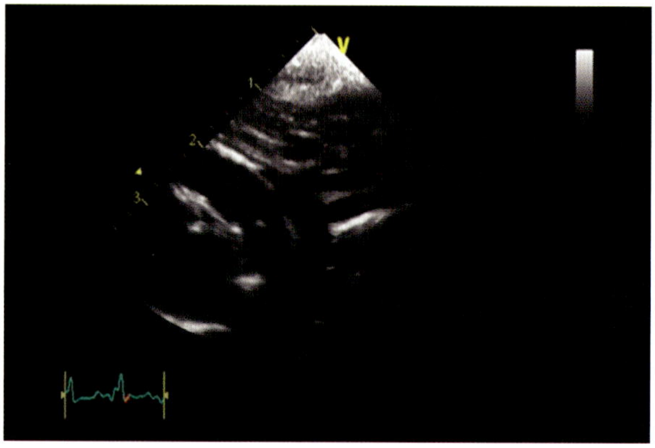

FIGURE and VIDEO 13-53. A ductal cut view using 2D imaging from a 30-week preterm infant with mild respiratory distress syndrome at 4 hours of life.

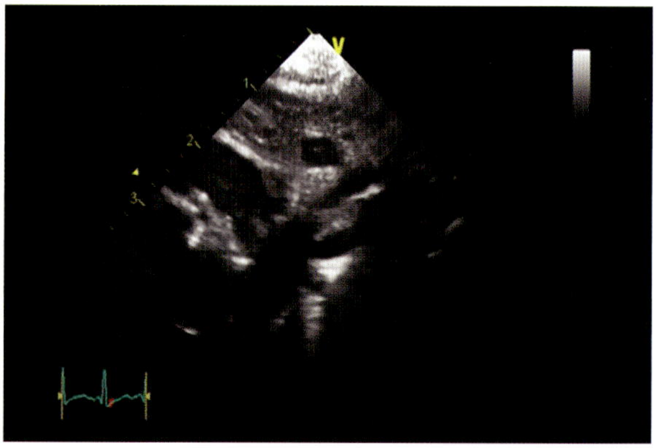

FIGURE and VIDEO 13-55. A ductal cut view using 2D imaging from an infant with prolonged premature rupture of membrane.

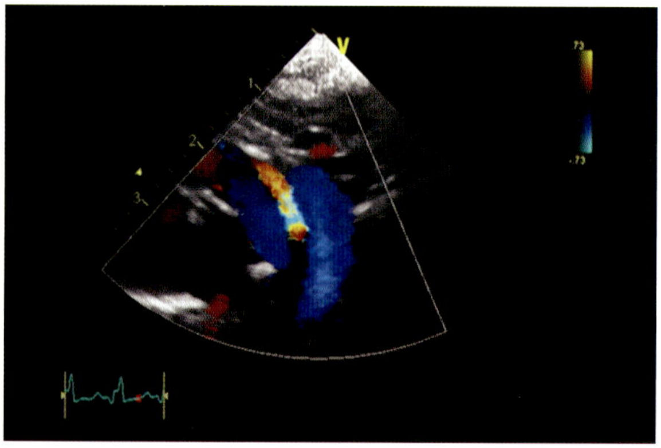

FIGURE and VIDEO 13-54. A ductal cut view using color flow Doppler from a 30-week preterm infant with mild respiratory distress syndrome at 4 hours of life.

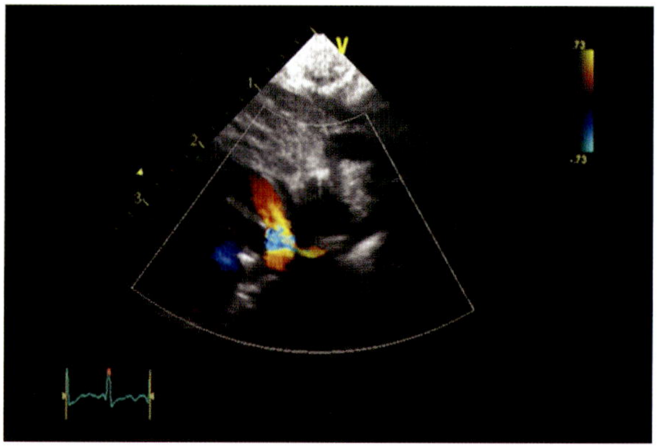

FIGURE and VIDEO 13-56. A ductal cut view using color flow Doppler from an infant with prolonged premature rupture of membrane.

Figures and Videos 13-53 and 13-54 show the ductal cut views using 2D and color flow Doppler from a 30-week preterm infant with mild RDS at 4 hours of life. Figures and Videos 13-55 and 13-56 show the same views from an infant with PROM. The spectral Doppler tracing from this PDA is shown in Figure 13-57. This PDA is bidirectional, but the right-to-left component can be difficult to visualize; cine loop with frame-by-frame evaluation is helpful to visualize the right-to-left component. Figure and Video 13-58 shows the color flow Doppler of the ductal cut view from the recipient infant of TTTS. The PW Doppler trace of this PDA is shown in Figure 13-59. Note that this PDA is large and flow is completely left to right and low velocity. Figure and Video 13-60 shows the color flow Doppler of the PDA from an infant with severe oligohydramnios at 13 hours of life. In this case, the PDA flow is mostly right to left.

Coronal Plane "Crab View"

This view is used to identify the pulmonary veins draining into the left atrium. Certain pulmonary veins can also be identified with other echocardiographic views throughout the echocardiogram. Total anomalous pulmonary venous return (TAPVR) is a congenital cardiac defect that can easily be confused with PPHN. Other signs of TAPVR that should be recognizable to the clinician performing the echocardiogram include a small left atrium and left

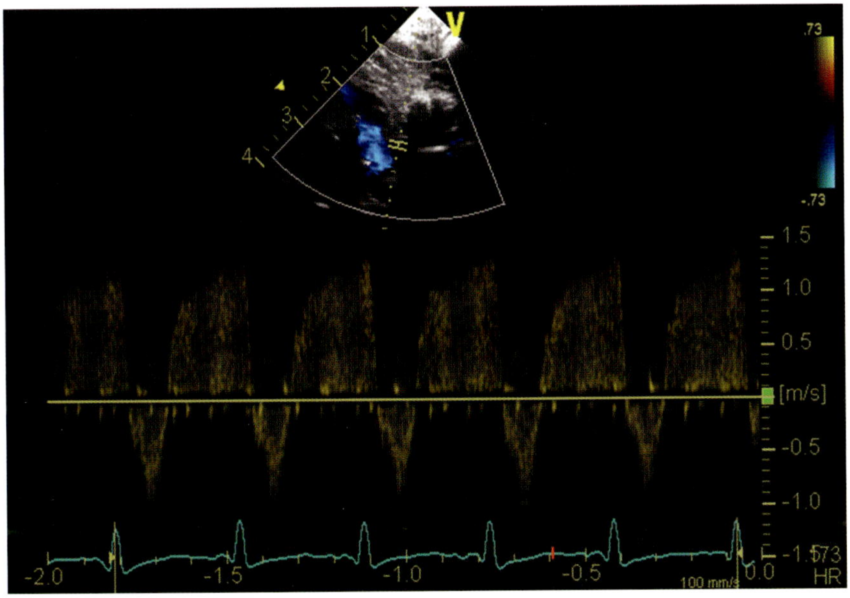

FIGURE 13-57. A spectral Doppler tracing of PDA in the same patient as in Figures and Videos 13-55 and 13-56. The PDA flow is bidirectional but the right-to-left component can be difficult to visualize; cine loop with frame-by-frame evaluation is helpful to visualize the right-to-left component.

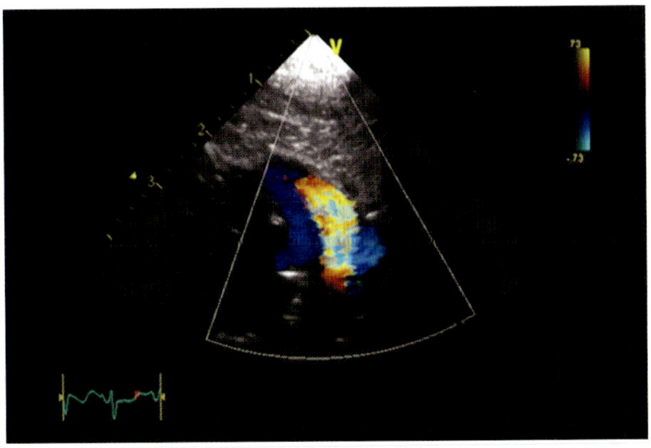

FIGURE and VIDEO 13-58. A color flow Doppler of the ductal cut view from the recipient infant of twin-to-twin-transfusion. Note that this PDA is large, and flow is completely left to right and low velocity.

ventricle, and pure right-to-left shunting through the foramen ovale. If TAPVR is a possibility, a complete pediatric echocardiogram should be obtained and interpreted by a pediatric cardiologist.

Figure and Video 13-61 shows this view using color Doppler to identify the four pulmonary veins.

Coronal Plane Branch Pulmonary Artery View

The PDA can often be identified in this view as well as the prior views. Spectral Doppler (PW/CW) in the left pulmonary artery can be helpful in determining the significance of a PDA or in identifying more severe cases of PPHN. The diameter of each branch pulmonary artery has been evaluated as a marker for predicting outcome in congenital diaphragmatic hernia.

Figure and Video 13 62 shows the branch pulmonary artery from the ductal cut view. Figure 13-63 shows a PW Doppler spectral tracing of the left pulmonary artery, obtained from the ductal cut view. Of note, the Doppler evaluation can be performed from multiple views, as long as the angle of insonation is minimized to ensure an accurate tracing.

Subcostal Window

Inferior Vena Cava and Descending Aorta View

In the initial cross section view, the descending aorta and inferior vena cava are identified relative to the liver and vertebrae, allowing for the identification of problems with abdominal situs (see Chapter 3).

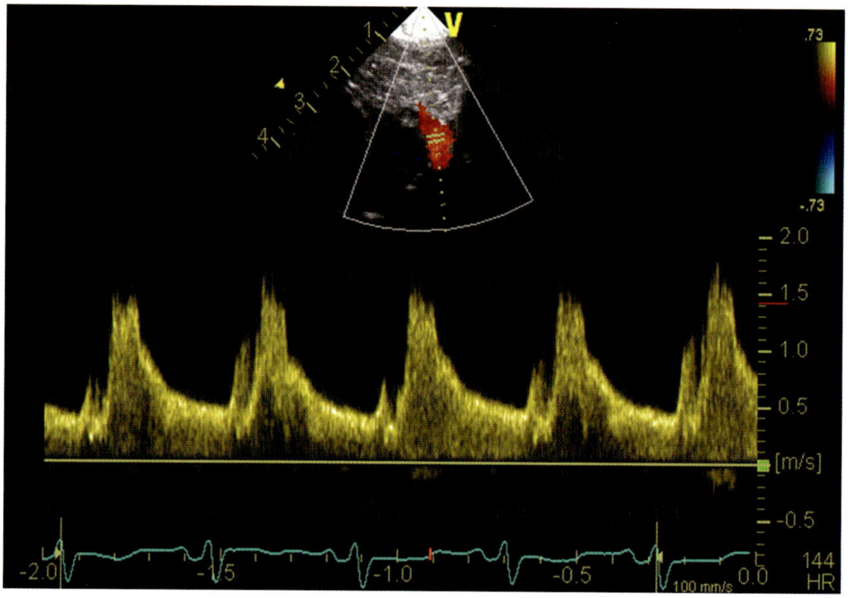

FIGURE 13-59. A PW Doppler tracing of the PDA in same patient as in Figure and Video 13-58. Note that flow is completely left to right and low velocity.

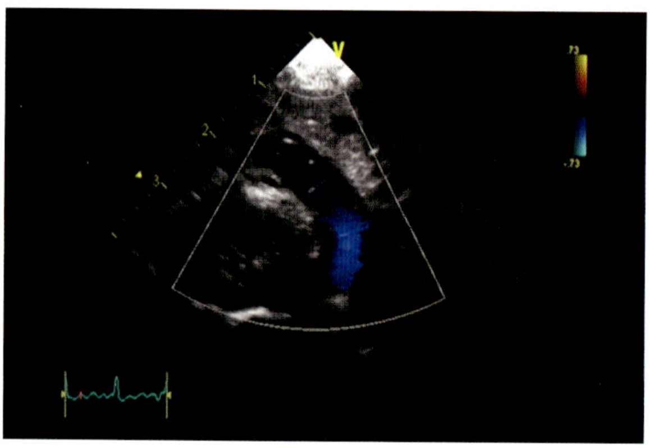

FIGURE and VIDEO 13-60. A color flow Doppler of the PDA from an infant with severe oligohydramnios at 13 hours of life. Note that the PDA flow is mostly right to left.

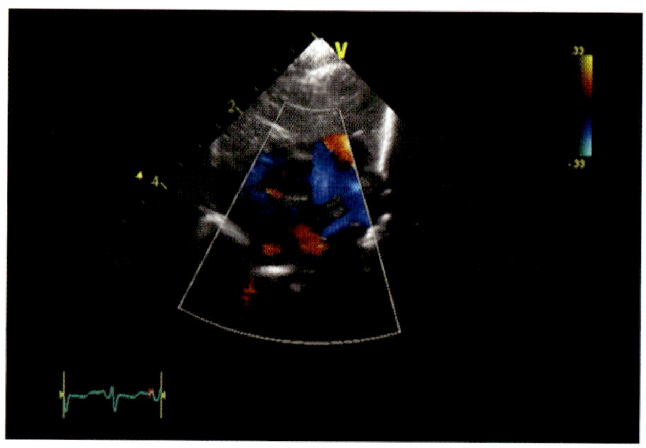

FIGURE and VIDEO 13-61. A coronal plane "crab view" using color Doppler to identify the four pulmonary veins.

Coronal Posterior View

This is the best view to evaluate flow across the atrial septum. The foramen ovale is frequently patent in the newborn period and can have a significant amount of flow across it. Color flow Doppler (with the scale reduced to venous flow settings) can help determine the size of the PFO and the direction of flow. PW Doppler can also help determine the direction of flow and can give an indication of the inter-atrial pressure differences. The direction of flow across the atrial septum is an important component of the evaluation of hypoxemia. In PPHN the shunt is usually bidirectional. A pure right-to-left shunt is a possible sign of congenital heart disease, especially TAPVR. Some preterm infants will have a large left-to-right atrial shunt, which can lead to increased pulmonary blood flow, and eventually might contribute to pulmonary edema.

Figures and Videos 13-64 and 13-65 show the atrial septum using 2D imaging and color flow Doppler from an infant with PPROM. The flow across the PFO is bidirectional.

Coronal Mid-Section and Coronal Anterior Views

From the subcostal window a sweep through the base of the heart can show the major vessels from the superior vena cava to the aorta to the pulmonary artery. These are excellent views for confirming the normal position of the great vessels.

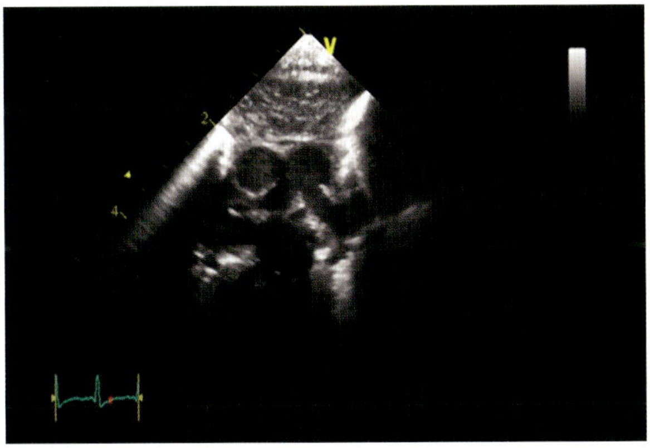

FIGURE and VIDEO 13-62. A 2D imaging of branch pulmonary artery from ductal cut view.

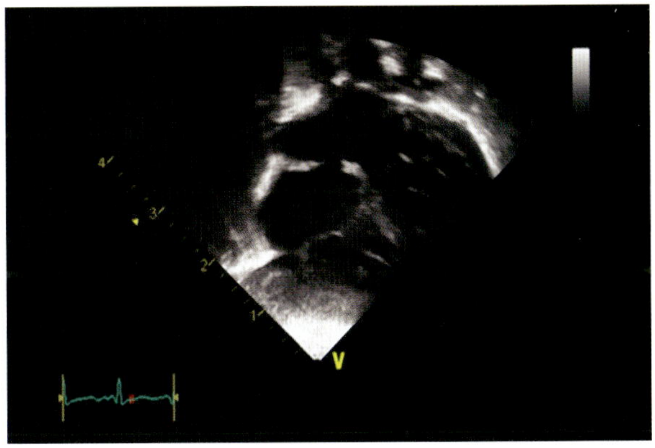

FIGURE and VIDEO 13-64. A 2D imaging of the atrial septum in coronal posterior view from an infant with prolonged premature rupture of membrane.

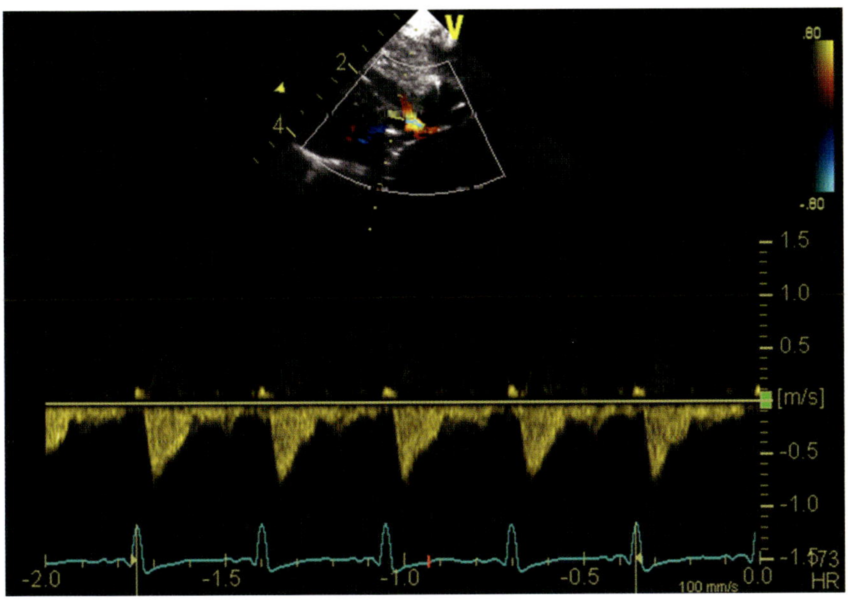

FIGURE 13-63. A PW Doppler spectral tracing of the left pulmonary artery, obtained from the ductal cut view.

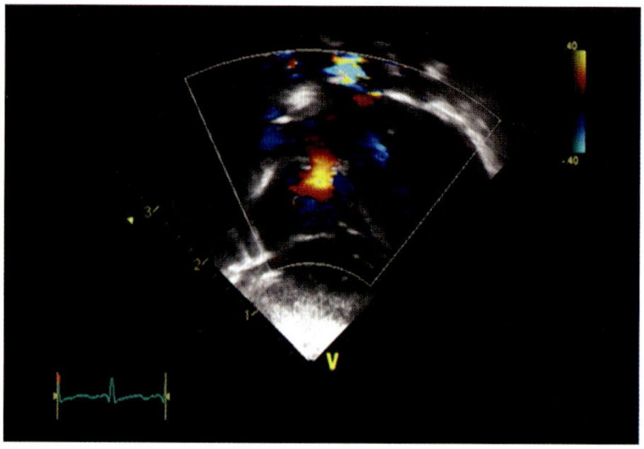

FIGURE and VIDEO 13-65. A color Doppler imaging of the atrial septum in coronal posterior view from an infant with prolonged premature rupture of membrane. The flow across the patent foramen ovale is bidirectional.

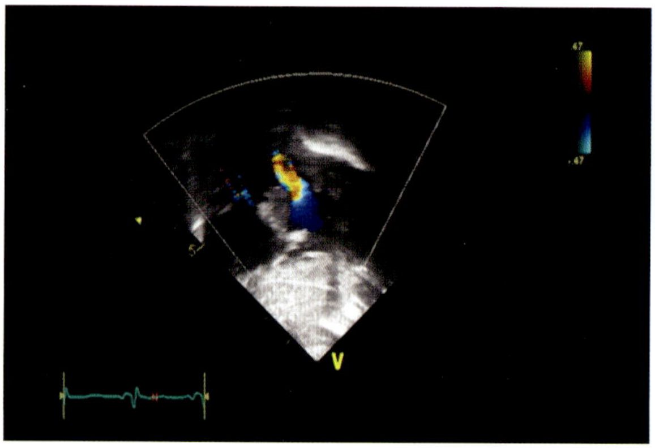

FIGURE and VIDEO 13-66. A color Doppler imaging of the pulmonary artery from the subcostal view. This image was taken from an infant with fetal closure of the ductus arteriosus.

Figure and Video 13-66 shows the pulmonary artery visualized from the subcostal view using color Doppler. This image was taken from an infant with fetal closure of the ductus arteriosus.

Global Assessment

After completing the imaging and performing the desired measurements, the clinician will find it helpful to review the findings in a systematic fashion to determine the significance of these findings. Beginning with the anatomy, the clinician must ensure that all structures were evaluated and appeared normal. The Doppler assessment at each valve, PDA, PFO, descending aorta, and abdominal vessels should be considered. Calculations of the left ventricular output, right ventricular output, and SVC flow should also be considered in the assessment of the overall assessment of the cardiovascular function. It is critical for the clinician to remember that the ventricular outputs in the transitioning neonatal heart do not represent systemic and pulmonary blood flow accurately due to PDA and PFO shunts. SVC flow can be a useful indicator of systemic blood flow, and left pulmonary artery blood flow velocity may be used as an indication of pulmonary blood flow. Each of these two measurements is a representation of systemic and pulmonary flow respectively, although they are not quantitatively complete measures, as they are evaluating only a portion of the full amount.

SUMMARY

Hypoxemia is one of the most frequent problems encountered in the neonatal intensive care unit. We have reviewed how echocardiography can be helpful in the management of infants with hypoxemia. This includes evaluating the cause of hypoxemia and identifying the level of illness of the infant. While more work is needed on how echocardiography can help guide specific therapies, it is clear that echocardiography can be used to follow the disease process over time in a population that frequently displays dynamic physiologic changes over several hours to days. The neonatologist can use echocardiography in conjunction with all of the other clinical findings available to make the most informed management decisions possible.

REFERENCES

1. Mahle WT, Newburger JW, Matherne GP, et al. Role of pulse oximetry in examining newborns for congenital heart disease: a scientific statement from the AHA and AAP. *Pediatrics*. 2009;124:823–836.
2. Mahle WT, Martin GR, Beekman RH 3rd, et al. Endorsement of Health and Human Services recommendation for pulse oximetry screening for critical congenital heart disease. *Pediatrics*. 2012;129:190–192.
3. de Wahl Granelli A, Wennergren M, Sandberg K, et al. Impact of pulse oximetry screening on the detection of duct dependent congenital heart disease: a Swedish prospective screening study in 39 821 newborns. *BMJ*. 2009;338:a3037.
4. Ewer AK, Middleton LJ, Furmston AT, et al. Pulse oximetry screening for congenital heart defects in newborn infants (PulseOx): a test accuracy study. *Lancet*. 2011;378:785–794.

5. Shivananda S, Ahliwahlia L, Kluckow M, Luc J, Jankov R, McNamara P. Variation in management of persistent pulmonary hypertension of the newborn: A survey of physicians in Canada, Australia, and New Zealand. *Am J Perinatol.* 2012;29:519–526.

6. Johnson GL, Cunningham MD, Desai NS, Cottrill CM, Noonan JA. Echocardiography in hypoxemic neonatal pulmonary disease. *J Pediatr.* 1980;96:716–720.

7. Walther FJ, Benders MJ, Leighton JO. Early changes in the neonatal circulatory transition. *J Pediatr.* 1993;123:625–632.

8. Evans N, Kluckow M, Currie A. Range of echocardiographic findings in term neonates with high oxygen requirements. *Arch Dis Child Fetal and Neonatal Ed.* 1998;78:F105–F111.

9. Halliday H, Hirschfeld S, Riggs T, Liebman J, Fanaroff A, Bormuth C. Respiratory distress syndrome: echocardiographic assessment of cardiovascular function and pulmonary vascular resistance. *Pediatrics.* 1977;60:444–449.

10. Randala M, Eronen M, Andersson S, Pohjavuori M, Pesonen E. Pulmonary artery pressure in term and preterm neonates. *Acta Pædiatr.* 1996;85:1344–1347.

11. Evans NJ, Archer LNJ. Doppler assessment of pulmonary artery pressure and extrapulmonary shunting in the acute phase of hyaline membrane disease. *Arch Dis Child.* 1991;66:6–11.

12. Seppanen MP, Kaapa PO, Kero PO, Saraste M. Doppler-derived systolic pulmonary artery pressure in acute neonatal respiratory distress syndrome. *Pediatrics.* 1994;93:769–773.

13. Evans N, Kluckow M. Early determinants of right and left ventricular output in ventilated preterm infants. *Arch Dis Child.* 1996;74:F88–F94.

14. Gutgesell HP, Speer ME, Rosenberg HS. Characterization of the cardiomyopathy in infants of diabetic mothers. *Circulation.* 1980;61:441–450.

15. Reller MD, Tsang RC, Meyer RA, Braun CP. Relationship of prospective diabetes control in pregnancy to neonatal cardiorespiratory function. *J Pediatr.* 1985;106:86–90.

16. Walther FJ, Siassi B, King J, Wu PYK. Cardiac output in infants of insulin-dependent diabetic mothers. *J Pediatr.* 1985;107:109–114.

17. Seppänen MP, Ojanperä OS, Kääpä PO, Kero PO. Delayed postnatal adaptation of pulmonary hemodynamics in infants of diabetic mothers. *J Pediatr.* 1997;131:545–548.

18. Vela-Huerta M, Aguilera-López A, Alarcón-Santos S, Amador N, Aldana-Valenzuela C, Heredia A. Cardiopulmonary adaptation in large for gestational age infants of diabetic and nondiabetic mothers. *Acta Pæditrica.* 2007;96:1303–1307.

19. Katheria A, Leone T. Altered transitional circulation in infant of diabetic mothers with strict antenatal obstetric management: a functional echocardiography study. *J Perinatol.* 2012;32:508–513.

20. Gewilling M, Brown SC, De Catte L, et al. Premature foetal closure of the arterial duct: clinical presentations and outcome. *Eur Heart J.* 2009;30:1530–1536.

21. Korhonen KO, Seppanen MP, Kero PO, Kaapa PO. Delayed adaptation of the pulmonary hemodynamics in infants with mild to moderate meconium aspiration syndrome. *J Pediatr.* 1999;134:355–357.

22. Skinner JR, Hunter S, Poets CF, Milligan DWA, Southall D, Hey EN. Haemodynamic effects of altering arterial oxygen saturation in preterm infants with respiratory failure. *Arch Dis Child Fetal Neonatal Ed.* 1999;80:F81–F87.

23. Bard H, Belanger S, Fouron JC. Comparison of effects of 95% and 90% oxygen saturations in respiratory distress syndrome. *Arch Dis Child.* 1996;75:F94–F96.

24. De Waal KA, Evans N, Osborn DA, Kluckow M. Cardiorespiratory effects of changes in end expiratory pressure in ventilated newborns. *Arch Dis Child Fetal Neonatal Ed.* 2007;92:F444–F448.

25. Kluckow M, Evans N. Low superior vena cava flow and intraventricular haemorrhage in preterm infants. *Arch Dis Child Fetal Neonatal Ed.* 2000;82:188–194.

26. Osborn DA, Evans N. Randomized trial of high-frequency oscillatory ventilation versus conventional ventilation: effect on systemic blood flow in very preterm infants. *J Pediatr.* 2003;143:192–198.

27. Hamdan AH, Shaw NJ. Changes in pulmonary artery pressure in infants with respiratory distress syndrome following treatment with surfactant. *Arch Dis Child.* 1995;72:F176–F179.

28. Kaapa P, Seppanen M, Kero P, Saraste M. Pulmonary hemodynamics after synthetic surfactant dosing. *J Pediatr.* 1993;123:115–119.

29. Bloom MC, Roques-Gineste M, Fries F, Lelong-Tissier MC. Pulmonary haemodynamics after surfactant replacement in severe neonatal respiratory distress syndrome. *Arch Dis Child.* 1995;73:F95–F98.

30. Sehgal A, Mak W, Dunn M, et al. Haemodynamic changes after delivery room surfactant administration to very low birth weight infants. *Arch Dis Child Fetal Neonatal Ed.* 2010;95:F345–F350.

CHAPTER 14

Aneurysm of Ductus Arteriosus, Cardiomyopathies, and Aortopulmonary Collaterals*

Ruben J. Acherman and William N. Evans

- **SECTION 1: ANEURYSM OF DUCTUS ARTERIOSUS**
  - Introduction
  - Echocardiography
  - Follow-up
- **SECTION 2: CARDIOMYOPATHIES**
  - Introduction
  - Dilated Cardiomyopathy
  - Hypertrophic Cardiomyopathy
  - Restrictive Cardiomyopathy
  - Arrhythmogenic Right ventricular Cardiomyopathy
  - Non-Compaction Cardiomyopathy
- **SECTION 3: SYSTEMIC TO PULMONARY COLLATERALS**
  - Introduction
  - Clinical Features
  - Echocardiographic Evaluation
- **REFERENCES**

SECTION 1: ANEURYSM OF DUCTUS ARTERIOSUS

Introduction

Current echocardiographic imaging demonstrates aneurysmal dilation of the ductus arteriosus in more than 8% of full-term newborns.[1,2] An aneurysm of the ductus arteriosus (ADA) manifests as a saccular dilation originating from the ductus arteriosus's descending aortic origin. An ADA may occur from an in utero process, result from a postnatal complication after a surgical or transcatheter closure of a patent ductus arteriosus, or occur secondarily from ductal endarteritis.[3,4] Proposed in utero mechanisms for an ADA include narrowing or tortuosity of the fetal ductus arteriosus with poststenotic dilatation,[5] increased fetal ductal flow, or abnormal intimal cushion formation secondary to abnormal elastin expression.[6]

Echocardiography

Either a prenatal or postnatal echocardiogram can demonstrate an ADA. In our experience, a prenatal echocardiogram more often proves a fetal ADA in the mid to late 3rd trimester rather than earlier in gestation. A fetal ADA is usually associated with increased ductal tortuosity, ductal narrowing (Figure 14-1), a variable degree of

*Videos can be accessed at http://PracticalNeonatalEcho.com.

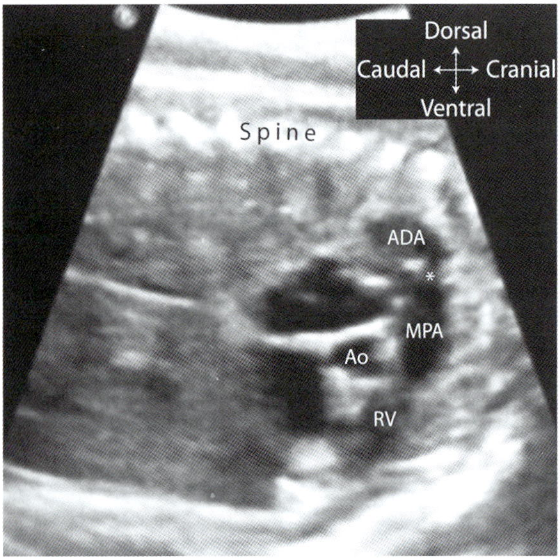

FIGURE 14-1. Fetal echocardiogram. This sagittal short axis view shows the narrowed passage* from the main pulmonary artery (MPA) to the aneurysm of the ductus arteriosus (ADA). Abbreviation: Ao, aortic valve; RV, right ventricular outflow.

ventricular asymmetry with right ventricular dominance, and an increased ductal flow velocity. In most cases, the neonatal ADA is an incidental finding noted during an echocardiogram performed for unrelated reasons. In some cases, a neonatal ADA is suspected because a chest radiograph demonstrates a left upper mediastinal mass. On rare occasion an ADA is discovered during evaluations for perinatal distress, pulmonary hypertension, dyspnea, stridor, hoarseness, severe perinatal hypoxia, or neonatal thromboembolic events.

In the neonate, the high-parasternal short-axis echocardiographic view visualizes the ADA just to the left of the main and left pulmonary arteries (Figure and Video 14-2). The ADA may be patent in the early neonatal evaluations with a narrowed pulmonary artery end and a wide-open aortic end. If the ductus is patent, color Doppler usually demonstrates a characteristic horizontal jet, as opposed to the almost vertical jet in the usual patent ductus arteriosus (Figure and Video 14-2). The horizontal ductal jet prevents accurate flow velocity measurement that is needed for estimating the pressure gradient between the aorta

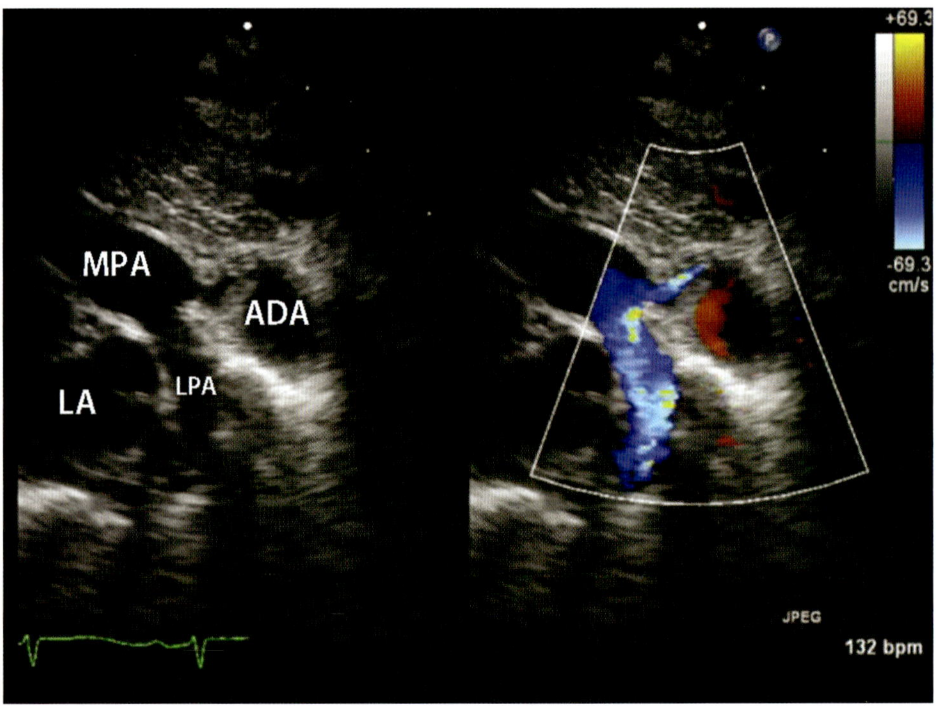

FIGURE and VIDEO 14-2. Two-dimensional high parasternal short axis showing the aneurysmal ductus arteriosus (ADA) to the left of the main pulmonary artery (MPA). The blue jet is almost horizontal due to left to right ductal shunt.

and the pulmonary artery.[5] With color Doppler, a low Nyquist frequency allows visualization of the low blood-flow velocities inside the ADA. Echocardiographic imaging may demonstrate thrombus formation inside the ADA (Figure and Video 14-3). Echocardiography can also rule out potential thrombus migration that can propagate into the descending aorta or the pulmonary arteries.

Follow-up

Most neonatal ADAs resolve spontaneously within the first 2 months of age.[1,2] In a work by Jan and colleagues, the ADA resolved as the ductus constricted in 70% of the cases; nevertheless, the echocardiogram showed thrombus formation inside the ADA in 30 percent of cases that ADA eventually resolved.[1] The natural history of an uncomplicated ADA persisting beyond 2 months of age is unknown. A few case reports in newborns, children, and adults have emphasized the rare, yet serious, complications associated with an ADA. Reported complications include spontaneous rupture, thromboembolism, erosion into airways or esophagus, and infection. Complications may arise at any age; a recent report accounts a case of fetal demise from thrombosis of an ADA.[7] Many of the reported complications occurred in previously undiagnosed patients. Some ADAs are diagnosed only at autopsy, following death from unrelated reasons.

All neonatal ADAs require serial echocardiograms. Surgical repair is recommended for ADAs persisting beyond the neonatal period. Surgical repair is also recommended in cases where a large ADA does not appear to be involuting, when there is migration of thrombus into pulmonary arteries or descending aorta, when there is evidence of thromboembolism, and where ADAs are compromising adjacent structures, and in patients with Marfan syndrome or other connective tissue disorders. Most authors recommend cardiopulmonary bypass for surgical resection. In those with a history of an ADA surgically repaired, follow-up is needed, as such patients may develop other cardiac lesions associated with connective tissue disorders.[6]

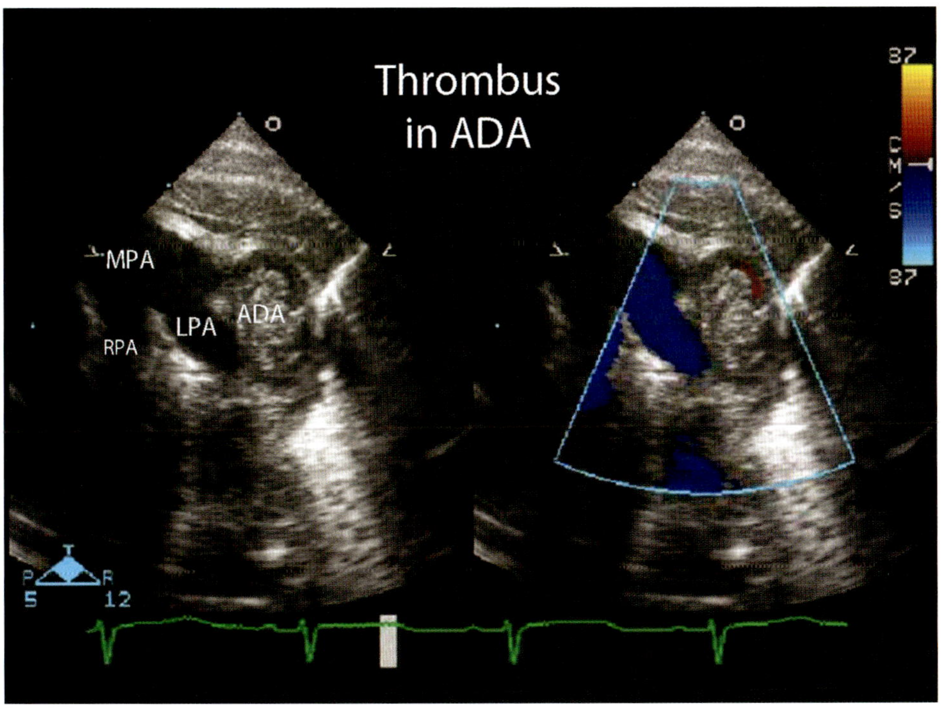

FIGURE and VIDEO 14-3. Two-dimensional high parasternal short axis view showing the thrombosed aneurysmal ductus arteriosus (ADA) to the left of the main (MPA) and left pulmonary artery (LPA). RPA, indicates right pulmonary artery.

SECTION 2: CARDIOMYOPATHIES

Introduction

Cardiomyopathies, or diseases of the myocardium, often cause both systolic and diastolic ventricular dysfunction. Most cardiomyopathies result in generalized myocardial disease and include dilated, hypertrophic, and restrictive forms.[8] Occasionally, myocardial abnormalities are localized, rather than diffuse, such as in arrhythmogenic right ventricular cardiomyopathy (ARVC) and noncompaction cardiomyopathy. Noncompaction cardiomyopathy detection has increased via echocardiography and magnetic resonance imaging (MRI); nonetheless, the World Health Organization does not include noncompaction cardiomyopathy in its classification schema.[9] The Pediatric Cardiomyopathy Registry estimates the annual pediatric incidence of all forms of cardiomyopathy at 1.13 per 100,000. Dilated cardiomyopathy is the most frequent at 0.54 per 100,000, followed by hypertrophic cardiomyopathy at 0.47 per 100,000. The overall incidence is significantly higher in infants <1 year of age at 8.34 per 100,000 than in older pediatric patients.[10]

Although "dilated cardiomyopathy" and "hypertrophic cardiomyopathy" imply primary myocardial disease, clinicians often use the terms to describe ventricular hypertrophy or dilatation of unclear etiology. We prefer using specific terminology such hypertrophic cardiomyopathy of the infant of diabetic mother or the left ventricular dysfunction and dilatation from perinatal asphyxia.

Dilated Cardiomyopathy

Dilated cardiomyopathy usually implies global systolic dysfunction and dilation of the left ventricle; however, the condition may also involve the right ventricle. Patients may present with symptoms and signs of congestive heart failure, arrhythmias, and thromboembolic events, especially from left ventricular mural thrombi. Occasionally, a prenatal echocardiogram detects fetal-cardiac systolic dysfunction, accompanied by a spectrum of fetal heart failure and hydrops.

Echocardiographic findings include increased left ventricular end-systolic and end-diastolic diameters, resulting in a reduced shortening fraction. The normally bullet-shaped left ventricle acquires a globular-spherical shape (Figures 14-4 and 14-5). The atria may also dilate, especially with atrioventricular valve regurgitation. Mitral valve annulus dilates with progressive left ventricular enlargement, leading to mitral valve regurgitation from poor leaflet coaptation (Figure and Video 14-6). Flow stasis may encourage intracardiac thrombus formation (Figure and Video 14-7).

Acute pharmacological support may require diuretics, dobutamine, dopamine, epinephrine, milrinone, and anticoagulants. Patients in significant distress will require

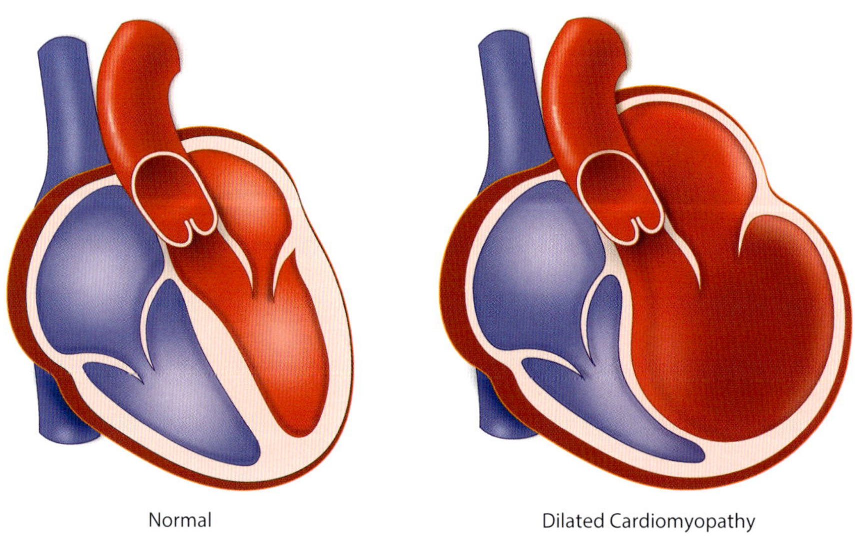

FIGURE 14-4. Dilated Cardiomyopathy: Note the normal bullet shaped left ventricle. In dilated cardiomyopathy the left ventricle is dilated, with a globular-spherical shape.

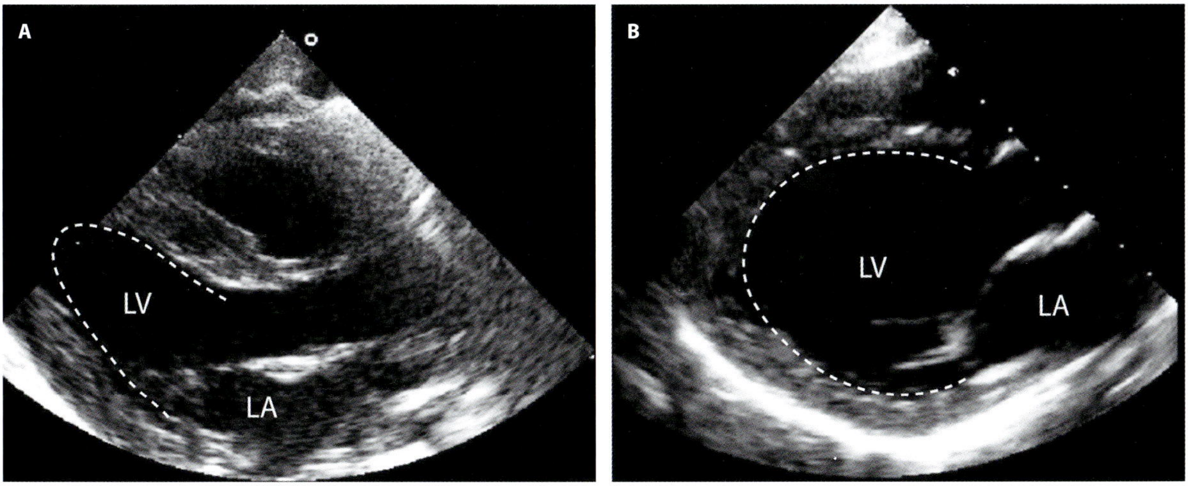

FIGURE 14-5. Dilated Cardiomyopathy: A, shows a normal long axis view with the "bullet" shaped left ventricle outlined by the dashed line. **B**, demonstrates the long axis in a patient with dilated cardiomyopathy, the dashed line outlines the globular dilated left ventricle and the dilated left atrium. Abbreviations: LA, left atrium; LV, left ventricle.

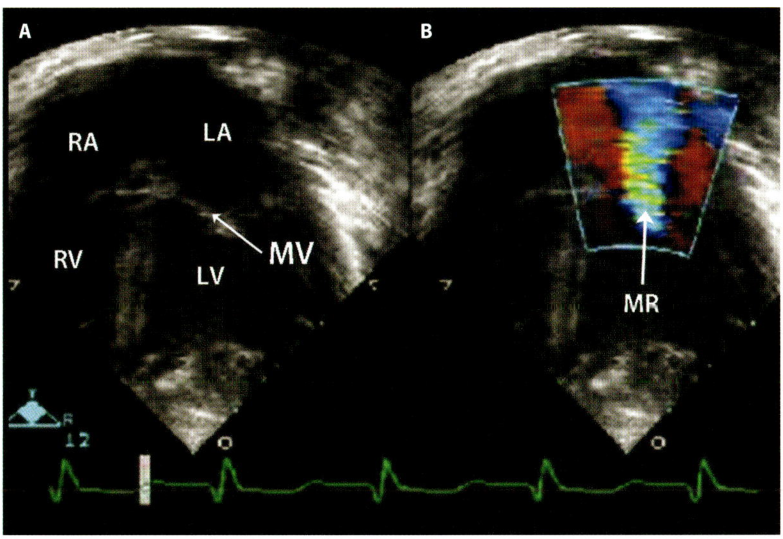

FIGURE and VIDEO 14-6. Dilated Cardiomyopathy: Long axis view in a patient with dilated cardiomyopathy. In A, the arrow points the non- compacted mitral valve leaflets. In B, color Doppler demonstrates the mitral valve regurgitation in blue (MR). Abbreviations: LA, left atrium; LV, left ventricle.

assisted ventilation. Patients not responding to supportive therapy may need cardiac transplant. Mechanical assist devices such as extracorporeal membrane oxygenation can serve as a bridge to transplant. Chronic therapy usually includes diuretics, digoxin, ACE inhibitors, and beta-blockers. Measuring B-type natriuretic peptide, which the ventricles secrete under stress, helps guide therapy.

Familial dilated cardiomyopathy occurs in about 20 to 50% of cases. All 1st-degree relatives require regular echocardiographic screening.

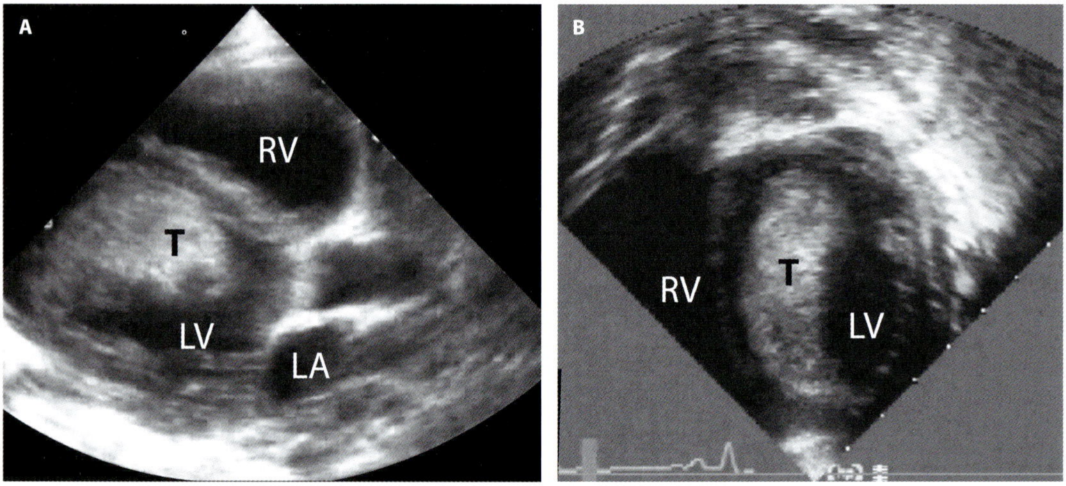

FIGURE and VIDEO 14-7. **Dilated Cardiomyopathy:** Thrombus formation (T) inside a dilated left ventricle (LV). **A**, long axis view; **B**, apical view. Abbreviations: LA, left atrium; RV, right ventricle.

Dilated Cardiomyopathy in Specific Diseases

Perinatal Asphyxia

Severe perinatal asphyxia may cause ventricular dysfunction and dilatation, likely from myocardial ischemia. Echocardiographic findings may include decreased fractional shortening, dilated ventricles, and mitral and tricuspid valve regurgitation. Tricuspid valve regurgitation may result from ischemia or necrosis of the papillary muscles and may be accentuated by coexistent pulmonary hypertension. Other than those with severe myocardial damage, most patients stabilize and improve their ventricular function after several days of supportive care.

Systemic Hypertension

Severe systemic hypertension may cause neonatal myocardial dysfunction with echocardiographic features similar to those in dilated cardiomyopathy. Echocardiography must include evaluation of the aortic arch for ruling out coarctation of the aorta, and evaluation of the abdominal descending aorta to rule out thrombi, especially in neonates with a history of having had an umbilical artery catheter. Frequently, myocardial dysfunction improves following hypertension treatment.

Structural Cardiovascular Disease

The left ventricular outflow, the descending aorta, the aortic arch, and the origin of the coronary arteries need careful assessment during echocardiographic evaluation of the infant with dilated cardiomyopathy. Aortic valve stenosis and coarctation of the aorta are frequent causes of left ventricular dysfunction and dilatation in the newborn. Anomalous origin of the left coronary artery is a rare congenital condition, which usually manifests later in infancy after the pulmonary vascular resistance decreases. With decreasing pulmonary vascular resistance, the left coronary artery blood flows retrograde into the pulmonary artery, leading to myocardial ischemia.

Myocarditis

Many viruses can cause myocarditis, including enterovirus, adenovirus, cytomegalovirus, echovirus, respiratory syncytial virus, influenza, mumps, and rubella. Viral transmission can occur transplacentally or postnatally. The echocardiogram usually reveals left-ventricular dilatation and systolic dysfunction. Nonetheless, in fulminant myocarditis, the ventricular function is often decreased without chamber dilatation. Pericardial effusion is common.

Treatment includes similar pharmacological supportive care that we noted above with dilated cardiomyopathy. Intravenous immunoglobulin may be of benefit, although validation studies are lacking.[11–13] Anecdotal evidence largely accounts for the use of steroids. Fortunately, most pediatric patients improve; however, a substantial number die or develop persistent dilated cardiomyopathy, which can lead to heart transplantation.[14]

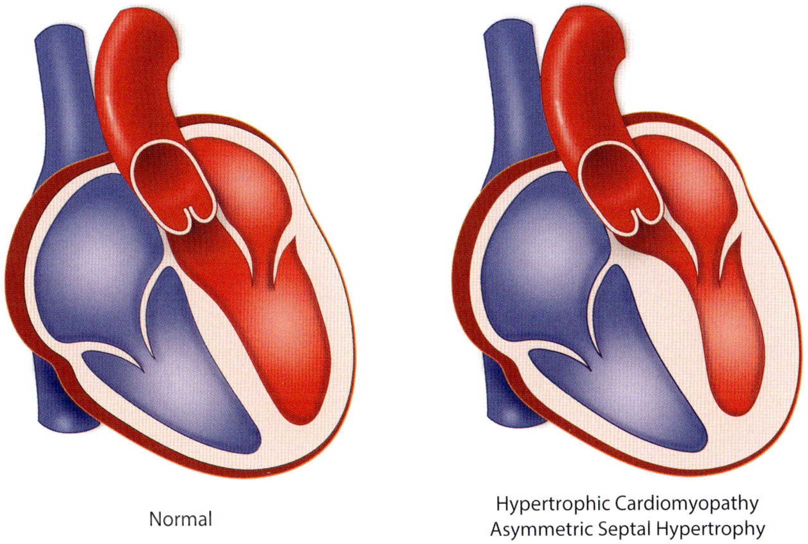

FIGURE 14-8. Asymmetric Septal Hypertrophy: The hypertrophy is more severe in the septum than in the free walls.

Sepsis

The cause of the sepsis related myocardial dysfunction is unclear. Possibly, dysfunction occurs from circulating myocardial depressants such as endotoxins, tumor necrosis factor, and interleukin. The echocardiographic findings may be indistinguishable from dilated cardiomyopathy. The echocardiogram should rule out intra-cardiac vegetations or masses. The presentation, clinical, and laboratory findings can assist in making a diagnosis.

Hypertrophic Cardiomyopathy

Myocardial hypertrophy in hypertrophic cardiomyopathy is not from outflow obstruction or systemic diseases. Studies have revealed several causative autosomal-dominant gene mutations. Symptoms and signs relate to decreased cardiac output and occasionally complicating arrhythmias. Ventricular hypertrophy may affect the normal hemodynamics via two principle mechanisms.

1. Outflow obstruction that limits cardiac output by blocking the exit of blood from the ventricle.
2. Abnormal diastolic function that limits cardiac output by impeding inflow to the ventricular cavity.

Asymmetric septal hypertrophy (ASH) is the most common phenotype. Septal hypertrophy is more severe than that of the free walls (Figure and Video 14-8). ASH frequently causes left ventricular outflow obstruction, systolic anterior motion (SAM) of the mitral valve, and mitral valve regurgitation. When the hypertrophied septum bulges in systole, the left ventricular outflow narrows, producing obstruction to the flow. The Venturi effect from the outflow jet sucks the mitral valve leaflets (systolic anterior motion), further obstructing the outflow and causing mitral valve regurgitation (Figure and Video 14-9 and Figure 14-10).

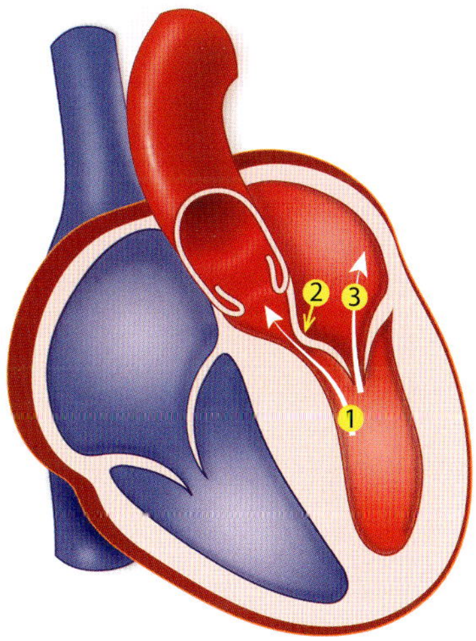

FIGURE 14-9. Mitral Valve Systolic Anterior Motion: The outflow jet Venturi effect (1) sucks the mitral valve leaflets (2), further obstructing the outflow and causing mitral valve regurgitation (3).

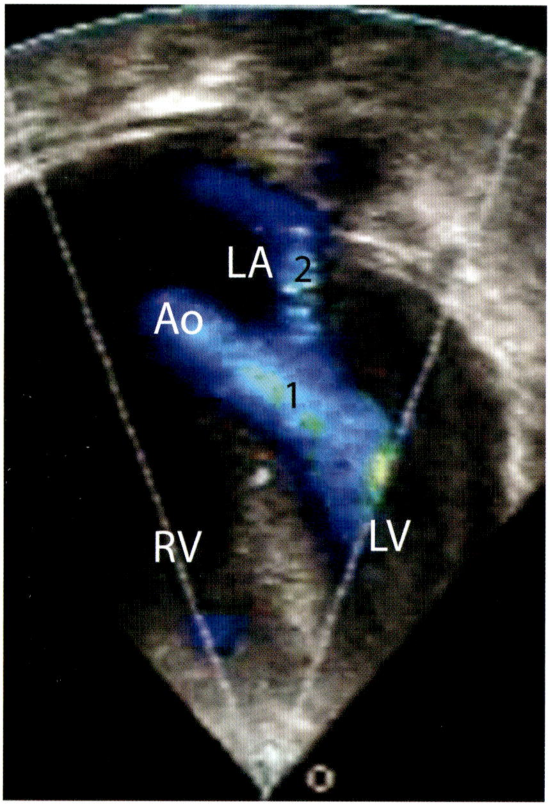

FIGURE 14-10. Subaortic Stenosis and Mitral Valve Regurgitation: Apical 5-chamber view in a patient with asymmetric septal hypertrophy. Color Doppler demonstrates the acceleration of flow in the subaortic area (1), and the mitral valve regurgitation, and the mitral valve regurgitation (2). Abbreviations: Ao, ascending aorta; LA, left atrium; LV, left ventricle; RV, right ventricle.

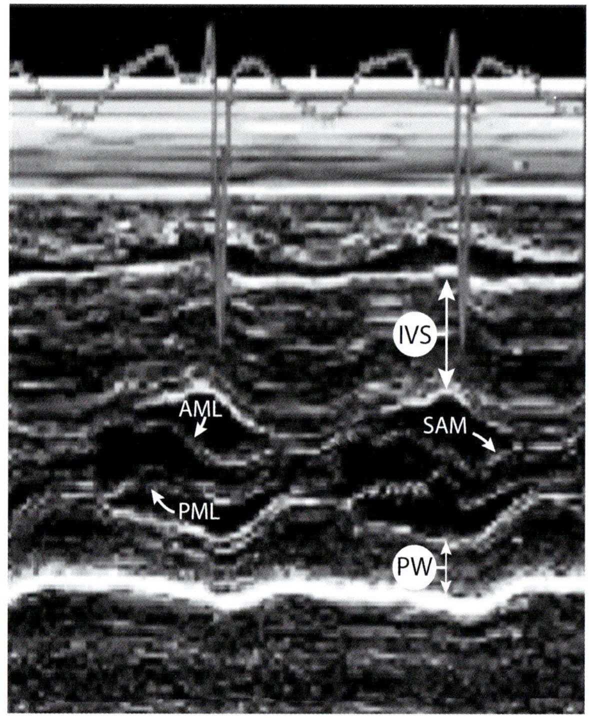

FIGURE 14-11. Hypertrophic Cardiomyopathy: M-mode tracing across the ventricles showing the hypertrophy of the interventricular septum (IVS), and the mitral valve systolic anterior motion (SAM) toward the IVS. Abbreviations: AML, anterior mitral leaflet; PML, posterior mitral leaflet; PW, left ventricular posterior wall.

The two-dimensional (2D) echocardiogram demonstrates the ventricular hypertrophy and can also evaluate the mitral valve for SAM. M-mode is useful for measuring wall thickness and documenting SAM (Figure 14-11). The systolic function is often normal to hyperdynamic. Color Doppler helps evaluate outflow obstruction and valve regurgitation. Spectral Doppler aids in quantifying the degree of stenosis and evaluating diastolic function. In hypertrophic cardiomyopathy, abnormal relaxation is responsible for diastolic abnormalities. Mitral valve-inflow Doppler can detect impaired myocardial relaxation by recording a reduced early rapid filling (E) and an increased flow velocity during atrial contraction (A) (Figure 14-12). We suggest more extensive references for a discussion of using tissue Doppler and speckle tracking for assessing diastolic dysfunction.

Other hypertrophic cardiomyopathy phenotypes include concentric, apical, and free-wall forms. In the concentric form, one or both ventricles may demonstrate uniform hypertrophy rather than ASH (Figures 14-13 and 14-14). Diastolic dysfunction may be the only hemodynamic abnormality. The apical form, usually of the left ventricle, produces a midcavitary obstruction that forms an apical pouch. The midcavitary obstruction causes suprasystemic pressure in the apical pouch, producing an apical aneurysm (Figure 14-15). The 2D long-axis view may miss an apical hypertrophic cardiomyopathy, because apical hypertrophy may be only visible from an apical four-chamber view.

Acutely, an esmolol infusion may improve cardiac output negatively impacted by outflow obstruction and diastolic dysfunction. Inotropes are often contraindicated because they may increase outflow obstruction and worsen diastolic function. Chronic therapy usually includes oral β-blockers, mainly propranolol in newborns. In the neonate, patients rarely need surgical

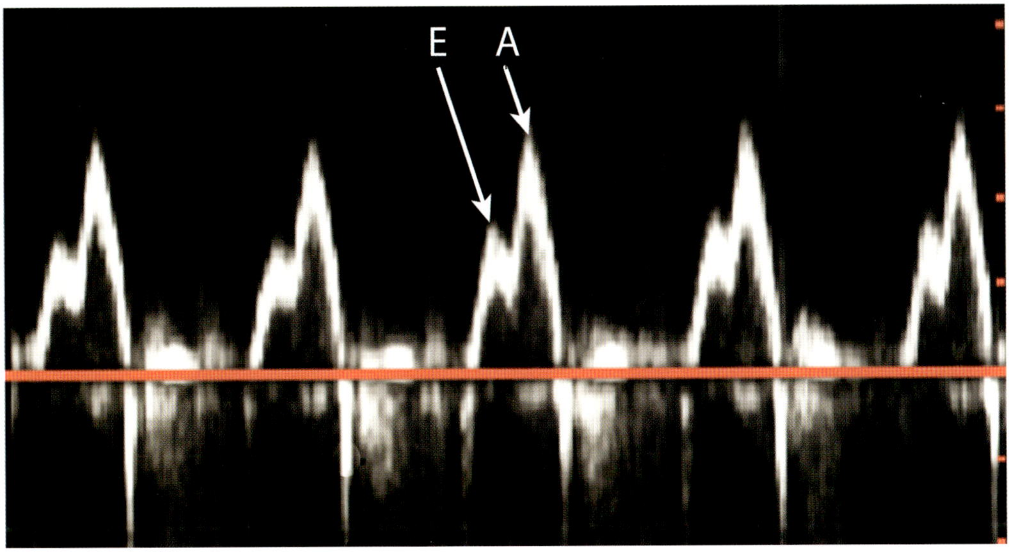

FIGURE 14-12. Mitral Valve Inflow Doppler in Hypertrophic Cardiomyopathy: Mitral valve inflow pulsed Doppler interrogation shows reduced early rapid filling (E) and an increased flow velocity during atrial contraction (A).

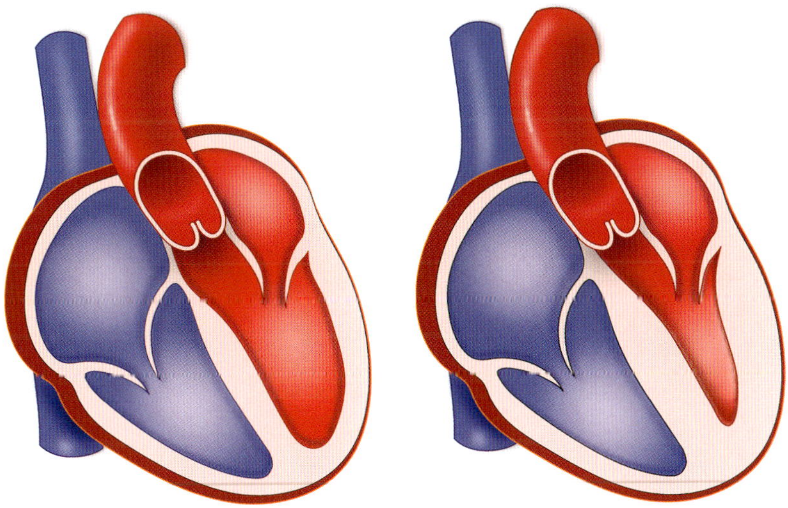

FIGURE 14-13. Concentric Hypertrophy: There is uniform wall hypertrophy.

myectomy, but the procedure should be considered in severe cases. Severe cases, not responding to medical treatment or not candidates for myectomy, may need cardiac transplantation.

All 1st-degree relatives of a patient with hypertrophic cardiomyopathy require regular echocardiographic screening.

Hypertrophic Cardiomyopathy in Specific Diseases

Hypertrophic Cardiomyopathy of the Infant of a Diabetic Mother

Maternal diabetes is the most frequent cause of ventricular hypertrophy during the perinatal period. The hypertrophy, resulting from the trophic response to fetal hyperinsulinemia, is usually mild to moderate and devoid of serious hemodynamic impairment.

Most affected infants are asymptomatic. Clinical presentation may include a systolic murmur from outflow obstruction and mild tachypnea. Occasionally, severe cases present with findings of poor cardiac output from significant diastolic dysfunction or outflow obstruction. Severe cases may require medical therapy.

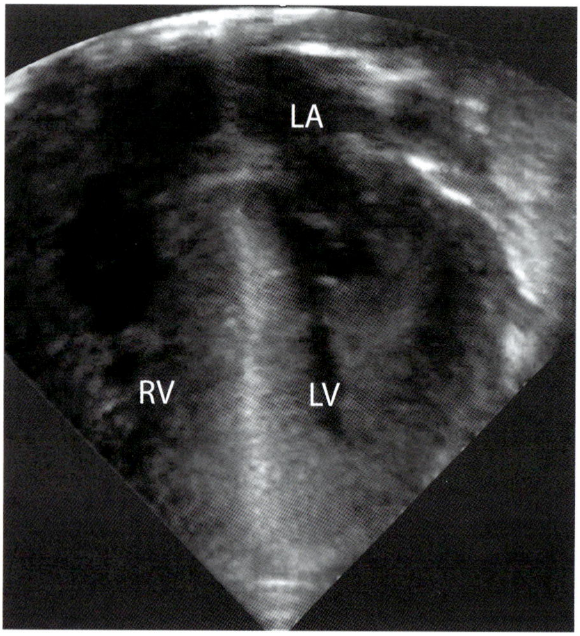

FIGURE 14-14. Concentric Hypertrophy: four-chamber view showing severe concentric left ventricular hypertrophy. Abbreviations: LA, left atrium; LV, left ventricle; RV, right ventricle.

The hypertrophy may be asymmetric or concentric, with echocardiographic findings identical to the ones we delineated above for hypertrophic cardiomyopathy. The hypertrophic cardiomyopathy of the infant of diabetic mother resolves spontaneously within few months of life. All affected patients need to be followed until the hypertrophy resolves.

Hypertrophic Cardiomyopathy in Storage Diseases

Glycogen storage diseases are inherited disorders characterized by accumulation of glycogen in liver, skeletal muscle, and cardiac muscle. Rarely, patients with the infantile form of the glycogen storage disease type II (Pompe disease) present with severe neonatal hypertrophic cardiomyopathy (Figure 14-16). The echocardiographic and clinical findings are identical to those in concentric hypertrophic cardiomyopathy.[15]

Hypertrophic Cardiomyopathy in Noonan Syndrome

Noonan syndrome includes unusual facial characteristics, cardiac, and extracardiac defects. The syndrome may be familial, with autosomal dominant inheritance in about 50% of the cases. The RAF1 gene mutation causes only 3 to 10% cases of Noonan syndrome, but hypertrophic cardiomyopathy is present in 95% of RAF1 gene-mutation

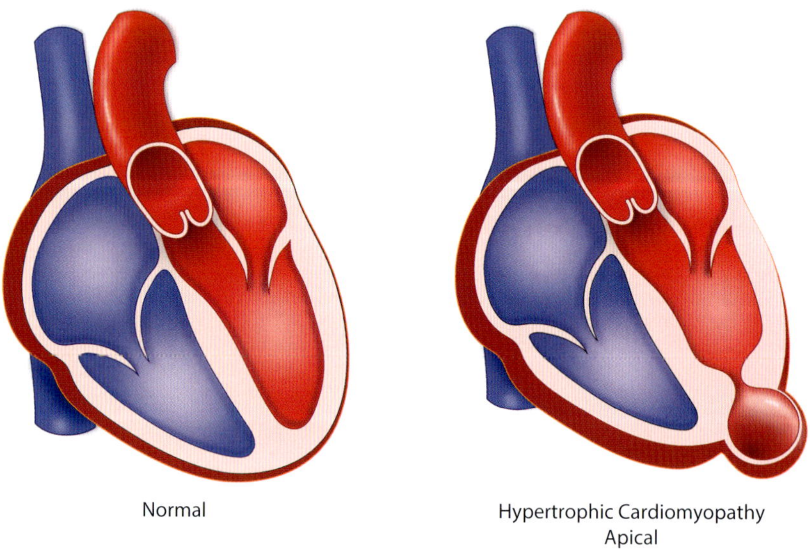

FIGURE 14-15. Apical Hypertrophy: The mid-cavitary obstruction causes supra-systemic pressure in the apical pouch, producing an apical aneurysm.

positive patients.[16] The clinical and echocardiographic findings of hypertrophic cardiomyopathy in Noonan syndrome are identical to those we described for hypertrophic cardiomyopathy.

Restrictive Cardiomyopathy

Restrictive cardiomyopathy is rare, composing 2 to 5% of pediatric cardiomyopathies.[17] Diagnosis usually occurs beyond the neonatal period. Nevertheless, there is a recent report of a fetus with a history of pericardial effusion and abnormal venous Doppler profiles that was diagnosed with restrictive cardiomyopathy shortly after birth.[18]

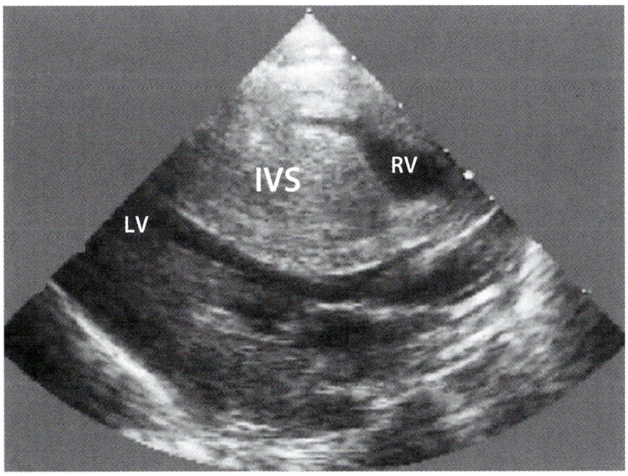

FIGURE and VIDEO 14-16. Concentric Hypertrophy: Pompe' disease.

Echocardiographic findings include normal or near-normal ventricular systolic function with abnormal diastolic function. The atria are severely dilated, and the ventricles appear underfilled, giving the four-chamber view the "Mickey Mouse" appearance (Figure 14-17 and Figure and Video 14-18). Elevated venous pressure dilates the inferior vena cava and hepatic veins. Pericardial effusion may be present. Impaired diastolic function causes the spectral Doppler inflow patterns to show a reduced early rapid filling (E) and an increased flow velocity during atrial contraction (A). Pulmonary artery hypertension may result from increased pulmonary venous pressure.

Pediatric restrictive cardiomyopathy carries a poor prognosis with a high incidence of sudden death. Heart transplantation is the only effective treatment.

Arrhythmogenic Right Ventricular Cardiomyopathy

Progressive fibrofatty replacement of the right ventricular myocardium results in arrhythmogenic right ventricular cardiomyopathy (dysplasia). Presentation includes ventricular arrhythmias, congestive heart failure, left bundle branch block, and sudden death. Some publications include ARVC as a cause of sudden infant death, including a 4-month infant.[19,20] In 30% of the cases, ARVC is familial with autosomal dominant-incomplete penetrance heredity.

In adults, the echocardiographic finding with the greatest sensitivity is dilation of the right ventricular outflow, best seen in the four-chamber view. The echocardiogram

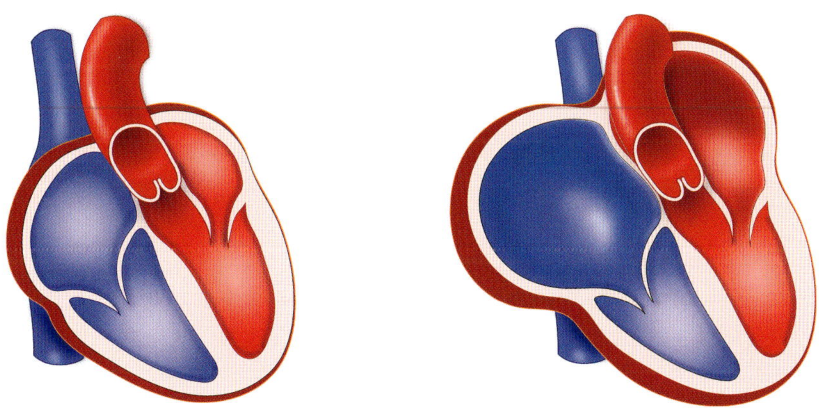

FIGURE 14-17. Restrictive Cardiomyopathy: The atria are severely dilated, giving the four-chamber view the "Mickey mouse" appearance.

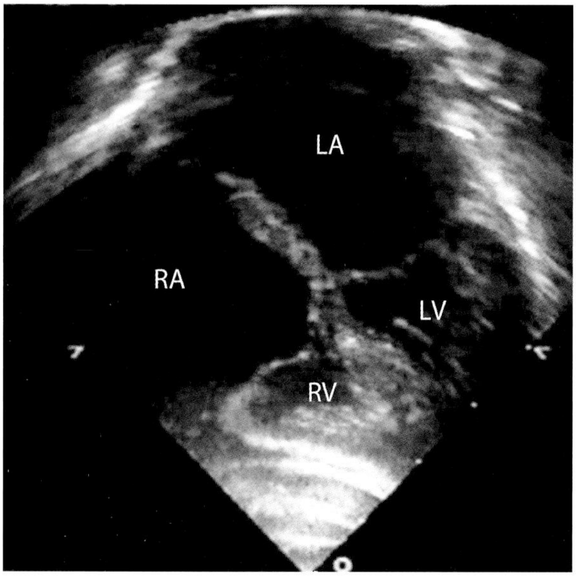

FIGURE 14-18. Restrictive Cardiomyopathy: Echocardiogram showing severe bilateral atrial dilatation. Abbreviations: LA, left atrium; LV, left ventricle; RA, right atrium; RV, right ventricle.

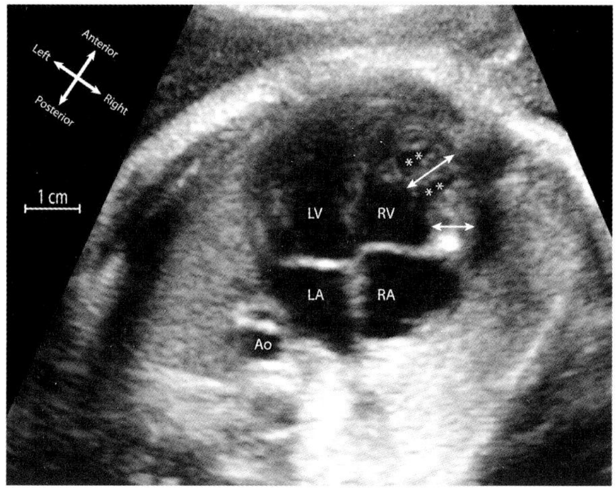

FIGURE 14-19. Fetal Right Ventricular Noncompaction: Fetal four-chamber view. The right ventricular (RV) wall is hypertrophied (arrows) with deep recesses (asterisks). Abbreviations: Ao, descending aorta; LA, left atrium; RA, right atrium; S, spine. [Reproduced with permission from Acherman RJ, Evans WN, Schwartz JK, et al. Right ventricular noncompaction associated with long QT in a fetus with right ventricular hypertrophy and cardiac arrhythmias, *Prenat Diagn* 2008 June;28(6):551–553].

may also show global right ventricular dilation and systolic dysfunction. Management of ARVC includes antiarrhythmic medications, implantable cardiac electronic devices, and heart transplant.

Noncompaction Cardiomyopathy

Myocardial noncompaction, a disorder of the embryonic endomyocardial morphogenesis, is usually sporadic but may be familial. In the general population, the prevalence is estimated at 0.05%. In up to 26% of cases, noncompaction is associated with structural congenital cardiac abnormalities.[21–23] In adult patients, studies show noncompaction limited to the left ventricle occurs in 62%, and noncompaction affecting both ventricles occur in 38%. Isolated right ventricular noncompaction is rare (Figure 14-19).[24]

Echocardiography is the best tool to detect myocardial noncompaction. Echocardiographic abnormalities include prominent ventricular trabeculae with deep intertrabecular recesses and the presence of blood flow filling the recesses, visualized by color Doppler imaging (Figures 14-19 and 14-20).[25] Systolic and diastolic functions may be abnormal.

Therapy includes medical management of heart failure and associated arrhythmias, anticoagulation, and the use of pacemakers and implantable defibrillators. Cardiac transplantation is indicated for refractory congestive heart failure. This condition has been diagnosed prenatally and in the early neonatal period.[26]

SECTION 3: SYSTEMIC TO PULMONARY COLLATERALS

Introduction

Patent ductus arteriosus is the most common cause of an extracardiac, left-to-right shunt. However, pathological systemic-to-pulmonary artery collaterals (SPC), either congenital or acquired, can also be sources of extracardiac left-to-right shunting. A compilation of older, angiography-based studies describe acquired SPC in 26 infants requiring prolonged ventilatory support; surgical ligation was performed in 1 and coil embolization in 3, leading to clinical improvement in all 4.[27–29]

Early in human development, the segmental arteries, branches of the dorsal aorta, are the only source of pulmonary blood flow (Figure 14-21A). At about 5 to 6 weeks of gestation, the lungs have two sources of blood flow: from the dorsal aorta through the segmental arteries and from the right ventricle through the pulmonary arteries (Figure 14-21B). After the involution of the segmental arteries, at the 7th week of gestation, the pulmonary arteries become the sole source of pulmonary blood flow[30]

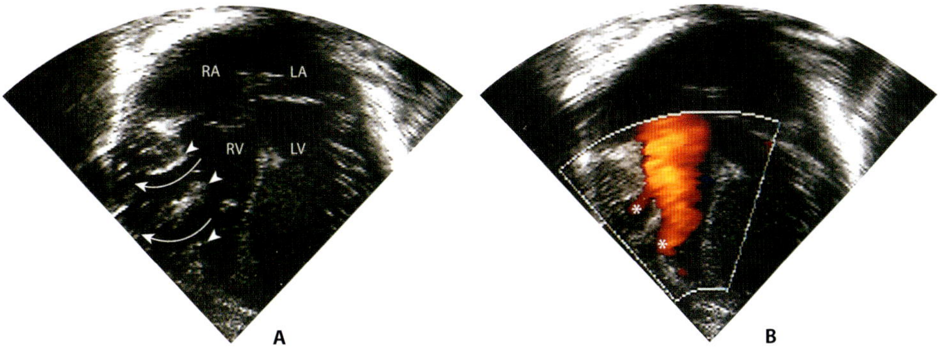

FIGURE 14-20. Right Ventricular Noncompaction: Postnatal echocardiogram, from the same patient in Figure 14-14, showing in **A** the prominent right ventricular trabeculations (arrowheads) and deep intertrabecular recesses (arrows). In **B** the color Doppler fills the intertrabecular recesses (asterisks). Abbreviations: LA, left atrium; LV, left ventricle; RA, right atrium; RV, right ventricle. [Reproduced with permission from Acherman RJ, Evans WN, Schwartz JK, et al. Right ventricular noncompaction associated with long QT in a fetus with right ventricular hypertrophy and cardiac arrhythmias, *Prenat Diagn* 2008 June;28(6):551–553].

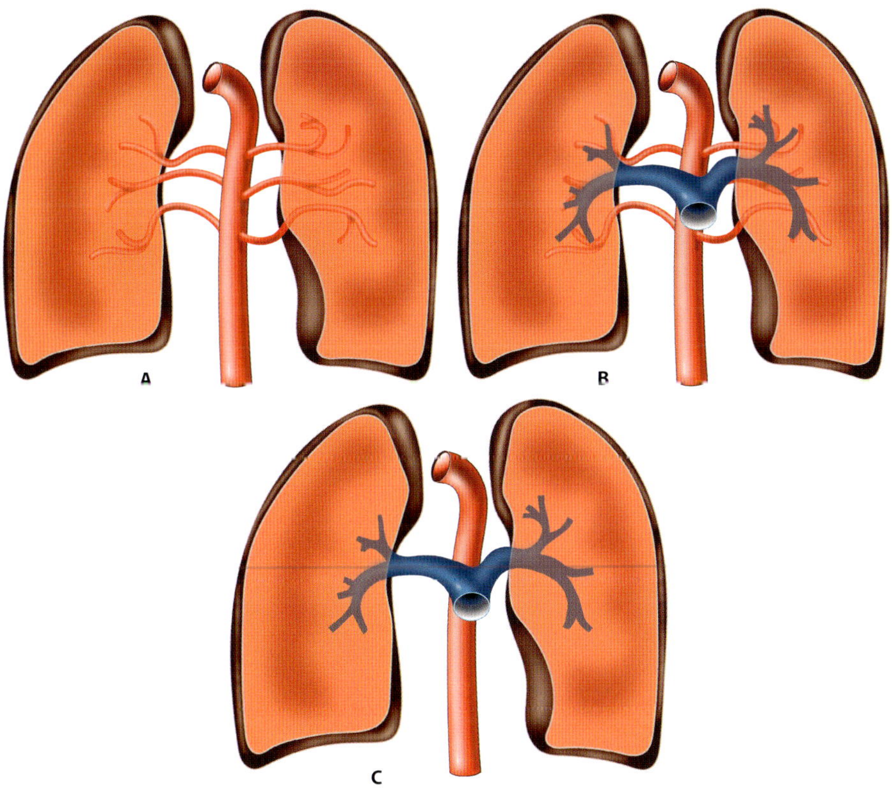

FIGURE 14-21. Source of Pulmonary Blood Flow: A, Early in human development, the segmental arteries, branches of the dorsal aorta, are the only source of pulmonary blood flow. **B**, At 5 to 6 weeks of gestation, the lungs have two sources of blood flow, the segmental arteries, and the pulmonary arteries. **C**, After the involution of the segmental arteries, at the 7th week of gestation, the pulmonary arteries become the sole source of pulmonary blood flow.

(Figure 14-21C). At the 9th to 12th weeks of gestation, the bronchial arteries derive mainly from the thoracic aorta and the first intercostals arteries. Accessory bronchial arteries originating from the brachiocepalic trunk and the subclavian arteries have also been described.[30] Although there is much variation, there are usually two bronchial arteries to the left lung and one to the right lung. The bronchial arteries supply blood to the bronchi, connective tissue of the lungs, visceral pleura, and the pericardium.[30,31] Pulmonary arteries supply terminal respiratory units.

Clinical Features

The SPC are communications between the systemic and pulmonary circulations. The congenital SPC are frequently persistent segmental arteries, often associated with congenital heart disease, typically pulmonary atresia with ventricular septal defect, but may be present without any concomitant cardiac or pulmonary disease. The acquired SPC are bronchopulmonary connections, usually associated with conditions generating alveolar hypoxia, like chronic pulmonary infections, tumors, bronchiectasis, pulmonary artery thrombosis, or during angiogenesis in granulation tissue.[31,32] There are normal anastomoses between the bronchial arteries and the peripheral branches of the pulmonary arteries, some supplying the visceral pleura of the lung; however, these anastomoses are clinically insignificant.[30-33] Prolonged alveolar and pulmonary interstitial hypoxia may stimulate the growth of the native bronchopulmonary connections and promote angiogenesis. The enlarged native connections and the newly formed vessels by angiogenesis are alternative paths of irrigation in case of persistent hypoxia.[32,33]

In 1994, Luna and colleagues first reported the detection of aortopulmonary collaterals in premature infants by color Doppler echocardiography.[34] A prospective echocardiographic evaluation in 196 very low birth weight infants reported a 66% incidence of SPC. Patients with SPC had significantly longer times on positive pressure ventilation and longer stays in the hospital. In most cases, the SPC resolved spontaneously; 10 patients required diuretics; 1 patient underwent cardiac catheterization and embolization of one collateral.[30] A more recent publication reports an infant without associated cardiac disease and with oxygen dependency. Echocardiography demonstrated SPC at 98 days of life. The patient underwent cardiac catheterization, angiography, and collateral embolization (Figure and Video 14-22), and 9 days after the procedure, the patient was weaned from supplemental oxygen.[35]

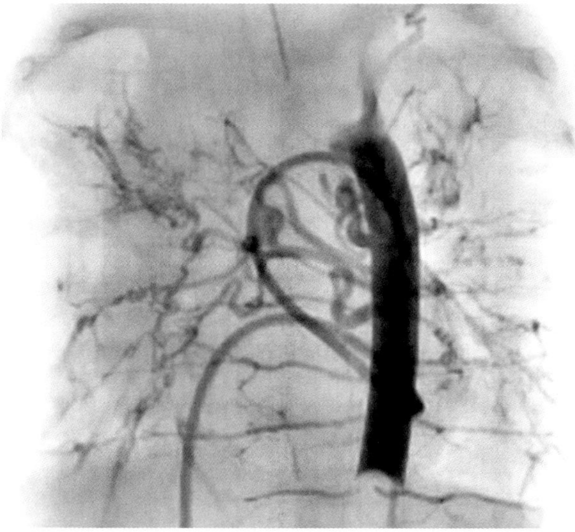

FIGURE and VIDEO 14-22. Systemic to pulmonary collaterals demonstrated by descending aortic angiography. Cine loop indicates course of the catheter from Inferior Vena Cava (1), Right Atrium(2), Left Atrium(3), Left Ventricle(4), and Arch of Aorta(5). Injection of contrast agent into the descending aorta reveals multiple sources of aortopulmonary collaterals.

Echocardiographic Evaluation

The acquired systemic-to-pulmonary artery collaterals are best visualized at their origin from the thoracic aorta and head and neck vessels by color Doppler imaging of the long axis of the aortic arch and its branches and proximal descending aorta. The aortic arch is best imaged from the suprasternal and high parasternal approaches. Color Doppler interrogation reveals abnormal sources of continuous flow originating from the undersurface of the distal aortic arch, the anterior wall of the proximal descending aorta, or the origin of the head and neck vessels (Figure and Video 14-22). The continuous flow from the SPC is easily differentiated from that of a patent ductus arteriosus; the SPC flow is not seen entering the intrapericardial pulmonary arteries. Pulsed Doppler interrogation shows continuous flow, consistent with systemic to pulmonary flow.

SPC should be searched for in premature infants, complicated by prolonged ventilation or the need for extended supplemental oxygen delivery. Echocardiographic examination with color Doppler, performed in premature infants to evaluate left-to-right shunts, should include careful search for systemic-to-pulmonary collaterals (Figures and Videos 14-23 and 14-24).

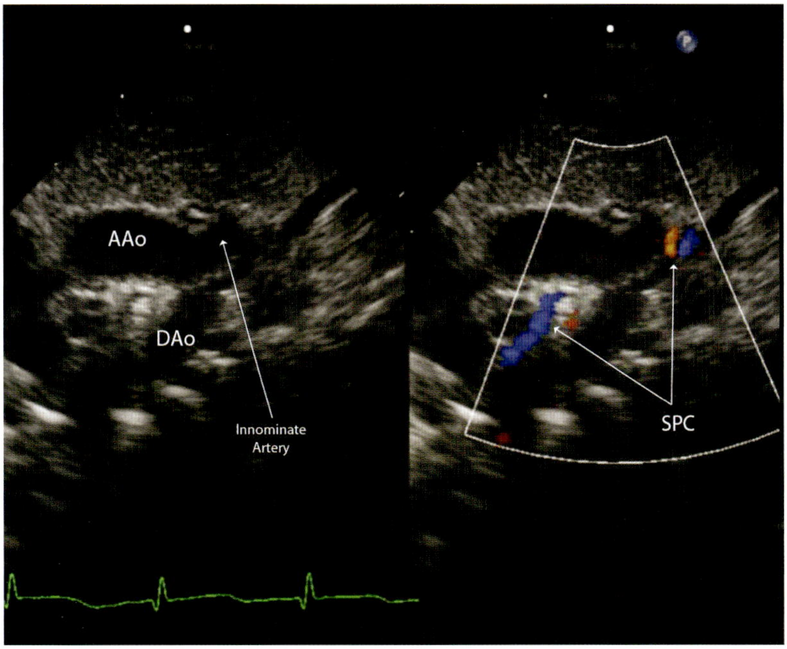

FIGURE and VIDEO 14-23. Systemic to pulmonary collateral originating from ascending and descending aorta. Abbreviations: AAo, ascending aorta; DAo, descending aorta; SPC, systemic to pulmonary collaterals.

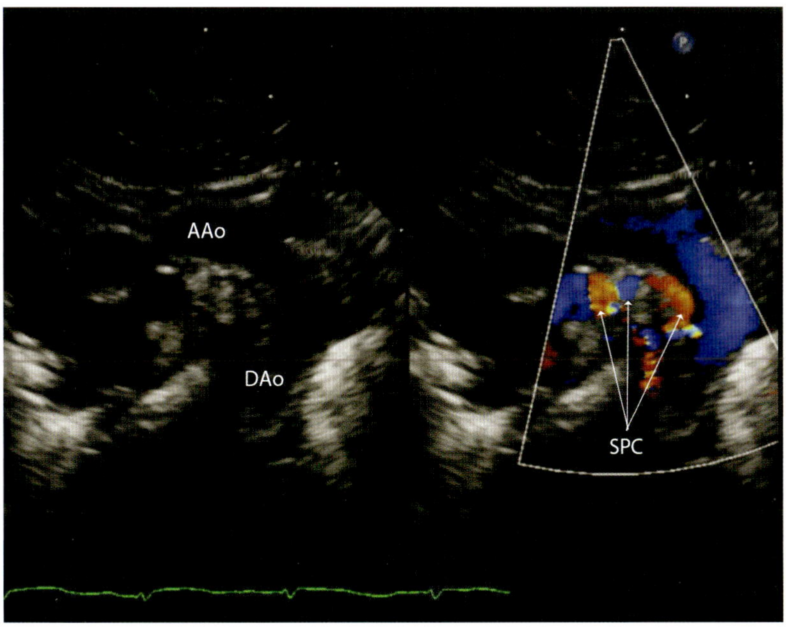

FIGURE and VIDEO 14-24. Systemic to pulmonary collateral originating from the descending aorta. Abbreviations: AAo, ascending aorta; DAo, descending aorta; SPC, systemic to pulmonary collaterals.

REFERENCES

1. Jan SL, Hwang B, Fu YC, Chai JW, Chi CS. Isolated neonatal ductus arteriosus aneurysm. *J Am Coll Cardiol.* 2002;39:342–347.
2. Tseng JJ, Jan SL. Fetal echocardiographic diagnosis of isolated ductusarteriosus aneurysm: a longitudinal study from 32 weeks of gestation to term. *Ultrasound Obstet Gynecol.* 2005;26:50–56.
3. Lund JT, Jensen MB, Hjelms E. Aneurysm of the ductus arteriosus: a review of the literature and the surgical implications. *Eur J Cardiothorac Surg.* 1991;5:566–570.
4. Shinkawa T, Yamagishi M, Shuntoh K, Fujiwara K, Watanabe T, Yoshida S. Infectious ductal aneurysm after coil embolization in an infant. *Ann Thorac Surg.* 2006 Jan;81:339–341.
5. Acherman RJ, Siassi B, Wells W, et al. Aneurysm of the ductus arteriosus: a congenital lesion. *Am J Perinatol.* 1998;15:653–659.
6. Dyamenahalli U, Smallhorn JF, Geva T, et al. Isolated ductusarteriosus aneurysm in the fetus and infant: a multi-institutional experience. *J Am Coll Cardiol.* 2000;36:262–269.
7. Sheridan RM, Michelfelder EC, Choe KA, et al. Ductus arteriosus aneurysm with massive thrombosis of pulmonary artery and fetal hydrops. *Pediatr Dev Pathol.* 2012;15:79–85.
8. Richardson P, McKenna W, Bristow M, et al. Report of the 1995 World Health Organization/International Society and Federation of Cardiology Task Force on the Definition and Classification of cardiomyopathies. *Circulation.* 1996;93:841–842.
9. Rosa LV, Salemi VM, Alexandre LM, Mady C. Noncompaction cardiomyopathy: a current view. *Arq Bras Cardiol.* 2011;97:e13–e19.
10. Wilkinson JD, Sleeper LA, Alvarez JA, Bublik N, Lipshultz SE; the Pediatric Cardiomyopathy Study Group. The Pediatric Cardiomyopathy Registry: 1995–2007. *ProgPediatrCardiol.* 2008 April;25(1):31–36.
11. Kim HJ, Yoo GH, Kil HR. Clinical outcome of acute myocarditis in children according to treatment modalities. *Korean J Pediatr.* 2010;53:745–752.
12. Robinson J, Hartling L, Vandermeer B, Crumley E, Klassen TP. Intravenous immunoglobulin for presumed viral myocarditis in children and adults. *Cochrane Database Syst Rev.* 2005 January 25;(1):CD004370.
13. Drucker NA, Colan SD, Lewis AB, et al. Gamma-globulin treatment of acute myocarditis in the pediatric population. *Circulation.* 1994;89:252–257.
14. Simpson KE, Canter CE. Acute myocarditis in children. *Expert Rev Cardiovasc Ther.* 2011;9:771–783.
15. Noori S, Acherman R, Siassi B, et al. A rare presentation of Pompe disease with massive hypertrophic cardiomyopathy at birth. *J Perinat Med.* 2002;30:517–521.
16. Allanson JE, Bohring A, Dörr HG, et al. The face of Noonan syndrome: Does phenotype predict genotype. *Am J Med Genet A.* 2010 August;152A(8):1960–1966.
17. Russo LM, Webber SA. Idiopathic restrictive cardiomyopathy in children. *Heart.* 2005;91:1199–1202.
18. Sekar P, Hornberger LK, Smallhorn JS. A case of restrictive cardiomyopathy presenting in fetal life with an isolated pericardial effusion. *Ultrasound Obstet Gynecol.* 2010;35:369–372.
19. Nucifora G, Benettoni A, Allocca G, Bussani R, Silvestri F. Arrhythmogenic right ventricular dysplasia/cardiomyopathy as a cause of sudden infant death. *J Cardiovasc Med (Hagerstown).* 2008;9:430–431.
20. Valdés-Dapena M, Gilbert-Barness E. Cardiovascular causes for sudden infant death. *PediatrPatholMol Med.* 2002;21:195–211.
21. Koh YY, Seo YU, Woo JJ, Chang KS, Hong SP. Familial isolated noncompaction of the ventricular myocardium in asymptomatic phase. *Yonsei Med J.* 2004;45:931–935.
22. Espinola-Zavaleta N, Soto ME, Castellanos LM, Jativa-Chavez S, Keirns C. Non-compacted cardiomyopathy: clinical echocardiographic study. *Cardiovasc Ultrasound.* 2006;4:35–49.
23. Lurie PR. The perspective of ventricular noncompaction as seen by a nonagenarian. *Cardiol Young.* 2008;18:243–249.
24. Hruda J, Sobotka-Plojhar MA, Fetter WP. Transient postnatal heart failure caused by noncompaction of the right ventricular myocardium. *PediatrCardiol.* 2005;26:452–454.
25. Jenni R, Oechslin E, Schneider J, Attenhofer JC, Kaufman PA. Echocardiographic and pathoanatomical characteristics of isolated left ventricular non-compaction: a step towards classification as a distinct cardiomyopathy. *Heart.* 2001;86:666–671.
26. Acherman RJ, Evans WN, Schwartz JK, et al. Right ventricular noncompaction associated with long QT in a fetus with right ventricular hypertrophy and cardiac arrhythmias. *PrenatDiagn.* 2008 June;28(6):551–553.
27. Ascher DP, Rosen P, Null DM, de Lemos RA. Systemic to pulmonary collaterals mimicking patent ductusarteriosus in neonates with prolonged ventilatory courses. *J Pediatr.* 1985;107:282–284.
28. Goodman G, Perkin R, Anas NG, Sperling DR, Hicks DA, Rowen M. Pulmonary hypertension in infants with bronchopulmonary dysplasia. *J Pediatr.* 1988;112:67–72.
29. Abman SH, Sondheimer HM. Pulmonary circulation and cardiovascularsequelae of bronchopulmonary dysplasia. In: Weir EK, ed. *The Diagnosis and Treatment of*

Pulmonary Hypertension. Mount Kisko, NY: Futura Publishing Inc; 1992:155–180.

30. Acherman RJ, Siassi B, Pratti-Madrid G, Luna C, Lewis AB, et al. Systemic to pulmonary collaterals in very low birth weight infants: color Doppler detection of systemic to pulmonary connections during neonatal and early infancy period. *Pediatrics*. 2000;105:528–532.
31. Do KH, Goo FM, Im JG, Kim KW, Chung JW, Park JH. Systemic arterial supply to the lungs in adults: spiral CT findings. *Radiographics*. 2001;21:387–402.
32. Botenga AS. The significance of broncho-pulmonary anastomoses in pulmonary anomalies: a selective angiographic study. *RadiolClin Biol*. 1969;38:309–328.
33. Shaughnessy RD, Reller MD, Rice MJ, McDonald RW. Development of systemic to pulmonary collateral arteries in premature infants. *J Pediatr*. 1997;131:763–765.
34. Luna CF, Acherman R, Ebrahimi M, Siassi B. Development of aortopulmonarycollateral circulation in infants with chronic lung disease. *Clin Res*. 1994;42:91. Abstract.
35. Evans WE, Acherman RJ, Collazos JC, Restrepo H, Mayman GA. Expedited Oxygen Wean after Coil Embolization of Systemic to Pulmonary Collaterals in a Premature Infant with Bronchopulmonary Dysplasia. *J Ultrasound Med*. 2007;26:695–697.

CHAPTER 15

Suspecting Congenital Heart Disease*

Bijan Siassi, Mahmood Ebrahimi, and Ruben J. Acherman

- **INTRODUCTION**
  - Review of Fetal and Transitional Physiology
- **CONGENITAL HEART DEFECTS**
- **CYANOSIS WITH DECREASED PULMONARY BLOOD FLOW**
  - Tetralogy of Fallot
  - Tetralogy of Fallot with Pulmonary Atresia
  - Pulmonary Atresia with Intact Ventricular Septum
  - Tricuspid Atresia
  - Ebstein's Anomaly
- **CYANOSIS WITH INCREASED PULMONARY BLOOD FLOW**
  - Transposition of Great Arteries
  - Persistent Truncus Arteriosus
- **CYANOSIS WITH PULMONARY EDEMA**
  - Total Anomalous Pulmonary Venous Return
- **CARDIOGENIC SHOCK**
  - Hypoplastic Left Heart Syndrome
- **HEART FAILURE WITH DIFFERENTIAL CYANOSIS**
  - Coarctation of the Aorta
  - Interruption of the Aortic Arch
- **ACYANOTIC CONGENITAL HEART DISEASE**
  - Atrioventricular Septal Defect
  - Ventricular Septal Defect
  - Atrial Septal Defect
- **PATENT DUCTUS ARTERIOSUS**
- **REFERENCES**

INTRODUCTION

Although prenatal detection of congenital heart defects (CHDs) is attempted during routine fetal ultrasonography, it is estimated that, at present, only 36% of CHDs are detected antenatally, with a wide variation among different localities and states.[1] Since the incidence of CHDs is approximately 8 per 1000 live births, and only a third are detected prior to birth, the proposition to perform echocardiography in all neonates for detecting CHDs[2] is a huge and costly undertaking in absence of appropriate infrastructure and adequate funding. However, the initial echocardiogram obtained in any neonate (for any indication) should be as complete as possible and interpreted by a pediatric cardiologist who is competent in the interpretation of echocardiograms, or alternately, if it is performed by a non-cardiologist physician, the physician should have enough training to at least *suspect* the presence of a CHD, which will then require referral to the pediatric cardiology service for further evaluation and management. Understanding fetal and transitional circulatory physiology, as it is affected by a CHD, is essential in anticipating the presentation of a CHD in the neonate. It is important to remember that CHDs that would have

*Videos can be accessed at http://PracticalNeonatalEcho.com.

significantly affected fetal systemic or placental circulation would likely have led to a fetal demise. Therefore, almost all critical congenital cardiac defects (CCHDs) that present at the time of birth were compatible with a fetal circulation that had adjusted to provide normal or near normal fetal systemic and placental circulation in utero; in the few instances in which fetal circulation is compromised, it is not to such degree as to cause fetal demise prior to birth.

Review of Fetal and Transitional Physiology

In fetuses with a normal heart, the right and left ventricles work in parallel; thus, fetal cardiac output is nearly equal to the combined output of both ventricles and approximates 430 ml/kg/min.[3] The right ventricle is dominant, accounting for approximately 56% of total cardiac output and pumps against a slightly greater resistance than the left ventricle (Figures 15-1 and 15-2). The fetal circulation in cases of aortic or pulmonary atresia are illustrated for comparison. In each case, the fetal systemic and placental circulations are preserved because of increases in the right or the left ventricular flow which will carry the function of combined ventricular outputs (Figure 15-3). Immediately following birth, ventilation of lungs, in association with increased arterial oxygen tension, leads to a sharp decrease in pulmonary vascular resistance and a marked increase in pulmonary blood flow. At the same time, separation of umbilico-placental circulation decreases inferior vena cava flow which in conjunction

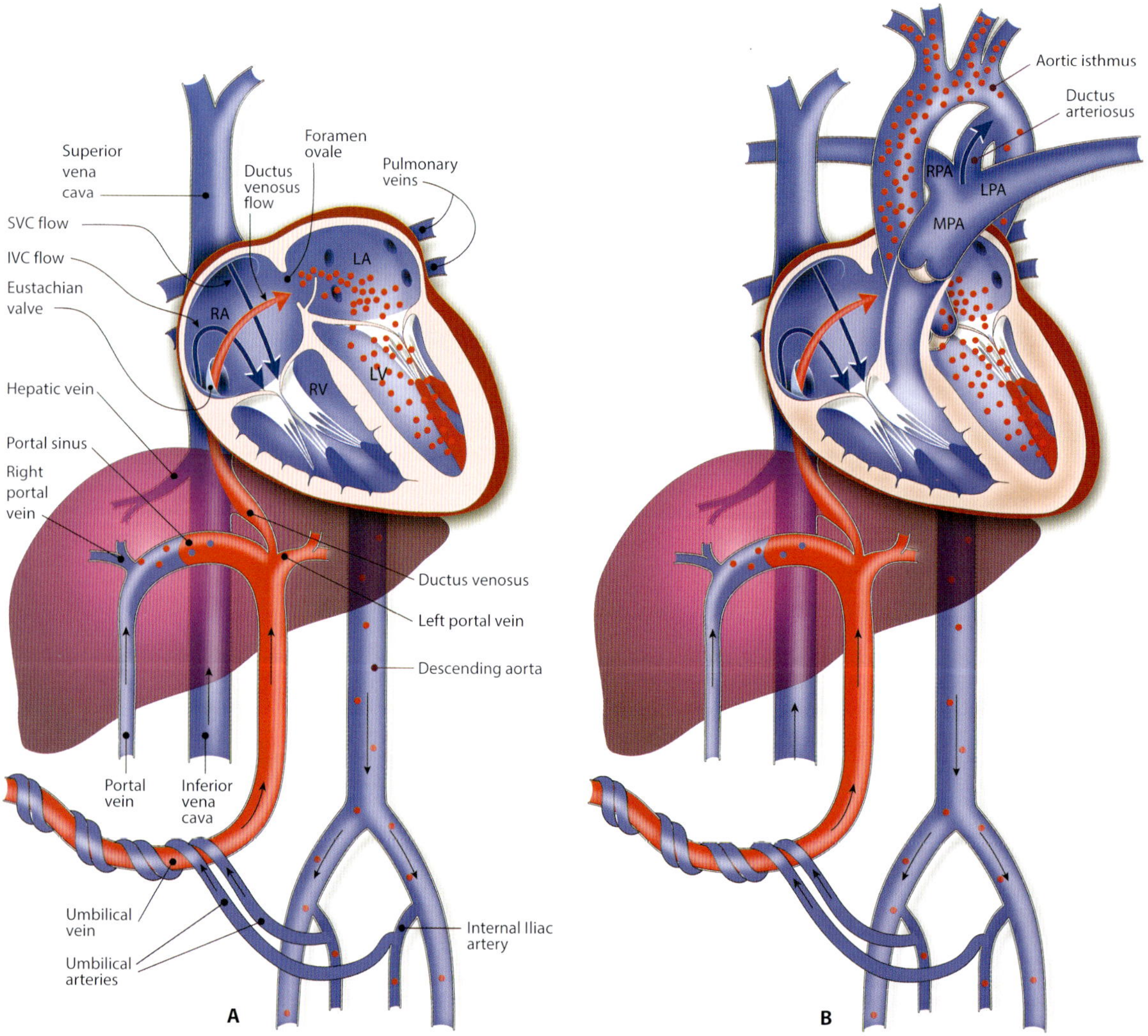

FIGURE 15-1. Figure A and B Fetal Circulation.

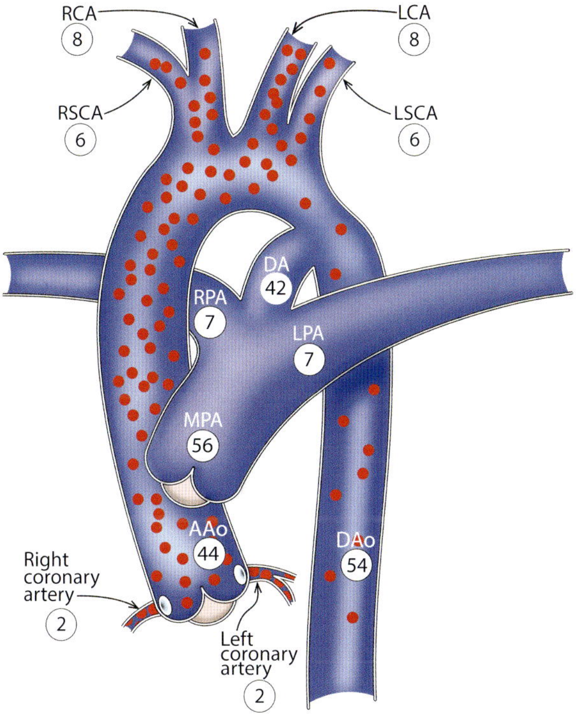

FIGURE 15-2. Systemic and placental circulation in fetuses with normal heart.

with increased pulmonary flow and venous return to the left atrium, results in the functional closure of the foramen ovale. Closure of ductus arteriosus during the first 48 hours of life,[4] completes separation of the pulmonary and systemic circulations. Postnatally, the two ventricles work in series, so neonatal cardiac output represents the volume of blood pumped by either the right or left ventricle, *not* the combined output of the two ventricles (Figures 15-4 and 15-5). The presentation of a CCHD during the early neonatal period depends upon:

- The status of the patent ductus arteriosus (PDA) that is widely patent initially, but develops signs of constriction and closure beyond 12 hours of life.
- Patent foramen ovale (PFO) that usually remains patent, and, depending upon the pressure relationship between the right and left atria, either shunts right to left or left to right. Restriction of flow at the PFO often contributes to the clinical presentation of CHD.
- Decreasing pulmonary vascular resistance. This will lead to increased pulmonary blood flow, further aggravating clinical symptomatology.

With few exceptions, neonates with CCHDs have minimal symptoms and appear deceptively healthy during the first 12 hours of life, which is mainly due to the presence of

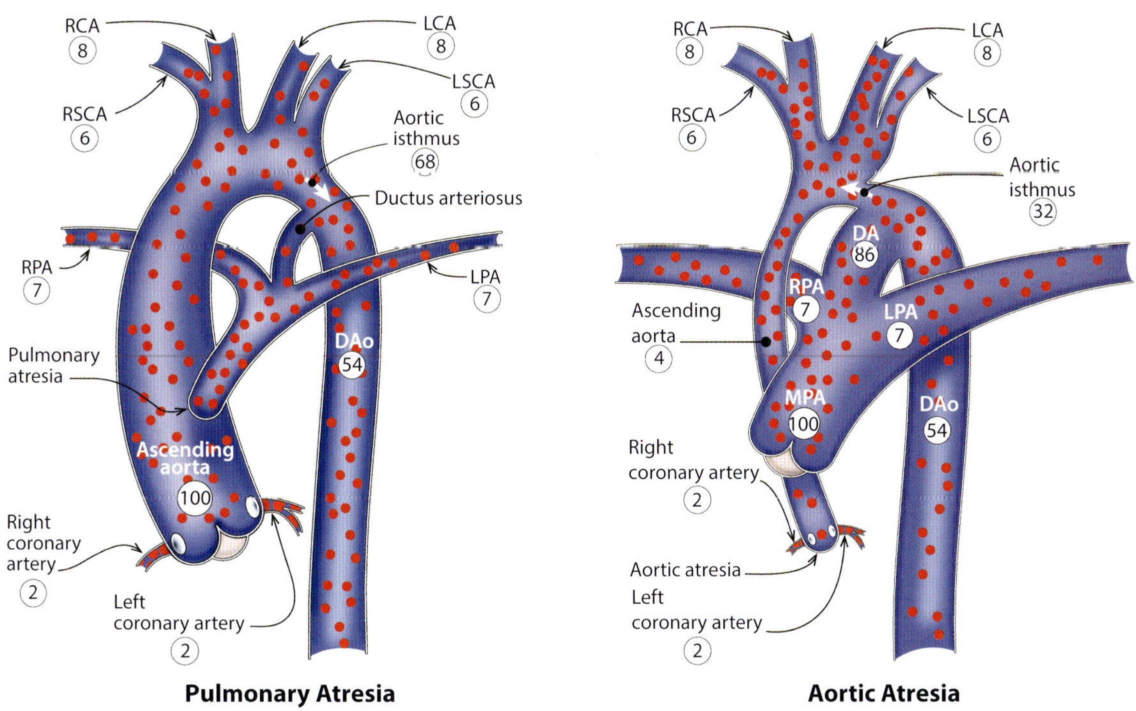

FIGURE 15-3. Systemic and placental circulation in fetuses with aortic or pulmonary atresia.

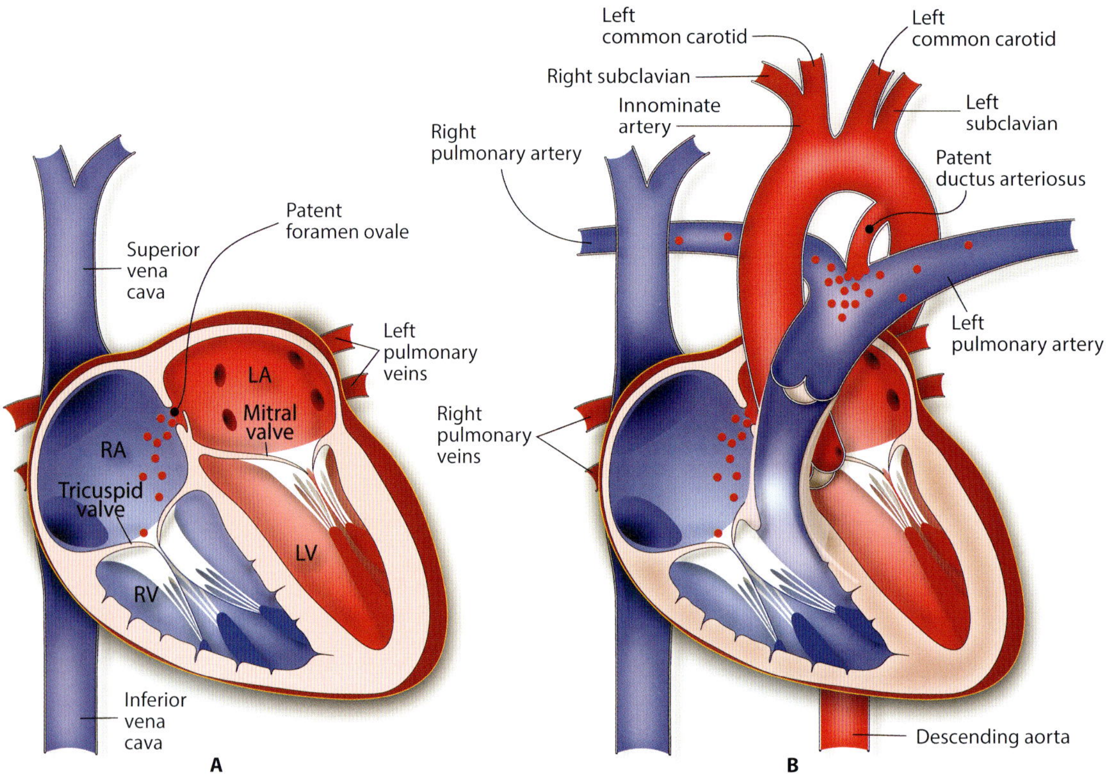

FIGURE 15-4. Newborn circulation during first 72 hours of life.

patent fetal channels (PFO, PDA) and the persistence of a relatively high pulmonary vascular resistance. The exceptions are heart failure that is already present prior to birth (such as in fetuses with tachyarrhythmia who generally have normal hearts), fetuses with cardiomyopathies, and fetuses with Ebstein's malformation of the tricuspid valve. In the latter instance, when the Ebstein's anomaly is severe enough, it can lead to fetal demise or severe heart failure at any gestational age. Other examples of neonates with symptomatic CCHDs include hypoplastic left heart syndrome (HLHS) and D-transposition of the great arteries (D-TGA) with a restrictive foramen ovale or intact atrial septum, or obstructed total anomalous pulmonary venous return (TAPVR). All of these forms of CCHDs can present immediately at birth, requiring vigorous resuscitation that is usually not effective, and they will likely require immediate transfer to the nearest pediatric cardiac center.

CONGENITAL HEART DEFECTS

It is customary to divide CHDs in two broad categories: cyanotic and acyanotic heart defects. Typically, cyanotic defects present with hypoxemia as the presenting symptom, and acyanotic defects with no symptoms or congestive heart failure/respiratory distress. However, some forms of CCHDs can present with overlapping symptoms of both respiratory distress and varying degrees of cyanosis, and others can manifest both prominent cyanosis as well as cardiogenic shock as the presenting symptomatology. With expanded use of pulse oximetry and echocardiography in the newborn, a significant number of these infants are being diagnosed before developing life-threatening symptomatology.

The following sections discuss various forms of CHDs that may be encountered in the newborn period. The transitional circulation in neonates with CHDs will be briefly described as it pertains to each defect. The typical echocardiographic findings for each type of CHD will also be described briefly. These will be given as a guide to the examiner as how to *suspect* the presence of cardiac defects. A more detailed description of the clinical features, echocardiographic findings, clinical course, and treatments of these infants is well beyond the scope of this chapter and the present book. For more information, consult other, more comprehensive references.[5,6]

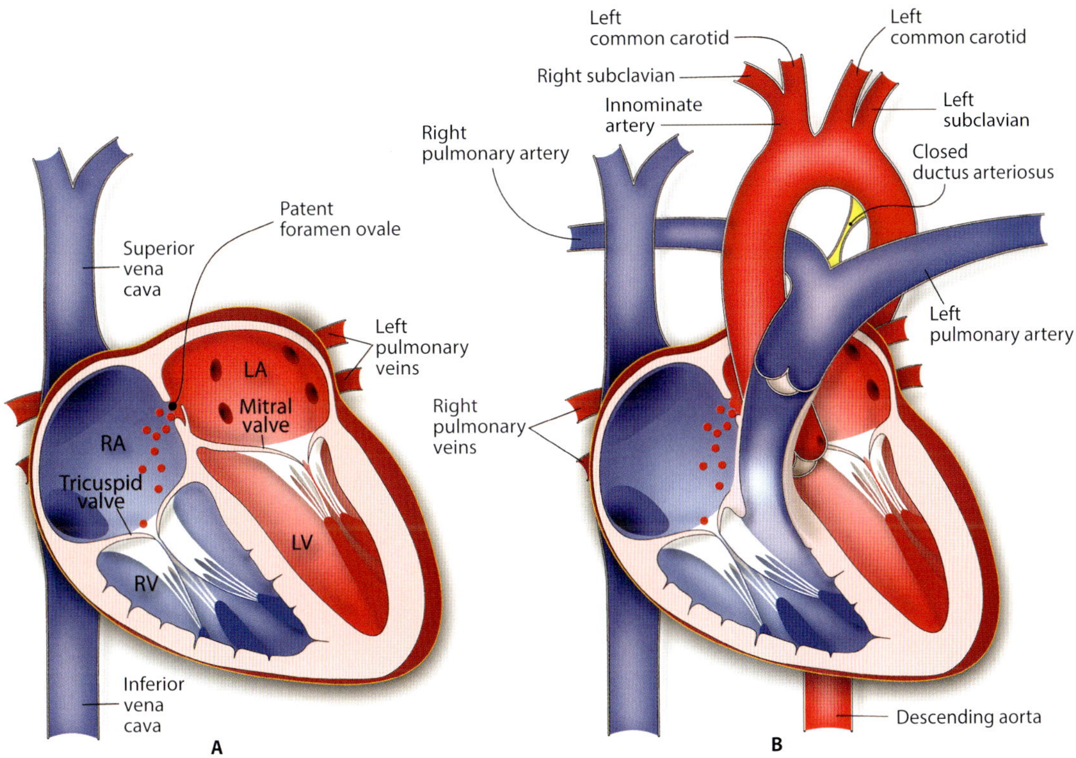

FIGURE 15-5. Newborn circulation beyond 72 hours of life.

CYANOSIS WITH DECREASED PULMONARY BLOOD FLOW

Tetralogy of Fallot

The four classical findings in tetralogy of Fallot include pulmonary valvar and infundibular stenosis, often including a small pulmonary valve annulus; malaligned ventricular septal defect (VSD) that is subaortic and generally extends into membranous septum; overriding of the aorta over the VSD; right ventricular hypertrophy. Since neonates are born with right ventricular hypertrophy, the latter is not a distinguishing feature of this defect in the neonate (Figure 15-6). In tetralogy of Fallot, the VSD is large and unrestrictive; therefore, the symptomatology is mainly related to the degree and severity of infundibular and valvar pulmonary stenosis. Severe stenosis leads to a large right-to-left shunt, with increasing severity of cyanosis, unless compensated for by the presence of a PDA with left-to-right shunting that will augment pulmonary blood flow and improve the systemic oxygen saturation. Conversely, mild stenosis can result in a large left-to-right shunt, which can lead to pulmonary over circulation and congestive heart failure. This

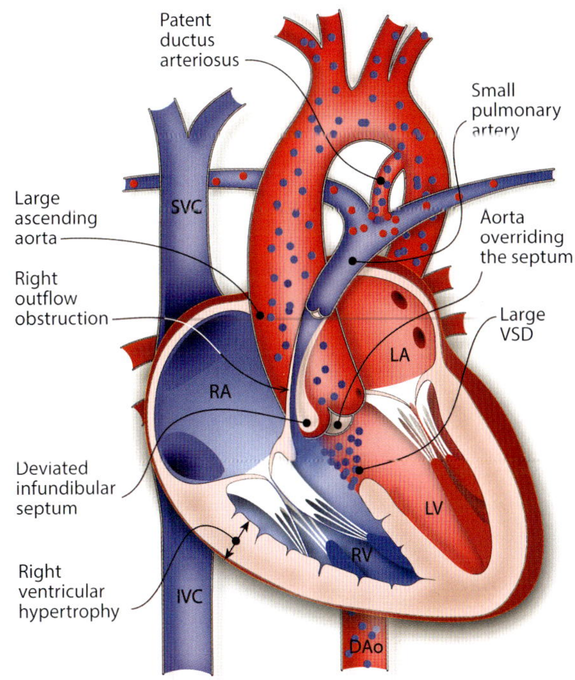

FIGURE 15-6. Tetralogy of Fallot.

is aggravated further in the presence of a PDA, which increases the amount of left-to-right shunting into the pulmonary arteries. Therefore, the spectrum of clinical symptomatology in tetralogy of Fallot ranges from the non-cyanotic neonate with congestive heart failure to a ductal-dependent cyanotic lesion with critical cyanosis upon closure of the PDA.

Echocardiography

Parasternal long axis reveals a large VSD, with the aorta overriding the VSD, and a large aortic valve annulus. Right-to-left, left-to-right, or bidirectional shunting can be noted across the VSD (Figure and Video 15-7). Parasternal short axis at the base of the heart or parasternal long axis of the right ventricular outflow tract and pulmonary artery demonstrate infundibular and valvar pulmonary stenosis, with a small pulmonary annulus, and turbulent flow through pulmonary valve (Figure and Video 15-8). With the use of two-dimensional (2D) imaging and color flow Doppler, parasternal short axis at the base and suprasternal ductal cut can visualize the presence and the size of a PDA. Associated defects can be investigated through other appropriate views.[7]

Tetralogy of Fallot with Pulmonary Atresia

This condition, also known as pulmonary atresia with VSD, represents an extreme form of tetralogy of Fallot in which the pulmonary outflow tract is completely atretic, and there is obligatory pure right-to-left shunting through the VSD. Pulmonary blood flow will be entirely dependent upon the size of left to right shunting through a PDA (Figure 15-9) or aortopulmonary collateral flow (see Chapter 14). If pulmonary blood flow is dependent solely upon a PDA, any constriction or closure of the ductus will lead to profound cyanosis.

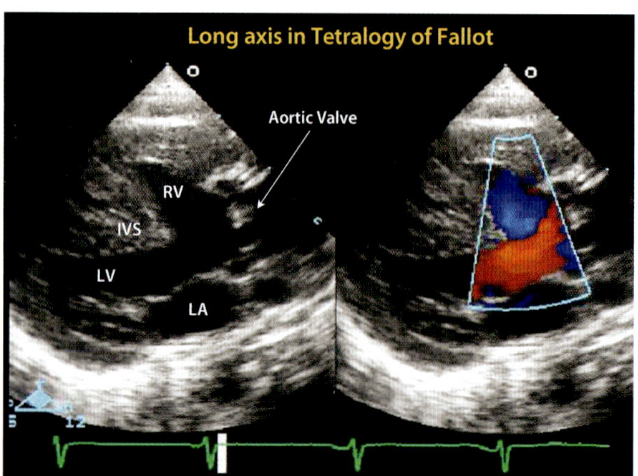

FIGURE and VIDEO 15-7. Parasternal long axis view of tetralogy of Fallot. Right ventricle, RV, Interventricular septum, IVS, Left atrium, LA, Left ventricle LV.

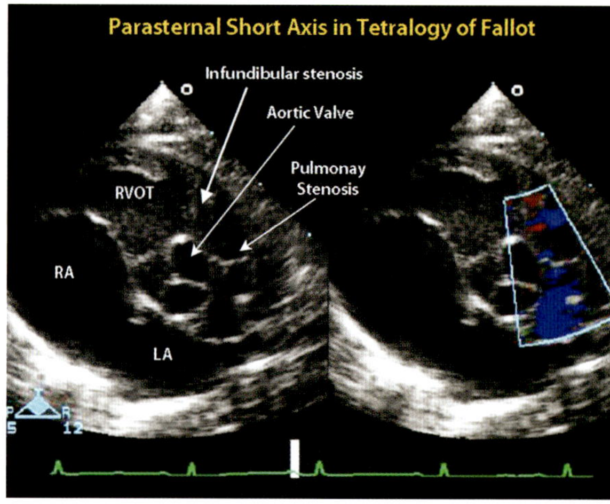

FIGURE and VIDEO 15-8. Parasternal short axis view of tetralogy of Fallot. Abbreviations: RVOT, right ventricular outflow tract; RV, right ventricle; RA, right atrium; LA, left atrium.

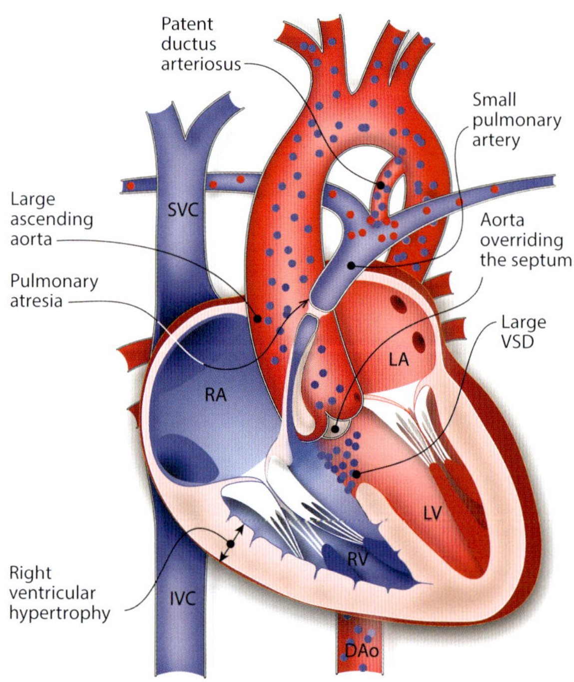

FIGURE 15-9. Tetralogy of Fallot with pulmonary atresia.

Echocardiography

The echocardiographic findings are the same as in tetralogy of Fallot with pulmonary stenosis, except that there is no flow through the atretic pulmonary outflow tract. The branch pulmonary arteries (and main pulmonary artery, if present) are filled in retrograde fashion through a PDA. Parasternal long- and short-axis and suprasternal aortic arch and ductal cut imaging will delineate the typical findings (Figures and Videos 15-10 and 15-12). The presence of aortopulmonary collaterals can be suspected or surmised by visualization of one or more collateral vessels arising from the descending aorta and/or aortic arch, and displaying a continuous arterial spectral Doppler waveform. In the most extreme cases of multiple aortopulmonary collateral arteries (also known as MAPCAs), confluent central branch pulmonary arteries might not be visible.

Pulmonary Atresia with Intact Ventricular Septum

Most infants with this condition have a hypoplastic right ventricle and diminutive tricuspid valve in association with pulmonary atresia (Figure 15-13). However, a few can have a normal or massively enlarged right ventricular cavity, and present with severe tricuspid regurgitation leading to both fetal and neonatal heart failure. In any case, all neonates with pulmonary atresia and intact ventricular septum have a ductal-dependent pulmonary circulation, and cyanosis increases markedly with ductal constriction or closure.

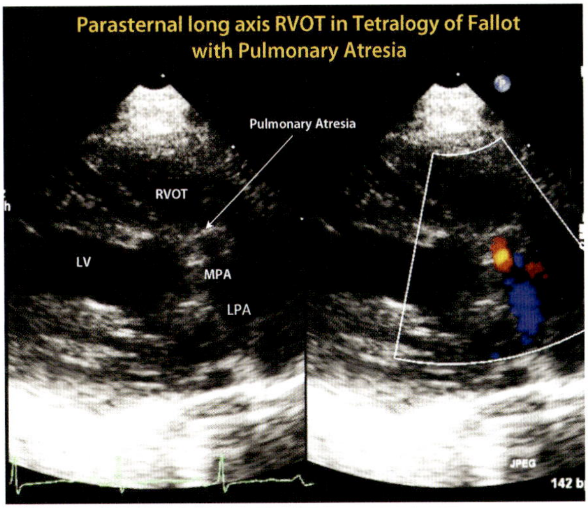

FIGURE and VIDEO 15-11. Parasternal long axis Right Ventricular outflow view of Tetralogy of Fallot with pulmonary Atresia. Distal main pulmonary artery, MPA, is visualized with PDA shunting left to right and no antegrade flow through an atretic pulmonary valve.

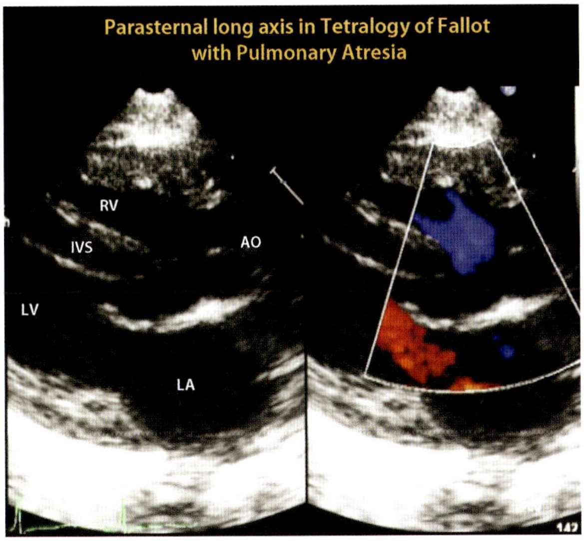

FIGURE and VIDEO 15-10. Parasternal long axis view of Tetralogy of Fallot with pulmonary atresia. Abbreviations: RV, right ventricle; IVS, interventricular septum; Ao, oorta; LA, left atrium.

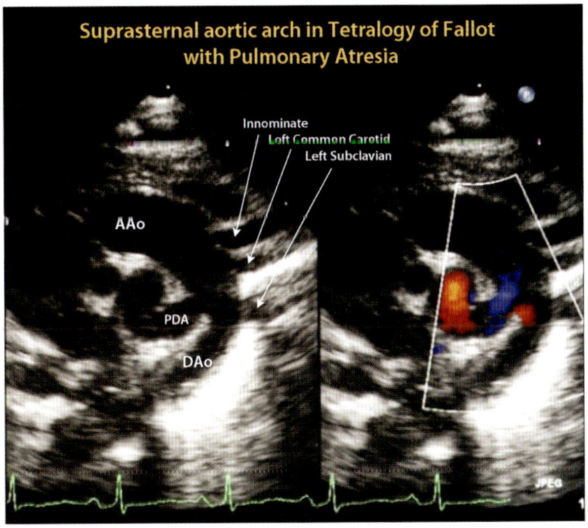

FIGURE and VIDEO 15-12. Suprasternal aortic arch view of tetralogy of Fallot with pulmonary atresia. It indicates PDA arising from transverse arch of aorta opposite left carotid artery with left to right shunt and no antegrade flow through an atretic pulmonary valve. Abbreviations: AAo, ascending aorta; DAo, descending aorta.

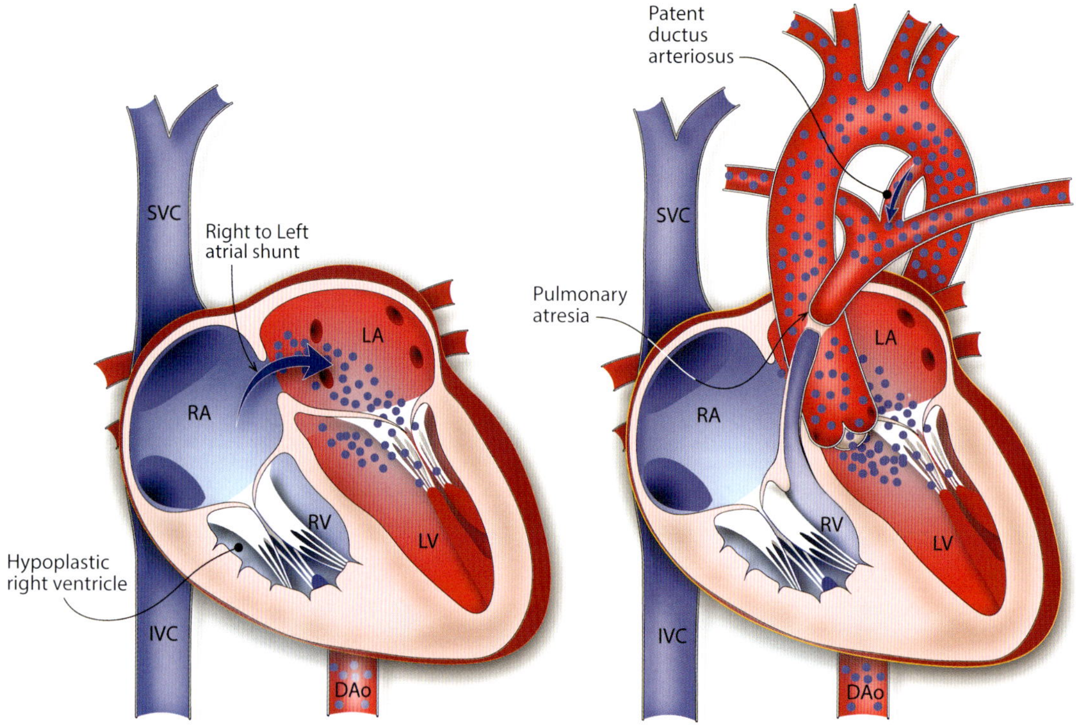

FIGURE 15-13. Diagram of pulmonary atresia and intact ventricular septum.

Echocardiography

Apical four-chamber view demonstrates the size of the right ventricle and tricuspid valve in comparison to the left ventricle and mitral valve (Figure and Video 15-14). The right ventricle is heavily trabeculated and small indentations in the ventricular septum or free wall of right ventricle might be indicative of the ventriculo-coronary artery fistulae that can be encountered in this condition. Parasternal long-axis right ventricular outflow or parasternal short-axis at base demonstrate pulmonary valve atresia and retrograde filling of the main pulmonary artery via a PDA (Figure and Video 15-15). The presence and size of the PDA is best viewed from the suprasternal aortic arch and ductal cut (Figure and Video 15-16). The PDA is often tortuous and has an abnormal takeoff opposite the left common carotid artery (and a vertical orientation) from the transverse aortic arch. The atrial septal communication is best viewed from subcostal coronal posterior or sagittal bicaval view. The large right to left atrial shunt constitutes total cardiac output, and

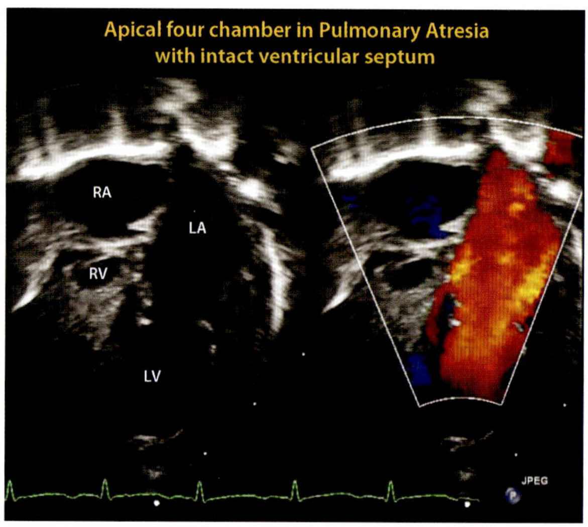

FIGURE and VIDEO 15-14. Apical four-chamber view of pulmonary atresia with intact ventricular septum. Note hypoplastic right ventricle and large right to left shunt through an atrial septal defect.

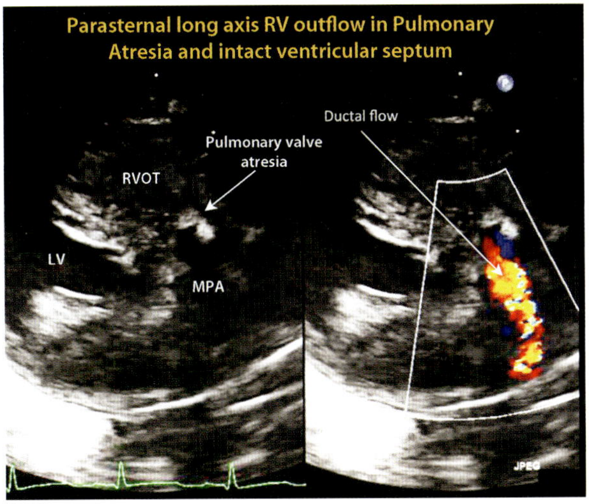

FIGURE and VIDEO 15-15. Parasternal long axis, right ventricular outflow view of pulmonary atresia with intact ventricular septum. Note no antegrade flow through an atretic pulmonary valve and a large left to right shunt through PDA which provides the only source for pulmonary circulation.

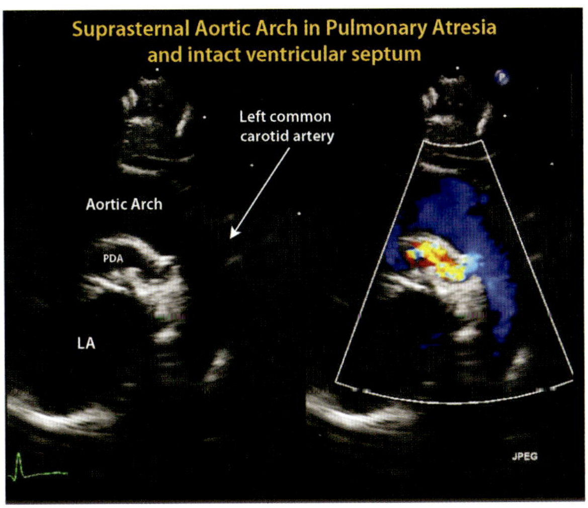

FIGURE and VIDEO 15-16. Suprasternal aortic arch view in pulmonary atresia with intact ventricular septum. Note PDA arises opposite the left carotid artery from transverse aortic arch.

unobstructed shunting is only possible through a widely stretched PFO or good sized atrial septal defect.

Tricuspid Atresia

In this condition, there is congenital absence or agenesis of the tricuspid valve. The inflow portion of the right ventricle is absent and the right ventricular cavity is decreased in size, whereas the left ventricle is enlarged and hypertrophic. During fetal life, the left ventricle carries the majority of total fetal cardiac output; postnatally, it carries most of the pulmonary and systemic circulation. There is an obligatory right to left shunt that equals systemic flow through a stretched PFO or an atrial septal defect. An associated muscular VSD of variable size is commonly present (Figure 15-17). The great arteries are usually normally related, but less commonly they can be transposed. With normally related great arteries, the degree of cyanosis and ductal dependency is related to the degree of obstruction to blood flow through the VSD as well as the degree of pulmonic or subpulmonic stenosis. When there is severe flow restriction through the VSD and/or pulmonary artery, the PDA becomes the major conduit of flow to the lungs, and its constriction or closure will lead to progressively severe cyanosis. In contrast, in neonates with no flow restriction through the VSD or pulmonary valve, there can be increased flow to the lungs and congestive heart failure may be the consequence.

Echocardiography

The apical four-chamber view is usually diagnostic for tricuspid atresia. The VSD and atrial communication can also be seen in this view (Figure and Video 15-18). However, the size of the VSD, atrial shunt, and the relationship of the great arteries can best be evaluated by other views described in their appropriate sections. A detailed discussion of the variation in anatomy and associated defects with tricuspid atresia is beyond the scope of this review.

Ebstein's Anomaly

Prominent features of this anomaly include displacement of the septal and posterior leaflets of tricuspid valve into the cavity of the right ventricle. The degree of displacement ranges from minimal to extremely severe. The degree of tricuspid valve displacement is usually associated with the severity of valvar insufficiency, and the clinical presentation depends upon the degree of insufficiency. There can be minimal cardiac symptoms (with mild tricuspid insufficiency) to marked cardiomegaly with massive enlargement of the right atrium and heart failure in the fetus and newborn (with severe tricuspid insufficiency). Enlargement of right atrium is partially due to tricuspid insufficiency and also due to the addition of the atrialized segment of the right ventricle as part of enlarged right atrium (Figure 15-19). Newborns with congestive heart failure and severe tricuspid insufficiency usually have a

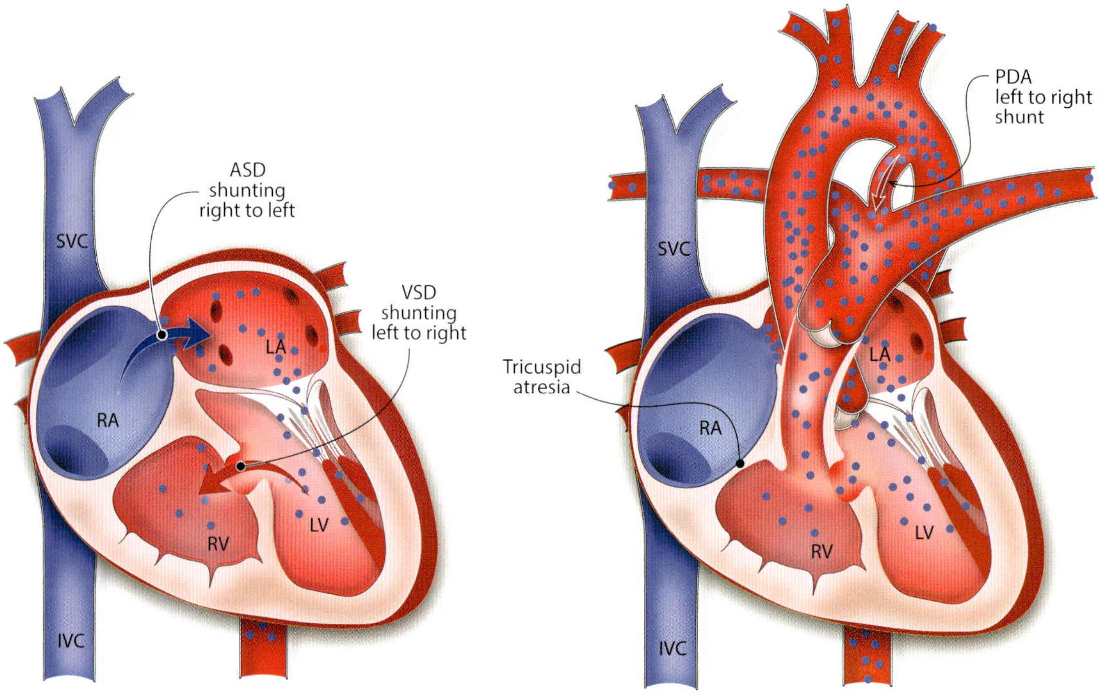

FIGURE 15-17. Tricuspid atresia with ventricular septal defect. Abbreviations: SVC, Superior Vena Cava, IVC, Inferior Vena Cava.

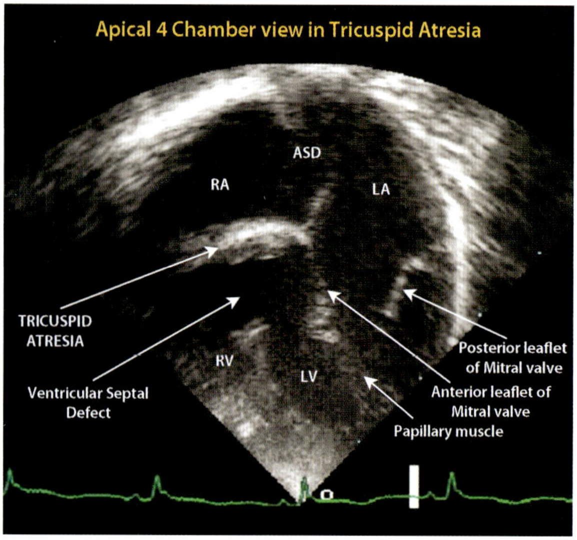

FIGURE and VIDEO 15-18. Apical four-chamber view of tricuspid atresia with ventricular septal defect.

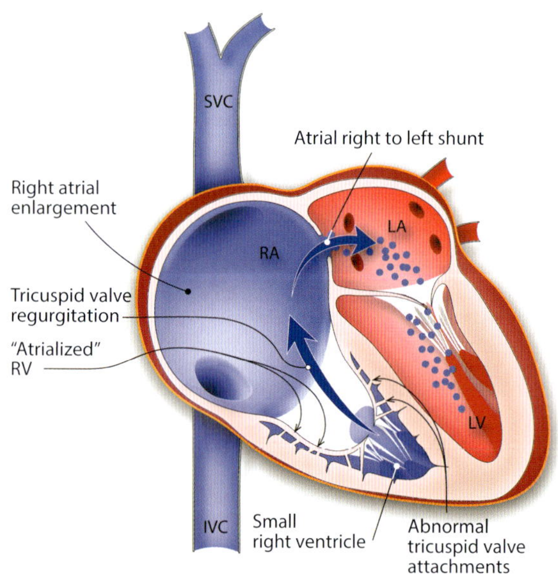

FIGURE 15-19. Diagram of Ebstein's anomaly of the tricuspid valve. Markedly enlarged RA including the atrialized portion of RV is displayed. Right to left atrial shunting leading to various degrees of cyanosis may be present.

right to left shunt through a PFO or an atrial septal defect, as well as decreased right ventricular output through the pulmonary valve, and decreased pulmonary blood flow unless augmented by a PDA with left-to-right shunting (ductal-dependent cyanotic CHD). Fortunately, in most cases, with the decrease in pulmonary vascular resistance after birth, the severity of tricuspid insufficiency diminishes, leading to improvement in right ventricular output and improved systemic arterial oxygen saturation.

Echocardiogram

The apical four-chamber view or its modifications are best for visualization of the displacement of tricuspid septal leaflet attachments as well as the degree and severity of tricuspid regurgitation via color flow Doppler (Figure and Video 15-20). Atrial septal anatomy and the presence of a PFO or atrial septal defect are best visualized via the subcostal sagittal bicaval or coronal views. Color flow and pulse wave Doppler will indicate the presence of right to left or left-to-right shunting (Figure and Video 15-21). The PDA is best visualized from parasternal short axis at the base or a suprasternal ductal cut. The pulmonary valve is best visualized from parasternal long-axis RV outflow view and its patency can be evaluated by color flow Doppler. A detailed analysis of defects associated with Ebstein's anomaly is beyond the scope of this review.

CYANOSIS WITH INCREASED PULMONARY BLOOD FLOW

Transposition of Great Arteries

The most common type of transposition is D-transposition of great arteries (D-TGA), in which the aorta arises from the right ventricle and the pulmonary artery from the left ventricle. In most cases of D-TGA, the aorta is located to the right of pulmonary artery (Figure 15-22). Since the pulmonary and systemic circulation function in parallel, D-TGA is the only cardiac condition in which the amount of pulmonary blood flow has no direct relationship with the degree of cyanosis. Admixture of blood between the two circulations (which occurs at level of the PDA , PFO, and VSD if present) determines the degree of cyanosis. The flow through PDA (and VSD) is usually from systemic to pulmonary circulation, whereas the flow through the PFO is from the pulmonary to systemic circulation. In the absence of other defects, any narrowing or closure of either of these shunts will lead to severe, life threatening cyanosis.

The other form of transposition, L-Transposition of great arteries (L-TGA) is a rare condition that generally does not result in cyanosis. In this anomaly, the atria are connected to the inappropriate ventricles (known as atrioventricular discordance), and the ventricles in turn are connected to the inappropriate great arteries (known as ventriculo-arterial discordance). This places the morphologic right ventricle (connected to the left atrium) to the left of the morphologic left ventricle (connected to the right atrium). The aorta arises from the morphologic right ventricle and is positioned to the left of the pulmonary artery that arises from the morphologic left ventricle. This "double discordance" results in physiologic correction, with pulmonary venous blood directed to the aorta, and systemic venous blood directed to the pulmonary artery. Therefore, such patients are rarely cyanotic. Hence, L-TGA is often termed "congenitally corrected transposition of great arteries."

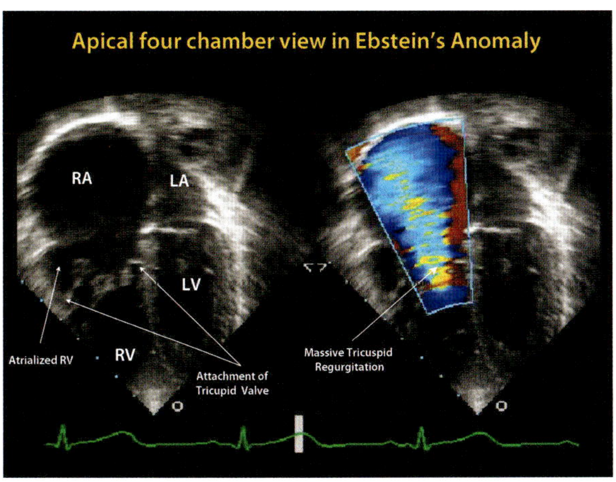

FIGURE and VIDEO 15-20. Apical four-chamber view of Ebstein's anomaly of the tricuspid valve.

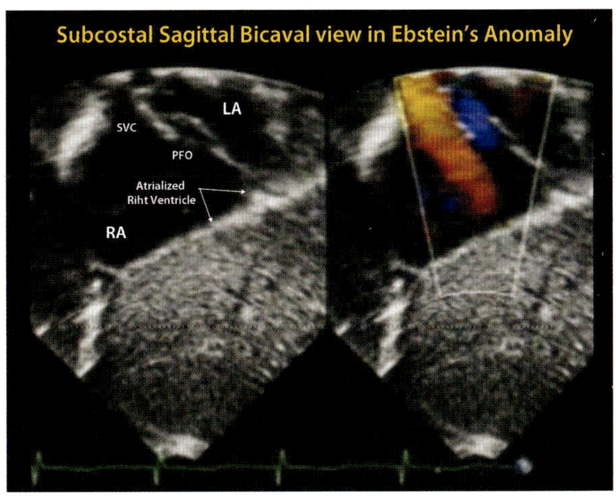

FIGURE and VIDEO 15-21. Subcostal sagittal bicaval view of the atrial septum in a patient with Ebstein's anomaly of the tricuspid valve. Note atrialized portion of RA.

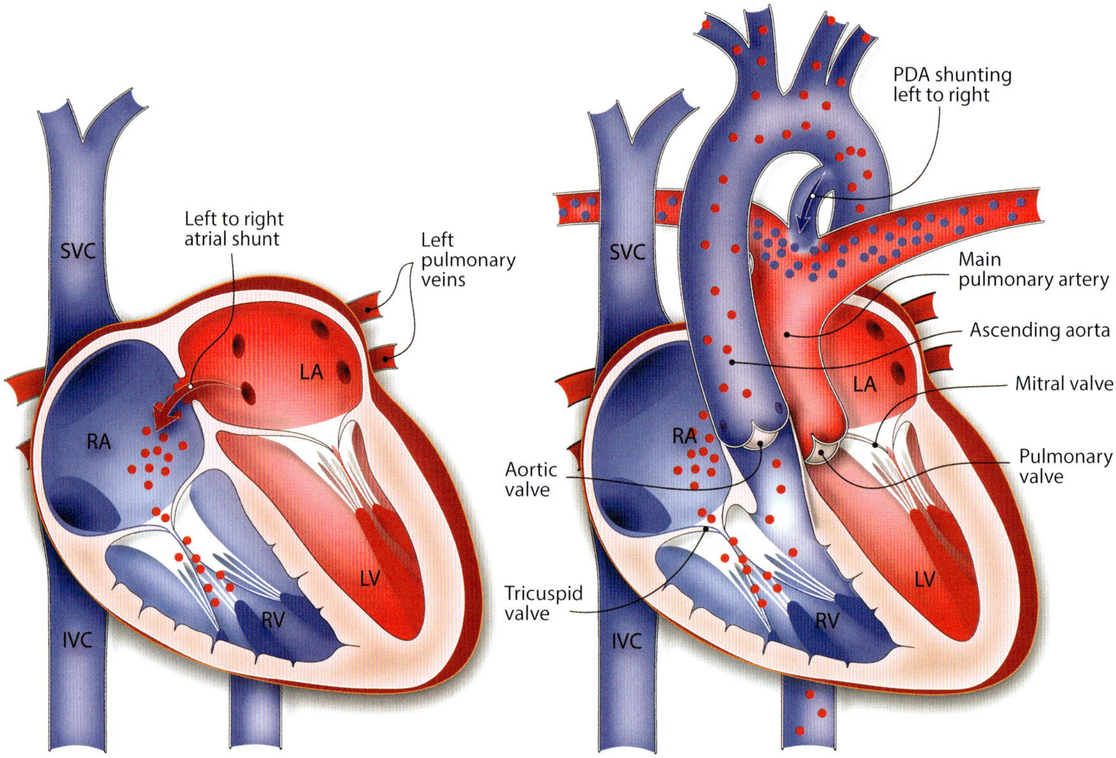

FIGURE 15-22. Diagram of D-transposition of the great arteries, atrial septal defect and patent ductus arteriosus.

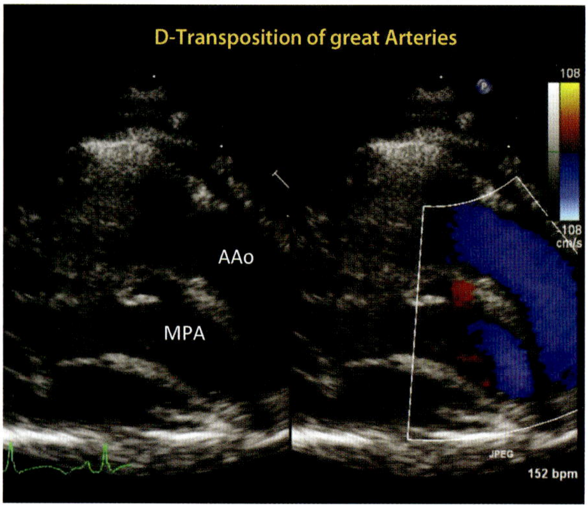

FIGURE and VIDEO 15-23. Parasternal long axis view of D-transposition of the great arteries. Note parallel course of Aorta and MPA.

Echocardiography

Standard parasternal long-axis and parasternal long-axis RV outflow views are often diagnostic of D-TGA. The aorta and pulmonary artery are seen to course parallel to each other (Figure and Video 15-23). Subcostal coronal and sagittal views will demonstrate a PFO or atrial septal defect, and the direction of shunting can be demonstrated by color flow Doppler (Figure and Video 15-24). The suprasternal aortic arch and ductal cuts will delineate the size and flow through the PDA if it is still patent (Figure and Video 15-25). A detailed analysis of all the defects associated with D-TGA (including coronary artery variations) is possible by echocardiography, but it is beyond the scope of this chapter. Also, the echocardiographic features of L-TGA will not be discussed in this chapter; refer to other references for a more detailed discussion on the echocardiographic evaluation of both D-TGA and L-TGA.

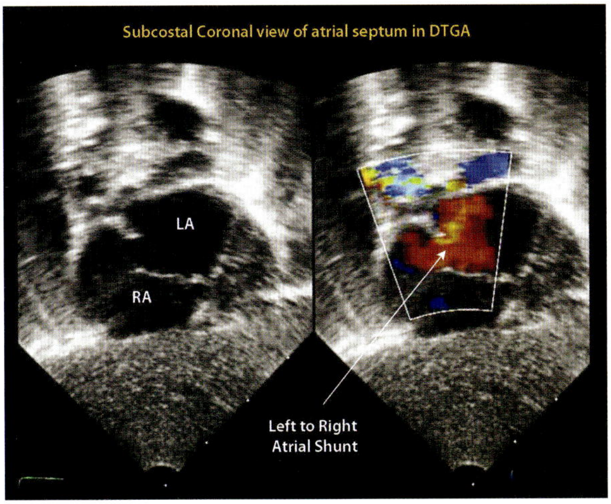

FIGURE and VIDEO 15-24. Subcostal coronal posterior view of D-transposition of the great arteries and an atrial septal defect with left to right shunting.

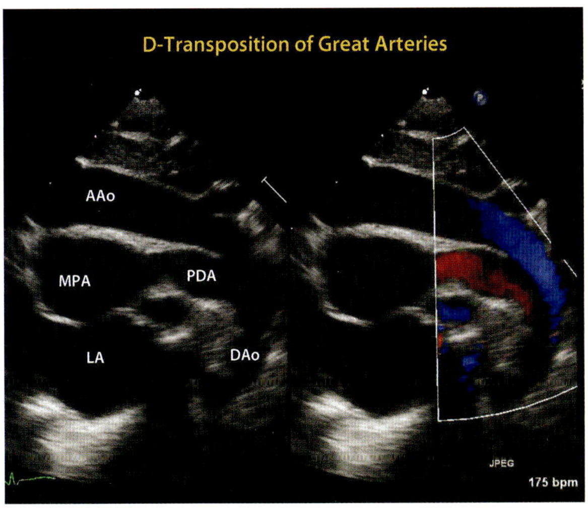

FIGURE and VIDEO 15-25. Suprasternal ductal cut in D-transposition of the great arteries with left to right shunting through a large patent ductus arteriosus.

Persistent Truncus Arteriosus

In this anomaly, a single arterial trunk supplies systemic, pulmonary, and coronary circulations. Almost always, a subaortic VSD is present. The most common type of Truncus Arteriosus is Type A1 of Van Praagh, in which the main pulmonary artery arises from the side of the trunk above the truncal valve (Figure 15-26). The other types are less common and will not be discussed further. Since there is usually unrestricted blood flow through pulmonary

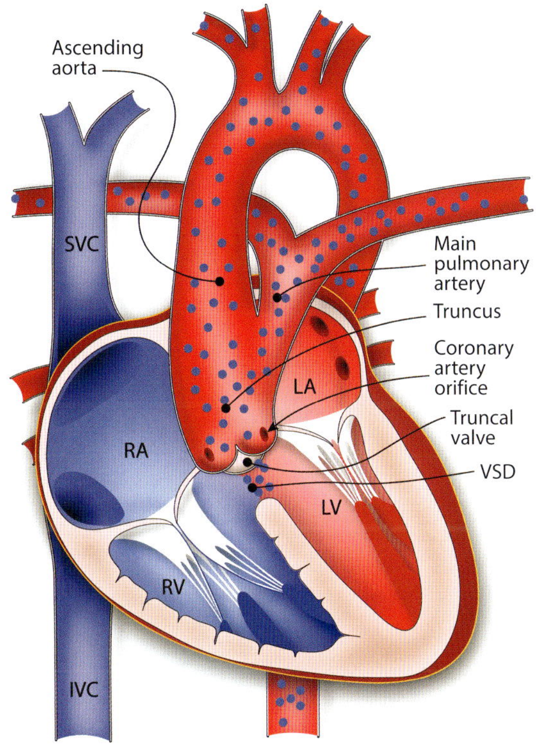

FIGURE 15-26. Diagram of truncus arteriosus with MPA arising from ascending trunk close to the truncal valve.

circulation, congestive heart failure is the usual consequence during the first 6 months of life, which, if not treated, will lead to the patient's demise. With increasing flow through the lungs, cyanosis becomes less prominent, and congestive heart failure becomes the predominant feature.

Echocardiography

Parasternal long axis, particularly with views directed toward showing right ventricular outflow, will reveal the arterial trunk overriding a subaortic VSD. No right ventricular outflow or main pulmonary artery can be identified in the usual location (Figure and Video 15-27). Subcostal coronal or sagittal LV-aorta views can demonstrate the presence of the main pulmonary artery arising from the side of arterial trunk (Figure and Video 15-28). The presence of atrial shunting though either a PFO or atrial septal defect can be evaluated from the subcostal coronal posterior view (Figure and Video 15-29). Echocardiography is also helpful in determining the origin of the pulmonary arteries from the ascending aorta in other less common types of truncus arteriosus; however, it is beyond the scope of the present discussion.

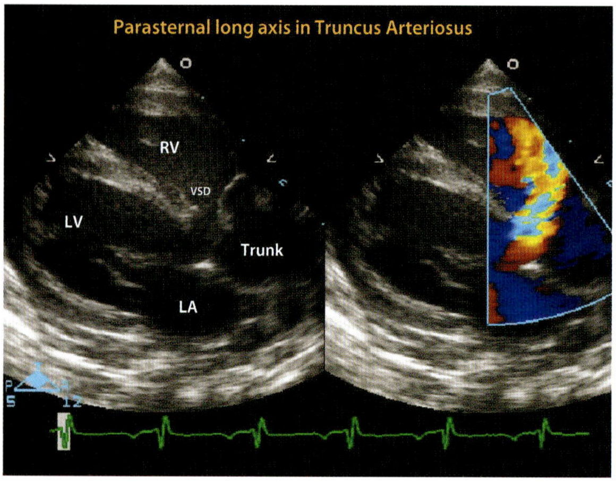

FIGURE and VIDEO 15-27. Parasternal long axis view in truncus arteriosus with the trunk overriding the interventricular septum, and a large ventricular septal defect.

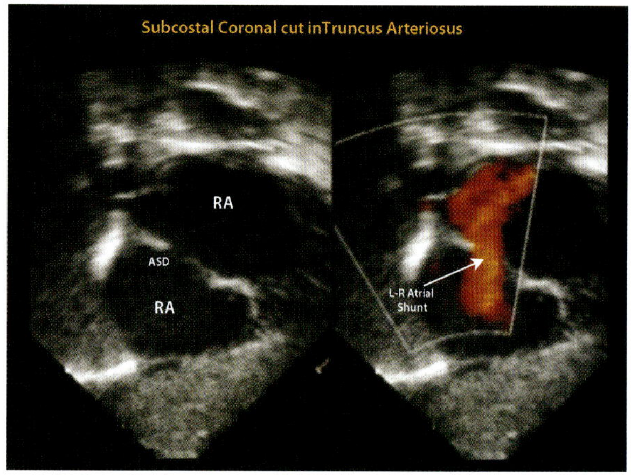

FIGURE and VIDEO 15-29. Subcostal coronal posterior view of the atrial septum in truncus arteriosus with a small atrial septal defect.

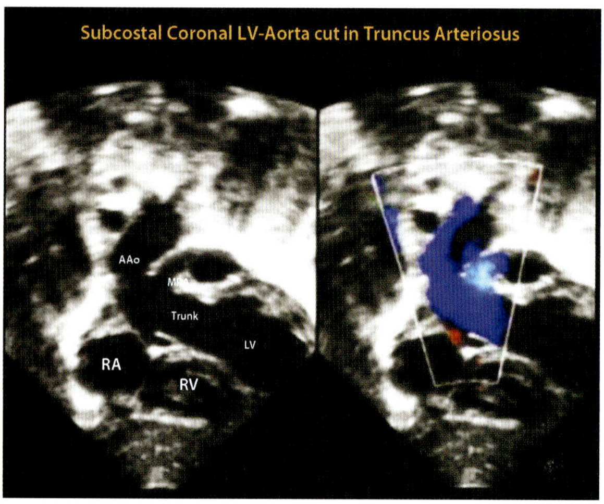

FIGURE and VIDEO 15-28. Subcostal coronal midsection view of truncus arteriosus, with the main pulmonary artery arising from the side of the ascending aorta.

CYANOSIS WITH PULMONARY EDEMA

Total Anomalous Pulmonary Venous Return

In total anomalous pulmonary venous return (TAPVR), all pulmonary veins bypass the left atrium and drain directly into a systemic vein or chamber, thereby returning directly or indirectly to the right atrium (Figure 15-30). Such patients are cyanotic because of the obligate mixing of systemic and pulmonary venous blood. An atrial defect is generally required for right-to-left shunting, in order to provide adequate blood to the left ventricle and aorta.

In the absence of pulmonary venous obstruction, pulmonary flow is increased, minimizing the degree of cyanosis. However, the excess pulmonary blood flow can eventually cause heart failure that usually occurs beyond the neonatal period. In neonates with obstruction to pulmonary venous return, which commonly accompanies the infradiaphragmatic type of TAPVR, the pulmonary venous obstruction leads to pulmonary edema, and hypoxemia and respiratory distress occur shortly after birth. In such patients, if the diagnosis of TAPVR is not initially suspected, it is common for the respiratory distress to be mistakenly attributed to aspiration or congenital infection, without any evidence for either one. Suspecting and diagnosing TAPVR by echocardiography can be daunting if attention is not paid to a few obvious details. The most important clue to the presence of TAPVR is detailed imaging of the atrial septum, which will demonstrate in all cases a large right-to-left shunt at atrial level. In TAPVR, pulmonary venous drainage should be evaluated by echocardiography, although visualization of the patterns of pulmonary venous return in TAPVR can be challenging.

Echocardiography

Subcostal coronal and sagittal imaging are useful to delineate the atrial septum, using color flow Doppler to determine the direction of atrial shunting. This is the most important aspect of suspecting the presence of TAPVR. Subcostal coronal imaging will outline an enlarged right atrium with a large right to left shunt across a stretched PFO or atrial septal defect, into a small left atrium. The confluence of pulmonary veins separated from

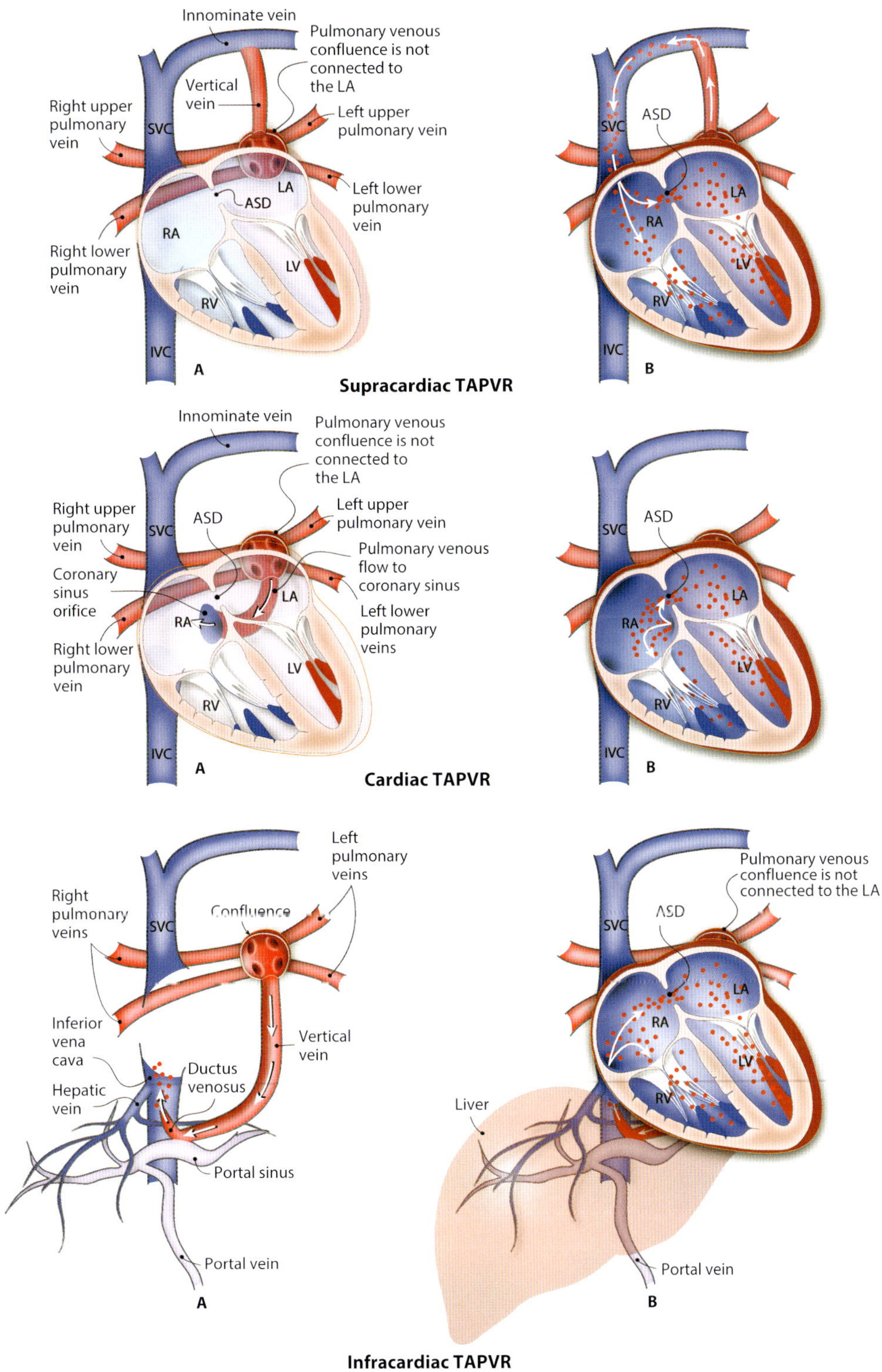

FIGURE 15-30. The three common variations of total anomalous pulmonary venous return: infracardiac, cardiac, and supracardiac.

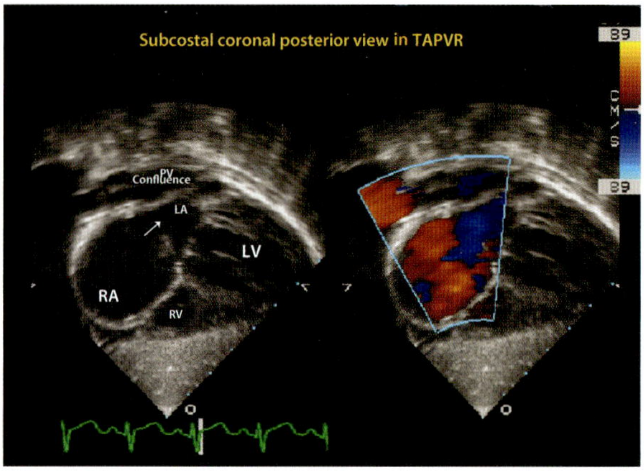

FIGURE and VIDEO 15-31. Subcostal coronal view of the right and left atria and the confluence of pulmonary veins posterior to the left atrium in a patient with total anomalous pulmonary venous return. Abbreviation: PV, Pulmnary veins.

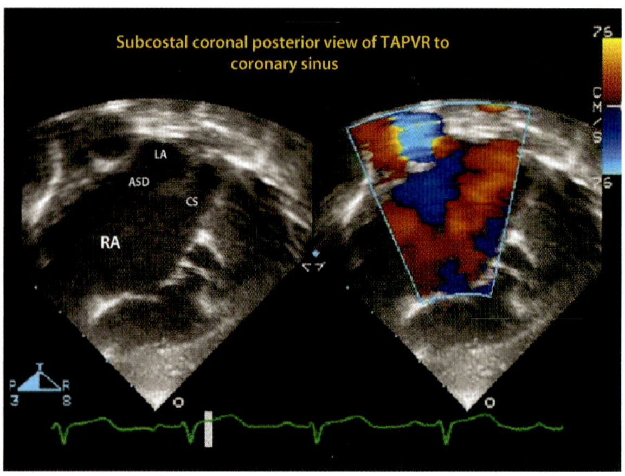

FIGURE and VIDEO 15-32. Subcostal coronal view showing total anomalous pulmonary venous return to the coronary sinus. Abbreviation: CS, Coronary sinus.

the left atrium can be visualized with careful examination (Figure and Video 15-31). TAPVR to the coronary sinus can pose a special challenge since a large amount of flow appears to come from the left atrium toward the right atrium. However, after careful evaluation, this flow is identified as coming through an enlarged CS to empty into the right atrium, with a concomitant right to left shunt through the atrial septal defect into the left atrium (Figure and Video 15-32). Tracing an ascending or descending vertical vein is possible by suprasternal or subcostal imaging (Figure and Video 15-33). It is imperative to perform careful subcostal imaging below the diaphragm (Subcostal cross-section and sagittal views of the IVC), in order to rule out infradiaphragmatic TAPVR.

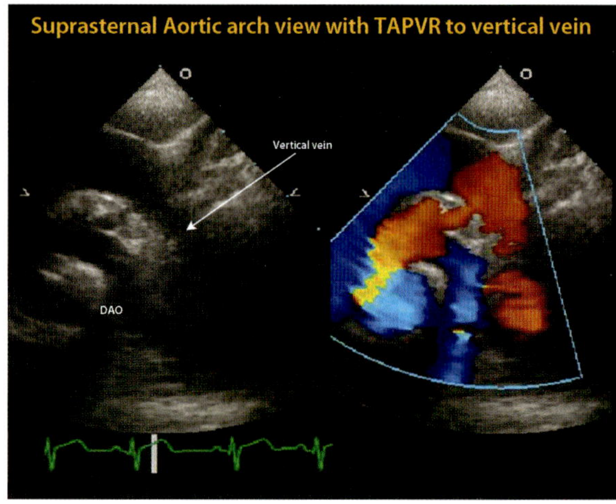

FIGURE and VIDEO 15-33. Suprasternal aortic arch view showing the vertical vein in total anomalous pulmonary venous return. Abbreviation: DAo, Descending aorta.

CARDIOGENIC SHOCK

Hypoplastic Left Heart Syndrome

The hallmarks of hypoplastic left heart syndrome (HLHS) include aortic atresia or stenosis, left ventricular hypoplasia, PDA, and an enlarged right ventricle (Figure 15-34). Because of the inadequacy of the left-sided structures to accommodate fully the systemic cardiac output, there needs to be partial or total rerouting of returning pulmonary blood flow across the PFO by left-to-right shunting, and the right ventricle becomes the systemic pump. Systemic arterial blood flow is therefore dependent partially or totally upon a right-to-left ductal shunt. If the PFO becomes restrictive, severe cyanosis and pulmonary congestion ensue, whereas if the PDA becomes restrictive, shock and severe congestive heart failure will occur. Even if both the PDA and PFO stay widely patent, with a decrease in pulmonary vascular resistance the pulmonary blood flow will increase at the expense of systemic blood flow, leading to pulmonary congestion and systemic hypo perfusion.

Echocardiography

Hypoplasia of the left ventricle, mitral valve and relative hypoplasia of the left atrium are visualized from the apical four-chamber view (Figure and Video 15-35). Subcostal coronal and sagittal views will show the patency of the atrial septum and the shunt across it (Figures and Videos 15-36 and 15-37). The presence of aortic atresia and the size of the ascending aorta are best visualized from the suprasternal aortic arch view (Figure and Video 15-38). A further detailed analysis of the echocardiographic findings in HLHS is beyond the scope of this chapter.

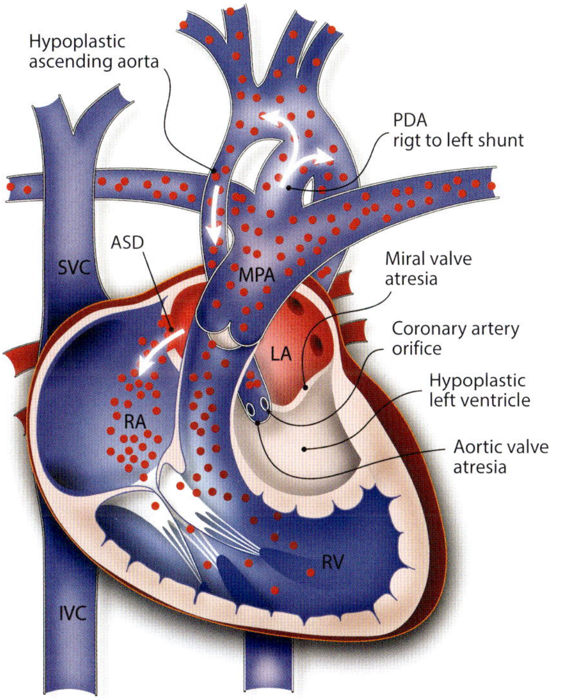

FIGURE 15-34. Hypoplastic left heart syndrome consisting of aortic atresia, hypoplastic left ventricle, hypoplasia of ascending aorta, large ductus arteriosus with right to left shunting.

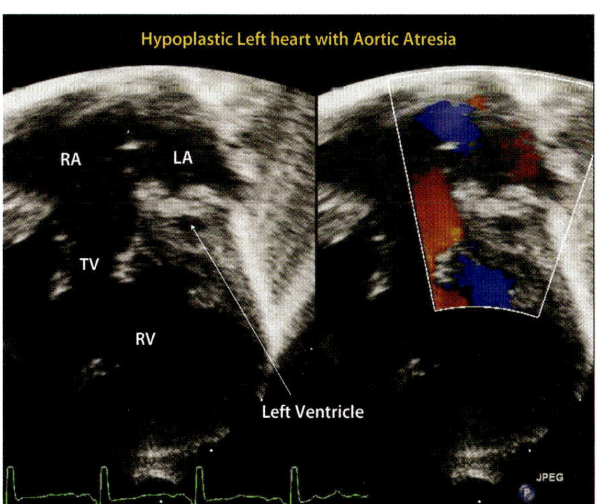

FIGURE and VIDEO 15-35. Apical four-chamber in hypoplastic left heart syndrome. Note enlarged RV, Hypoplastic LV and small LA.

HEART FAILURE WITH DIFFERENTIAL CYANOSIS

Coarctation of the Aorta

Coarctation of the aorta in newborns is generally preductal or juxta ductal in location. The status of ductal patency has a significant effect on clinical symptomatology. In severe forms of coarctation, right to left shunting through the PDA to the descending aorta leads to differential cyanosis, with decreased arterial oxygen saturation in the legs as compared to the arms (Figure 15-39). Closure of the ductus arteriosus increases the severity of obstruction in juxtaductal coarctation and

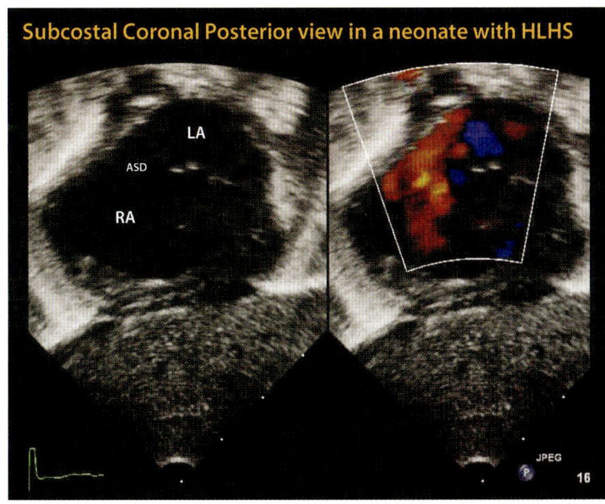

FIGURE and VIDEO 15-36. Subcostal coronal posterior imaging of the atrial septum in hypoplastic of the left heart syndrome. Note right to left atrial shunting.

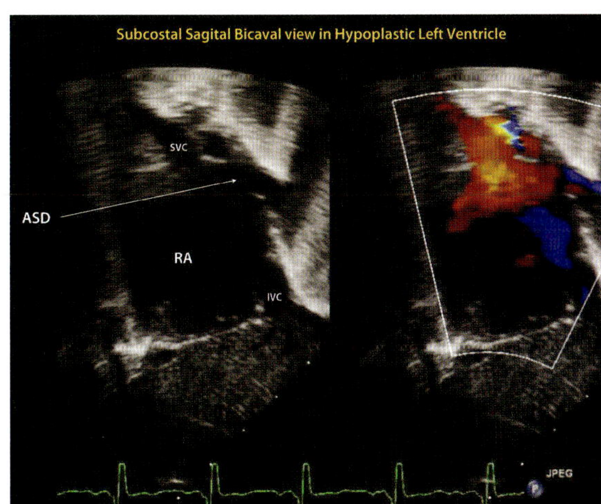

FIGURE and VIDEO 15-37. Subcostal sagittal bicaval view in hypoplastic left heart syndrome, showing the atrial shunt.

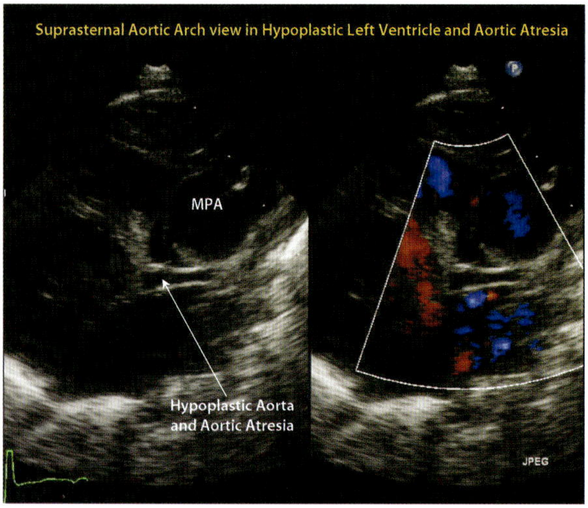

FIGURE and VIDEO 15-38. Suprasternal aortic arch in a neonate with hypoplastic left heart syndrome. Note atreti aortic valve and AAo measuring 2 mm in diameter.

eliminates the supplemental flow to the lower part of the body, which can lead to more severe heart failure. Coarctation of aorta is often associated with other cardiac anomalies.

Echocardiography

Coarctation of aorta is best evaluated by suprasternal aortic arch and ductal cuts. The descending aorta appears to be "kinked" at the site of coarctation and color flow turbulence often is an early sign of constriction (Figure and Video 15-40).

Interruption of the Aortic Arch

The most common type of interruption of the aortic arch (Type A) involves the segment of the arch between the left subclavian artery and PDA (Figure 15-41). Other types proximal to this site are less common. The PDA is the only means of blood supply to the parts of the body beyond the interruption. The ascending aorta is small as compared to the main pulmonary artery, and there may be hypoplasia of segments of the transverse arch. Commonly, a VSD is present. Differential cyanosis is often detected by pulse oximetry, but the difference might become less obvious as the result of torrential pulmonary blood flow that, through mixing from the left to right atrial (and ventricular) shunting, will increase the pulmonary artery and descending aortic oxygen saturations. Heart failure is the preponderant clinical sign.

Echocardiography

Suprasternal aortic arch and ductal cuts usually reveal the presence and severity of aortic interruption (Figure and Video 15-42). A suprasternal "crab view" usually reveals a side-by-side comparison of the cross sections of aorta and pulmonary artery (Figure and Video 15-43). Other associated defects are detected using appropriate views.

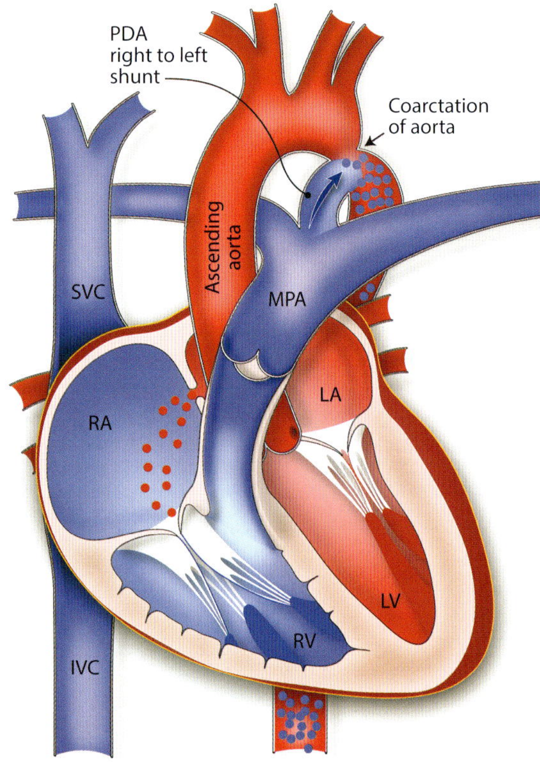

FIGURE 15-39. Diagram of coarctation of the aorta with juxtaductal shelf of coarctation.

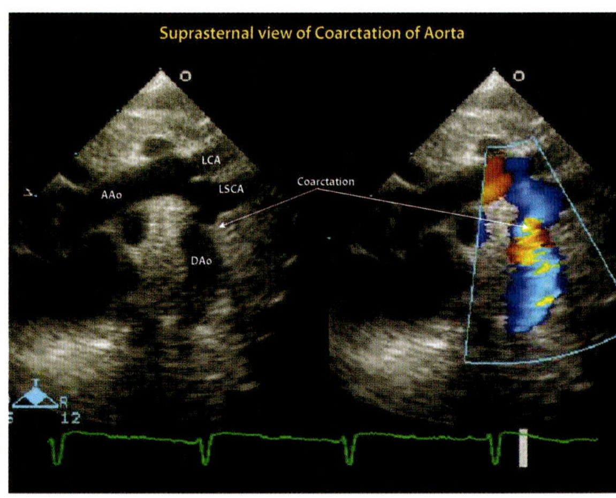

FIGURE and VIDEO 15-40. View of suprasternal aortic arch and descending aorta in coarctation of the aorta. Abbreviations: LSCA, left subclavian artery, LCA, left carotid artery.

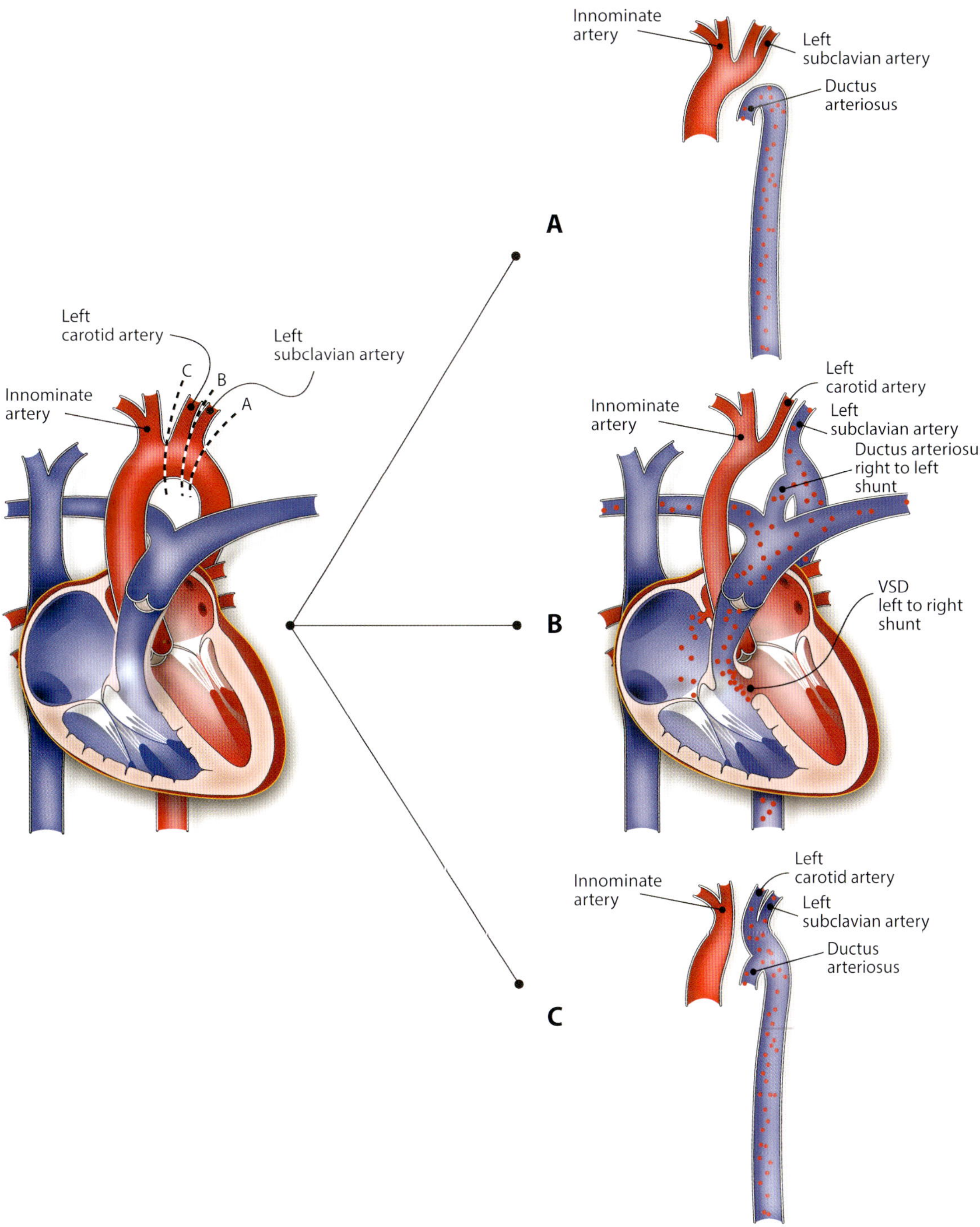

FIGURE 15-41. Various types of interruption of the aortic arch. Right to left shunting through PDA significantly contributes to systemic circulation. **A**. Interruption between left subclavian artery and PDA. **B**. Interruption between left carotid artery and left subclavian artery **C**. Interruption between left carotid artery and the innominate artery.

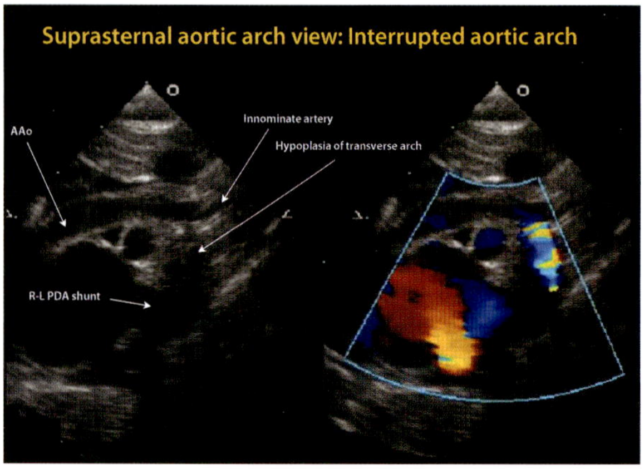

FIGURE and VIDEO 15-42. Suprasternal aortic arch in interruption of the aortic arch type A. Note hypoplasia of transverse arch.

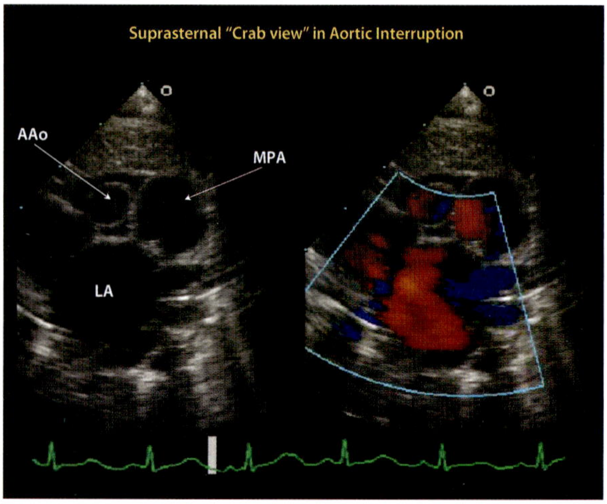

FIGURE and VIDEO 15-43. Suprasternal crab view in aortic arch interruption. Note enlarged cross section of MPA in comparison to AAo.

ACYANOTIC CONGENITAL HEART DISEASE

Atrioventricular Septal Defect

Also known as an atrioventricular canal or endocardial cushion defect, this congenital cardiac anomaly is commonly found in neonates with Trisomy 21. The site of the defect is at the atrioventricular septum or crux of the heart. Associated defects include a large inlet VSD, ostium primum atrial septal defect, and a large common atrioventricular valve (Figure 15-44). Usually, symptoms develop beyond the neonatal period. Transient cyanosis noted shortly after birth in infants with Trisomy 21 is frequently

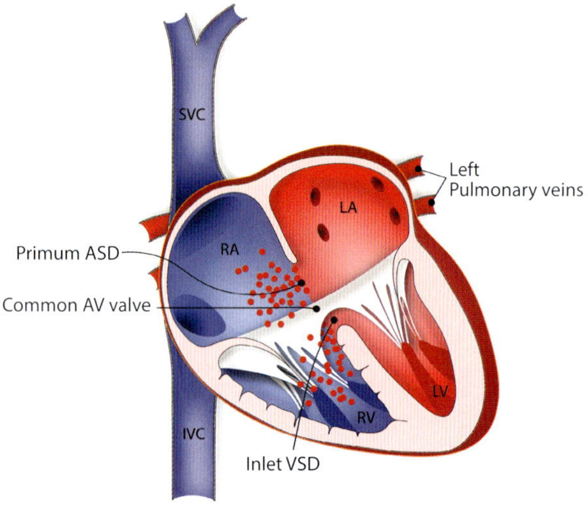

FIGURE 15-44. Complete atrioventricular septal defect. The common atrioventricular valve is divided into anterior and posterior components.

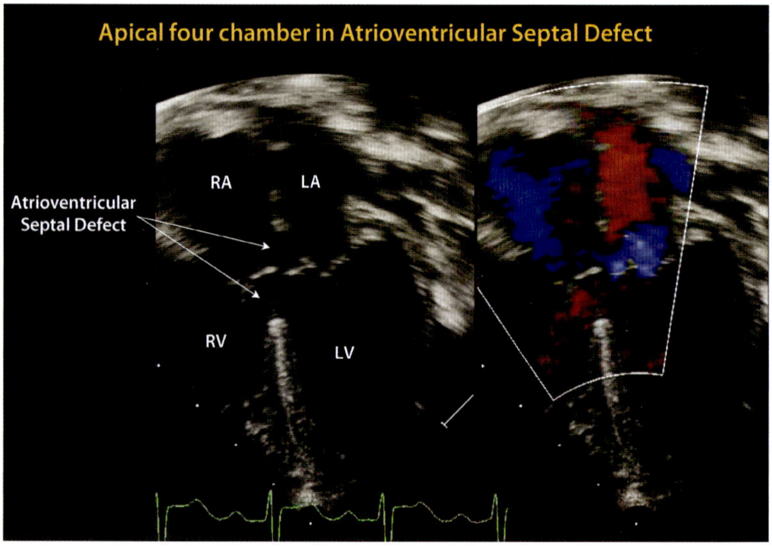

FIGURE and VIDEO 15-45. Apical four-chamber view in atrioventricular septal defect. Ostium secundum ASD in addition to atrioventricular septal defect is present.

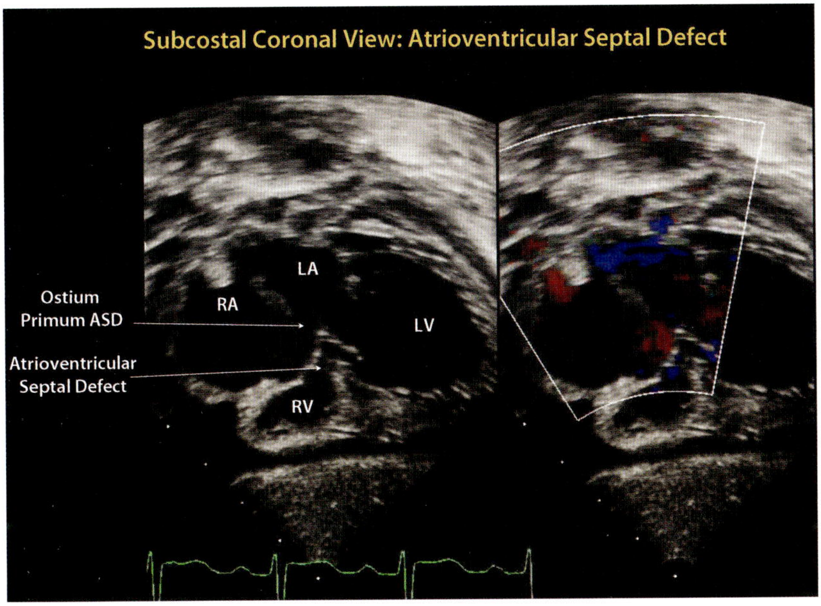

FIGURE and VIDEO 15-46. Subcostal coronal view in atrioventricular septal defect. Note ostium secundum defect in addition to ostium primum defect.

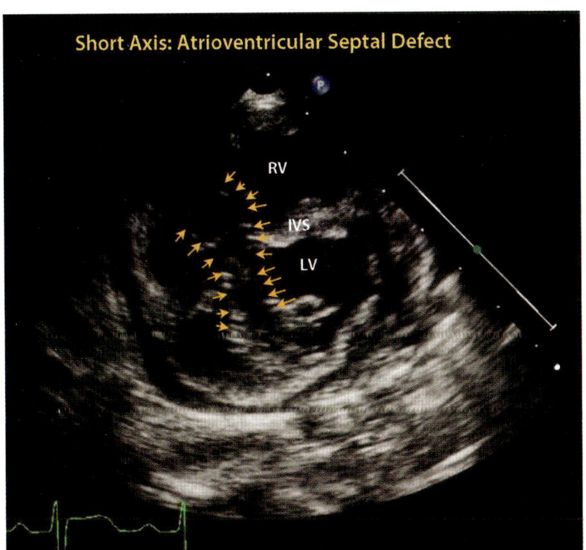

FIGURE and VIDEO 15-47. Parasternal short axis view in atrioventricular septal defect showing common atrioventricular valve. The edges of the common valve are marked by arrows.

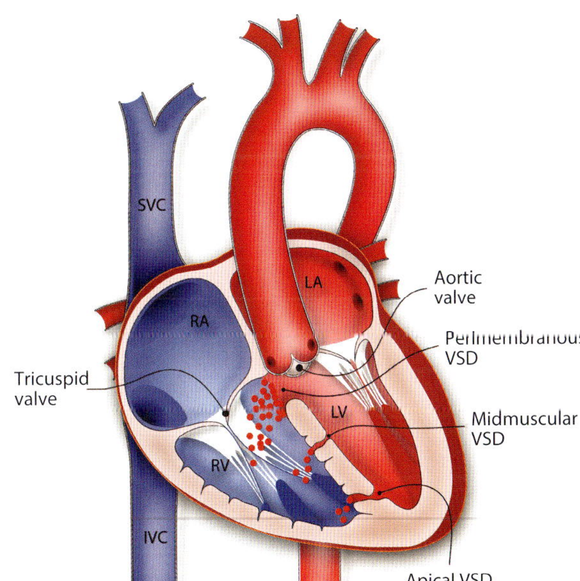

FIGURE 15-48. Perimembranous and muscular ventricular septal defects.

related to pulmonary hypertension and polycythemia. A heart murmur is often the presenting sign.

Echocardiography

The atrioventricular septal defect is well-visualized from the apical four-chamber view (Figure and Video 15-45). In the subcostal coronal view, the atrial septum and ostium primum atrial septal defect is well-seen (Figure and Video 15-46). Parasternal short axis at the base of the heart reveals a large common atrioventricular valve that crosses the ventricular septum and is well-balanced over both ventricles (Figure and Video 15-47).

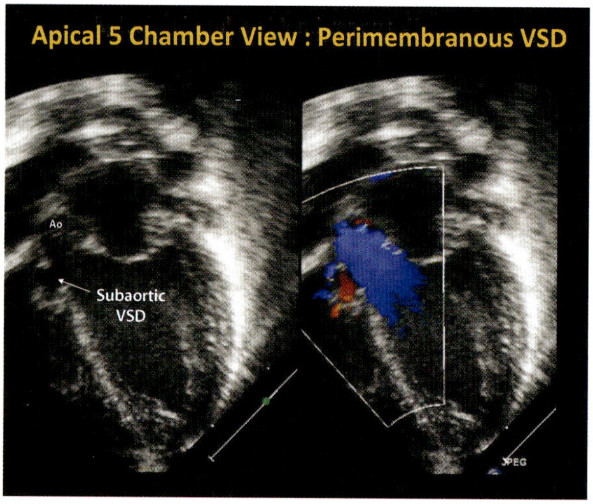

FIGURE and VIDEO 15-49. Apical four-chamber view showing perimembranous ventricular septal defect.

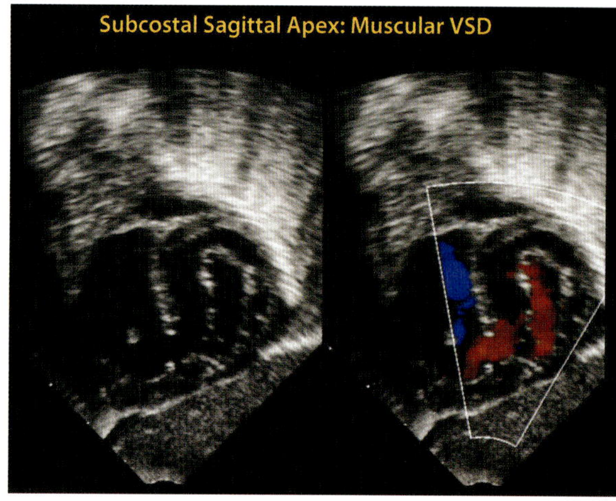

FIGURE and VIDEO 15-51. Subcostal sagittal showing an apical muscular ventricular septal defect.

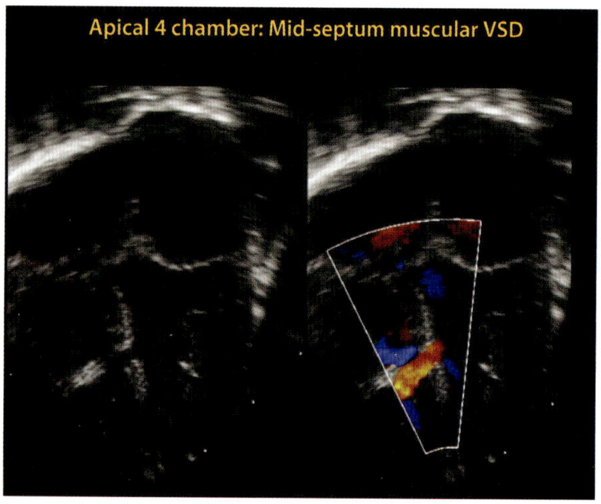

FIGURE and VIDEO 15-50. Apical four-chamber mid-septal muscular ventricular septal defect.

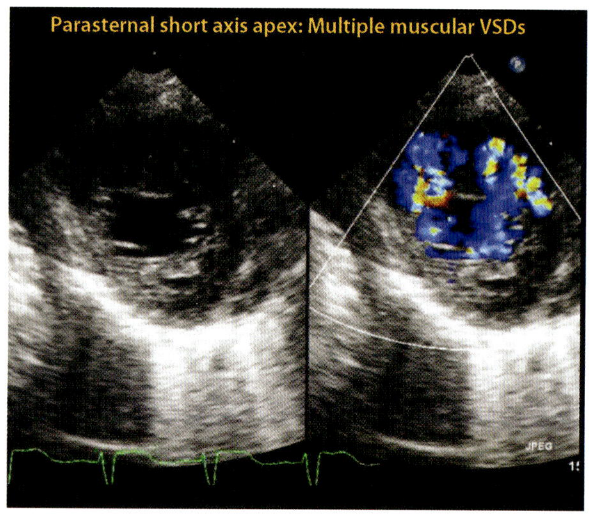

FIGURE and VIDEO 15-52. Parasternal short axis apex view of multiple muscular ventricular septal defects ("Swiss cheese") with bidirectional shunting.

Ventricular Septal Defect

VSDs are the most common congenital cardiac defects. However, most neonates with a VSD—except for rare exceptions—remain asymptomatic during the neonatal period. VSDs can be present in any part of ventricular septum (Figure 15-48). A heart murmur is prominent and might be the only presenting sign.

Echocardiography

Except for the suprasternal window, scans obtained from all other echocardiographic windows are helpful in determining the location of the VSDs throughout the interventricular septum. Exploring interventricular septum through PLAX and PSAX views and looking for left-to-right shunt by color flow Doppler will usually indicate the location of VSD (Figures and Videos 15-49 to 15-52).

Atrial Septal Defect

Isolated atrial septal defects are usually completely silent during the first year of life. However, if echocardiography is performed for any reason, they can be identified, provided appropriate views of atrial septum as well as color flow Doppler are obtained. There are three main types of atrial septal defects characterized by their distinct locations on the atrial septum: ostium primum, ostium secundum, and sinus venosus defects (Figure 15-53).

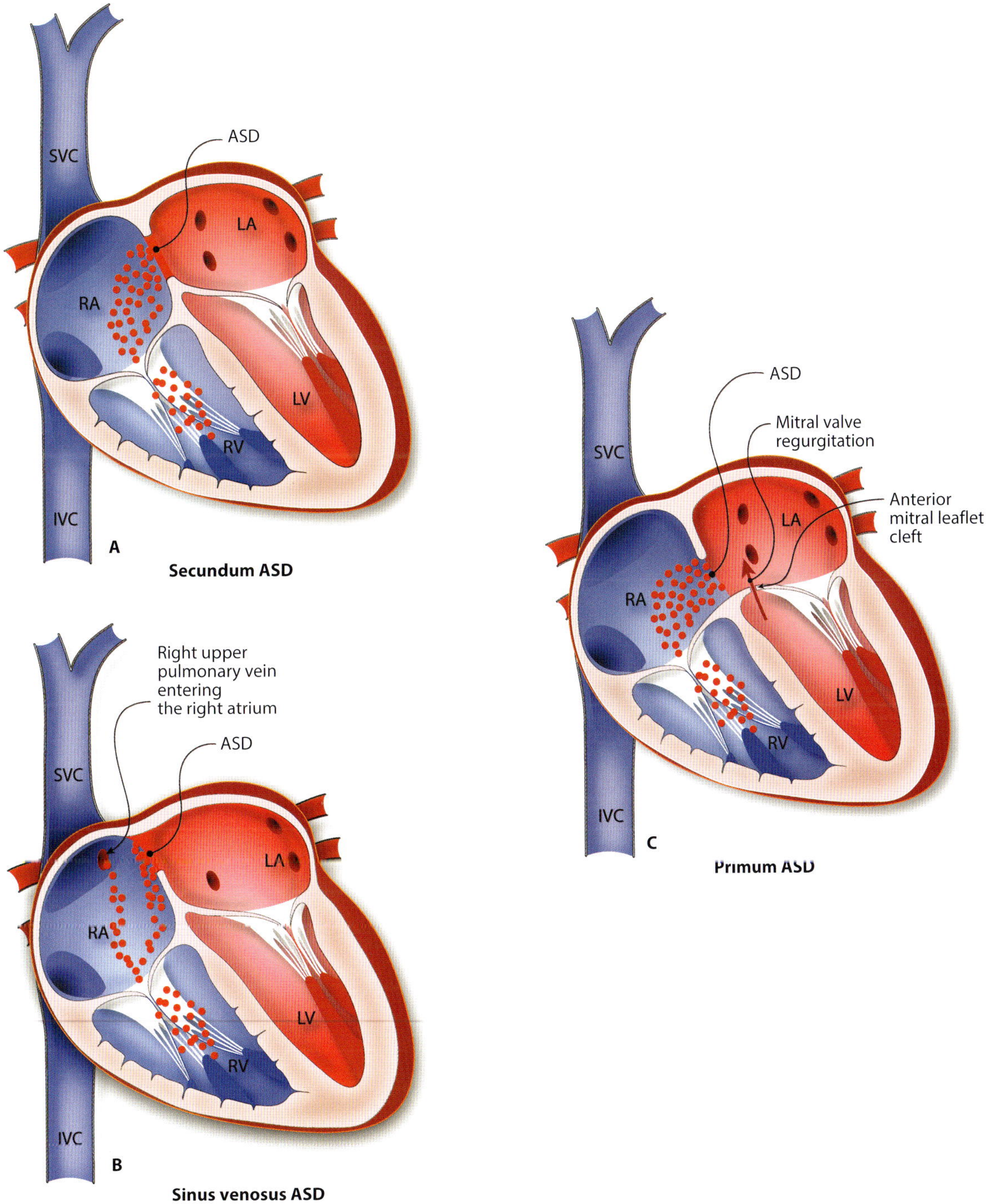

FIGURE 15-53. Ostium primum, ostium secundum and sinus venosus atrial septal defects. Ostium secundum defect is in the central segment of atrial septum, Ostium primum is located in septum primum segment of atrial septum and sinus venosus ASD is located at the mouth of superior vena cava often involving anomalous drainage of right pulmonary veins to RA.

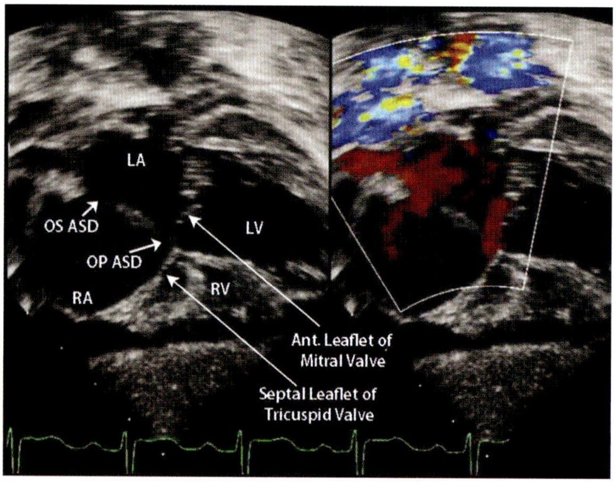

FIGURE and VIDEO 15-54. Ostium primum and ostium secundum atrial septal defects.

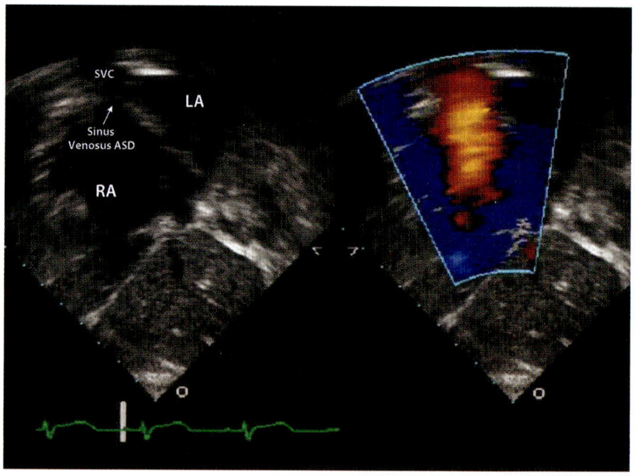

FIGURE and VIDEO 15-56. Sinus venosus atrial septal defect.

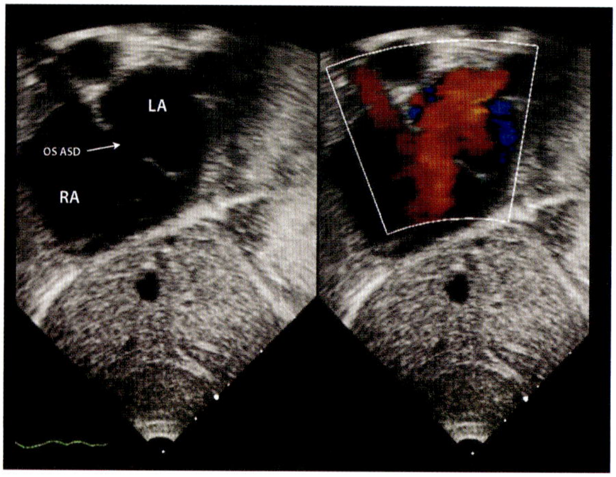

FIGURE and VIDEO 15-55. Ostium secundum atrial septal defect.

Echocardiography

Subcostal coronal and sagittal imaging can visualize the three types of atrial septal defects (Figures and Videos 15-54 to 15-56).

PATENT DUCTUS ARTERIOSUS

Full-term neonates with PDA as a congenital cardiac defect are usually asymptomatic during the neonatal period. The echocardiographic features of a PDA in these patients do not differ from those in premature neonates; these are described in detail in Chapter 11.

REFERENCES

1. Freidberg MK, Silverman NH, Moon-Grady AJ, et al. Prenatal detection of congenital heart disease. *J Pediatr.* 2009;155:26–31.
2. Wang NK, Shen CT, Lin MS. Result of echocardiographic screening in 10,000 newborn. *Acta Paediatr Taiwan.* 2007;48:7–9.
3. Mielke G, Benda N. Cardiac output and central blood flow distribution in the human fetus. *Circulation.* 2001;103:1662–1668
4. Gentile R, Stevenson G, Dooley, et al. Pulsed Doppler echocardiographic determination of time of ductal closure in normal newborn infants. *J Pediatr.* 1981;98:443–448.
5. Freedom RM, Benson LN, Smallhorn JF. *Neonatal Heart Disease.* London: Springer-Verlag; 1992.
6. Allen HD, Shaddy RE, Penny DJ, Feltes TF, Ceta F. *Moss and Adams' Heart Disease in Infants, Children, and Adolescents: Including the Fetus and Young Adults.* 9th ed. Philadelphia, PA: Wolters Kluwer; 2016.
7. Lai Wyman W, Mertens LL, Cohen MS, Geva T. *Echocardiography in Pediatric and Congenital Heart Disease: From Fetus to Adult.* 2nd ed. Hoboken, NJ: Wiley-Blackwell; 2016.

CHAPTER 16

Overview of Fetal Echocardiography*

Ruben J. Acherman, and William N. Evans

- PRENATAL DETECTION OF CONGENITAL HEART DISEASE
  - Current Status
  - Screening Fetal Echocardiogram
  - Normal Screening Fetal Echocardiogram
- EVALUATION OF FETAL CARDIOVASCULAR SYSTEM
  - Spectral Doppler in Evaluation of Fetal Growth Restriction
  - Umbilical Artery Flow
  - Middle Cerebral Artery Flow
  - Inferior Vena Cava and Hepatic Veins Flow
  - Ductus Venosus Flow
  - Umbilical Vein Flow
  - Fetal Anemia
  - Fetal Heart Failure
  - Fetal Cardiac Arrhythmias
  - 2D Imaging
  - M-mode Echocardiography
  - Pulsed Doppler
- REFERENCES

PRENATAL DETECTION OF CONGENITAL HEART DISEASE

Current Status

Most infants born with serious congenital heart disease undergo rapid evaluation and life-saving treatment. Most fetuses with significant cardiac malformations, however, are not diagnosed prenatally. Those not diagnosed prenatally cannot receive state-of-the-art fetal cardiology evaluation and treatment, a situation tantamount to sending a cyanotic newborn home without the benefit of currently available diagnostic and treatment methods.

Cardiac malformations are the most frequent anomalies of human development. Cardiac defects occur in about 8/1000 live births. Among congenital abnormalities tabulated in the United States, cardiac malformations are the number one cause of death. Even today, 1 out of 10 infants dying from congenital heart disease do so without diagnosis until autopsy, a sobering fact that universal fetal cardiac evaluation could alter. Nonetheless, fetal cardiac evaluations are currently limited to those women who are referred because of risk factors for fetal heart disease (Table 16-1). Studies, however, show that most newborns with congenital heart disease are born to women without risk factors[1]; hence, most infants with congenital heart disease are not diagnosed prenatally.

The first reports on the use of ultrasound to evaluate the fetal heart appeared in the 1960s and 1970s. The work by Kleinman and colleagues, first published in 1988,[2] marked the beginning of modern fetal echocardiography

*Videos can be accessed at http://PracticalNeonatalEcho.com.

TABLE 16-1. Risk Factors for Fetal Heart Disease and Current Indications for Fetal Echocardiography

Maternal
Suspected fetal cardiac anomaly during obstetric ultrasound
Maternal Diabetes
Phenylketonuria
Methylene tetrahydrofolate reductase (MTHFR) gene mutations
Medications
Alchol
Illicit drugs
Infections
Autoimmune diseases
Maternal congenital heart disease
Maternal obesity
Pregnancies of assisted reproductive technology
Familial
Congenital heart disease
Nonchromosomal syndromes
Fetal
Increased nuchal transluscency thickness
Single umbilical artery
Chromosomal abnormalities
Hydrops fetalis
Cardiac arrhythmias
Extracardiac abnormalities
Monochorionic placentation
Abnormal first trimester markers

and the birth of fetal cardiology as a new super specialty of pediatric cardiology. Thus, prenatal cardiac diagnosis has been possible for over 30 years. With today's clinical knowledge and technical advancements, the prenatal diagnosis of serious congenital heart diseases by fetal echocardiogram approaches 100%. Because of limitations placed on the use of fetal cardiac evaluation, these advancements have not improved the general prenatal detection of serious cardiac abnormalities.[3]

Most pregnant women undergo only a general obstetric ultrasound which, following the joint recommendations by the American Institute of Ultrasound in Medicine, the American College of Radiology, and the American College of Obstetrics and Gynecologists, includes a limited evaluation of the 4 chambers of the heart, and if possible, a view of the outflows.[4] By following these current strategies, we and other investigators have shown that ⅔ of fetuses with serious congenital heart diseases remain undiagnosed.[3,5] Primarily for financial reasons, most fetuses still do not undergo a useful cardiac evaluation.

Screening Fetal Echocardiogram

We have previously proposed universal screening fetal-cardiac evaluation as the best method for detecting serious cardiac malformations prenatally.[3] In our opinion, a screening fetal echocardiogram, as proposed by Yagel and colleagues,[6] should replace the current four-chamber view strategy. The screening evaluation includes five axial slices of the fetal abdomen and chest obtained by sliding the transducer cephalad beginning from the upper abdomen view (Figure 16-1). The five axial slices include (1) upper abdomen to evaluate abdominal situs (Figure 16-1A); (2) four-chamber view to evaluate cardiac chambers, atrial septum, ventricular septum, and atrioventricular valves (Figure 16-1B); (3) left outflow (Figure 16-1C); (4) right outflow (Figure 16-1D); and (5) the three-vessel trachea view (Figure 16-1E). A more detailed fetal echocardiogram than these five axial views is reserved for patients with risk factors, and those with clear or suspected abnormalities noted in screening fetal echocardiograms. Experienced specialists should perform the detailed fetal echocardiographic studies.

Normal Screening Fetal Echocardiogram

The description of normal findings in the screening fetal echocardiogram's slices are as follows. Deviations from normalcy require further evaluation by detailed fetal echocardiographic study.

1. Upper Abdomen

The upper abdomen slice evaluates the abdominal situs (Figure 16-2). In the normal situs solitus, the stomach is on the left side of the abdomen, the descending aorta is to the left of the spine, the inferior vena cava is anterior and to the right of the aorta, and the umbilical vein turns toward the right into the portal sinus; when visible, the gallbladder is to the right of the umbilical vein.

2. Four-chamber View

The four-chamber view is obtained from a transverse slice of the fetal chest slightly above the upper abdomen. Before concentrating on the intracardiac anatomy, the examiner should pay attention to the position of the heart within the chest, the cardiac axis, the cardiac size, and the structures surrounding the heart.

Cardiac position. The heart is normally positioned toward the left chest, and in the four-chamber view, the left lung usually appears slightly smaller than the right (Figure 16-3). The right ventricular free wall is in contact with the anterior chest wall (Figure 16-3 and Figure and Video 16-7). Mass effect on either side of the chest, from diaphragmatic

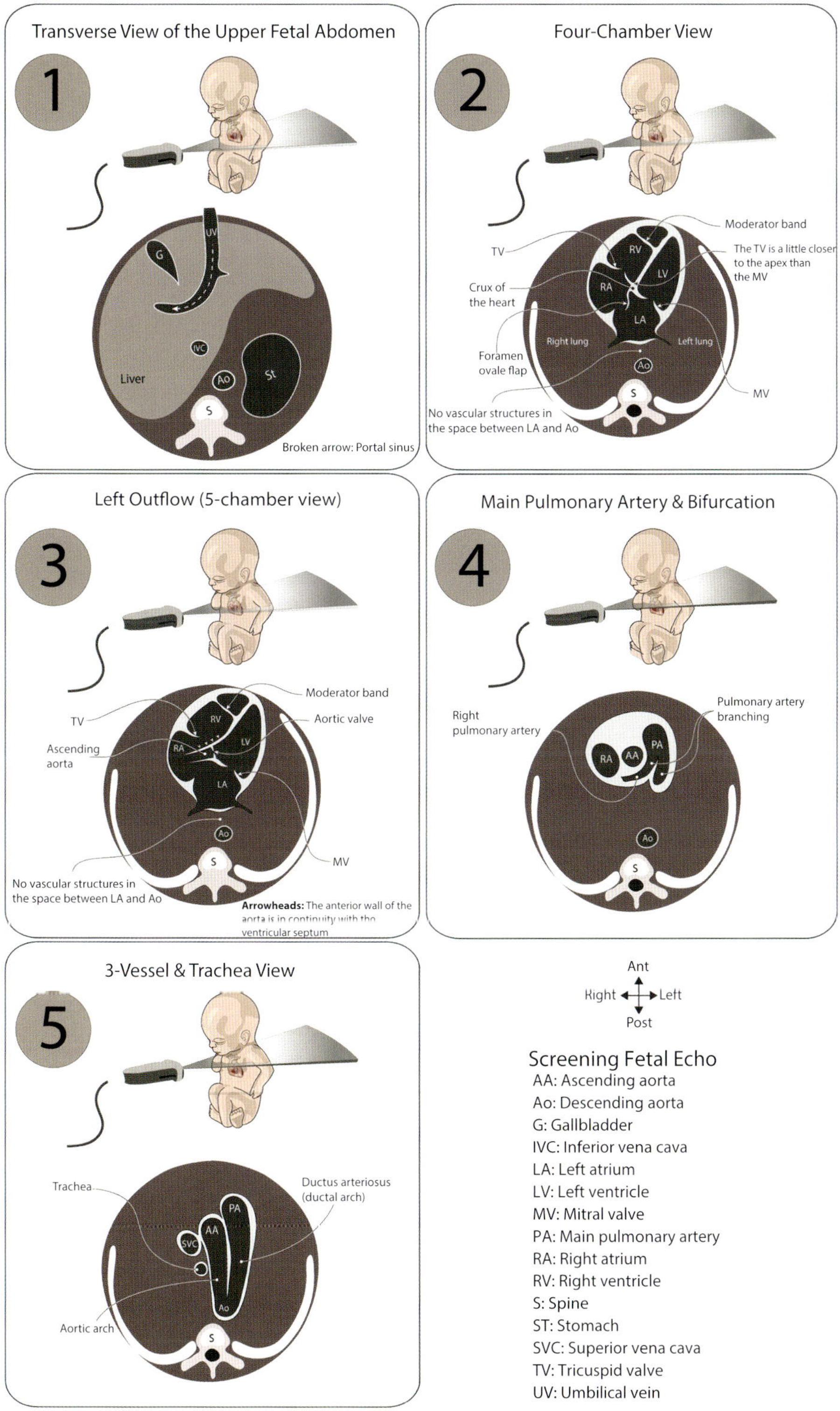

FIGURE 16-1. Screening fetal echo (Reproduced with permission from Evans WN, Acherman RJ, Luna CF: *Simple & Easy Pediatric Cardiology*. Las Vegas: Childrens Heart Center Press.)

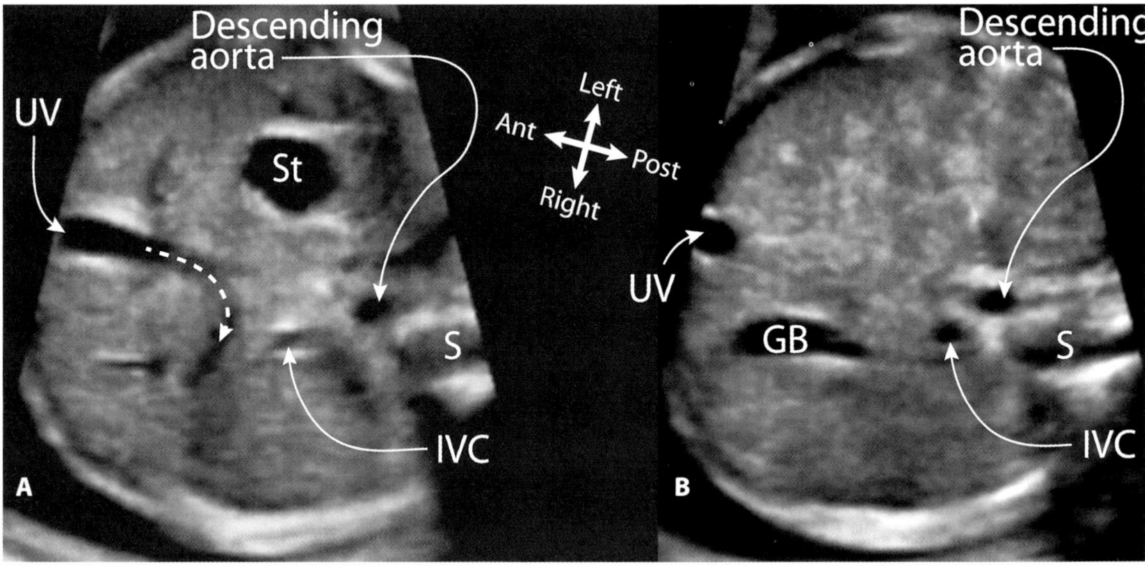

FIGURE 16-2. Abdominal situs. Transverse slice of the upper fetal abdomen demonstrating a normal abdominal situs. In **A,** the stomach (ST) is on the left side of the abdomen, the descending aorta (Ao) is to the left of the spine (S), the inferior vena cava (IVC) is anterior and to the right of the aorta; the dashed arrow shows the umbilical vein (UV) turning to the right into the portal sinus. In **B,** the normal gallbladder (GB) is to the right of the umbilical vein (UV).

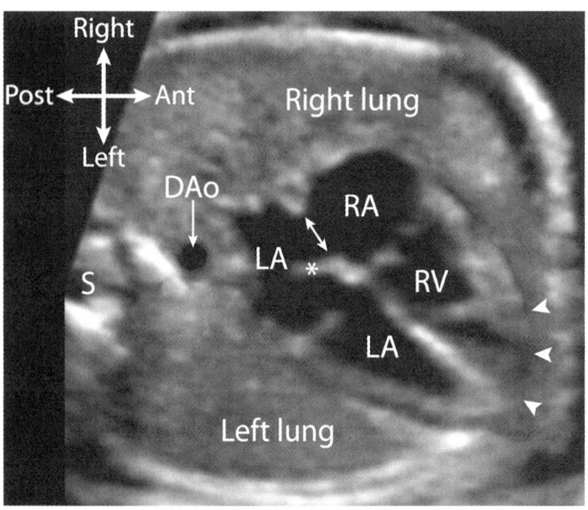

FIGURE 16-3. Position of the heart in the chest. Transverse slice of the fetal chest at the level of the four-chamber view. The heart is positioned toward the left chest, and the left lung appears slightly smaller than the right. The arrowheads show the right ventricular free wall in contact with the anterior chest wall. The double-headed arrow shows the foramen ovale. The foramen ovale flap (*) is opened toward the left atrium (LA). The descending aorta (DAo) is anterior to the spine (S) and posterior to the left atrium. Abbreviations: LV, left ventricle; RA, right atrium; RV, right ventricle.

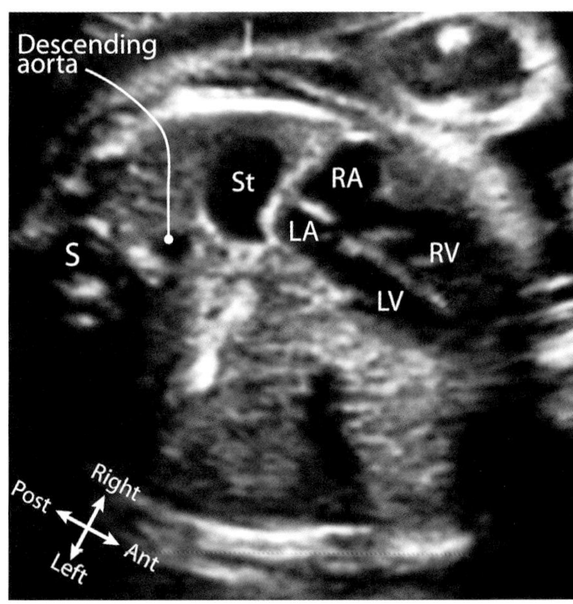

FIGURE 16-4. Fetal heart in the right chest. The heart is pushed against the right chest wall in this fetus with a left diaphragmatic hernia. The descending aorta is pushed to the right of the spine (S). The stomach (St) is behind the heart. Abbreviations: LA, left atrium; LV, left ventricle; RA, right atrium; RV, right ventricle.

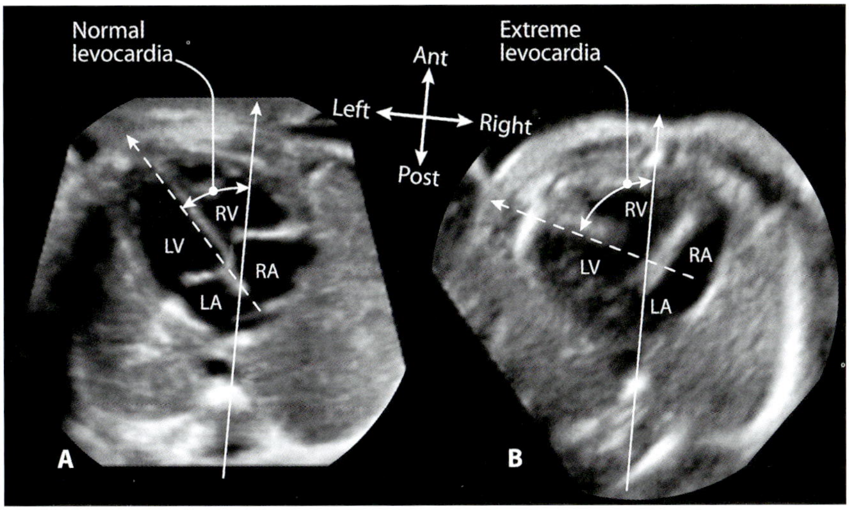

FIGURE 16-5. Levocardia. The degree of levocardia is measured by the angle between the ventricular septum (dashed arrows) and the midline of the chest (arrows). Figure A demonstrates a normal levocardia of 35°. Figure B demonstrates a case of extreme levocardia of about 80°. Abbreviations: LA, left atrium; LV, left ventricle; RA, right atrium; RV, right ventricle.

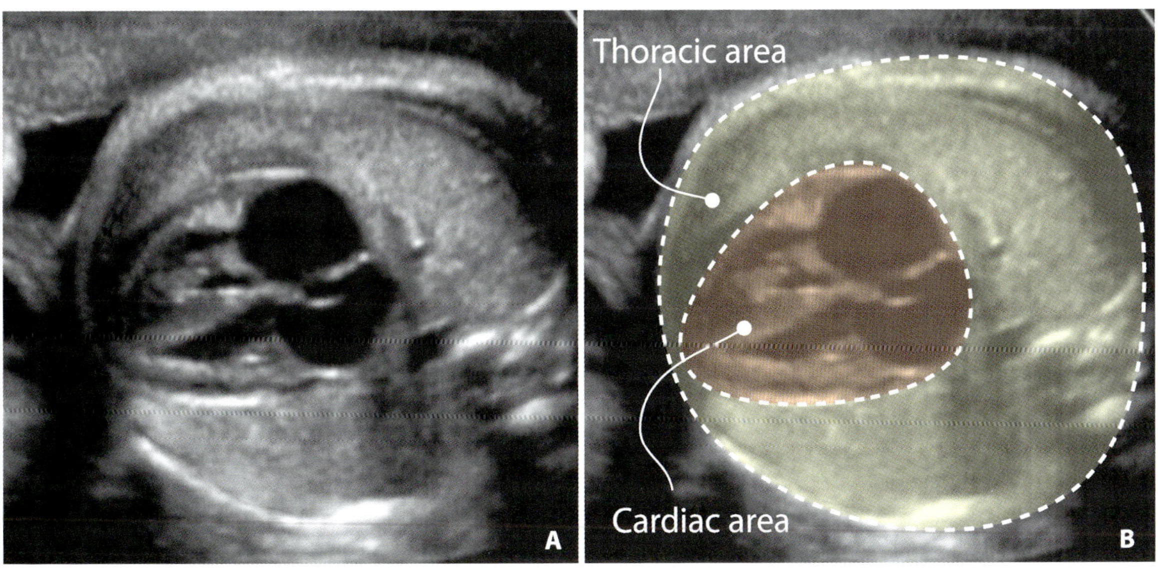

FIGURE 16-6. Cardiothoracic ratio. The normal cardiac area is about 1/3 of the chest area. In the four-chamber view the normal heart fits about 3 times in the normal chest.

hernias, tumors, or pleural effusions, may deviate the heart toward the contralateral chest side (Figure 16-4). Mass impingement on cardiovascular structures may significantly affect hemodynamics and cause hydrops.

Cardiac axis. The normal angle between the ventricular septum and the midline of the chest is about 45° (Figure 16-5). Extreme levocardia with angles above 50° (Figure 16-5) and dextrocardia are associated with increased incidence of congenital heart disease.

Cardiac size. The normal cardiac area is about 1/3 of the chest area (Figure 16-6). Modern ultrasound equipment software facilitates measurements of heart and chest areas

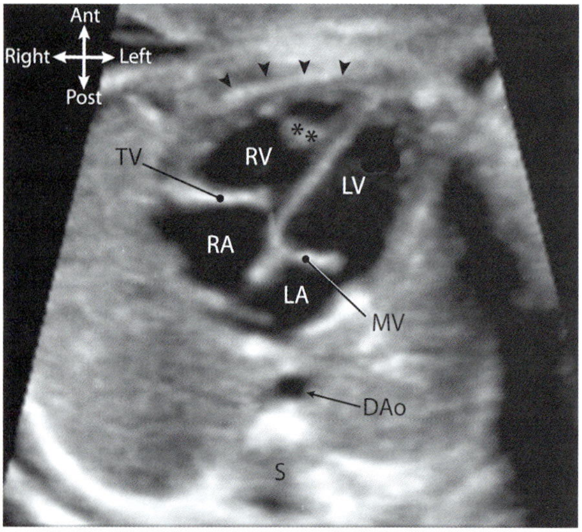

FIGURE and VIDEO 16-7. **Fetal four-chamber view.** The descending aorta (DAo) is anterior to the spine (S); the left atrium (LA) is anterior to the descending aorta. Note the normal echogenicity of the lungs. The black arrowheads show the right ventricular free wall in contact with the anterior chest wall. The tricuspid valve (TV) is slightly closer to the cardiac apex than the mitral valve (MV). The moderator band (**) is in the right ventricle (RV). Abbreviations: LV, left ventricle; RA, right atrium.

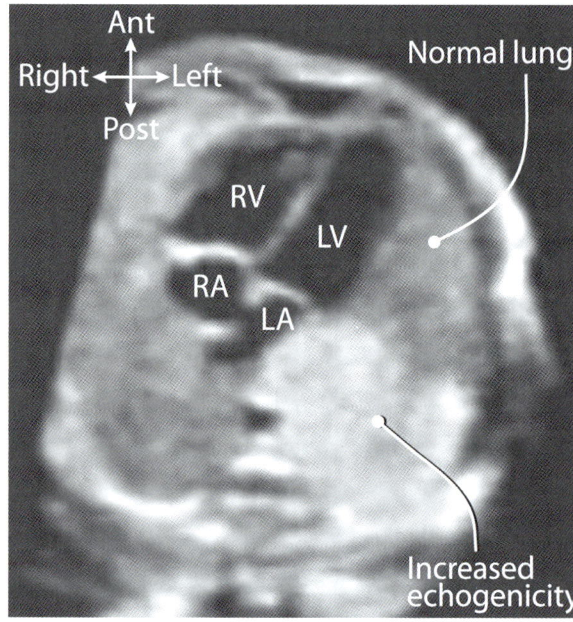

FIGURE 16-8. **Increased lung echogenicity.** An area of increased echogenicity in the posterior left lung of this patient with a pulmonary sequestration. Abbreviations: LA, left atrium; LV, left ventricle; RA, right atrium; RV, right ventricle.

to calculate the cardiac/thoracic ratio. Area cardiothoracic ratios above 35% indicate cardiomegaly.

Structures surrounding the heart. The descending aorta is anterior and to the left of the spine, and the left atrium is anterior to the descending aorta (Figure and Video 16-7). The echogenicity of the lungs is homogeneous. Areas of significant increased or decreased echogenicity may represent masses and deserve careful evaluation (Figure 16-8).Areas of absent echogenicity indicate the presence of abdominal viscera within the chest, cysts, or effusions.

The cardiac four-chamber view. The four-chamber shows the two atria, two ventricles, two atrioventricular valves, and atrial and ventricular septae (Figure 16-9).

Both atria are about the same size. The atrial septum contains the foramen ovale. The foramen ovale flap normally opens toward the left atrium; the foramen ovale flap excursion is normally 50% of the left atrial width or less. Exaggerated foramen ovale flap excursion, also known as atrial septal aneurysm or foramen ovale aneurysm, is associated with fetal arrhythmias, congenital heart diseases, and increased incidence of postnatal atrial septal defects.[7–9] The normal tricuspid valve is slightly closer to the apex than the mitral valve. Both ventricles are about the same size, but the right ventricle contains the moderator band (Figure 16-9). Large ventricular septaldefects are seen with twodimensional (2D) imaging (Figure 16-10). Smaller defects are visualized only with the help of color Doppler.

3. Left Outflow

Angling cephalad from the four-chamber view the aorta appears exiting the left ventricle. The anterior wall of the aorta is in continuity with the interventricular septum. The aortic valve is seen opening and closing between the left ventricle and the ascending aorta (Figure and Video 16-11).

4. Right Outflow

The right ventricular outflow lies immediately cephalad to the left outflow. The right outflow is usually seen together with the ascending aorta and the superior vena cava (Figure 16-12). The ascending aorta is immediately to the right of the right outflow, and the superior vena cava is just to the right of the ascending aorta. Increased distance between the ascending aorta and the superior vena cava in

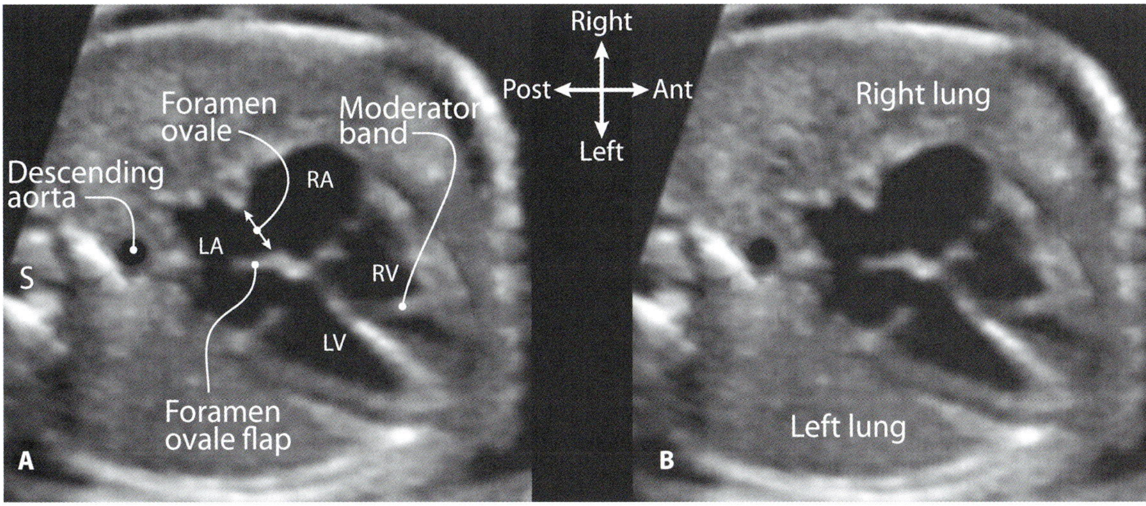

FIGURE 16-9. Normal four-chamber view. Abbreviations: LA, left atrium; LV, left ventricle; RA, right atrium; RV, right ventricle; S, spine.

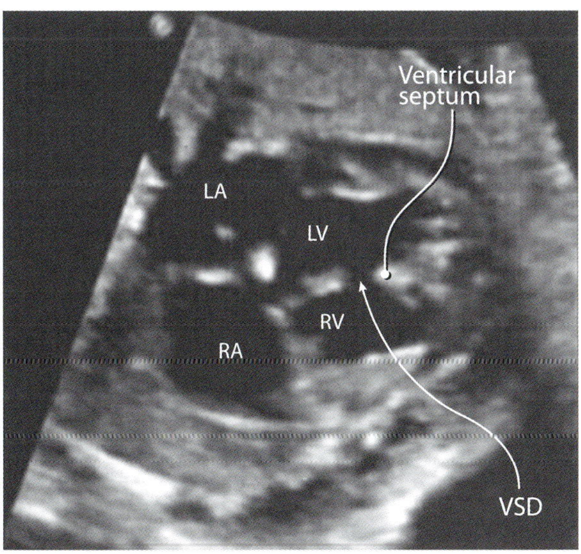

FIGURE 16-10. Large ventricular septal defect. Abnormal four-chamber view demonstrating a large mid-muscular ventricular septal defect (VSD). Abbreviations: LA, left atrium; LV, left ventricle; RA, right atrium; RV, right ventricle.

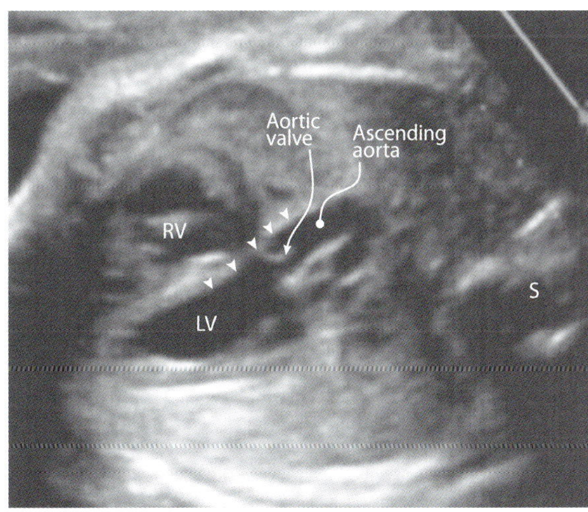

FIGURE and VIDEO 16-11. Normal left ventricular outflow tract. The left ventricular outflow is shown with the ascending aorta anterior wall in continuity with the ventricular septum (white arrowheads). Abbreviations: LV, left ventricle; RV, right ventricle.

the three-vessel view may indicate the presence of a right diaphragmatic hernia[10] (Figure 16-13).

5. Three-Vessel and Trachea View

Slightly cephalad from the right outflow plane we find the three-vessel and trachea view. This view is ideal to evaluate the size and position of the aortic arch. The trachea is normally to the right of the aortic arch (Figure 16-14). In cases of right aortic arch, the trachea is to the left of the aortic arch. A right aortic arch with a left ductus arteriosus form a vascular ring, with the trachea seen between the aortic and ductal arches (Figure 16-15).

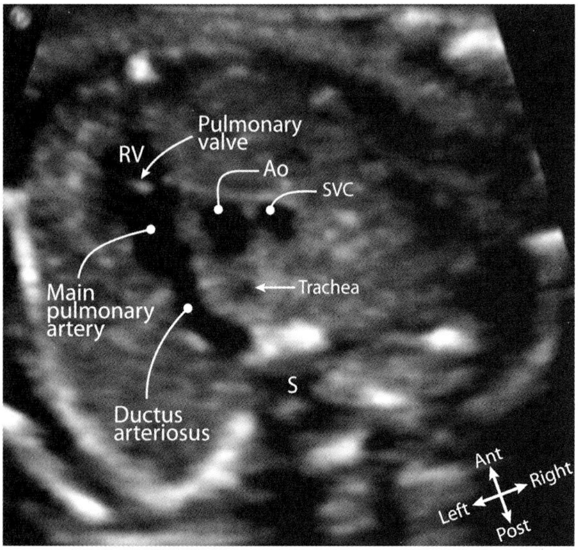

FIGURE 16-12. Normal right ventricular outflow tract. The right ventricular outflow (RV) is shown with the main pulmonary artery and the ductus arteriosus. The main pulmonary artery is anterior and to the left of the ascending aorta (Ao). The ductus arteriosus is to the left of the trachea. The ascending aorta is to the left of the superior vena cava (SVC). Note that normally the ascending aorta and superior vena cava are close to each other. Abbreviation: S, spine.

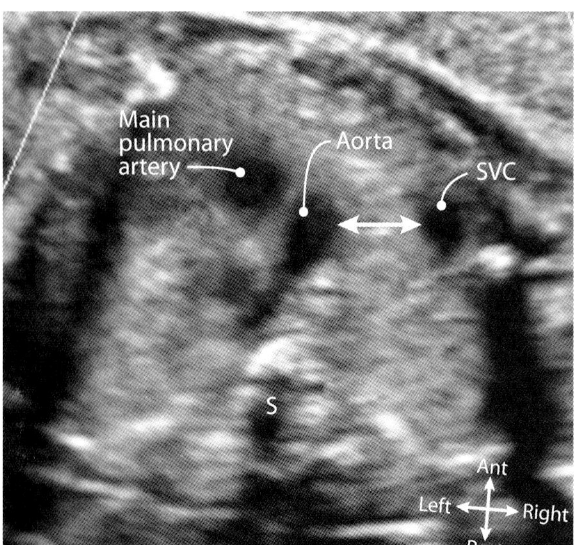

FIGURE 16-13. Abnormal ascending aorta-superior vena cava separation. The double-headed arrow shows the abnormal large separation between the ascending aorta and the superior vena cava (SVC) in this fetus with a right diaphragmatic hernia. Abbreviation: S, spine.

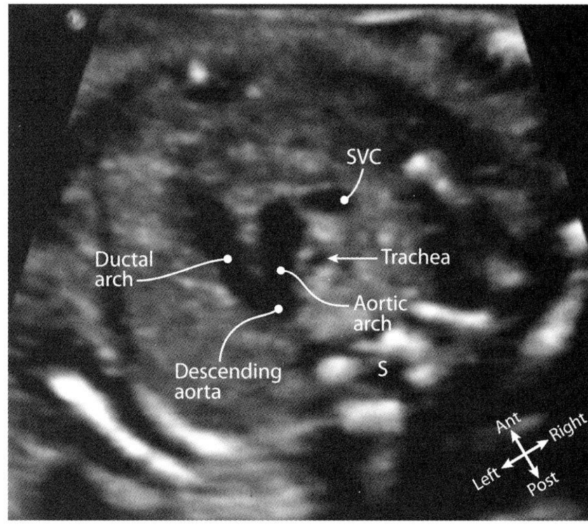

FIGURE 16-14. The three-vessel and trachea view. This normal three-vessel and trachea view shows the "V" formed by the ductal and aortic arches as they join at the descending aorta. Normally both arches are to the left of the trachea. Note the normal position of the superior vena cava (SVC) close to the ascending aorta. Abbreviation: S, spine

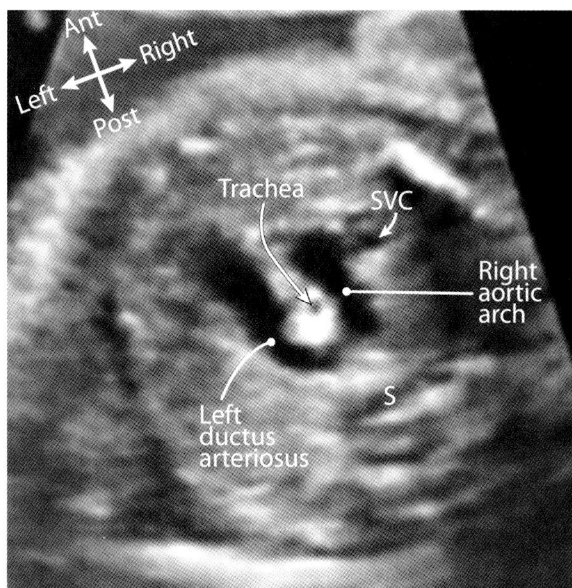

FIGURE 16-15. Vascular ring. The trachea is surrounded by the right aortic arch and the left ductal arch in this fetus with a vascular ring. Abbreviations: S, spine; SVC, superior vena cava.

EVALUATION OF FETAL CARDIOVASCULAR SYSTEM

Spectral Doppler in Evaluation of Fetal Growth Restriction

Basic knowledge of fetal circulation is fundamental to understanding Doppler echocardiographic interrogation of both normal and abnormal fetal-flow pathways. Figure 16-16 diagrams fetal circulation. The diagram on the left shows the fetal heart a bit more posterior than the figure on the right. Hence, the figure on the left better demonstrates the function of the foramen ovale, and the diagram on the right is better for showing the function of the ductus arteriosus.

Deoxygenated fetal blood passes through the placenta's capillary bed and picks up oxygen from maternal

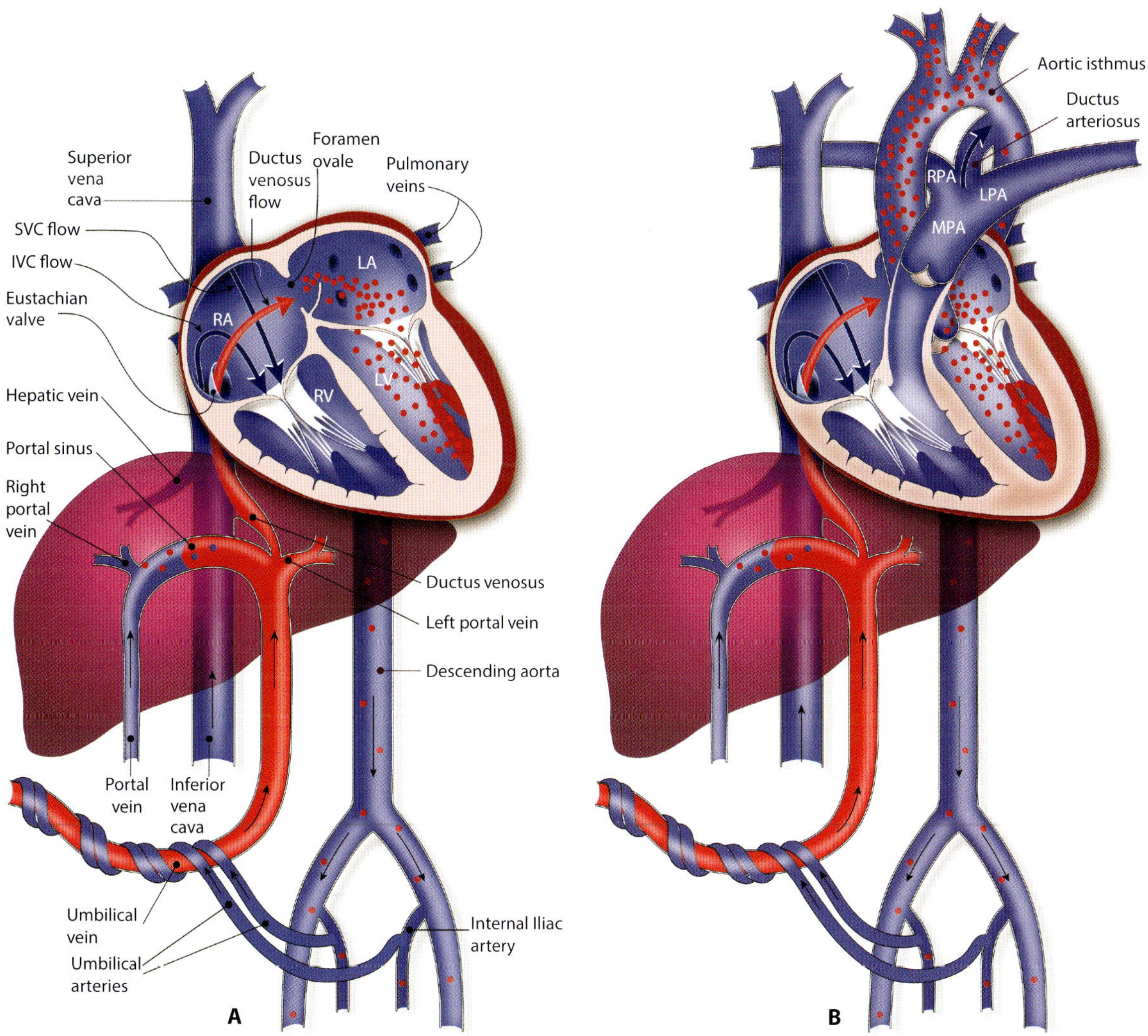

FIGURE 16-16. Fetal circulation. The diagram on the left shows the fetal heart a bit more posterior than the figure on the right. Hence, the figure on the left better demonstrates the function of the foramen ovale, and the diagram on the right is better for showing the function of the ductus arteriosus. Reproduced with permission from Evans WN, Acherman RJ, Luna CF: *Simple & Easy Pediatric Cardiology*. Las Vegas: Childrens Heart Center Press.)

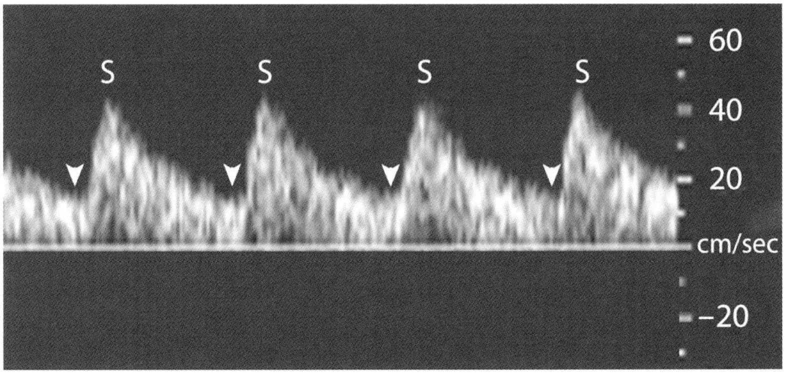

FIGURE 16-17. Normal umbilical artery flow. Normal umbilical artery pulsed Doppler. The white arrowheads show the normal diastolic flow velocity. Abbreviation: S, peak systolic flow.

blood. Deoxygenated fetal blood has a PaO2 in the low 20s. However, the "oxygenated" blood the umbilical vein conveys back to the fetal heart has a PaO2 of only about 35 mm Hg. About 50% of the oxygenated blood returning from the placenta to the fetus, via the umbilical vein, enters the inferior vena cava through the ductus venosus. The ductus venosus produces a jet directing the flow into the left atrium through the foramen ovale. Besides directing the blood from the umbilical vein to the heart, the ductus venosus restricts the volume of blood entering the fetal heart, preventing cardiac overload. The oxygenated blood in the left atrium then enters the left ventricle. From there, the left ventricle pumps the oxygenated blood principally to the brain and the coronary arteries, with a minimal portion of this blood crossing the aortic isthmus into the descending aorta. The fetal right ventricle primarily receives desaturated venous blood from the superior and inferior vena cavas. Because of high fetal pulmonary vascular resistance, only about 10% of right ventricular ejection enters the collapsed fetal lung's pulmonary circulation; the remainder of the right ventricular ejection traverses the ductus arteriosus into the descending aorta. The two umbilical arteries, branches of the internal iliac arteries, take a portion of the oxygen-depleted blood back to the placenta for oxygenation.

Diagnosis and management of fetal-growth restriction decreases fetal and neonatal morbidity and mortality. Fetal Doppler helps to differentiate a healthy, small for gestational age fetus from a growth-restricted fetus.[11] Umbilical artery, middle cerebral artery, umbilical vein, inferior vena cava, and ductus venosus flow Doppler are useful for monitoring growth-restricted fetuses.[12–14] In growth-restricted fetuses, arterial Doppler changes occur before those in the venous channels, and venous Doppler changes precede abnormalities on cardiotocography. In addition, recent studies report fetal aortic isthmus flow changes, fetal cardiac diastolic dysfunction, and elevated fetal B-type natriuretic peptide are associated with poor perinatal outcome in intrauterine growth restriction; however, these latter methods are still under evaluation.[13,14]

Umbilical Artery Flow

Normally, the umbilical arteries demonstrate forward flow throughout systole and diastole (Figure 16-17). The systolic-diastolic ratio (S/D) is normally less than 3 in the 3rd trimester. With placental insufficiency and increasing placental resistance, there is decreased, absent, or reversed end diastolic flow in the umbilical arteries, resulting in an elevated S/D ratio (Figure 16-18). Absent or reversed end diastolic flow is associated with poor perinatal outcome.

Middle Cerebral Artery Flow

Growth-restricted fetuses have limited oxygen and nutrient supply, leading the fetal cardiovascular physiology to redistribute flow to vital organs. Doppler evaluation of the middle cerebral artery (Figure 16-19) may detect increased diastolic velocities that indicate decreased cerebral vascular resistance (the so-called brain sparing effect; Figure 16-20). In more severe cases, there is a

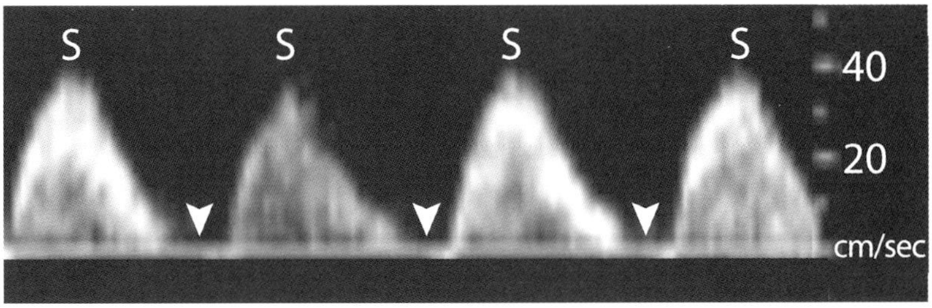

FIGURE 16-18. Abnormal umbilical artery flow. The white arrowheads show the absent diastolic flow. Abbreviation: S, peak systolic flow velocity.

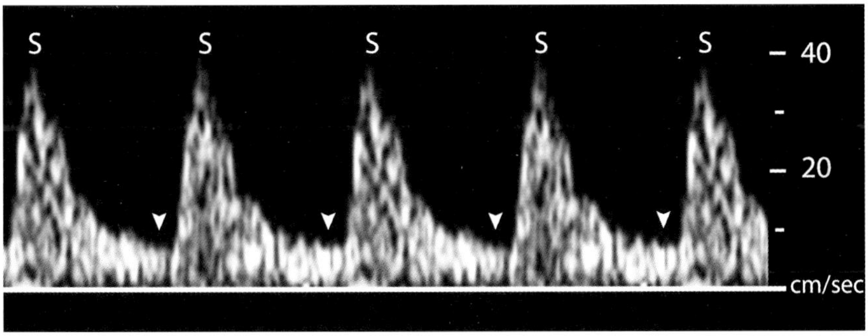

FIGURE 16-19. Normal middle cerebral artery flow. Normal umbilical artery pulsed Doppler. The white arrowheads show the normal diastolic flow. Abbreviation: S, peak systolic flow velocity.

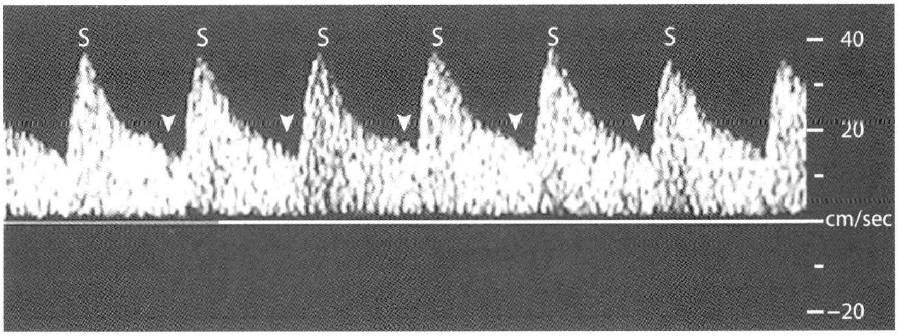

FIGURE 16-20. Abnormal middle cerebral artery flow. The white arrowheads show the increased diastolic flow. Abbreviation: S, peak systolic flow velocity.

pseudo-normalization of the middle cerebral artery Doppler where the diastolic velocity decreases, resembling normal flow. This pseudo-normalization occurs because there is inadequate fetal-cardiovascular reserve to maintain favorable redistribution of flow to the brain.

Inferior Vena Cava and Hepatic Veins Flow

The normal inferior vena cava and the hepatic vein Doppler waveforms consist of an initial forward wave during ventricular systole, a second forward wave during diastole that is less prominent that than the forward wave during systole, and a third retrograde wave during atrial contraction (Figure 16-21). Systemic venous Doppler abnormalities may be consequences of deteriorating systemic or placental resistance and increased right atrial pressure. With increased right atrial pressure, there is an increase in the velocity and duration of the retrograde inferior vena cava and hepatic venous flows during atrial contraction (Figure 16-22).

Ductus Venosus Flow

The Doppler profile of the ductus venosus flow consists of two peaks of antegrade flow: the first during systole and the second during early diastole. A nadir of flow occurs during atrial contraction (Figure 16-23). With increasing venous pressure, the ductus venosus flow velocity, during atrial contraction, progressively decreases and even may reverse during more adverse conditions (Figure 16-24).

Umbilical Vein Flow

The normal umbilical vein flow is continuous (Figure 16-25). Venous pulsations in the umbilical vein flow may result from increased venous pressure and from the tricuspid valve regurgitation secondary to right ventricular dilatation (Figure 16-26).

Fetal Anemia

Fetal anemia causes increased cardiac output without redistribution of blood flow. The increased cardiac output generates increased venous and arterial flow velocities.

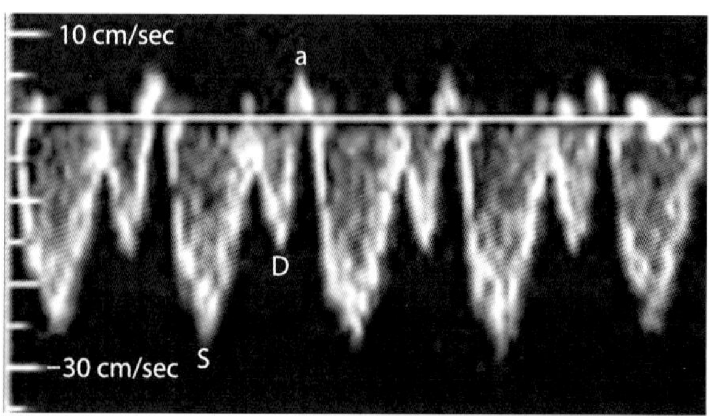

FIGURE 16-21. Normal inferior vena cava flow. Note that the normal retrograde flow during atrial contraction (a) is of short duration and low velocity, about 5 cm/sec. Abbreviations: S, systolic flow velocity; D, early diastolic peak flow velocity.

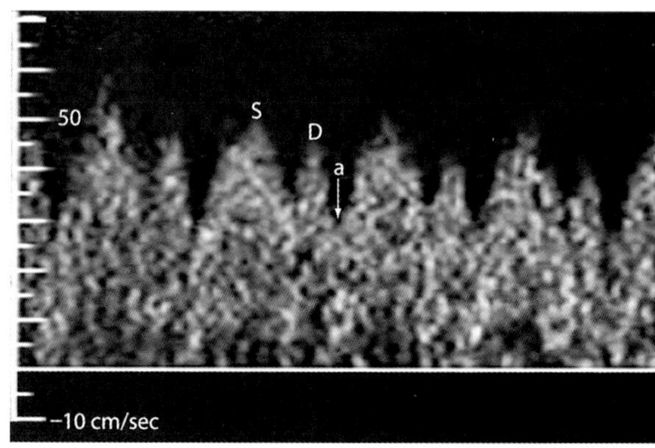

FIGURE 16-23. Normal ductus venosus flow. The figure demonstrates the normal antegrade and relatively high-velocity flow during atrial contraction (a) in the normal ductus venosus. Abbreviations: S, systolic flow velocity; D, early diastolic peak flow velocity.

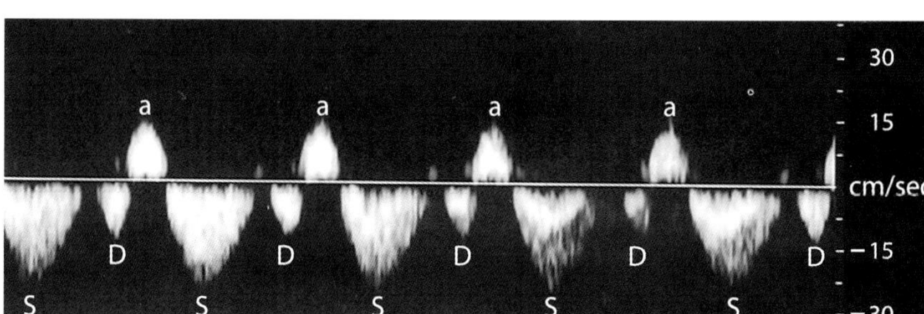

FIGURE 16-22. Abnormal inferior vena cava flow. Note that the abnormal retrograde flow during atrial contraction (a) is of long duration and high velocity, about 15 cm/sec. Abbreviations: S, systolic flow velocity; D, early diastolic peak flow velocity.

Doppler studies show a relationship between flow velocities and fetal hematocrit. The Doppler flow velocities in the fetal aorta and middle cerebral arteries are helpful monitors in the anemic fetus. Monitoring these Doppler flows helps determine when the fetal hemoglobin should be checked by cordocentesis and when to perform intrauterine transfusion. In fetal anemias, serial Doppler evaluations of the middle cerebral artery have led to a more than 70% reduction in the number of invasive tests.[15,16]

Fetal Heart Failure

Fetal heart failure may result in fetal hydrops (Figure 16-27) and death. The fetus with effusions and suspected cardiomegaly need, at a minimum, evaluation of the cardiothoracic ratio (Figures 16-26, 16-28, and 16-29), color Doppler of the cardiac valves, and spectral Doppler of the umbilical vein, ductus venosus, and umbilical artery. A fetal cardiothoracic ratio ≥ 0.35 constitutes cardiomegaly. Refer to the "Spectral Doppler in Evaluation

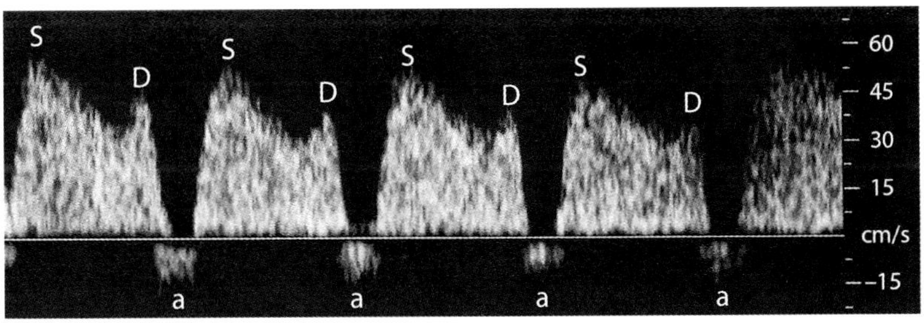

FIGURE 16-24. Abnormal ductus venosus flow. The flow during atrial contraction is retrograde in this abnormal ductus venosus Doppler. Abbreviation: S, systolic flow velocity; D, early diastolic peak flow velocity.

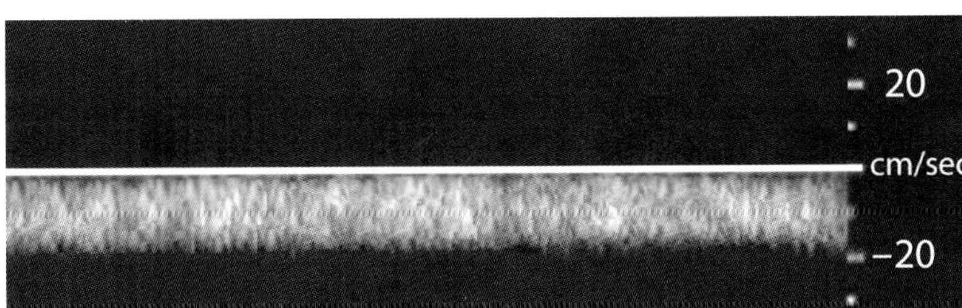

FIGURE 16-25. Normal umbilical vein flow. Low flow velocity unchanged throughout the cardiac cycle.

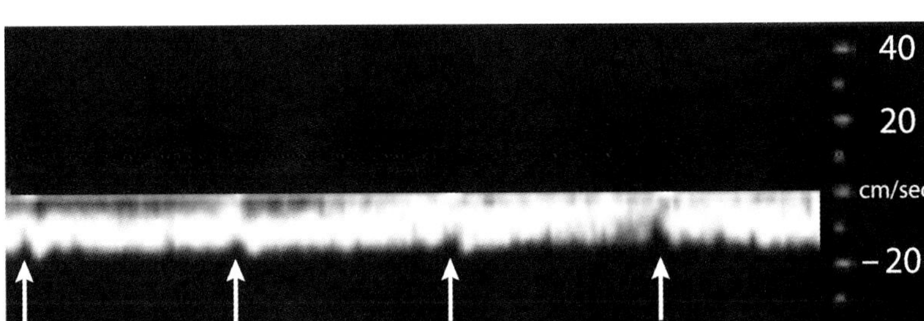

FIGURE 16-26. Abnormal umbilical vein flow. The arrows show the abnormal pulsations in the umbilical vein flow.

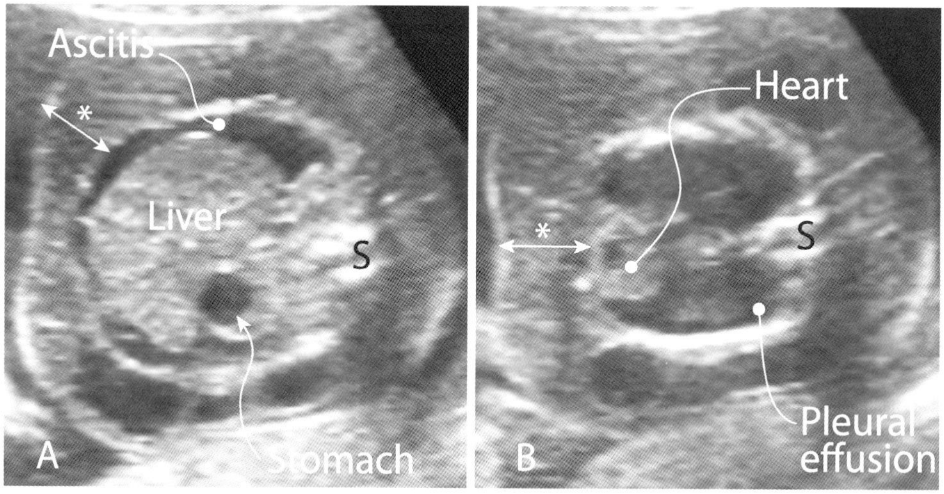

FIGURE 16-27. Hydrops fetalis. Figure A shows a transverse slice across the abdomen of a hydropic fetus. Figure B is a transverse slice of the chest in the same fetus. The double-headed arrow (*) shows the thickened edematous skin. Abbreviation: S, spine.

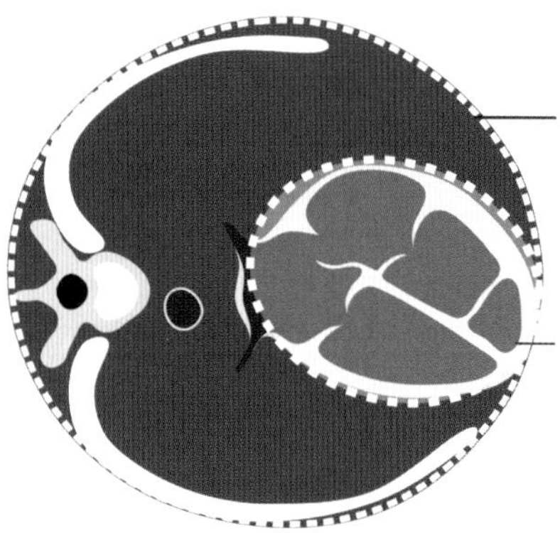

FIGURE 16-28. Fetal cardiothoracic ratio. The areas of the heart and thorax are measured and expressed as a ratio. Note that the normal heart area is about 1/3 of the chest area. (Adapted with permission from Acherman RJ, Evans WN, Luna CF, et al. Fetal bradycardia. A practical approach. *Fetal Matern Med Rev*. August 2007;18(3):225–255)

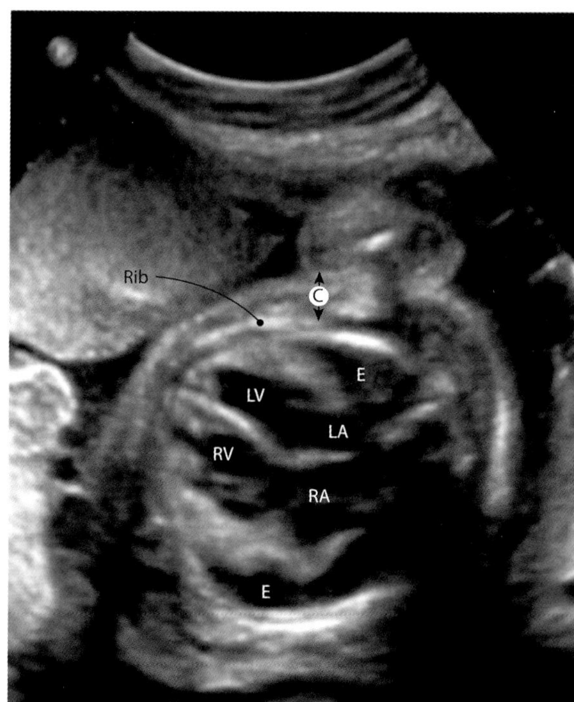

FIGURE 16-29. Cardiomegaly in a fetus with severe anemia. Note the enlarged heart, pleural effusions (E), and thickened chest wall (C) from edema. Abbreviations: LA, left atrium; LV, left ventricle; RA, right atrium; RV, right ventricle.

of Fetal Growth Restriction" section for the normal venous and arterial flow profiles and changes associated with increased resistance and increased venous pressure.

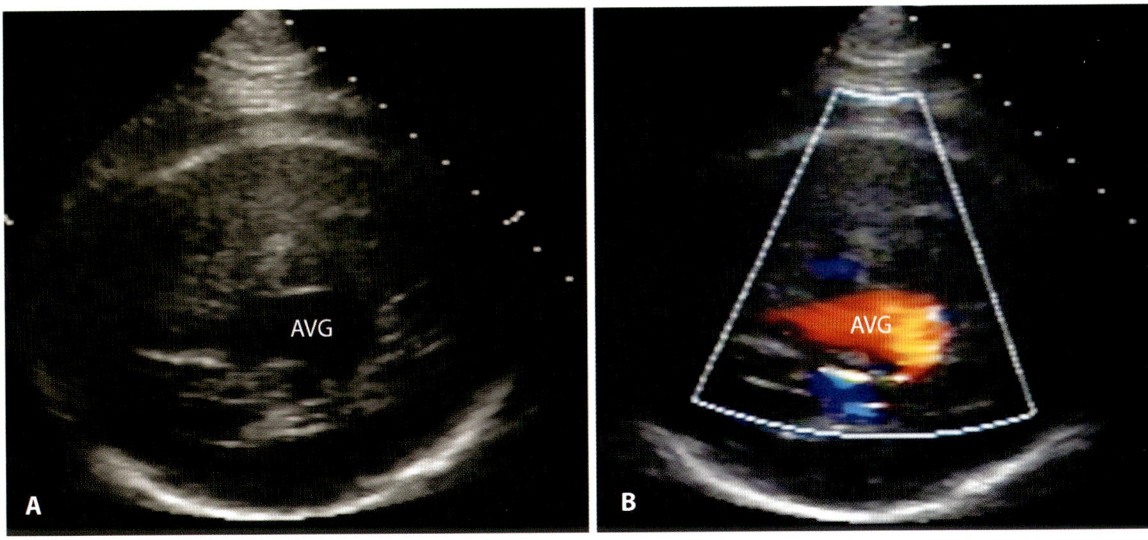

FIGURE 16-30. Vein of Galen malformation. A. Transverse scan of the fetal head showing a central hypoechoic image corresponding to an aneurysm of the vein of Galen (AVG). **B**. Color Doppler of the same structure showing blood flow in the aneurysm.

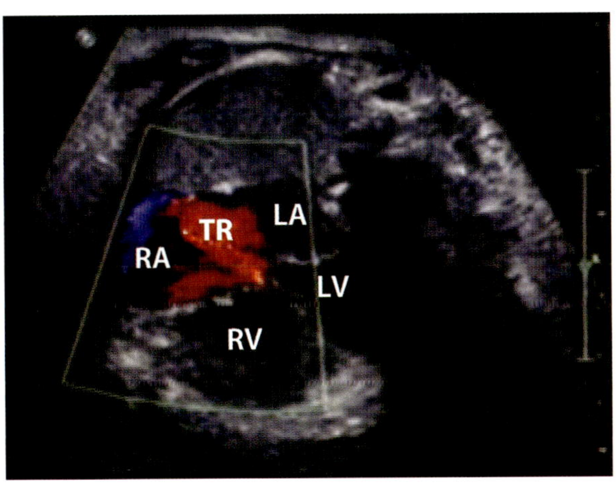

FIGURE and VIDEO 16-31. Tricuspid valve regurgitation. Color Doppler interrogation of the fetal four-chamber view demonstrating significant tricuspid valve regurgitation (TR). The enlarged right atrium impinges in the left atrium (LA). Abbreviations: LV, left ventricle; RV, right ventricle.

As in postnatal life, fetal heart failure has numerous etiologies. Prognosis depends on the cause, response to therapy, and timing of delivery. Significant sustained fetal bradycardia or tachycardia may conduce to fetal heart failure. Fetal anemia was discussed above, but increased middle cerebral artery flow velocity suggests anemia. Arteriovenous malformations are rare but should be suspected in the fetus with cardiomegaly and effusions of unclear etiology. Color Doppler interrogation of the brain, liver, umbilical vein and placenta helps identify arteriovenous malformations (Figure 16-30). Valvar regurgitation is easily detected by color Doppler (Figure and Video 16-31). Significant valvar regurgitation, especially of the tricuspid and pulmonary valves, is not an infrequent cause of fetal heart failure. Primary myocardial disease, particularly with decreased systolic function, may cause fetal heart failure. Fetal heart failure may also be due to myocarditis or dilated cardiomyopathy. The absence of the ductus venosus may lead to congestive heart failure from volume overload; the overload may be the result of an abnormal direct, unrestricted connection between the umbilical vein and the systemic venous system or the right atrium. However, areas of stenosis within the umbilical venous pathway may mitigate volume overload[17,18]

Fetal Cardiac Arrhythmias

Fetal cardiac-rhythm evaluation requires all echocardiographic modalities including M-mode, Doppler, and 2D imaging. Consult other references for fetal electrocardiography and magnetocardiography, as these techniques are not usually available in most clinical settings.

2D Imaging

Two-dimensional imaging permits evaluation of the heart size (see cardiothoracic ratio above), systolic function, effusions, cardiac structure, myocardial appearance, and abdominal situs. All these characteristics may affect, or be affected by, cardiac rhythm abnormalities. Examples include bradycardia related to left atrial isomerism,[19] cardiac arrhythmias, and long QT syndrome associated with myocardial noncompaction,[20,21] and the association of premature atrial contractions and supraventricular tachycardia with atrial septal aneurysms.[22] Ultrasound imaging also guides the direct delivery of medications to the fetus with arrhythmias (Figure 16-32).

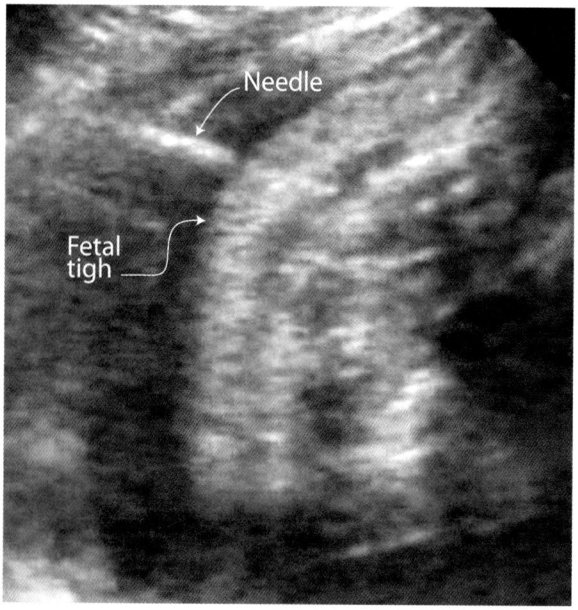

FIGURE 16-32. Intramuscular digoxin injection. The needle is seen entering the fetal thigh to deliver the medication in a fetus with supraventricular tachycardia.

M-mode Echocardiography

M-mode echocardiography is useful for evaluating cardiac systolic function and for diagnosing an arrhythmia mechanism. The M-mode cursor is placed across the atrial and ventricular walls to display the movement of both chambers. Chamber movements are used to time atrial and ventricular systole. The atrial appendages and lateral ventricular walls are typically areas of maximal wall motion (Figure 16-33).

Pulsed Doppler

There are several techniques for recording atrial and ventricular events simultaneously. In the five-chamber view, the cursor is placed between the mitral valve inflow and the left ventricular outflow (Figure 16-34). In normal 1:1 atrioventricular conduction, systolic antegrade flow through the subaortic area follows each atrial contraction.

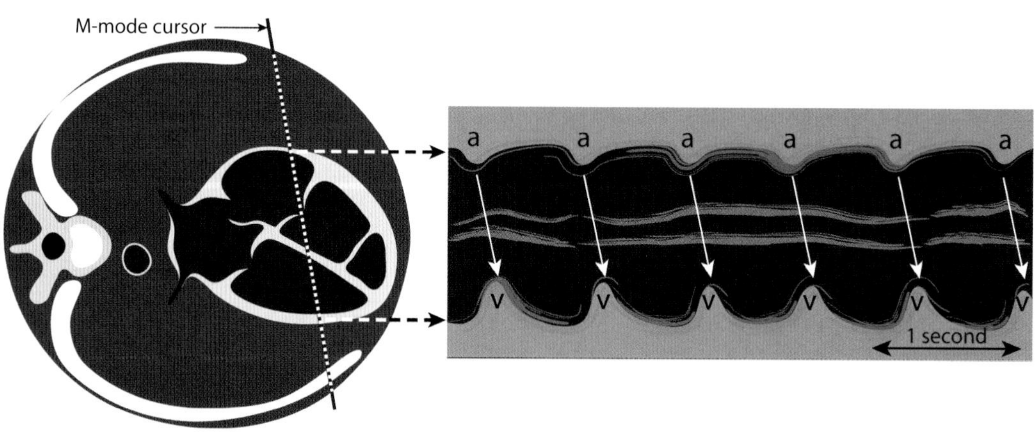

FIGURE 16-33. Fetal M-mode echocardiographic tracing demonstrating normal 1:1 atrioventricular conduction from the four-chamber view. The M-mode cursor is across the right atrial wall to display the atrial contractions (a) and across the left ventricular wall to display the ventricular contractions (v). In 1:1 atrioventricular conduction, every atrial contraction (a) is followed by a ventricular contraction (v). (Reproduced with permission from Acherman RJ, Evans WN, Luna CF, et al. Fetal bradycardia. A practical approach. *Fetal Matern Med Rev.* August 2007;18(3):225–255)

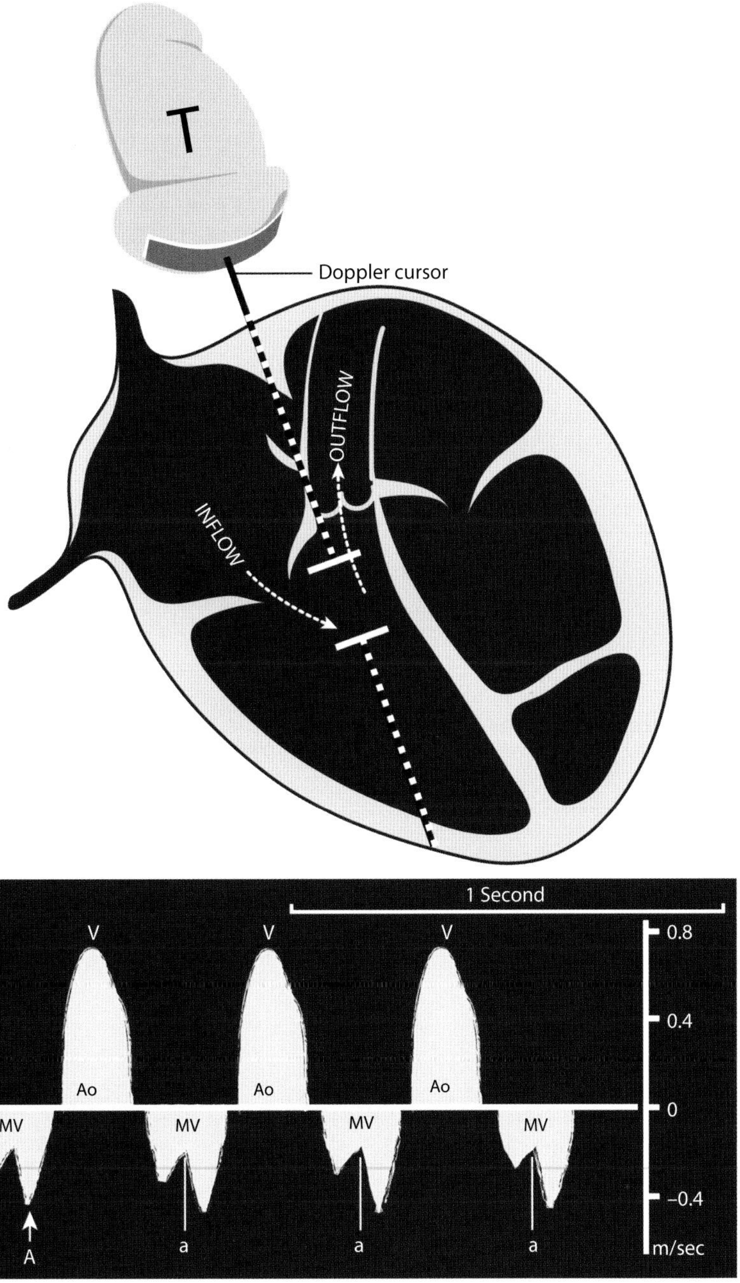

FIGURE 16-34. Fetal pulsed Doppler tracing demonstrating normal 1:1 atrioventricular conduction from the five-chamber view. The Doppler cursor is between the mitral valve inflow and the left ventricular outflow. The Doppler sample-volume gate is opened to record the inflow and outflow simultaneously. In this view, mitral valve inflow (MV) flows away from the transducer (T) and records below the baseline. The aortic outflow (Ao) flows toward the transducer (T) and records above the baseline. The aortic outflow represents the ventricular contraction (v). The mitral valve inflow has an early wave (E) and a late wave during atrial contraction (A). The beginning of the mitral-valve A wave marks the beginning of the atrial contraction (a). In 1:1 atrioventricular conduction, each atrial contraction (a) is followed by a ventricular contraction (v). (Reproduced with permission from Acherman RJ, Evans WN, Luna CF, et al. Fetal bradycardia. A practical approach. *Fetal Matern Med Rev*. August 2007;18(3):225–255.)

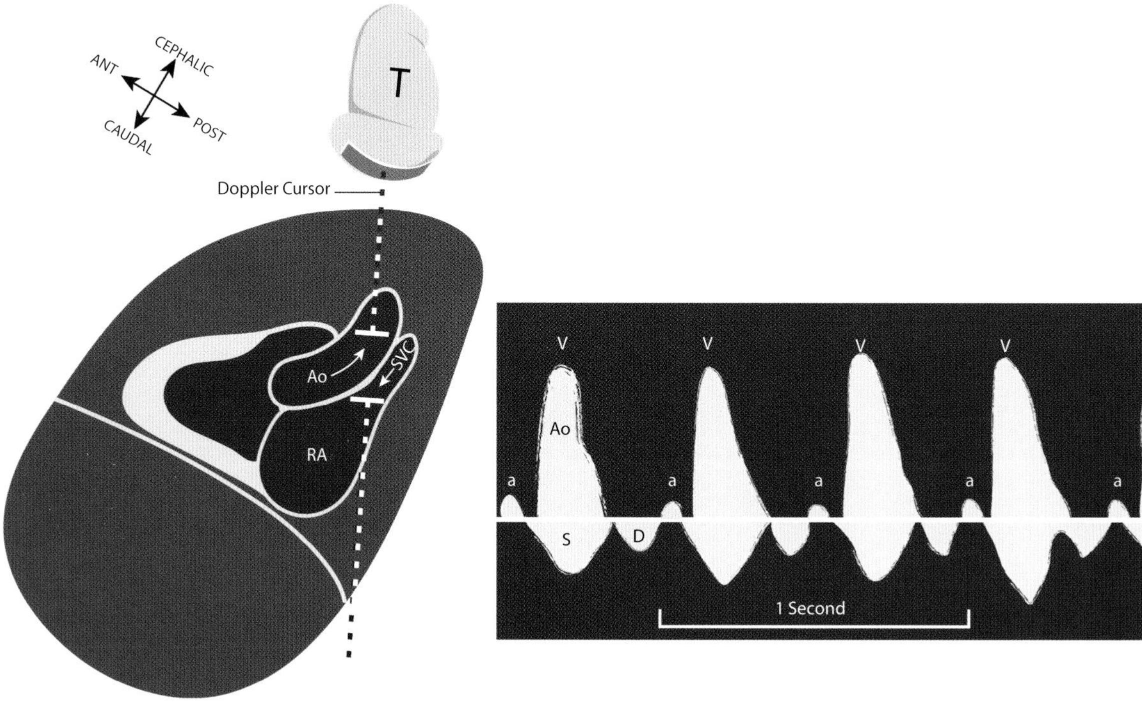

FIGURE 16-35. Fetal pulsed Doppler tracing demonstrating normal 1:1 atrioventricular conduction parasagittal view. The Doppler cursor is between the superior vena cava and the ascending aorta. The Doppler sample-volume gate is opened to record both flows simultaneously. The aortic flow (Ao) streams toward the transducer (T) and records above the baseline. The superior vena cava flow has three waves. The first two waves represent systolic (S) and diastolic (D) antegrade flow that stream away from the transducer (T) and record below the baseline. The third superior vena cava wave occurs during atrial contraction (a), flows toward the transducer (T), and records above the baseline. In 1:1 atrioventricular conduction, each atrial contraction (a) is followed by a ventricular contraction (v). (Reproduced with permission from Acherman RJ, Evans WN, Luna CF, et al. Fetal bradycardia. A practical approach. *Fetal Matern Med Rev*. August 2007;18(3):225–255.)

Alternatively, the cursor can be placed to simultaneously record the superior vena cava and ascending aorta (Figure 16-35), the inferior vena cava and abdominal aorta, or the pulmonary artery branch and pulmonary vein. The pulsed Doppler sample-volume gate size is adjusted to include both targeted flows.

REFERENCES

1. Stümpflen I, Stümpflen A, Wimmer M, Bernasheck G. Effect of detailed fetal echocardiography as part of routine prenatal ultrasonographic screening on detection of congenital heart disease. *Lancet*. 1996;348:854–857.
2. Kleinman CS, Hobbins JC, Jaffe CC, Lynch DC, Talner NS. Echocardiographic studies of the human fetus: prenatal diagnosis of congenital heart disease and cardiac dysrhythmias. *Pediatrics*. 1980;65:1059–1067.
3. Acherman RJ, Evans WN, Luna CF, et al. Prenatal detection of congenital heart disease in southern Nevada: the need for universal fetal cardiac evaluation. *J Ultrasound Med*. 2007;26:1715–1719.
4. American Institute of Ultrasound in Medicine. *AIUM Practice Guideline for the Performance of Obstetric Ultrasound Examinations*. Laurel, MD: American Institute of Ultrasound in Medicine; 2007. Available at: http://www.aium.org/publications/guidelines/obstetric.pdf.
5. Friedberg MK, Silverman NH, Moon-Grady AJ, et al. Prenatal detection of congenital heart disease. *J Pediatr*. 2009;155:26–31.
6. Yagel S, Cohen SM, Achiron R. Examination of the fetal heart by five short-axis views: a proposed screening method for comprehensive cardiac evaluation. *Ultrasound Obstet Gynecol*. 2001;17:367–369.

7. Rice MJ, McDonald RW, Reller MD. Fetal atrial septal aneurysm: a cause of fetal atrial arrhythmias. *Am Coll Cardiol.* 1988;12:1292–1297.
8. Ozcelik N, Atalay S, Tutar E, Ekici F. Prevalence of interatrial septal aneurysm in newborns and their natural course. *Pediatr Cardiol.* 2006;27:343–346.
9. Freedom RM, Rowe RD. Aneurysm of the atrial septum in tricuspid atresia: diagnosis during life and therapy. *Am J Cardiol.* 1976;38:265–267.
10. Luna CF, Acherman RJ, Rollins RC, Castillo WJ, Berthoty DP, Evans WN. Laterally displaced superior vena cava on the fetal 3-vessel view from a right diaphragmatic hernia. *J Ultrasound Med.* 2011;30:1161–1162.
11. Soothill PW, Bobrow CS, Holmes R. Small for gestational age is not a diagnosis. *Ultrasound Obstet Gynecol.* 1999;13:225–228.
12. Craigo SD, Beach ML, Harvey-Wilkes KB, D'Alton ME. Ultrasound predictors of neonatal outcome in intrauterine growth restriction. *Am J Perinatol.* 1996;13:465–471.
13. Cruz-Martínez R, Figueras F, Benavides-Serralde A, Crispi F, Hernandez-Andrade E, Gratacós E. Sequence of changes in myocardial performance index in relation with aortic isthmus and ductus venosus Doppler in fetuses with early-onset intrauterine growth restriction. *Ultrasound Obstet Gynecol.* 2011;38:179–184.
14. Crispi F, Comas M, Hernández-Andrade E, et al. Does pre-eclampsia influence fetal cardiovascular function in early-onset intrauterine growth restriction? *Ultrasound Obstet Gynecol.* 2009;34:660–665.
15. Delle Chiaie L, Buck G, Grab D, Terinde R. Prediction of fetal anemia with Doppler measurement of the middle cerebral artery peak systolic velocity in pregnancies complicated by maternal blood group alloimmunization or parvovirus B19 infection. *Ultrasound Obstet Gynecol.* 2001;18:232–236.
16. Mari G. Middle cerebral artery peak systolic velocity for the diagnosis of fetal anemia: the untold story. *Ultrasound Obstet Gynecol.* 2005;25:323–330.
17. Acherman RJ, Evans WN, Galindo A, et al. Diagnosis of absent ductus venosus in a population referred for fetal echocardiography: association with a persistent portosystemic shunt requiring postnatal device occlusion. *J Ultrasound Med.* 2007;26:1077–1082.
18. Acherman RJ, Rollins RC, Castillo WJ, Evans WN. Stenosis of alternative umbilical venous pathways in absence of the ductus venosus. *J Ultrasound Med.* 2010;29:1227–1231.
19. Acherman RJ, Evans WN, Luna CF, et al. Fetal bradycardia. A practical approach. *Fetal Matern Med Rev.* 2007;18:225–255.
20. Acherman RJ, Evans WN, Schwartz JK, et al. Right ventricular noncompaction associated with long QT in a fetus with right ventricular hypertrophy and cardiac arrhythmias. *Prenat Diagn.* 2008;28:551–553.
21. Drago F, Stefano Silvetti M, Annichiarico M, et al. Biventricular pacing in an infant with noncompaction of the ventricular myocardium, congenital AV block, and prolonged QT interval. *J Interv Card Electrophysiol.* 2010;28:67–70.
22. Papa M, Fragasso G, Camesasca C, et al. Prevalence and prognosis of atrial septal aneurysm in high-risk fetuses without structural heart defects. *Ital Heart J.* 2002;3:318–321.

Index

Page references followed by f indicate figures; those followed by t indicate tables.

A

Abdominal situs, 260, 262f
Acoustic impedance, 2
Acyanotic congenital heart disease, 254–258
  atrial septal defect, 256, 257f–258f, 258
  atrioventricular septal defect, 254–255, 254f–255f
  ventricular septal defect, 255f–256f, 256
Afterload, 154, 154f
Aliasing, 10, 11f, 13, 13f
Amplification, 22–23
Analog-to-digital converter (ADC), 24
Aneurysm of ductus arteriosus (ADA), 217–219
  echocardiography, 217–219, 218f–219f
  follow-up, 219
  overview, 217–219
Angle correction, 14, 15f
Anterior cerebral artery, measurement of blood flow in, 114–116, 114f, 115t, 116f
Aortic regurgitation, 91, 92f
Aortic valve stenosis/atresia, 88, 237f
Apical window, 46f–48f
Arrhythmogenic right ventricular cardiomyopathy, 227–228
Artifacts, 7–8, 8f
Asphyxia, 156–158, 157f
Atrial septal defect, 256, 257f–258f, 258
Atrial shunting through PFO during transitional circulation, 143–144
  left-to-right shunting through a PFO in healthy preterm neonates, 143
  left-to-right shunting through PFO in healthy full-term neonates, 143, 144f
  left-to-right shunting through PFO in premature neonates with PDA or chronic lung disease, 143–144, 144f–145f
Atrioventricular septal defect, 254–255, 254f–255f
a-wave, 140, 140f
Axial resolution, 5, 5f

B

Bandwidth, 21
Bernoulli equation, simplified, 87

C

Cardiac chambers, heart valves, and great vessels
  2D echocardiography, 36–40, 36f–37f
    imaging planes of heart, 37–38, 38f–40f
    location of heart valves and great vessels, 37, 37f
Cardiac output, determinants of, 152–154, 152f
  afterload, 154, 154f
  contractility, 154
  preload, 152–153, 153f
Cardiac tamponade and pericardial effusion, 158–159, 158f–159f
Cardiogenic shock, 155–158, 250–251
  asphyxia, 156–158, 157f
  hypoplastic left heart syndrome, 250–251, 251f–252f
  myocardial dysfunction and postnatal cardiovascular maladaption, 156, 156f
  sepsis, 158
Cardiomegaly in fetus with severe anemia, 272f
Cardiomyopathies, 220–228
  arrhythmogenic right ventricular cardiomyopathy, 227–228
  dilated cardiomyopathy, 220–222, 220f–222f
    in perinatal asphyxia, 222
    in systemic hypertension, 222
  hypertrophic cardiomyopathy, 223–225, 223f–226f
    infants of a diabetic mother, 225–226
    Noonan syndrome, 226–227
    storage diseases, 226, 227f
  myocarditis, 222
  noncompaction cardiomyopathy, 228, 228f–229f
  overview, 220
  restrictive cardiomyopathy, 227, 227f–228f
  sepsis, 223
  structural cardiovascular disease, 222
Case studies and report generation, with virtual neonatal echocardiography training simulator (VNETS), 68
Celiac artery blood flow
  PDA, hemodynamic effects of, 163
Cerebral blood flow
  estimation, 110–116, 111f–112f, 112t–113t, 114f
  PDA
    hemodynamic effects of, 162–163
    ligation, effects of, 165
Circumferential fiber shortening, velocity of, 125–126
Coarctation of the aorta
  heart failure with differential cyanosis, 251–252, 252f
Color-flow, pulsed-wave, and continuous-wave Doppler in assessment of regurgitant flow and measurement of pressure gradients, 85–99
  Doppler display modalities, 87
  Doppler principle, 86–87, 86f
  overview, 85–86
  pulmonary arterial pressure determination, 92–98
    direction and velocity of blood flow through a patent ductus arteriosus assessment, 94, 95f–96f
    flow velocity through a ventricular septal defect, 94, 96, 97f–98f
    peak velocity of tricuspid regurgitation measurement, 92–94, 93f–95f
  simplified Bernoulli equation, 87
  valvar pathology, 87–91
    valvar regurgitation/insufficiency, 90–91, 91f–92f
    valvar stenosis/atresia, 88–90, 89f–90f

Color-flow aliasing, 13, 14f
Color-flow Doppler, 11–14, 13f–14f
evaluation of shunts through the PFO, 141, 143, 143f
virtual neonatal echocardiography training simulator (VNETS), 64, 65f, 66
Compensation, 23, 23f
Compression, 23, 24f
Congenital heart defects, 238
Congenital heart disease, suspected, 235–258
acyanotic congenital heart disease, 254–258
atrial septal defect, 256, 257f–258f, 258
atrioventricular septal defect, 254–255, 254f–255f
ventricular septal defect, 255f–256f, 256
cardiogenic shock, 250–251
hypoplastic left heart syndrome, 250–251, 251f–252f
congenital heart defects, 238
cyanosis with decreased pulmonary blood flow, 239–245
Ebstein's anomaly, 243, 244f–245f, 245
pulmonary atresia with intact ventricular septum, 241–243, 242f
tetralogy of Fallot, 239–240, 239f
tetralogy of Fallot with pulmonary atresia, 240–241, 240f–241f
tricuspid atresia, 243, 244f
cyanosis with increased pulmonary blood flow, 245–248
persistent truncus arteriosus, 247, 247f–248f
transposition of great arteries, 245–246, 246f–247f
cyanosis with pulmonary edema, 248–250
total anomalous pulmonary venous return (TAPVR), 248, 249f–250f, 250
full-term neonates with PDA as congenital cardiac defect, 258
heart failure with differential cyanosis, 251–252
coarctation of the aorta, 251–252, 252f
interruption of the aortic arch, 252, 253f–254f
overview, 235–238
review of fetal and transitional physiology, 236–238, 236f–239f
Continuous-wave Doppler, 11, 12f, 87
Continuous-wave, pulsed-wave, and color-flow Doppler in assessment of regurgitant flow and measurement of pressure gradients, 85–99
Doppler display modalities, 87
Doppler principle, 86–87, 86f
overview, 85–86
pulmonary arterial pressure determination, 92–98
direction and velocity of blood flow through a patent ductus arteriosus assessment, 94, 95f–96f
flow velocity through a ventricular septal defect, 94, 96, 97f–98f
peak velocity of tricuspid regurgitation measurement, 92–94, 93f–95f
simplified Bernoulli equation, 87
valvar pathology, 87–91
valvar regurgitation/insufficiency, 90–91, 91f–92f
valvar stenosis/atresia, 88–90, 89f–90f
Continuous-wave and pulsed-wave Doppler in assessment and measurement of cardiac and systemic blood flow, 101–120
left ventricular output, 102–104
technique, 102–104, 103f–104f
mitral and tricuspid flow Doppler, 109–110
technique, 109–110, 110f
overview, 101–102
regional and organ blood flow, 110–116, 111f
anterior cerebral artery, 114–116, 114f, 115t, 116f
cerebral blood flow, 110–116, 111f–112f, 112t–113t, 114f
renal artery, 118, 118t, 119f
technique, 118
right ventricular output, 104–106
technique, 104–106, 105f–107f
superior mesenteric artery (SMA), 116, 117t, 118f
superior vena cava flow, 106–109, 107t
technique, 106–109, 108f–109f
Contractility, 154
Contrast resolution, 6–7
Control panel, 21–22, 22f
"Crab view (coronal plane), 210–211, 212f
Cross-sectional neonatal cardiac anatomy using 2D echocardiography, 33–60
cardiac chambers, heart valves, and great vessels, 36–40, 36f–37f
imaging planes of heart, 37–38, 38f–40f
location of heart valves and great vessels, 37, 37f
cross-sectional neonatal anatomy, 33–36
cardiac orientation in the fetus, 34–36, 34f–35f
changes in cardiac orientation during gestation, 34–36
differences between neonatal and adult hearts, 36, 36f
obtaining neonatal echocardiograms, 39
display of 2D images, 39
preparing infant for echocardiography, 39, 40f
selection and manipulation of appropriate probe, 39, 40f
obtaining specific sector scans, 39–60
apical window, 46f–48f
infradiaphragmatic subcostal views, 54f–55f
parasternal long axis (PLAX), 41f–43f
parasternal short axis (PSAX), 43f–45f
subcostal coronal views, 49f–50f
subcostal sagittal views, 50f–53f
suprasternal window: innominate, right subclavian and right carotid arteries, 59f–60f
suprasternal window: left atrium and pulmonary veins, 58f–59f
suprasternal window: superior vena cava, aortic arch, ductal cut, 56f–57f
overview, 33–34, 60
c-wave, 140, 140f
Cyanosis in newborn infants without congenital heart disease. *See* Desaturation and cyanosis in newborn infants without congenital heart disease
Cyanosis secondary to persistent prominent Eustachian valve, 147–148, 147f–149f
Cyanosis with decreased pulmonary blood flow, 239–245
Ebstein's anomaly, 243, 244f–245f, 245
pulmonary atresia with intact ventricular septum, 241–243, 242f
tetralogy of Fallot, 239–240, 239f
tetralogy of Fallot with pulmonary atresia, 240–241, 240f–241f
tricuspid atresia, 243, 244f

Cyanosis with increased pulmonary blood flow, 245–248
  persistent truncus arteriosus, 247, 247f–248f
  transposition of great arteries, 245–246, 246f–247f
Cyanosis with pulmonary edema, 248–250
  total anomalous pulmonary venous return (TAPVR), 248, 249f–250f, 250

D
Demodulation, 24, 24f
Depth gain compensation (DGC) control, 6–7
Desaturation and cyanosis in newborn infants without congenital heart disease, 191–215
  differentiating primary cause of hypoxemia, 192–193
  echocardiographic evaluation of therapeutic responses, 194–195
    oxygen, 194
    surfactant, 194–195
    ventilation, 194
  echocardiographic findings in specific causes of hypoxemia, 193–194
    fetal ductus arteriosus closure, 193
    infants of diabetic mothers, 193
    meconium aspiration syndrome, 193–194
    respiratory distress syndrome, 193
  overview, 191–192, 214
  systematic approach to performing echocardiogram, 195–214
    apical window, 205–207, 206f–209f
    parasternal short-axis views, 202–205, 203f–206f
    parasternal window, 195–201, 195f–203f
    subcostal window, 211–214, 213f–214f
    suprasternal window, 207–211, 209f–213f
Detail resolution, 5–6
Dextrocardia, 263
DGC (depth gain compensation) control, 6–7
Diabetic mothers, infants of, 193
  hypertrophic cardiomyopathy, 225–226
Diameter measurement in assessment of cardiac output, 78–79
  LVOT diameter measurement, 78, 78f
  RVOT diameter measurement, 78–79, 79f
  velocity time integral (VTI), 79
Diastolic function assessment, 128–134
  mitral and tricuspid flow Doppler, 129–130, 129f
  pulmonary vein Doppler, 132, 134, 134f
  tissue Doppler, 130, 131t, 132f, 133t
Digoxin injection, intramuscular, 274f
Dilated cardiomyopathy, 220–222, 220f–222f
  in perinatal asphyxia, 222
  in systemic hypertension, 222
Display, 26, 27
Disturbed flow, 10
Doppler controls, 30–31
Doppler display modalities, 87
Doppler echocardiography, 8–18
  color flow imaging (color Doppler), 11–14, 13f–14f
  continuous-wave (CW) Doppler, 11, 12f
  overview, 8–9
  pitfalls of, 14–18
    angle correction, 14, 15f
    improper gain settings for Doppler measurement, 15–16
    Nyquist limit, transducer frequency, and depth setting, 16–18, 16f–18f
  pulsed-wave (PW) Doppler, 9–11, 9f–11f
Doppler equation, 8
Doppler principle, 8, 86–87, 86f
Doppler shift, 86, 86f
Doppler spectral display, 9, 9f
Dropout artifacts, 7, 8f
Ductus arteriosus, aneurysm of, 217–219
  echocardiography, 217–219, 218f–219f
  follow-up, 219
  overview, 217–219

E
Ebstein's anomaly, 243, 244f–245f, 245
Echocardiogram, systematic approach to performing, 195–214
  apical window, 205–207, 206f–209f
  parasternal short-axis views, 202–205, 203f–206f
  parasternal window, 195–201, 195f–203f
  subcostal window, 211–214, 213f–214f
  suprasternal window, 207–211, 209f–213f
Echocardiographic scanners and transducers, 19–31
  controls of echocardiographic modalities, 29–31
    Doppler controls, 30–31
    M-mode controls, 30
    two-dimensional controls, 29–30, 29f
  integrated system, 26–29, 28f
  main unit, 21–27, 21f
    amplification, 22–23
    compensation, 23, 23f
    compression, 23, 24f
    control panel, 21–22, 22f
    demodulation, 24, 24f
    display, 26, 27
    memory and storing images, 24–26, 26f
    pulse generator, 22
    receiver, 22
    reject, 24, 25f
  overview, 19, 20f
  transducers, 19–21, 20f–21f
Echocardiographic simulators in training for neonatal echocardiography, 61–69
  EchoCom-training simulator, 62
  overview, 61–62
  virtual neonatal echocardiography training simulator (VNETS), 62–68, 63f–64f, 65t
    case studies and report generation, 68
    color flow echocardiography, 64, 65f, 66
    complete 2D echocardiography, 64, 66f
    M-mode echocardiography, 68, 69f
    spectral Doppler echocardiography, 66–68, 68f
Echocardiography, basic principles of, 1–18
  Doppler echocardiography. *See* Doppler echocardiography
  image creation, 2–3, 2f
  M-mode (motion mode) echocardiography, 3–4, 3f–4f
  overview, 1–2, 2t
  three-dimensional (3D) echocardiography, 4–5
  two-dimensional (2D) echocardiography, 4–8
    artifacts, 7–8, 8f
    image resolution, 5–7, 5f–7f
    optimizing quality of images, 5–8

Echocardiography, fetal, overview of, 259–277
evaluation of fetal cardiovascular system, 267–276
2D imaging, 274, 274f
ductus venosus flow, 270, 270f–271f
fetal anemia, 270–271
fetal cardiac arrhythmias, 273–274
fetal heart failure, 271–273, 272f–273f
inferior vena cava and hepatic veins flow, 269–270, 270f
middle cerebral artery flow, 268–269, 269f
M-mode echocardiography, 274, 274f
pulsed Doppler, 274, 275f–276f, 276
spectral Doppler in evaluation of fetal growth restriction, 267–268, 267f
umbilical artery flow, 268, 268f–269f
umbilical vein flow, 270, 271f
prenatal detection of congenital heart disease, 259–266
current status, 259–260, 260t
normal screening fetal echocardiogram, 260–266, 261f–266f
Echocardiography of atrial septum
shunts through a patent foramen ovale (PFO), 141–143
color-flow and pulsed-Doppler evaluation of shunts through the PFO, 141, 143, 143f
2D echocardiography of the foramen ovale, 141, 141f–142f
EchoCom-training simulator, 62
Edler, Dr. Inge, 71–72
Ejection fraction (EF), 124
Eustachian valve, 140

F
Fetal and transitional physiology, 236–238, 236f–239f
Fetal ductus arteriosus closure, 193
Flap valve, 140
Foramen ovale, 140, 140f
anatomy and physiology of, 139–140
developmental anatomy, 139–140, 140f
Eustachian valve, 140
interatrial pressure differences during normal transitional circulation, 140, 140f
flow pattern at
estimating pulmonary artery pressure, 182–183, 183f–184f

G
Gain control, 6
Global myocardial function assessment, 134–136
myocardial performance index (MPI), 134–136, 135f–136f

H
Heart failure, shock, and myocardial dysfunction, 151–160
blood pressure and flow, 151–152
cardiac output, determinants of, 152–154, 152f
afterload, 154, 154f
contractility, 154
preload, 152–153, 153f
cardiogenic shock, 155–158
asphyxia, 156–158, 157f
myocardial dysfunction and postnatal cardiovascular maladaption, 156, 156f
sepsis, 158
hypovolemic shock, 158–159
hypovolemia, 158
pericardial effusion and cardiac tamponade, 158–159, 158f–159f
overview, 151
vasodilatory shock, 154–155
echocardiography findings, 155, 155f
Heart failure with differential cyanosis, 251–252
coarctation of the aorta, 251–252, 252f
interruption of the aortic arch, 252, 253f–254f
Hertz, Hellmuth, 71
High pulse repetition frequency (PRF) PW Doppler, 17–18, 18f
Hydrops fetalis, 272f
Hypertension, systemic
dilated cardiomyopathy, 222
Hypertrophic cardiomyopathy, 223–225, 223f–226f
infant of a diabetic mother, 225–226
Noonan syndrome, 226–227
storage diseases, 226, 227f
Hypoplastic left heart syndrome
cardiogenic shock, 250–251, 251f–252f
Hypovolemic shock, 158–159
hypovolemia, 158
pericardial effusion and cardiac tamponade, 158–159, 158f–159f
Hypoxemia, echocardiographic findings in, 193–194
fetal ductus arteriosus closure, 193
infants of diabetic mothers, 193
meconium aspiration syndrome, 193–194
respiratory distress syndrome, 193

I
Image resolution
two-dimensional (2D) echocardiography, 5–7, 5f–7f
Infradiaphragmatic subcostal views, 54f–55f
Interatrial shunts in neonates with congenital heart defects, 148
Interruption of the aortic arch
heart failure with differential cyanosis, 252, 253f–254f

L
LA/Ao (left atrium to aortic root) ratio, 77, 171–172, 172f
LA (left atrial) dimensions and volume, 2D assessment of, 81–83, 82f
LA area, 83
LA linear dimensions, 82–83
LA volume, 83
Laminar flow, 10
Large unrestrictive PDA, 94
Large VSD, 96
Lateral gain compensation (LGC), 30
Lateral resolution, 5f, 6
Left-to-right shunting through a PFO in healthy preterm neonates, 143
Left-to-right shunting through PFO in healthy full-term neonates, 143, 144f
Left-to-right shunting through PFO in premature neonates with PDA or chronic lung disease, 143–144, 144f–145f
Left ventricular output
pulsed-wave and continuous-wave Doppler, 102–104
technique, 102–104, 103f–104f
Levocardia, 263, 263f
LGC (lateral gain compensation), 30
Log compression or dynamic range control, 6
LVIDD (left ventricular internal diameter at the end of diastole), 152–153
LV (left ventricular) mass assessment
M-mode echocardiography and 2D cardiac measurements, 77, 81, 81f–82f

LV (left ventricular) systolic function assessment
M-mode echocardiography and 2D cardiac measurements, 76–77, 76t
limitations, 77
LVOT diameter measurement, 78, 78f

M
Main unit. *See* Echocardiographic scanners and transducers, main unit
Matrix (image plane), 25
Mechanical transducer, 4
Meconium aspiration syndrome, 193–194
Memory and storing images, 24–26, 26f
Middle cerebral artery, 110–111, 112f, 112t–113t, 114f
Mitral and tricuspid flow Doppler, 109–110
diastolic function assessment, 129–130, 129f
technique, 109–110, 110f
Mitral and tricuspid valve annular dimensions
M-mode echocardiography and 2D cardiac measurements, 83, 83f
Mitral regurgitation, 90, 91
Mitral valve stenosis/atresia, 88
M-mode (motion-mode) controls, 30
M-mode (motion mode) echocardiography, 3–4, 3f–4f
virtual neonatal echocardiography training simulator (VNETS), 68, 69f
M-mode (motion mode) echocardiography and 2D cardiac measurements, 71–84
2D assessment of left atrial dimensions, 81–83, 82f
LA area, 83
LA linear dimensions, 82–83
LA volume, 83
2D assessment of LV mass, 81, 81f–82f
diameter measurement in assessment of cardiac output, 78–79
LVOT diameter measurement, 78, 78f
RVOT diameter measurement, 78–79, 79f
velocity time integral (VTI), 79
LA size and LA:AO ratio assessment, 77
LV mass assessment, 77
LV systolic function assessment, 76–77, 76t
limitations, 77
measurements obtained, 77–78
mitral and tricuspid valve annular dimensions, 83, 83f
M-mode echocardiography, 71–73, 72f–73f
obtaining M-mode images, 73–74, 74f–75f
pericardial effusion assessment, 77
Simpson's method for LV ejection fraction, 79–80, 80f
uses of M-mode echocardiography, 73
visual estimation of systolic function based on 2D echocardiography, 80–81
wall thickness assessment, 74, 75f, 76t
Myocardial dysfunction, shock, and heart failure, 151–160
blood pressure and flow, 151–152
cardiac output, determinants of, 152–154, 152f
afterload, 154, 154f
contractility, 154
preload, 152–153, 153f
cardiogenic shock, 155–158
asphyxia, 156–158, 157f
myocardial dysfunction and postnatal cardiovascular maladaption, 156, 156f
sepsis, 158
hypovolemic shock, 158–159
hypovolemia, 158
pericardial effusion and cardiac tamponade, 158–159, 158f–159f
overview, 151
vasodilatory shock, 154–155
echocardiography findings, 155, 155f
Myocardial dysfunction and postnatal cardiovascular maladaption, 156, 156f
Myocardial performance index
estimating pulmonary artery pressure, 187–188, 188f
Myocarditis, 222

N
Neonatal and adult hearts, differences between
2D echocardiography, 36, 36f
Neonatal cardiac anatomy, cross-sectional, using 2D echocardiography, 33–60
cardiac chambers, heart valves, and great vessels, 36–40, 36f–37f
imaging planes of heart, 37–38, 38f–40f
location of heart valves and great vessels, 37, 37f
cross-sectional neonatal anatomy, 33–36
cardiac orientation in the fetus, 34–36, 34f–35f
changes in cardiac orientation during gestation, 34–36
differences between neonatal and adult hearts, 36, 36f
obtaining neonatal echocardiograms, 39
display of 2D images, 39
preparing infant for echocardiography, 39, 40f
selection and manipulation of appropriate probe, 39, 40f
obtaining specific sector scans, 39–60
apical window, 46f–48f
infradiaphragmatic subcostal views, 54f–55f
parasternal long axis (PLAX), 41f–43f
parasternal short axis (PSAX), 43f–45f
subcostal coronal views, 49f–50f
subcostal sagittal views, 50f–53f
suprasternal window: innominate, right subclavian and right carotid arteries, 59f–60f
suprasternal window: left atrium and pulmonary veins, 58f–59f
suprasternal window: superior vena cava, aortic arch, ductal cut, 56f–57f
overview, 33–34, 60
Noncompaction cardiomyopathy, 228, 228f–229f
Noonan syndrome, 226–227
Normal screening fetal echocardiogram, 260–266, 261f–266f
Nyquist limit, 9–10, 11f–12f, 16–18, 16f–18f

O
Ostium primum, 140

P
Parasternal long axis (PLAX), 41f–43f
Parasternal short axis (PSAX), 43f–45f
Patent ductus arteriosus (PDA), 161–176
as congenital cardiac defect in full-term neonates, 258
echocardiographic evidence of a hemodynamically significant PDA, 165–174

Patent ductus arteriosus (PDA) (*Cont.*)
indicators of hemodynamic significance of a PDA, 170–174, 171f–173f
limitations, 170, 170f
measurement, 168
technique, 166–168, 166f–169f
estimating pulmonary artery pressure, 94, 95f–96f, 179–181, 181f–183f
hemodynamic effects, 162–163
cardiac function, 162
cerebral blood flow, 162–163
pulmonary blood flow, 162
renal blood flow, 163
superior mesenteric and celiac artery blood flow, 163
hemodynamic effects of PDA ligation, 163–165
blood flow to other organs, effects on, 165
cardiac effects, 163, 164f–165f
cerebral blood flow effects, 165
overview, 161–162
Patent foramen ovale (PFO), shunts through, 139–149
anatomy and physiology of foramen ovale, 139–140
developmental anatomy, 139–140, 140f
Eustachian valve, 140
interatrial pressure differences during normal transitional circulation, 140, 140f
atrial shunting during transitional circulation, 143–144
left-to-right shunting fhrough PFO in healthy full-term neonates, 143, 144f
left-to-right shunting through a PFO in healthy preterm neonates, 143
left-to-right shunting through PFO in premature neonates with PDA or chronic lung disease, 143–144, 144f–145f
echocardiography of atrial septum, 141–143
color-flow and pulsed-Doppler evaluation of shunts through the PFO, 141, 143, 143f
2D echocardiography of the foramen ovale, 141, 141f–142f
interatrial shunts in neonates with congenital heart defects, 148
left-to-right shunt volume estimation, 144–146
diameter of color flow Doppler, 145–146, 146f
pulmonary to systemic flow ratios, 144–145
overview, 139
right-to-left shunt through foramen ovale, 146–148
cyanosis secondary to persistent prominent Eustachian valve, 147–148, 147f–149f
detection of right-to-left atrial shunting, 146, 146f
transient right-to-left atrial shunt secondary to crying, Valsalva maneuver, and deep inspiration, 146–147
PDA (patent ductus arteriosus). *See* Patent ductus arteriosus (PDA)
Pericardial effusion, 158–159, 158f–159f
assessment with M-mode echocardiography and 2D cardiac measurements, 77
Perinatal asphyxia and dilated cardiomyopathy, 222
Persistent pulmonary hypertension in newborn infants: assessment of pulmonary artery pressure, 177–190
estimating pulmonary artery pressure, 178–181
flow pattern at patent foramen ovale, 182–183, 183f–184f
interventricular septum position, 186–187, 187f
myocardial performance index, 187–188, 188f
patent ductus arteriosus, 179–181, 181f–183f
pulmonary artery flow pattern, 186, 187f
right ventricular function, 187
systolic time intervals, 183–186, 185f
tricuspid annular plane systolic excursion (TAPSE), 188
tricuspid regurgitation jet, 178–179, 179f–180f
overview, 177–178, 189
Persistent truncus arteriosus, 247, 247f–248f
PFO (patent foramen ovale), shunts through. *See* Patent foramen ovale (PFO), shunts through
Phased-array transducer, 4
Piezoelectric properties, 2
PLAX (parasternal long axis), 41f–43f
PPHN (persistent pulmonary hypertension of the newborn). *See* Persistent pulmonary hypertension in newborn infants: assessment of pulmonary artery pressure
Preload, 152–153, 153f
PRF (pulse repetition frequency), 3, 9
PSAX (parasternal short axis), 43f–45f
Pseudonormalization of E/A, 129
Pulmonary arterial pressure determination, 92–98
direction and velocity of blood flow through a patent ductus arteriosus assessment, 94, 95f–96f
flow velocity through a ventricular septal defect, 94, 96, 97f–98f
peak velocity of tricuspid regurgitation measurement, 92–94, 93f–95f
Pulmonary artery flow pattern
estimating pulmonary artery pressure, 186, 187f
Pulmonary atresia, 237f
with intact ventricular septum, 241–243, 242f
Pulmonary vein Doppler
diastolic function assessment, 132, 134, 134f
Pulmonic regurgitation, 91
Pulmonic valve stenosis/atresia, 88
Pulsed-wave (PW) Doppler, 9–11, 9f–11f, 87
Pulsed-wave, continuous-wave, and color-flow Doppler in assessment of regurgitant flow and measurement of pressure gradients, 85–99
Doppler display modalities, 87
Doppler principle, 86–87, 86f
overview, 85–86
pulmonary arterial pressure determination, 92–98
direction and velocity of blood flow through a patent ductus arteriosus assessment, 94, 95f–96f
flow velocity through a ventricular septal defect, 94, 96, 97f–98f
peak velocity of tricuspid regurgitation measurement, 92–94, 93f–95f
simplified Bernoulli equation, 87
valvar pathology, 87–91
valvar regurgitation/insufficiency, 90–91, 91f–92f
valvar stenosis/atresia, 88–90, 89f–90f
Pulsed-wave and continuous-wave Doppler in assessment and

measurement of cardiac and systemic blood flow, 101–120
left ventricular output, 102–104
technique, 102–104, 103f–104f
mitral and tricuspid flow Doppler, 109–110
technique, 109–110, 110f
overview, 101–102
regional and organ blood flow, 110–116, 111f
anterior cerebral artery, 114–116, 114f, 115t, 116f
cerebral blood flow, 110–116, 111f–112f, 112t–113t, 114f
renal artery, 118, 118t, 119f
technique, 118
right ventricular output, 104–106
technique, 104–106, 105f–107f
superior mesenteric artery (SMA), 116, 117t, 118f
superior vena cava flow, 106–109, 107t
technique, 106–109, 108f–109f
Pulse generator, 22
Pulse repetition frequency (PRF), 3, 9
PZT, 19

Q

Quality of images, optimizing
two-dimensional (2D) echocardiography, 5–8

R

Range ambiguity, 11
Read magnification, 26
Receiver, 22
Receiving gate, 10
Reflection, sound wave, 2, 2f
Regional and organ blood flow
pulsed-wave and continuous-wave Doppler, 110–116, 111f
anterior cerebral artery, 114–116, 114f, 115t, 116f
cerebral blood flow, 110–116, 111f–112f, 112t–113t, 114f
Rejection, 24, 25f
Renal artery
pulsed-wave and continuous-wave Doppler in assessment and measurement of cardiac and systemic blood flow, 118, 118t, 119f
technique, 118
Renal blood flow
PDA, hemodynamic effects of, 163
Respiratory distress syndrome, 193
Restrictive cardiomyopathy, 227, 227f–228f
Right-to-left shunt through foramen ovale, 146–148
cyanosis secondary to persistent prominent Eustachian valve, 147–148, 147f–149f
detection of right-to-left atrial shunting, 146, 146f
transient right-to-left atrial shunt secondary to crying, Valsalva maneuver, and deep inspiration, 146–147
transitory shunt secondary to crying, Valsalva maneuver, and deep inspiration, 146–147
Right ventricular function
estimating pulmonary artery pressure, 187
Right ventricular output
pulsed-wave and continuous-wave Doppler in assessment and measurement of cardiac and systemic blood flow, 104–106
technique, 104–106, 105f–107f
RVOT diameter measurement, 78–79, 79f

S

Sample volume, 9
Scattering, sound wave, 2, 2f
Sepsis, 158, 223
Septum position, interventricular
estimating pulmonary artery pressure, 186–187, 187f
Septum primum, 139–140
Septum secundum, 140
Shock, myocardial dysfunction, and heart failure, 151–160
blood pressure and flow, 151–152
cardiac output, determinants of, 152–154, 152f
afterload, 154, 154f
contractility, 154
preload, 152–153, 153f
cardiogenic shock, 155–158
asphyxia, 156–158, 157f
myocardial dysfunction and postnatal cardiovascular maladaption, 156, 156f
sepsis, 158
hypovolemic shock, 158–159
hypovolemia, 158
pericardial effusion and cardiac tamponade, 158–159, 158f–159f
overview, 151
vasodilatory shock, 154–155
echocardiography findings, 155, 155f
Shortening fraction, 121–123, 122f–124f
Shunts through a patent foramen ovale (PFO), 139–149
anatomy and physiology of foramen ovale, 139–140
developmental anatomy, 139–140, 140f
Eustachian valve, 140
interatrial pressure differences during normal transitional circulation, 140, 140f
atrial shunting during transitional circulation, 143–144
left-to-right shunting through a PFO in healthy preterm neonates, 143
left-to-right shunting through PFO in healthy full-term neonates, 143, 144f
left-to-right shunting through PFO in premature neonates with PDA or chronic lung disease, 143–144, 144f–145f
echocardiography of atrial septum, 141–143
color-flow and pulsed-Doppler evaluation of shunts through the PFO, 141, 143, 143f
2D echocardiography of the foramen ovale, 141, 141f–142f
interatrial shunts in neonates with congenital heart defects, 148
left-to-right shunt volume estimation, 144–146
diameter of color flow Doppler, 145–146, 146f
pulmonary to systemic flow ratios, 144–145
overview, 139
right-to-left shunt through foramen ovale, 146–148
cyanosis secondary to persistent prominent Eustachian valve, 147–148, 147f–149f
detection of right-to-left atrial shunting, 146, 146f
transient right-to-left atrial shunt secondary to crying, Valsalva maneuver, and deep inspiration, 146–147
Simplified Bernoulli equation, 87
Simpson's method, 79–80, 80f, 125, 125f–126f
Small restrictive PDA, 94
Small restrictive VSD, 96
SMA (superior mesenteric artery). *See* Superior mesenteric artery (SMA)

Spectral Doppler echocardiography, 87
virtual neonatal echocardiography training simulator (VNETS), 66–68, 68f
Storage diseases, 226, 227f
Stress-velocity index, 126
Structural cardiovascular disease, 222
Subcostal coronal views, 49f–50f
Subcostal sagittal views, 50f–53f
Superior mesenteric artery (SMA)
PDA, hemodynamic effects of, 163
pulsed-wave and continuous-wave Doppler in assessment and measurement of cardiac and systemic blood flow, 116, 117t, 118f
Superior vena cava flow
pulsed-wave and continuous-wave Doppler in assessment and measurement of cardiac and systemic blood flow, 106–109, 107t
technique, 106–109, 108f–109f
Suprasternal window
innominate, right subclavian and right carotid arteries, 59f–60f
left atrium and pulmonary veins, 58f–59f
superior vena cava, aortic arch, ductal cut, 56f–57f
Suspecting congenital heart disease. *See* Congenital heart disease, suspected
Systemic to pulmonary collaterals, 228–231
clinical features, 230, 232f
echocardiographic evaluation, 230, 231f
overview, 228, 229f, 230
Systolic function, visual estimation of based on 2D echocardiography, 80–81
Systolic function assessment, 121–128
ejection fraction (EF), 124
linear left ventricular minor-axis dimensions, 124
modified Simpson's biplane method, 125, 125f
shortening fraction, 121–123, 122f–124f
stress-velocity index, 126
velocity of circumferential fiber shortening, 125–126
wall stress (WS), 127–128, 128f
Systolic time intervals
estimating pulmonary artery pressure, 183–186, 185f

T

TAPSE (tricuspid annular plane systolic excursion)
estimating pulmonary artery pressure, 188
TAPVR (total anomalous pulmonary venous return), 248, 249f–250f, 250
TDI (tissue Doppler imaging), 31
Temporal (time) resolution, 7
Tetralogy of Fallot, 239–240, 239f
with pulmonary atresia, 240–241, 240f–241f
Three-dimensional (3D) echocardiography, 4–5
Time-gain compensation (TGC), 7, 25
Tissue Doppler
diastolic function assessment, 130, 131t, 132f, 133t
Total anomalous pulmonary venous return (TAPVR), 248, 249f–250f, 250
Training for neonatal echocardiography using simulators, 61–69
EchoCom-training simulator, 62
overview, 61–62
virtual neonatal echocardiography training simulator (VNETS), 62–68, 63f–64f, 65t
case studies and report generation, 68
color flow echocardiography, 64, 65f, 66
complete 2D echocardiography, 64, 66f
M-mode echocardiography, 68, 69f
spectral Doppler echocardiography, 66–68, 68f
Transducers, 2, 19–21, 20f–21f
Transposition of great arteries, 245–246, 246f–247f
Tricuspid atresia, 243, 244f
Tricuspid regurgitation, 90, 92f–93f, 273f
jet, 178–179, 179f–180f
measurement of peak velocity of, 92–94, 93f–95f
Tricuspid valve stenosis/atresia, 88
Turbulent flow, 10
Two-dimensional (2D) controls, 29–30, 29f
Two-dimensional (2D) echocardiography, 4–8
artifacts, 7–8, 8f
image resolution, 5–7, 5f–7f
neonatal cardiac anatomy.*See* Cross-sectional neonatal cardiac anatomy using 2D electrocardiography
optimizing quality of images, 5–8

U

Ultrasound, 1–2, 2t

V

Valvar pathology, 87–91
valvar regurgitation/insufficiency, 90–91, 91f–92f
valvar stenosis/atresia, 88–90, 89f–90f
Valvar regurgitation/insufficiency, 90–91, 91f–92f
Valvar stenosis/atresia, 88–90, 89f–90f
Variance, 10
Vasodilatory shock, 154–155
echocardiography findings, 155, 155f
Vein of Galen malformation, 273f
Velocity aliasing, 10, 11f, 13, 13f
Velocity time integral (VTI), 79
Ventricular septal defect, 255f–256f, 256
flow velocity through, pulmonary arterial pressure determination, 94, 96, 97f–98f
Virtual neonatal echocardiography training simulator (VNETS), 62–68, 63f–64f, 65t
case studies and report generation, 68
color flow echocardiography, 64, 65f, 66
complete 2D echocardiography, 64, 66f
M-mode echocardiography, 68, 69f
spectral Doppler echocardiography, 66–68, 68f
v-wave, 140, 140f

W

Wall stress (WS), 127–128, 128f, 154, 154f
Wall thickness assessment, 74, 75f, 76t
Write magnification, 25–26

Z

Zero line shift, 17, 17f